Disability in American Life

Disability in American Life

AN ENCYCLOPEDIA OF CONCEPTS, POLICIES, AND CONTROVERSIES

VOLUME 2: M–Z

Tamar Heller, Sarah Parker Harris, Carol J. Gill, and Robert Gould, Editors

Foreword by Andy Imparato

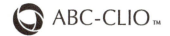

An Imprint of ABC-CLIO, LLC

Santa Barbara, California • Denver, Colorado

Library of Congress Cataloging-in-Publication Data

Names: Heller, Tamar, editor. | Harris, Sarah Parker, editor. |
    Gill, Carol J., editor. | Gould, Robert (Robert P.), editor; foreword by Andy Imparato.
Title: Disability in American life : an encyclopedia of concepts, policies,
    and controversies / Tamar Heller, Sarah Parker Harris, Carol J. Gill, and
    Robert Gould, Editors.
Description: Santa Barbara, California : ABC-CLIO, [2019] | Includes
    index.
Identifiers: LCCN 2018014155 (print) | LCCN 2018015805 (ebook) | ISBN
    9781440834233 (eBook) | ISBN 9781440834226 (set : alk. paper) | ISBN
    9781440848803 (volume 1) | ISBN 9781440848810 (volume 2)
Subjects: | MESH: Disabled Persons | United States | Encyclopedias
Classification: LCC HV1553 (ebook) | LCC HV1553 (print) | NLM HV1553 | DDC
    362.403—dc23
LC record available at https://lccn.loc.gov/2018014155

ISBN: 978-1-4408-3422-6 (set)
        978-1-4408-4880-3 (vol. 1)
        978-1-4408-4881-0 (vol. 2)
        978-1-4408-3423-3 (ebook)

23 22 21 20 19   1 2 3 4 5

This book is also available as an eBook.

ABC-CLIO
An Imprint of ABC-CLIO, LLC

ABC-CLIO, LLC
130 Cremona Drive, P.O. Box 1911
Santa Barbara, California 93116-1911
www.abc-clio.com

This book is printed on acid-free paper ∞
Manufactured in the United States of America

Contents

M

Madness, Mad Studies, and Psychiatric Survivors

Conversations about mental illness and difference have become part of the U.S. cultural landscape. Go to the TED Talks Web site, and you'll find a curated playlist of presentations on "All Kinds of Minds." Listen to an interview with HBO show *Girls'* creator Lena Dunham, and she will speak openly about her time in therapy and the need for new national perspectives on what it means to be mentally ill. Google "mad pride," and you'll discover that the *New York Times* has covered it. Each of these examples shows that mental difference is less of a taboo topic than it used to be and that many people—not only professionals and experts—are pushing our society to rethink what it means to be "mentally ill."

Approaches to "Mental Illness"

One of the clearest ways to understand emerging alternative views of what most people know as "mental illness" is to articulate how the alternatives differ from psychiatry. While historically psychiatry has viewed mental distress as pathological and abnormal, activists and scholars who challenge these views argue that different mental experiences, states, and functions shape individuals' lives and form a defining feature of humanity. In other words, uncommon mental functioning is not negative for all people or in all situations. Also, while psychiatry views psychiatrists and medical professionals as the authorities on diagnosing and treating mentally ill patients,

alternative views find value, expertise, and authority in those same patients. The individual, not the psychiatrist, is the chief authority on what one's experience means and what type of response to distress would be beneficial. Not surprisingly, then, critics of psychiatry are vehemently against forced drugging, electroshock, and incarceration of those in mental distress.

Psychiatric Survivors

Activists and scholars with alternative views of mental illness go by many names and work in many fields. Many activists identify themselves as "consumers/survivors/ex-patients" or as part of the "mad pride movement." And some scholars choose to locate their work within "mad studies" to signal their opposition to psychiatry. Taken together, these scholars and activists will be referred to here as *psychiatric survivors*. Psychiatric survivors define themselves and articulate their views in opposition to psychiatry, and although alternative voices are emerging, mainstream American culture in the 21st century still accepts psychiatry as the authority on "mental illness." One of the chief fights that psychiatric survivors face is demonstrating that psychiatry is not a purely objective or scientific account of human mental difference. Furthermore, the concept of "mental illness," which likens physical ailments to those of a mental or emotional nature, is not a scientific fact. It is only one of many frameworks that can and historically have been used to make sense of different mental experiences and issues. For example, a person who hears voices would be diagnosed by a psychiatrist using the *Diagnostic and Statistical Manual of Mental Disorders* (DSM-V), but what if the voices were helpful or comforting to that person? What if the person did not understand the voices to indicate an illness but instead viewed them as part of what made that person unique? What message does it send a person that his or her personality and life experiences need to be altered by taking medication?

Activism and Challenges to Psychiatry

At their core, psychiatric survivors take issue with the illness model of mental difference and with the authority of psychiatry. Scholars Peter Beresford and Peter Campbell explain that psychiatric survivors hold the opinion that psychiatry's methods result in greater harm than help:

> A mental illness diagnosis and use of mental health services, although sometimes helpful in easing confusion and distress, effectively mark out the individual as a citizen of lesser value. This is confirmed by their arrival at the bottom of the pile—isolated, distrusted, largely unemployed and dependent on the welfare system. (2004, 327)

As a result of the stigmatized place in society that mental patients occupy, survivors "talk back," as Linda Morrison terms it, to psychiatry. Many psychiatric survivors adopt an oppositional position that challenges psychiatry, instead of being compliant patients. If we were to visualize this theoretical concept through a workers' rights analogy, we might imagine that psychiatric survivors have moved beyond protesting (standing on a picket line) and have decided to reject the system altogether (they have found a new job or become entrepreneurs).

Rejecting the Role of the Patient. Psychiatric survivors cite multiple reasons for rejecting the role of the patient, including that psychiatry provides them limited help and that it is not scientifically valid. Peter Beresford and Peter Campbell write that "mental health workers, led by psychiatrists, will very often think of psychotic behaviour and perceptions as primarily symptoms of illness. They will dismiss the content of psychosis as meaningless or of only negative value" (333). For those people who have not experienced psychosis, it might seem natural that it would be undesirable and devoid of meaning. However, those with firsthand experience of psychosis have found meaning and, for some, an identity defined by the experience. Furthermore, in-depth critiques of psychiatry's credibility contend that the criteria it uses to diagnose patients are a result of invalid scientific claims. In most cases, there is no physical proof (for example, a broken bone) that would confirm a psychiatrist's diagnosis because most diagnoses are given to patients solely on the basis of the patients' own words. As a result, psychiatric survivors have expressed skepticism about any connection between a diagnosis (such as bipolar disorder I or II) and any mental or emotional state that an individual actually experiences. After all, until 1973 psychiatrists diagnosed homosexuality as a mental disorder, which raises the question of which current diagnoses will one day seem preposterous.

Creative Maladjustment. These critiques of psychiatry define the groundwork for psychiatric survivors' activism and lead to their involvement in protests against the American Psychological Association (APA) and what they understand to be human rights violations, including forced electroshock therapy. However, in the 21st century especially, not only have psychiatric survivors been oppositional, but they have also nurtured a community with a positive *creative maladjustment* identity, which is a term borrowed from Dr. Martin Luther King Jr. Creative maladjustment urges people to embrace a minority identity that stands for justice and equal rights. The psychiatric survivor movement does not ask individuals to develop a firm stance on issues like electroshock therapy or prescription medication but is instead active in forming compassionate and safe communities where psychiatric survivors can find support and define their individual identities and needs. These communities have in-person gatherings but are increasingly digital in nature. Some of the most developed online communities feature discussion boards and resources in the form of knowledge banks and e-books.

Mad Studies: An Academic Pursuit

The term "mad studies" refers to an emerging academic field of study composed of activists and scholars who share similar critiques of psychiatry. This field is identifiable within at least the United States, Canada, and the United Kingdom. I use the term "mad studies" to refer to a constellation of approaches in higher education that have roots in psychiatric survivor activism. However, not all scholars would identify themselves as working within "mad studies" as much as they would within their own disciplines, including disability studies, medical humanities, rhetoric, and social work. In recent years, some schools outside of the United States, such as Ryerson University, the University of Toronto, and Lancaster University, have developed concentrations and degree programs in mad studies. But the standard in the United States is that mad studies classes are offered and research is published in a range of disciplines. The disparate approaches within mad studies are

in part due to its status as a "broad church of psychiatric survivors who fear endorsing one rigid understanding of mental difference that would 'divid[e]' rather than unit[e] survivors" (Beresford and Wallcraft 1997). These many approaches to critiquing psychiatry have been attractive to scholars and activists looking to escape psychiatry's dogma.

The term "mad" in mad studies and mad pride harkens back to beliefs about mental difference that came before the illness model and psychiatry. The term suggests that mental difference could be the result of many things, not just illness, and might be a gift or a challenge. While mad studies is distinct from any medical approach, such strong lines of distinction cannot be drawn between disciplines more theoretically similar to mad studies. For example, the relationship between mad studies and disability studies (or madness and disability themselves) is less clear. A perusal of the scholarship in disability studies will likely discourage a conclusive stance on whether or not madness can or should be considered a disability. In fact, madness both is and is not a disability.

Madness and Disability

Whether or not an individual identifies as mad or disabled, madness can be covered under the Americans with Disabilities Act (ADA). Thus, from a legal perspective, a connection exists. Similarly, students requesting accommodations for mental or emotional differences use the same channels as those with physical disabilities and are likely to work with school psychologists or other staff members on an individualized education plan (IEP) in K–12 settings, or in college, with the Office of Disability Services. Beresford, in particular, has noted that, regardless of how "we as disabled people or psychiatric system survivors may think of ourselves, we are still lumped together within the same externally imposed definitions, administrative categories and statistics . . . we are both subject to discrimination and oppression" (2000, 169). The choice to accept any identity is an individual one, but regardless of whether an individual identifies with the psychiatric survivor movement, the disability community, or neither, legal and bureaucratic systems frequently devise policies and procedures that consider mental illness to be a disability.

Considering Madness as a Disability. Aside from these legal groupings, some scholars and activists strategically ally mad studies and disability studies because both disciplines contend that mental and physical differences are defining features of humanity. So, differences are not necessarily negative deviations from the norm. Disability studies scholars writing about madness sometimes refer to it as a subset of the disability experience, terming it "mental disability." One argument for considering madness as a disability is that the motto of the disability rights movement, "Nothing about us without us," is useful for psychiatric survivors and disabled people alike. It applies to both groups' desire to be seen as authorities on their own experience and to be included in individual and large-scale policy decisions. When scholars and activists group nearly all mental and physical differences under the umbrella of "disability," this choice is a strong statement that they wish to unite people around an alternative view of human difference. From this perspective, then, making distinctions between different disabilities, illnesses, or diagnoses is not useful because it separates people instead of unites them. It also relies on medical professionals' labels of what is "wrong" with each person, when instead

disability activists and psychiatric survivors prefer to understand their madness or disabilities as part of their identities and not necessarily as a negative part of their lives.

An Uneasy Fit. Despite the overlaps between mad studies and disability studies, the two disciplines are an uneasy fit in some ways. A powerful rift between the approaches is that many psychiatric survivors do not identify as being disabled, and likewise, many disabled people do not identify as psychiatric survivors. More than a problem of recognition, members of both communities sometimes actively resist the other identity. Psychiatric survivors who view themselves as mentally different and celebrate their uniqueness might reject the label of disability or impairment and its implied pathology. On the other hand, a common trope in disability autobiography or personal narrative is to assert that physical disabilities or illnesses do not interfere with one's mental functioning. Such assertions along the lines of, "I may use a wheelchair, but my mental functioning is all there!" imply that impaired mental functioning is an undesirable state, which runs counter to the views of most psychiatric survivors.

Theoretical Rifts. The existing rifts between the disability and psychiatric survivor communities are also theoretical in nature. Foundational concepts in disability studies, like the social model of disability, do not account for mental difference. For example, the social model makes a chief distinction between impairment and disability: impairment is a limitation imposed by one's body, while disability is the limitation caused by a discriminatory and inaccessible society. When applied to mental difference, the social model loses utility because many psychiatric survivors do not believe they have any impairment. Furthermore, it is difficult to define and create an accessible society for psychiatric survivors, although it is an important undertaking. While curb cuts, ramps, and elevators can make a building accessible to wheelchair users, activists and researchers have yet to so clearly define what makes a building accessible to mentally different people. One new area of overlap with potential to gain traction is mad studies and *neurodiversity*, which is a term used by autistic self-advocates. Because both of these approaches involve seeing all human difference along a continuum, they reject identifying anyone in binary terms like impaired/able-bodied or abnormal/normal.

Conclusion

Activists and scholars committed to more positive and humane understandings of mental difference are a growing voice in academia, politics, and health care. They share a perspective that collectively values human difference. And despite the range of perspectives and disciplinary locations in which such redefinition of "mental illness" is taking place, mad studies is becoming a recognizable field of study within universities. Furthermore, psychiatric survivors are an identifiable activist movement gaining greater mainstream recognition and visibility in popular media.

Elizabeth Brewer

See also: Critical Disability Studies; Disability Studies; Mental Health Narratives; Social Model of Disability

Further Reading

Beresford, Peter. 2000. "What Have Madness and Psychiatric System Survivors Got to Do with Disability and Disability Studies." *Disability & Society* 15, no. 2: 167–172.

Beresford, Peter, and Peter Campbell. 2004. "Participation and Protest: Mental Health Service Users." In *Democracy and Participation: Popular Protest and New Social Movements,* edited by Malcolm J. Todd and Gary Taylor, 326–342. London: Merlin Press.

Beresford, Peter, and Jan Wallcraft. 1997. "Psychiatric System Survivors and Emancipatory Research: Issues, Overlaps and Differences." In *Doing Disability Research*, edited by Colin Barnes and Geof Mercer, 66–87. Leeds, UK: The Disability Press.

Morrison, Linda J. 2005. *Talking Back to Psychiatry: The Psychiatric Consumer/Survivor/Ex Patient Movement*. New York: Routledge.

Managed Long-Term Services and Supports (MLTSS)

Long-term services and supports (LTSS) are widely used by individuals with disabilities to help with their daily living needs. Medicaid is the main funding source for LTSS in the United States. States have flexibility in how they choose to provide LTSS. Managed long-term services and supports (MLTSS) as an option is growing in popularity. In MLTSS, states provide their LTSS programs using a managed care approach. In managed care, the state pays a managed care organization (MCO) a set amount of money per person per month (known as a capitated payment). The MCO then coordinates and pays for needed services within a contracted network of providers. As with many managed care programs, states turn to MLTSS because of potential improvements in quality of and access to services along with reduced cost to the state.

MLTSS is a growing trend in the United States. Individuals with disabilities are living longer lives, and more of the U.S. population is aging and experiencing disability. These changing U.S. demographics will increase the number of people using and expenditures on LTSS. MLTSS grew from eight states in 2004 to sixteen states by 2012, and more states are moving to MLTSS every year (Saucier et al. 2012). MLTSS also aims to produce cost savings. Money potentially gained from cost savings in MLTSS could provide additional LTSS for individuals waiting for services (President's Committee for People with Intellectual Disabilities 2012).

Background

To begin a MLTSS program, states apply to the Centers for Medicare and Medicaid Services (CMS) through a Section 1115 Demonstration Waiver or a 1915(b) Managed Care Waiver. States have many options in developing a MLTSS program. Some states use MLTSS to provide and coordinate all services, including health, mental health, and LTSS. In other states, MLTSS only involves coordinating LTSS. Further, states can decide whether to offer their MLTSS program statewide or just in certain areas. In some states, enrollment in MLTSS is mandatory, and in others, people with disabilities have the choice whether to enroll in MLTSS or stay with a fee-for-service LTSS program.

Various MCOs, including local or national private for-profit companies or local not-for-profit agencies, can provide MLTSS. Finally, states can require MLTSS enrollment for certain groups of people and exclude (or "carve out") other groups from MLTSS. Older adults (over age 65), persons with physical disabilities, and children with disabilities are common groups enrolled in MLTSS, while people with intellectual and developmental disabilities (IDD) have historically been carved out. In recent years, more states are also requiring people with IDD to enroll in MLTSS.

Quality of Care and MLTSS

Many states turn to MLTSS to improve quality of care by better coordinating needed supports and by improving access to services. Compared to individuals without disabilities, individuals with disabilities experience higher rates of chronic conditions, higher rates of mental health conditions, and more difficulty accessing services (President's Committee for People with Intellectual Disabilities 2012). In MLTSS, there are opportunities to better coordinate needed health, LTSS, and mental health services for individuals with disabilities. Care coordination and access to services in MLTSS may help reduce health disparities among individuals with disabilities. States are responsible for overseeing quality and costs in MLTSS and must report their outcomes back to CMS. However, the variety of options that states have for MLTSS programs makes it difficult to identify whether MLTSS is an effective approach for individuals with disabilities (Saucier et al. 2012).

Ongoing Issues in the Field

Despite the promises of MLTSS, there are several concerns about the use of MLTSS for people with disabilities. At times, MCOs may have little to no experience providing LTSS for people with disabilities. This lack of experience could result in services and supports not being accessible. In addition, there are concerns that MLTSS will result in a medical model approach to LTSS, less individualization of services, and less consumer choice (President's Committee for People with Intellectual Disabilities 2012). Individuals with disabilities can require daily support from a family caregiver, and it is uncertain whether MLTSS will adequately support these caregivers. Furthermore, there are concerns over who determines if a person needs LTSS and how much LTSS a person can get. For-profit MCOs have a conflict of interest; they may determine that an individual needs a lesser amount of services to reduce costs and potentially increase the MCO's profits.

Best Practices Guidance

The goals to control costs, increase access, and improve quality in MLTSS are not yet realized. Measures/indicators of each of these goals are still being developed. In May 2015, CMS proposed new MLTSS regulations that included ten best practices for states to address rapid MLTSS growth and concerns (CMS 2013). The following items are best practice recommendations from CMS that provide guidance to states considering adopting MLTSS for individuals with disabilities:

1. States should allow ample time for planning of MLTSS programs. This planning should provide for smooth transitions into MLTSS and time to include feedback from stakeholders on MLTSS.
2. Stakeholders of MLTSS should be involved in the planning, implementation, and evaluation of MLTSS programs. MLTSS programs need to provide stakeholders timely education on MLTSS programs so they can provide feedback.
3. MLTSS programs should support individuals with disabilities with achieving community inclusion and obtaining employment.
4. States should oversee the payment structures in MLTSS to make sure that managed care providers are meeting quality goals. This state oversight can include penalties and rewards for providers related to achieving goals.

5. MLTSS programs need to provide individuals with disabilities ongoing and accessible education regarding MLTSS.
6. MLTSS programs need to use a person-centered approach and promote self-direction of services.
7. Managed care providers need to provide integrated care by helping with care coordination across health, mental health, and LTSS. Individuals with disabilities should be able to access needed services and supports in a timely manner.
8. MLTSS programs should ensure a large, diverse, and qualified provider network to allow access to services.
9. States must provide protections for individuals with disabilities in MLTSS to ensure their health and welfare. These protections include access to a fair grievance process and systems in place to prevent abuse and neglect.
10. States need to complete quality oversight and improvements related to MLTSS. These quality efforts should address the needs of individuals with disabilities.

Summary and Conclusion

In summary, MLTSS is a newer approach that states use to provide LTSS to people with disabilities. It is rapidly growing in popularity among states because of the promise of decreasing cost while increasing access to and quality of LTSS. Very little is known about MLTSS in practice and its ability to achieve those goals.

Heather J. Williamson and Randall Owen

See also: Care-Coordination and the Medical Home; Health Insurance; Medicaid

Further Reading

Centers for Medicare and Medicaid Services. 2013. "CMS Guidance for States Using

1115 Demonstrations or 1915(b) Waivers for Managed Long Term Services and Supports Programs." http://www.medic aid.gov/Medicaid-CHIP-Program-Infor mation/By-Topics/Delivery-Systems /Downloads/1115-and-1915b-MLTSS -guidance.pdf.

Centers for Medicare and Medicaid Services. 2015. "Medicaid and CHIP Managed Care Proposed Rule CMS-2390-P." https:// www.cms.gov/Newsroom/MediaRelease Database/Fact-sheets/2015-Fact-sheets -items/2015-05-26.html.

President's Committee for People with Intellectual Disabilities. 2012. "Managed Long-Term Services and Supports." http://www .acl.gov/NewsRoom/Publications/docs /PCPID_FullReport2012.pdf.

Saucier, Paul, Jessica Kasten, Brian Burwell, and Lisa Gold. 2012. "The Growth of Managed Long-Term Services and Supports (MLTSS) Programs: A 2012 Update." Centers for Medicare & Medicaid Services. http://www.medicaid.gov/Medicaid -CHIP-Program-Information/By-Topics /Delivery-Systems/Downloads/MLTSSP _White_paper_combined.pdf.

Maternal and Child Health

Maternal and child health (MCH) is a discipline focused on analyzing and developing programs that protect the health and wellness of women, children, and families. The MCH focus is based on the assumption that the well-being of this particular group influences the health and wellness of future generations and, in turn, will affect future public health challenges for the entire health care system. MCH-specific programs include, but are not limited to, access to comprehensive prenatal and well-child care, prevention of infant mortality, newborn screenings, injury prevention, and services for children with special health care needs (Maternal and Child Health Bureau 2016). Federal and state funds contribute to these programs, including the Title V Maternal and Child Health Services Block Grant; Medicaid; the Children's Health Insurance Program; the Healthy Start Initiative; the Emergency Medical Services for Children Program; and the Special Supplemental Food Program for Women, Infants, and Children (WIC).

History of MCH

The Children's Bureau, created by President William Howard Taft in 1912, was the first system for MCH in the United States. The Children's Bureau focused exclusively on improving the lives of children and families (Administration for Children and Families 2015). This was the first federal agency within the U.S. government tasked with children's health issues, and the Children's Bureau set priorities in such areas as infant and maternal death, child labor, family economic security, and abused and neglected children. In 1921, the Sheppard-Towner Act, also known as the "maternity act," was passed with the direct purpose of reducing maternal mortality. Funds were appropriated for the creation of health clinics for women and children, the training of midwives, and education surrounding hygiene and nutrition. Although passage of the act represented growing federal support for MCH issues, it did not receive funding until after 1929 because of political opposition. To continue the progress made by the Sheppard-Towner Act, Title V of the Social Security Act was passed in 1935. Still in effect to this day through the Maternal and Child Health Services Block Grant, this legislation ensures that measures are taken to improve the lives of women, children, and youth, including children with special health care needs (CSHCN).

Goals of MCH

While MCH covers a wide range of topics and disciplines, public health professionals focus their efforts on several key issues, including the following:

- reduction of the fetal, infant, child, and adolescent death rate
- reduction of cesarean births among low-risk women
- reduction of low-birth-weight infants and preterm births
- increase in the proportion of pregnant women receiving early and adequate prenatal care
- improvement of health behaviors, such as abstinence from alcohol, cigarettes, and illicit drugs
- increase in the proportion of women receiving preconception care
- increase in the proportion of young children with autism spectrum disorder (ASD) and other developmental delays who are screened, evaluated, and enrolled in special services in a timely manner
- increase in the proportion of children, including those with special health care needs, who have access to a medical home

These goals are listed as key objectives within the Healthy People 2020 goals. Progress toward achievement of these goals requires addressing some of the key determinants adversely affecting the health status of children and their mothers. Access to health care services, chronic stress, educational inequities, nutrition, poor health-related behaviors, poverty, quality of the family environment, and racial and ethnic disparities are widely recognized factors that directly affect health outcomes and are key targets of MCH efforts.

Public health professionals are working to address persistent disparities and inequities in MCH by using a life-course perspective to understand health promotion and disease prevention. As more than half of pregnancies are unplanned, there has been a recent push for improved preconception health initiatives aimed at providing care for women prior to pregnancy. The life-course perspective is rooted in assessment of social determinants and health equity models, and it focuses on the social and economic factors that influence health and wellness throughout one's life.

MCH and Disability

As defined by the Maternal and Child Health Bureau, children with special health care needs (CSHCN) are children who "have or are at increased risk for a chronic physical, developmental, behavioral, or emotional condition and who also require health and related services of a type or amount beyond that required by children generally" (2008). Many programs for these children are funded through Title V programs as a means to facilitate systems of care that are family centered and community based. States are required to use at least 30 percent of Federal MCH Block Grant funds for services for CSHCN. State and federal performance measures for CSHCN focus on improving family-centered care, providing services for transition to adulthood, ensuring adequate insurance to cover necessary services, and implementing early and continuous childhood screenings.

Future of MCH

Although MCH professionals need specialized skills and knowledge to effectively navigate and use MCH services and systems, recent studies have shown that 80 percent of the public health workforce had not received formal training (Altarum Institute 2013). The Division of MCH Workforce Development, housed within the Health Resources and Services Administration's MCH Bureau, is tasked with providing education and training for future leaders in the MCH field. In collaboration with state MCH programs, academic institutions, and professional organizations, the division seeks to ensure that well-trained MCH leaders are present at local, state, and national levels.

In addition to the cultivation of leaders, advocacy for programs and services focused on improving the lives of mothers and their families is critical for the continued improvement of MCH. The Association of Maternal and Child Health Programs (AMCHP) advocates at the federal level for MCH programs and provides a forum for state leaders to improve policy, services, and systems of care for MCH populations. Additionally, state Title V profiles provide summaries of how the Title V MCH Block Grant works in each state and provide key MCH statistics that can be used when advocating for state-specific policies, programs, and services.

Alexandra Ibrahim

See also: Preventive Health Care; Public Health

Further Reading

Administration for Children and Families. 2015. "History." http://www.acf.hhs.gov /programs/cb/about/history.

Altarum Institute. 2013. "Improving Diversity in the Future Maternal and Child Health Workforce." http://altarum.org/our -work/improving-diversity-in-the-future -maternal-and-child-health-workforce.

Maternal and Child Health Bureau. 2008. "The National Survey of Children with Special Health Care Needs Chartbook 2005–2006." Rockville, MD: U.S.
Department of Health and Human Services, Health Resources and Services Administration.

Maternal and Child Health Bureau. 2016. "National Conference of State Legislatures." http://www.ncsl.org/research/health /maternal-and-child-health-overview.aspx.

Medicaid

In addition to providing assistance to low-income individuals, Medicaid serves as a major provider of primary and supplemental insurance for people with disabilities. People with disabilities compose a significant portion of the people receiving Medicaid services. More than 10 million people with disabilities are enrolled in the program, making up about 17 percent of all Medicaid enrollees (Klees, Wolfe, and Curtis 2015).

Background and History

For most of the 20th century, health insurance in the United States was primarily available as a benefit through regular full-time employment. Private health insurance was inaccessible for many people with disabilities who could not work or who were unemployed or underemployed. Additionally, many of the services and benefits offered by Medicaid that are critical to the management of various disability conditions may not be provided or economically accessible under traditional private insurance. Medicaid offers a broader array of medical and long-term service options than Medicare or employer-sponsored private insurance plans (Herz 2012). As a result, Medicaid has become an important and accessible source of health care coverage for the disability population in the United States (Musumeci 2014).

Medicaid is a federal-state partnership to provide public health assistance to vulnerable and economically disadvantaged populations. In an amendment to the Social Security Act of 1935, Medicaid was enacted in 1965 under President Lyndon B. Johnson as part of the Great Society programs to provide health care access to people who were indigent or poor (Iglehart and Sommers 2015; Paradise, Lyons, and Rowland 2015). Medicaid provides both acute and specialty medical care as well as *long-term services and supports* (LTSS) to 74.5 million Americans, serving approximately one out of every five people in the United States (Paradise, Lyons, and Rowland 2015; Centers for Medicare and Medicaid Services 2017).

Important Points to Understand about Medicaid

Means Testing. Medicaid is the third-largest federal domestic program in the United States (following Social Security and Medicare) and is the largest means-tested welfare program in the nation (Iglehart and Sommers 2015; Paradise, Lyons, and Rowland 2015). A *means test* is the determination of whether a person or family has the means to do without help from an assistance or welfare program, like Medicaid (Stevens and Stevens 2003). People who benefit from Medicaid are those who would otherwise not have the financial means to pay for their health care. Many Medicaid recipients have complex, chronic conditions, as well as significant social service needs (Mann 2013).

Eligibility and Enrollment. People who are eligible for and enrolled in the Medicaid program are known as enrollees. By federal law, states must provide access to basic medical services to certain populations, including low-income adults, low-income parents and children, low-income pregnant women, qualifying aging persons (*dually eligible* for

Medicare and Medicaid), and qualifying people with disabilities (National Health Policy Forum 2015). Other individuals may qualify for Medicaid benefits if variations in state eligibility guidelines expand coverage beyond that mandated by federal policy. Medicaid eligibility standards may be temporarily expanded to serve as a coverage safety net to mitigate the effects of economic recession or in response to emerging public health trends (Paradise, Lyons, and Rowland 2015).

Medicaid Program Structure. Medicaid programs are regulated in part at the federal level; however, their design, administration, and implementation are determined by each individual state. Each state has a unique Medicaid program, and states have authority to regulate the structure and standards of their Medicaid program within established federal mandates (Klees, Wolfe, and Curtis 2015). Consequently, one of the features of the Medicaid program at the national level is *interstate variation*, or differences across states (Paradise, Lyons, and Rowland 2015). These differences include specific eligibility criteria, state expenditures, and service cost rates. A state also determines the range of health care coverage, or the extent of services afforded by a health insurance or assistance policy. For example, a state may place limits on the amount and duration of services that will be paid by its Medicaid program, such as on the number of Medicaid-paid days of inpatient hospital care, physician visits, or medication prescriptions per month (Klees and Wolfe 2013).

As discussed later in the entry, state Medicaid plans have an institutional bias in that they *must* cover nursing home reimbursement and home health services, while home and community-based long-term services and supports are optional, provided through waivers or personal care services

(PCS) amendments to the Medicaid state plan (Reaves and Musumeci 2015).

Key Components of Medicaid

Medicaid Services. Under federal law, states are required to cover certain mandatory benefits for all program enrollees (Paradise 2015; Centers for Medicare and Medicaid Services 2015a). These benefits follow:

- inpatient and outpatient hospital services
- laboratory and X-ray services
- physician, midwife, and nurse practitioner services
- nonemergency transportation to medical care
- federally qualified health center (FQHC) and rural health clinic (RHC) services
- early and periodic screening, diagnosis, and treatment for individuals up to age 21
- family planning services and supplies
- freestanding birth center services
- nursing facility (NF) services for individuals up to age 21
- home health services for individuals qualified to receive NF care
- tobacco cessation counseling and pharmacotherapy for women who are pregnant
- parity between physical and mental health or substance abuse disorder benefits for those enrollees eligible under the Affordable Care Act

States may also elect to offer optional benefits and services to enrollees (Paradise 2015; Centers for Medicare and Medicaid Services 2015a). For example, prescription drugs are an optional benefit for state Medicaid programs. However, all states include prescription drugs as a covered service in their Medicaid benefit package. The optional benefits for states to elect for coverage include, but are not limited to, the following:

- prescription drugs
- dental care
- durable medical equipment (DME)
- personal care services
- home- and community-based services (HCBS)

Medicaid Financing. The Medicaid program is funded by a combination of both federal and state dollars. Though each state administers its own Medicaid program, the federal government must pay at least 50 percent of the costs for a state's expenditures on health care services to enrollees. The share of costs paid to an individual state by the federal government is calculated through a formula known as the federal medical assistance percentage (FMAP) (2014; Kaiser Commission on Medicaid and the Uninsured 2012). The remaining program costs, also called the nonfederal share, are paid for by the state. FMAPs are most commonly presented as a percentage rate (for example, a FMAP of 65 percent means that the federal government pays 65 percent of a state's Medicaid service costs). FMAPs are recalculated every three years to determine the amount of funding that will be provided by the federal government for a state's Medicaid program. Under law, a state FMAP may not be lower than 50 percent or greater than 82 percent (Centers for Medicare and Medicaid Services 2015b).

FMAPs are calculated on the basis of state average income per capita (or per person). FMAPs vary from state to state because of differences in average income levels and state-specific population needs (Kaiser Commission on Medicaid and the Uninsured 2012). States with lower per capita incomes have higher FMAPs, meaning that the federal government pays for a larger percentage of that state's Medicaid program, in an effort to ensure that federal contribution is fair across state Medicaid programs. This allows states with larger FMAPs to offer services comparable to states with lower FMAPs.

Medicaid Expenditures. Medicaid is a core source of health care financing in the United States (Paradise, Lyons, and Rowland 2015). Total Medicaid expenditures reached $498 billion in 2014, representing 15.4 percent of total U.S. health care spending (Medicaid and CHIP Payment and Access Commission [MACPAC] 2015). Hospital care (such as inpatient, outpatient, or emergency department care) is the most expensive Medicaid service, accounting for over 30 percent of program spending (MACPAC 2015). Medicaid finances over half of all U.S. health care spending in residential and personal care services (including services delivered under home and community-based service waivers, care provided in residential facilities for people with intellectual disabilities or mental health and substance abuse disorders, ambulance services, school health, and work-site health care), and these residential and personal care services makes up the second largest Medicaid expense (after hospital care), with over 16 percent of program funds spent in that area (MACPAC 2015). Additionally, Medicaid funds account for about 36 percent of all home health care in the United States, a quarter of total national spending on mental health services, and over one-fifth of total national spending on substance abuse treatment (MACPAC 2015; Substance Abuse and Mental Health Services Administration 2013). Medicaid is also the largest single funding source for nursing homes in the United States, providing coverage for 64 percent of all nursing home residents and funding about 30 percent of all nursing home care in the country (MACPAC 2015).

Dilemmas, Debates, and Unanswered Questions in Medicaid

Health Care Spending for People with Disabilities. Complex health care needs related to disability and the management of chronic health conditions may require more frequent use or more costly forms of medical and specialty care (Stanton and Rutherford 2006). People with disabilities may also require long-term care services and supports to meet their care needs. People with disabilities cost more than any other Medicaid enrollee group (such as adults, parents, children, or aging individuals) (Klees, Wolfe, and Curtis 2015). The need for disease monitoring and long-term care services is expected to increase as the aging and disabled Medicaid enrollee populations grow over time (Klees and Wolfe 2013).

Service delivery strategies, like *managed care*, have been implemented in many state Medicaid programs to coordinate care and control overall health care spending for all enrollees while improving access to quality services (Reaves and Musumeci 2015). Managed care continues to grow within the Medicaid program, and the term has also been applied to the delivery of LTSS (known as managed long-term services and supports, or MLTSS) (Paradise, Lyons, and Rowland 2015). Differences in state Medicaid plans and other factors have produced mixed results regarding managed care's impact on saving on costs, increasing service access, and meeting the complex needs of Medicaid enrollees.

Long-Term Care. Increased Medicaid spending for enrollees with disabilities may be related to the accessibility of certain long-term care options available through state programs. Nursing home care is a required benefit, making up a significant portion of total Medicaid expenditures (MACPAC 2015). However, long-term *home and community-based services and supports* (HCBS) are only optional benefits that a state Medicaid program may elect to provide through a waiver system offered to qualifying enrollees as an expansion of traditional Medicaid benefits. State optional

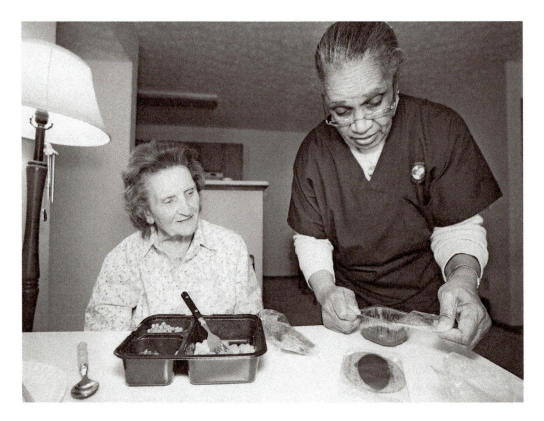

Caregiver Frances McDaniel helps Alice Terrell with her lunch at Terrell's home in Columbus, Ohio. Medicaid-funded supports allow many older adults and people with disabilities to remain in their homes, instead of moving into nursing homes or other institutions. (Neal C. Lauron/ MCT/MCT via Getty Images)

HCBS benefits entitle enrollees to services as available, and because of program economic constraints and enrollment caps, many enrollees remain on a needs-based waiting list for a period of time before services can be delivered under a HCBS waiver (Paradise, Lyons, and Rowland 2015).

Medicaid enrollees are federally entitled to immediate and unlimited nursing home care, and Medicaid reimbursement rates are financially desirable for the nursing facility industry (Grogan 2014). Medicaid policy has been characterized in the past as holding an institutional bias that mandates institutional placement and only makes home and community-based care an option (Reaves and Musumeci 2015). However,

research shows that home and community-based long-term services and supports save states money over time (Kaye, Harrington, and LaPlante 2010). Further, overall Medicaid spending on nursing home care has notably decreased since the 1990s and has increased since then for HCBS services (Reaves and Musumeci 2015). Medicaid remains an important source of home and community-based long-term services and supports that facilitate independent living and community integration for many people with disabilities.

Conclusion

As the largest health care program in the nation, Medicaid provides a critical health and social safety net for low-income populations. Over 20 percent of the U.S. population receives Medicaid benefits, and the program plays a major role in the delivery of both medical and long-term care services for more than 11 million people with disabilities. Medicaid spending constitutes a significant portion of overall national health expenditures, and the program is the largest sole payer of nursing home care in the United States. Medicaid spending is disproportionately dedicated to paying for services used by enrollees with disabilities, an issue that has prompted innovative approaches in delivery strategy and community-based services and supports. As the disability and aging populations grow, Medicaid must keep working toward providing consistent, high-quality health care services to its large population of enrollees with disabilities.

Anne M. Bowers

See also: Managed Long-Term Services and Supports (MLTSS); Personal Care Attendance Services; Poverty

Further Reading

Centers for Medicare & Medicaid Services. 2015a. "Benefits." https://www.medicaid.gov/medicaid-chip-program-information/by-topics/benefits/medicaid-benefits.html.

Centers for Medicare & Medicaid Services. 2015b. "Financing & Reimbursement." https://www.medicaid.gov/medicaid-chip-program-information/by-topics/financing-and-reimbursement/financing-and-reimbursement.html.

Centers for Medicare & Medicaid Services. 2017. "Medicaid & CHIP March 2017 Application, Eligibility, and Enrollment Data." https://www.medicaid.gov/medicaid/program-information.

Congressional Budget Office. 2014. "Budget and Economic Outlook: 2014–2024." https://www.cbo.gov/sites/default/files/113th-congress-2013-2014/reports/45010-Outlook2014_Feb_0.pdf.

Groganees, Barbara S., and Christian J. Wolfe. 2013. "Brief Summaries of Medicare & Medicaid: Title XVIII and Title XIX of the Social Security Act." Centers for Medicare & Medicaid Services. https://www.cms.gov/Research-Statistics-Data-and-Systems/Statistics-Trends-and-Reports/MedicareProgramRatesStats/Downloads/MedicareMedicaidSummaries2013.pdf.

Klees, Barbara S., Christian J. Wolfe, and Catherine A. Curtis. 2015. "Medicaid (Annual Statistical Supplement to the Social Security Bulletin, 2014)." Baltimore, MD: Centers for Medicare & Medicaid Services. https://www.ssa.gov/policy/docs/statcomps/supplement/2014/medicaid.pdf.

Mann, Cindy. 2013. "Targeting Medicaid Super-Utilizers to Decrease Costs and Improve Quality." Baltimore, MD: Centers for Medicare & Medicaid Services. https://www.medicaid.gov/federal-policy-guidance/downloads/cib-07-24-2013.pdf.

Medicaid and CHIP Payment and Access Commission (MACPAC). 2015. "MACStats: Medicaid and CHIP Data Book." https://www.macpac.gov/wp-content/uploads/2015/12/MACStats-Medicaid-and-CHIP-Data-Book-December-2015.pdf.

Musumeci, MaryBeth. 2014. "The Affordable Care Act's Impact on Medicaid Eligibility, Enrollment, and Benefits for People with Disabilities." Washington, DC: Kaiser Family Foundation. https://kaiserfamilyfoundation.files.wordpress.com/2014/04/8390-02-the-affordable-care-acts-impact-on-medicaid-eligibility.pdf.

National Health Policy Forum. 2015. "The Basics: Medicaid Eligibility and Benefits." https://www.nhpf.org/library/the-basics/Basics_Medicaid_02-02-15.pdf.

Paradise, Julia. 2015. "Medicaid Moving Forward." Washington, DC: Kaiser Family Foundation. http://kff.org/health-reform/issue-brief/medicaid-moving-forward/.

Paradise, Julia, Barbara Lyons, and Diane Rowland. 2015. "Medicaid at 50." Washington, DC: Kaiser Family Foundation. http://files.kff.org/attachment/report-medicaid-at-50.

Reaves, Erica L., and MaryBeth Musumeci. 2015. "Medicaid and Long-Term Services and Supports: A Primer." Washington, DC: Kaiser Family Foundation. http://kff.org/medicaid/report/medicaid-and-long-term-services-and-supports-a-primer/.

Stanton, Mark W., and Margaret K. Rutherford. 2006. "The High Concentration of U.S. Health Care Expenditures: Research in Action, Issue 19." Rockville, MD: Agency for Healthcare Research and Quality. http://archive.ahrq.gov/research/findings/factsheets/costs/expriach.

Substance Abuse and Mental Health Services Administration. 2013. "National Expenditures for Mental Health Services and Substance Abuse Treatment, 1986–2009." http://store.samhsa.gov/shin/content/SMA13-4740/SMA13-4740.pdf.

Medical Education

The current system of medical education generally does not prepare physicians to care for persons with disabilities. Shortcomings in physicians' knowledge, attitudes, and skills contribute to poorer health outcomes for persons with disabilities and undermine national efforts to address the health disparities of persons with disabilities.

For persons with disabilities, access to quality primary and specialty medical care, allied health services, and durable medical equipment depends upon finding physicians with the knowledge, attitudes, and skills to meet their needs. Nonetheless, many physicians complete their medical training with limited or no exposure to disability and are unprepared to care for patients with disabilities in medical practice. Gaps in physicians' preparedness compromise the delivery of quality health care and may jeopardize health status and quality of life. This realization led the Office of the Surgeon General (2002, 2005) and Institute of Medicine (2007) to issue policy recommendations to improve disability-related training for health care providers.

Barriers in Medical Education

Implementing the recommendations has been challenging. The complexity of medical education complicates efforts to modify training methods and curricula. Several distinct organizations influence what is included in the formal curriculum during the four years of medical school and the three or more years of residency training, depending upon specialty. Physicians in training are also exposed to a hidden curriculum—that is, messages about values and assumptions in their institutions that can support or undermine the formal curriculum (Hafferty 1998). Both the formal and hidden curricula are influenced by attitudes and assumptions about persons with disabilities within society at large. In addition, there is limited information about what physicians need to know to guide training initiatives, and uncertainty about the level of information that is appropriate at different levels and in different specialties. Some believe that physicians with specialized training in disability-related topics are best prepared to manage the health care of patients with disabilities. Examples include physical medicine and rehabilitation or a proposed new specialty in developmental medicine. This entry focuses on the disability-related training needs of physicians who do not specialize but care for patients with disabilities in the course of their medical practice, and it applies primarily to physicians who care for adults with disabilities.

Physicians caring for children with disabilities typically complete residency programs in pediatrics or family medicine, which offer specialized training to address needs specific to children and families.

Disability-Competent Care

While a number of medical schools, residency programs, and continuing medical education programs nationwide offer formal content on disability, curricula are often limited to brief, one-time occurrences and are typically elective rather than required experiences. These efforts are generally initiated by a small number of faculty who champion the needs of patients with disabilities, and they reach only a minority of physicians and physicians-to-be.

To replace the current piecemeal approach, medical educators and policy makers need a clear vision of the knowledge, attitudes, and skills that constitute core competencies for training physicians to care for persons with disabilities. Moreover, it is important that persons with disabilities be involved in this process. While physicians need technical competence, technical skills alone are not sufficient to provide quality care. Curriculum development efforts involving persons with disabilities highlight the importance of attitudes in informing physicians' knowledge and skills. A disability curriculum advisory committee in family medicine that included the voices of people with disabilities identified three key issues, each of which emphasized the importance of attitudes (Minihan et al. 2004):

1. All patients must be respected and valued. The curriculum must help counter the perception that persons with disabilities are "less than" persons without disabilities and less worthy and deserving of good health care.

2. Persons with disabilities have functional lives that matter. The curriculum must help students consider the impact of disability and its management on all aspects of patients' lives, including employment; household responsibilities; and family, social, and sexual relationships.

3. The physician-patient relationship must reflect a willingness to negotiate toward shared goals. The curriculum must stress the need for physicians to listen to and learn from their patients with disabilities to arrive at treatment plans that are realistic for patients and that conform to the highest patient care standards.

Persons with disabilities are an essential source of information for physicians, and communication skills are critical; for instance, physicians must work with patients who communicate atypically and may require accommodations or assistive technology.

Kirschner and Curry (2009) proposed six core competencies for training physicians to care for persons with disabilities. These core competencies, as reformulated by Iezzoni and Long-Bellil (2012, 138), follow:

- "Framing disability within the context of human diversity across the lifespan and within social and cultural environments;
- "Skills training for assessment of disability and functional consequences of health conditions, considering implications for treatment and management;
- "Training in general principles concerning etiquette for interactions with persons with disabilities;
- "Learning about roles of other health care professionals forming integrated teams to care for persons with disabilities;

- "Understanding legal requirements of the 1990 Americans with Disabilities Act for accommodating disability in health care settings, along with principles of universal design; and
- "Competency in patient-centered care approaches, including understanding patients' perceptions of quality of life."

A variety of health profession education organizations are working to develop disability-related competencies. Those organizations include the Alliance for Disability in Health Care Education; the American Academy of Developmental Medicine and Dentistry, through its National Curriculum Initiative in Developmental Medicine; and the Society of Teachers of Family Medicine.

Current Systems for Physician Education and Disability-Related Training

The organizations responsible for accreditation standards that determine curricular content in undergraduate and graduate medical education programs are the Liaison Committee on Medical Education (LCME) and the Accreditation Council for Graduate Medical Education (ACGME). Neither of these standards directly addresses disability-related training, although they do not preclude the inclusion of disability and even provide openings where this topic could be covered. The U.S. Medical Licensing Examination (USMLE or "boards"), which is the three-step examination that physicians-in-training must pass to be licensed to practice medicine, also influences curricular content. "If it's not on the boards, it isn't taught" is a common refrain. Some board examinations include content on disabling medical conditions, but there has been little effort to strengthen disability-related curricular content.

Kirschner and Curry (2009) have applied lessons from the concept of "universal design" in accessibility for the built environment to a universal approach to disability in medical education. They proposed integrating disability-related learning objectives within the standards, competencies, and curricular formats that are already in place to prepare physicians to practice medicine. This approach would ensure that every graduate of a medical school and residency program enters medical practice possessing core competencies in the care of patients with disabilities as a matter of routine. Training initiatives focused specifically on disability would only be provided to address identified gaps in the universal curriculum.

Teaching Strategies

To teach about disability, medical education programs use a variety of strategies, such as classroom-based exercises, clinical exercises, training with standardized patients, and sessions in community programs. Some programs have developed teaching skills using standardized patients with disabilities in a segregated disability curriculum, and these programs then employ the trainees to teach in the mainstream curriculum. Interacting with persons with disabilities within their own homes or in community-based clinical sites is particularly valuable. Additional recommendations offered by experienced medical educators include involving persons with disabilities as teachers, using cultural competency as a framework for teaching about disability, organizing longitudinal experiences, and providing opportunities to learn about interdisciplinary care-management approaches.

Self-awareness is critically important, and medical educators need to help students and trainees become aware of their own attitudes, including negative attitudes, about persons with disabilities. New media offer new ways to provide disability-related training. For example, a webinar series offered by the American Academy of Family Physicians offers continuing medical education credits.

With few exceptions, evaluation of the impact of disability-related training has been limited to assessments of students' attitudes and satisfaction measured immediately upon completion of the experience. Evidence on the long-term impact of training on clinical practice and health outcomes is still lacking, and it is an important future direction for research. Finally, senior physicians who serve as role models for students and early practitioners are important in the training of new physicians. An attending physician with positive attitudes toward patients with disabilities can be very influential as part of the training process.

Moving Forward

Policy influences outside of medical education, including laws and regulations, may be critical factors in ensuring that physicians are competent to care for patients with disabilities. Potential policies that require changes in physician preparation include amendments to the standards and core competencies issued by accrediting organizations and the content covered in the national boards. While the 1990 Americans with Disabilities Act (ADA) did not materially improve training of health care professionals, ADA-related lawsuits have led to improvements in access. The 2010 Patient Protection and Affordable Care Act (ACA) included a provision (Section 5307) that authorizes federal funding for training health care professionals in competencies related to "disability culture" and development of model curricula on the needs of people with disabilities, though no funding

was allocated to support implementation of this disability content. The National Council on Disability (2009) suggested curriculum requirements as a condition for receipt of federal funding of internship and residency programs in medical schools and other professional health care training institutions, as a mechanism for building a physician workforce that is competent to care for persons with disabilities.

Conclusion

Most physicians will likely care for patients with disabilities during their medical careers. Integrating disability-related learning objectives within the standards and competencies that currently govern medical education would ensure that graduates of medical schools and residency programs enter into medical practice possessing core competencies in the care of patients with disabilities. The likelihood that accrediting organizations and other associated entities would do this voluntarily in the foreseeable future is unlikely. Federal laws like the ADA and the ACA offer some hope for influencing medical education systems. A physician workforce that is competent to care for patients with disabilities is an important element of efforts to improve the health status of persons with disabilities, which is a national goal.

Paula M. Minihan

See also: Americans with Disabilities Act (ADA); Disability Studies; Disability Studies in Higher Education; Health Care Provider Activism

Further Reading

Hafferty, Frederick. 1998. "Beyond Curriculum Reform: Confronting Medicine's Hidden Curriculum." *Academic Medicine* 73: 403–407.

Iezzoni, Lisa, and Linda Long-Bellil. 2012. "Training Physicians about Caring for Persons with Disabilities: 'Nothing about Us without Us!' " *Disability and Health Journal* 5: 136–139.

Institute of Medicine. 2007. *The Future of Disability in America*. Washington, DC: National Academies Press.

Kirschner, Kristi, and Raymond Curry. 2009. "Educating Health Care Professionals to Care for Patients with Disability." *Journal of the American Medical Association (JAMA)* 302: 1334–1335.

Minihan, Paula, Ylisabyth Bradshaw, Linda Long, Wayne Altman, Sonya Perduta-Fulginiti, Jeanette Ector, Karen L. Foran, Lillian Johnson, Paul Kahn, and Robert Sneirson. 2004. "Teaching About Disability: Involving Patients with Disabilities as Medical Educators." *Disabilities Studies Quarterly* 24, no. 4. http://dsq-sds.org/article/view/883/1058

National Council on Disability. 2009. "The Current State of Health Care for People with Disabilities." https://www.ncd.gov/publications/2009/Sept302009.

U.S. Department of Health and Human Services Office of the Surgeon General. 2005. "The Surgeon General's Call to Action to Improve the Health and Wellness of Persons with Disabilities." https://www.ncbi.nlm.nih.gov/books/NBK44667/.

U.S. Public Health Service Office of the Surgeon General. 2002. "Closing the Gap: A National Blueprint for Improving the Health of Individuals with Mental Retardation." https://www.ncbi.nlm.nih.gov/books/NBK44346.

Medical Home. See Care Coordination and the Medical Home

Medical Model. See Social Model of Disability

Medical Paternalism

U.S. society greatly values individuality, independence, and autonomy. It is particularly important for patients to feel empowered, to have control when in such a vulnerable role, and to feel that their rights and opinions are being respected. Medical paternalism has changed over the years, largely in response to the patients' rights movement. This change has occurred as increasing numbers of "outsiders" are becoming involved in the process of medical practice (Rothman 2003). These outsiders hold medical professionals accountable for their actions as well as their inaction.

What Is Medical Paternalism?

Medical paternalism is the idea that doctors have expertise and, therefore, because of that expertise, have the authority to determine what is in the best interests of their patients. This concept is rooted in a medical model of disability that sees disability as something that is defective or broken within an individual and that needs to be treated and somehow fixed.

Key Concepts in Medical Paternalism

Medical paternalism is an extension of paternalism, wherein an authority figure determines what is in the best interests of others. Such paternalism may be played out within different contexts, such as in authoritarian governments or to varying degrees in different parenting approaches.

Autonomy. There has been much discussion, within intellectual disability research in particular, around the relationship between the notion of autonomy and medical paternalism. Van Hooren, Widdershoven, Candel, van den Borne, and Curfs theorize that there are four concepts of autonomy as it relates to medical paternalism: (1) the paternalistic model, (2) the informative model, (3) the interpretive model, and (4) the deliberative model:

1. **Paternalistic Model:** "The physician encourages the patient to consent to the medical intervention chosen by him. . . . Patient autonomy is conceived as patient assent to the physician's determinations of what is best. The conception of [competency] is the ability to cooperate."

2. **Informative Model:** "The objective . . . is for the physician to provide the patient with all the relevant information so that the patient can select the medical intervention [they] want. The physician then executes the selected interventions. In this model, the physician is a purveyor of technical expertise, providing the patient with the means to exercise control. The conception of patient autonomy is patient control over medical decision making. [Competency] is conceived as the ability to understand the provided information, to weigh this information against one's own values and to take decisions."

3. **Interpretive Model:** "The physician helps to elucidate the patient's values, and to make clear what [they] actually want . . . works with the patient to reconstruct the patient's goals and aspirations, commitments, and character. The physician is a counselor, engaging the patient in a joint process of understanding. Patient autonomy is viewed as self-understanding . . . and how the various medical options bear on her or his identity. The conception of [competency] is the ability to understand one's own values and to clarify the relevance of these values."

4. **Deliberative Model:** "This model sees the aim of the physician–patient interaction being to help the patient to determine and to choose the best values for her or his health, but unlike the interpretive model, the values of the patient not only need to be elucidated, they also are open for development and revision through moral discussion and deliberation. The physician can suggest that certain health related values are more worthy and should be aspired to. In this model, the physician's role is that of a teacher or friend. The conception of patient autonomy is moral self-development: the patient is empowered not simply to follow unexamined preferences or examined values, but to consider, through dialogue, alternative health-related values, their worthiness and their implications for treatment. [Competency] is conceived as the ability to learn and develop one's own values." (2006, 563)

Paternalistic models are familiar and have long been critiqued by disability studies. The informative model is similar to what we consider informed consent in the current medical paradigm, which struggles between medical paternalism and patient autonomy, which depend on judgments of competency. The other two models stem from the supposition that autonomy is a matter of self-realization. Rather than being contrasted with dependency, perhaps autonomy occurs in relation to other human beings. This relational model of autonomy focuses on the importance of social context. The researchers caution, however, that there is a risk of relational models functioning as disguised paternalism if one is not careful. In the interpretive model, physicians work with patients to achieve the patients' goals and give guidance. In the deliberative model, however, negotiation occurs between physician and patient. This model provides individuals with the opportunity to express their respective viewpoints in a balanced relationship and allows physician and patient to learn from each other.

History of the Patients' Rights Movement

In his book *Strangers at the Bedside*, David Rothman postulates that the issues of medical paternalism and autonomy came to fruition around the time of the civil rights movement, which bolstered society's response and maintained awareness of medical issues and patients' rights.

> The impact of these events . . . was to make the invisible visible. Outsiders to medicine . . . penetrated every nook and cranny, in the process giving medicine an exceptional prominence on the public agenda and making it the subject of popular discourse. This glare of the spotlight transformed medical decision making, shaping not merely the external conditions under which medicine would be practiced . . . but the very substance of medical practice—the decisions that physicians made at the bedside. (2003, 3)

Medical decisions were no longer private ones based on the trust built between a doctor and patient. Rather, these decisions became matters of public record and inquiry, as patients were encouraged to become active participants in their treatment.

The societal pressure to respond to ethical dilemmas in medicine was consistent with and strengthened by the contemporaneous social movements. Growing public awareness of the inhumane conditions in institutions and in medical research experienced by individuals with disabilities served as a catalyst for disability rights and the deinstitutionalization movement in the 1960s and 1970s. Since then, efforts have been made to move individuals with disabilities out of institutions and help them become integrated into the community. The power of these movements influenced the way in which society responded to medical paternalism, as well as the scale of the response.

Patient's Bill of Rights. In his book *The Rights of Patients*, George Annas remarked that "the patients rights movement is as slow as a glacier, equally relentless at changing the landscape, but ultimately healthy. That it is not as organized and identifiable as other consumer movements is explained by the fact that when individuals are sick or injured, they are not themselves" (1989, 1). This statement speaks to a critical disconnect between the patients' rights movement and the disability rights movement (DRM) at the time, for people with disabilities were fighting to be seen not as merely patients or consumers under the auspices of a medical model of disability but rather as individuals living with impairments who were being marginalized and disadvantaged by an inaccessible society that was disabling them and denying their civil rights. Conversely, the patients' rights movement was focused more specifically on ensuring that a balance in decision making was maintained within medical settings between individuals and medical professionals in a way that respected the rights and responsibilities of patients to make the ultimate decisions regarding their care and treatment. A key aspect of this argument became the concept of *informed consent*, that before making a medical decision an individual has the right to be fully informed about the acts that will be taken and any possible benefits or risks (such as side effects).

It was not until 1998 that the U.S. Advisory Commission on Consumer Protection and Quality in the Health Care Industry adopted the "Consumer Bill of Rights and Responsibilities," which has come to be known as the "Patient's Bill of Rights." There are eight components of this document:

1. information for patients
2. choice of providers and plans
3. access to emergency services
4. participation in treatment decisions
5. respect and nondiscrimination
6. confidentiality (privacy) of health information
7. complaints and appeals
8. consumer responsibilities

The passing of the Patient Protection and Affordable Care Act (ACA) in 2014 led to the addition of new rules for the Patient's Bill of Rights, aimed at keeping insurance companies from limiting the care an individual needs and removing insurance barriers between individuals and their doctors. Some of the protections in these rules include the following:

- ensuring coverage for people with preexisting conditions
- ensuring the right to choose a doctor
- ensuring fair treatment of emergency care
- making sure policies can't be canceled unfairly
- ending annual and lifetime limits
- enhancing access to preventive services
- ensuring the right to appeal health plan decisions
- ensuring health coverage for young adults
- ensuring protections under "grandfathered plans"

Providing coverage for individuals with *preexisting conditions* is an issue that has made a large impact on the disability community, ensuring that more individuals can access health insurance and care than ever before. Further, this topic has led to controversy regarding conservative efforts to repeal and replace the ACA under the Trump administration.

Dilemmas, Debates, and Unresolved Questions

There are many debates and controversies within the disability context where medical paternalism, or the idea that "doctors know best," becomes bioethical issues, such as when families and professionals have conflicting opinions on patient care. Fundamentally, these discussions center on the value of disabled lives within medical discourse and on the role of medical professionals.

Prenatal Testing, Genetic Screening, and Physician Prognostication. For example, what exactly is the role of medical professionals when conducting prenatal testing and genetic screening, what is their expertise when a disability is detected, and how does this diagnosis affect a family's medical decisions? Research has shown that as disability, intellectual disability in particular, becomes more severe, physician prognosis (what the physician expects to happen in the future) becomes more negative. Consequently, physicians overestimate the negative effects and underestimate the positive effects of disability (Blaymore Bier et al. 1996; Wolraich, Siperstein, and O'Keefe 1987). This combination can lead parents to decide to terminate pregnancies of children who physicians believe will have impairments, because of the belief that those children cannot have fulfilling or productive lives.

Organ Transplant Discrimination. The issue of negative prognostication comes to the forefront in debates regarding organ transplants for people with disabilities. There have been multiple news stories about people who need an organ transplant to live but who were denied or placed low on the waiting list because of their disability and the belief (based in medical model thinking) that someone without a disability was more deserving. One such case, involving an infant with an intellectual and developmental disability (IDD) who needed a heart transplant, prompted the Autistic Self Advocacy Network (ASAN) to create a policy brief on organ transplant discrimination in 2013 and a toolkit for advocates on ending organ transplant discrimination.

Euthanasia: Right to Live vs. Right to Die. One of the core debates throughout the history of medical paternalism has been that of euthanasia: whether it is morally ethical to end the life of a patient who is believed to be suffering, and whether that is a decision for a medical professional to make. This question was central to the genesis of the patients' rights movement during the case of Karen Ann Quinlan, who, in 1975, fell into a coma followed by a "persistent vegetative state" after an accidental overdose. Quinlan became the topic of a legal battle between her family, who requested she be removed from a ventilator so as not to prolong her suffering, and hospital officials, who argued that ending her life in this way would constitute murder on their part. In 1976, Quinlan was removed from the ventilator and, to much surprise, continued to breathe on her own. She lived nine more years in a nursing facility.

A similar, but very much different, case is that of Terri Schiavo, who, in 1990, fell into a coma followed by a "persistent vegetative state" after a cardiac arrest. Schiavo's case was complicated by the contentious relationship between her husband, Michael Schiavo, who had himself appointed as her guardian, and her family and physicians. There were concerns that her husband was

hoping to benefit financially from Schiavo's death and as such was not acting in her best interests. In 2003, after a lengthy legal battle, Schiavo's feeding tube was removed. Soon afterward, Florida governor Jeb Bush passed "Terri's Law," giving the governor authority to intervene in the case. The feeding tube was reinserted, and Schiavo was appointed a guardian *ad litem* and moved into hospice care. Part of the role of the guardian *ad litem* was to help determine what course of action was in Schiavo's best interests and to help make medical decisions. Terri's Law was eventually struck down as unconstitutional as disagreements and differing medical opinions regarding Terri's care continued, and the case was moved to federal jurisdiction because of an act of Congress under President George W. Bush in 2005, when the Senate unanimously passed a bill that came to be known as the "Palm Sunday Compromise." Schiavo had at that point become very much an object in a political issue in which her right to live was subject to another's decision about her best interests. Schiavo died in hospice in 2005 due to undetermined causes.

A more recent case that touches upon this issue is that of young Jerika Bolen, a 14-year-old girl with spinal muscular atrophy who had made the decision to hold a prom for herself before ending her life. She called the prom "Jerika's Last Dance" and raised $36,482 for it on a fund-raising Web site (gofundme.com). Bolen's mother supported her decision, bolstered by physicians' prognosis of Bolen's pain and suffering. However, disability advocacy groups in Wisconsin and around the country, such as Disability Rights Wisconsin and Not Dead Yet, mobilized in response to what they saw as the result of an ableist system that promotes medical model thinking and would allow a teenager to commit suicide.

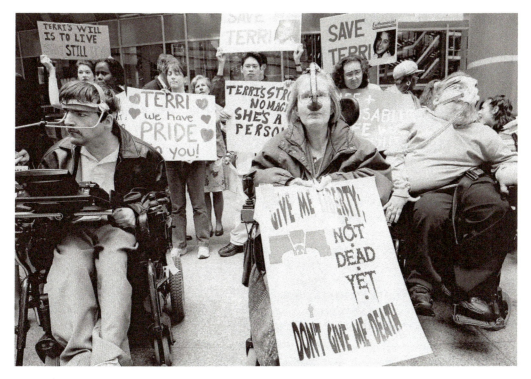

Disabled activists stage a protest calling for continued care and feeding of Terri Schiavo at the Thompson Center Plaza, in Chicago, Illinois, on March 29, 2005. Schiavo, the Florida woman who was severely brain-damaged, went more than 11 days without food or water after a judge ordered her feeding tube removed at her husband's request. (Scott Olson/Getty Images)

These disability organizations saw this promotion of assisted suicide for her as a clear case of discrimination and requested an investigation as to whether Bolen had been receiving "competent medical care, proper pain management advice for her circumstances and proper support for her emotional and mental health" (Broverman 2016). In particular, people with impairments similar to Bolen's wanted to make sure she was informed about the quality of life she could have if she were receiving adequate care and support. An investigation did not come. Instead, Bolen passed away as she had planned, in 2016. This was not a decision that a medical professional made directly. However, the physicians' prognosis (founded in the medical model of disability)

may likely have resulted in discriminatory care and support that led to the decision Bolen's mother supported.

Conclusion

In recent years, bioethical debates in disability studies have moved away from discussing medical paternalism. This move is perhaps due to divisions between the patients' rights movement and the disability rights movement. However, the current push against the repeal of the ACA is an issue that may benefit from uniting these histories and movements. Medical paternalism overlaps to a considerable degree with guardianship concerns, and given the increasing involvement of outsiders within medical settings, medical decisions cannot be said to be made simply between physician and patient. Rather, they occur in relation to other human beings and within social and governmental systems that may intervene in different ways. There remains a need for further theoretical development of medical paternalism in the modern age, as policy and technology have advanced.

Kate Caldwell

See also: Bioethics; Guardianship and Capacity; Medicalization; Social Model of Disability

Further Reading

Annas, George J. 1989. *The Rights of Patients: The Basic ACLU Guide to Patient Rights.* Carbondale: Southern Illinois University Press.

Blaymore Bier, Jo-Ann, Jill A. Liebling, Yesenia Morales, and Marianne Carlucci. 1996. "Parents' and Pediatricians' Views of Individuals with Meningomyelocele." *Clinical Pediatrics* 35, no. 3: 113–117.

Broverman, Aaron. 2016. "Paralyzed Teen Jerika Bolen Dies, as Planned." *New Mobility: The Magazine for Active Wheelchair Users,* September 23. http://www.newmobility.com/2016/09/paralyzed-teen-jerika-bolen-dies/.

Rothman, David J. 2003. *Strangers at the Bedside: A History of How Law and Bioethics Transformed Medical Decision Making.* New York: Aldine de Gruyter.

van Hooren, Rob H., Guy A. M. Widdershoven, Math Candel, Bart W. van den Borne, and Leopold M. G. Curfs. 2006. "Between Control and Freedom in the Care for Persons with Prader-Willi Syndrome: An Analysis of Preferred Interventions by Caregivers." *Patient Education and Counseling* 63, no. 1–2: 223–231.

Wolraich, Mark L., Gary N. Siperstein, and Paul O'Keefe. 1987. "Pediatricians' Perceptions of Mentally Retarded Individuals." *Pediatrics* 80, no. 5: 643–649.

Medicalization

Most broadly, medicalization refers to the process by which an experience or aspect of life comes to be understood as an individual medical problem and, as such, explained through medical knowledge and frameworks. This, in turn, initiates a series of solutions, interventions, and systems aimed at solving the problem.

What Is Medicalization? Why Is It Important?

Though this overview of medicalization is seemingly straightforward, several things about it are worth highlighting. First, and perhaps most important, medicalization is a *process.* This process occurs over time, involves many actors, and for that reason is connected to historical, cultural, societal, political, and economic contexts. It also reflects such processes as the struggle over professionalization (of medicine and other sciences), authority, and knowledge. Similarly, race, class, gender, sexuality, age, ethnicity, and disability all influence how and what experiences are understood as medical problems (when and for whom). Medicalization affects people differently depending on their positionality and the broader context in which the processes of medicalization occur. Medicalization is, in other words, much more than a moment in time when an individual person discovers and names a previously unknown or unidentified medical condition. Medicalization, rather, describes the bigger picture (and process) of how experiences become addressed as problems *and* the subsequent mobilization of knowledge, power, authority, and material resources toward managing that problem.

Second, medicalization identifies experiences or aspects of life thought to be (or understood as) *individual* problems in need of medical intervention. These problems are located within an individual's body or mind, and therefore, attempts at "solving the problem" are addressed on or in the individual or at the level of a collective group of individuals. For instance, the medicalization of disability, in particular, involves the identification of disability (through its varying medical diagnostic categories) as a problem rooted in the body or mind of an individual. As such, medicalization involves and relies on the individualization of disability and illness (making disability and illness problems of the individual). Importantly, this individualization still allows for groups of people who are understood as having impairments to be tied together and seen as groups who share in individual body or mind experience in the way that people who are blind or people with diabetes are discussed as a group. This can result in interventions that are targeted at the group (people with diabetes, for instance), but those interventions remain located within the bodies and minds of individuals rather than environments, social attitudes or structures, policies, etc.

This brings us to the third point; medicalization involves the identification of *problems* within the individual and the subsequent development of interventions or solutions aimed at fixing the identified problem. These interventions or solutions rely heavily, if not exclusively, on medicine and medical knowledge and involve classification systems that separate "normal" from "abnormal" or "functional" from "dysfunctional." These classifications are, in turn, connected to social values and, in many social contexts and historical moments, heavily inflected by and with morality. For instance, normal is valued as "good," whereas "abnormal" or "dysfunctional" carry valences of "bad"

or "immoral." In other words, the process of medicalization, despite assumptions of the objectivity and neutrality of medicine, is tied to systems of value that carry significant social, cultural, political, and economic consequences.

Historical Overview

The history of medicalization is closely tied to the history of medical knowledge and its professionalization. The late 18th and early 19th centuries saw a shift in the role of medicine within Western societies (which, in turn, also affected lands colonized by Western nation-states). Medicine, medical knowledge, and medical professionals gained a level of cultural and moral authority that previously had been held by religion and the church. This shift resulted from a confluence of factors. The scientific revolution fostered a greater belief in rationality and the promise of science and scientific reasoning. Industrialization and urbanization lead to rapid population growth in cities, which resulted in greater exposure to communicable diseases as well as growing rates of injuries due to industrial accidents. At the same time, technological, pharmaceutical, and medical advances led to a growing number of tools that helped to combat diseases and treat injuries. In short, medicine gained tools that made the practice of medicine more efficient and allowed medical practitioners to save and extend lives in unprecedented ways. This growing effectiveness helped to secure a popular belief and investment in medical knowledge and expertise.

Key Concepts in Medicalization

The development of mass communication technologies allowed for the dissemination of medical knowledge into the social and cultural spheres. This dissemination played a key role in popularizing the authority of medical knowledge and helped to lay the groundwork for the emerging *health care industry*. The health care industry is made up of a wide range of entities from hospitals, rehabilitation clinics, fitness facilities, pharmacies, and companies that make and sell products used to help secure and maintain health. This industry profits from and (therefore) perpetuates the medicalization of aspects of life by selling the promise of health, or the products that will help solve the problem of illness or disability. As such, medicalization cannot be understood outside of the economic structures that have given rise to and helped facilitate medicalization.

Medical Industrial Complex. Some activists and scholars use the term "medical industrial complex" to describe this broader industry connected to medicine and medicalization. Like any complex, the medical industrial complex is made up of smaller components like the medical profession, pharmaceutical companies, and the state. These smaller components are bound together within the complex by a particular set of ideas: that medical knowledge can and should have the capacity and authority to solve the problem of bodyminds (the body and the mind inseparable) deemed deviant, disabled, or sick.

This brings us to another key point that is central to the understanding of medicalization. Medical knowledge is not only specialized knowledge held by medical practitioners but a set of ideas that people, companies, and systems, in general, put into practice. Medicalization, then, might be thought of as the act of putting medical ways of viewing the body and mind into practice as well as the permeation of these ideas into the cultural, social, economic, and political spheres. The state, for instance,

adopts medicalized views of disability in the administration of services or support, which require extensive documentation by a physician or licensed medical authority to verify experiences of the body or mind.

Bodyminds. Processes of medicalization also often distinguish between bodies and minds. Despite critiques of this Cartesian dualism, medical knowledge still predominantly understands the mind and body to be two distinct systems that require two distinct knowledge bases. This continued distinction should be understood as an *effect* of medicalization itself, which divides professional authority of the mind and body into distinct disciplines, and does not consider the inherent aspect of the relationship between bodies and minds. Margaret Price (2015), for instance, uses the term "bodyminds" to call attention to the inseparability between them.

Part of what makes medicalization such a central and useful concept for disability studies is that it describes the degree to which the frameworks of understanding bodies and minds found within (and informed by) medicine extend into other spheres. It might be useful to think of this in terms of "who" medicalizes the patient and "where" medicalization occurs. In other words, as suggested, it is not just doctors, therapists, or rehabilitation professionals who medicalized patients within the clinic. Individuals (from friends and family to strangers) as well as social and cultural structures (from the education system to social support services and popular media) adopt and employ this framework of understanding human difference as a medical problem.

Interpersonal Interactions. Medicalization occurs even at the level of everyday interpersonal interactions. When strangers, for instance, ask people with disabilities,

"What's wrong with you?" they engage in the process of medicalization. In this scenario, the stranger views disability as something wrong (a problem). As many disabled people attest, these questions carry considerable meaning and are often experienced as microaggressions because they reflect a demand (and assumed right) to know the specific (medical) diagnosis of the disabled person. The medicalization of disability leads to the belief that upon knowing a person's diagnosis, we know all of the information, or the most important part, we need to know about the person.

Exploring what is behind the willingness of strangers to ask for disabled people's diagnoses reveals several important aspects of medicalization. First, it highlights the presumed neutrality of medicine and medical knowledge. Such questions are made possible by the presumption that asking for a diagnosis is seeking factual and therefore neutral information. This presumed neutrality, in other words, makes the question seem permissible. Disability studies has joined other critical disciplines to offer important interventions into this presumed neutrality of medicine by naming the medicalization of disability as a political issue and making clear that questions presuming that disability is wrong are far from neutral. This word choice further reveals the dominance or cultural authority of medical frameworks because it relies on the assumption that everyone understands disability as a medical problem and that everyone (including the disabled person) views disability as such, reflecting the extent to which medicalization pervades cultural and social spheres.

Such encounters also signal an investment within the authority and promise of medicine. The question "What's wrong with you?" is motivated, at least in part, by a belief that medicine can, does, and should cure all "problems" of the body and mind. This belief can lead to a demand to account for what has been done to try to solve (cure) the disability, and speakers often include such follow-up questions as "Have you tried seeing a specialist?" or "Can't they do anything about that?" Such questions, of course, differ in specific content and tone depending upon the disability, context, and positionality of the person asking. They are, for instance, often (but not exclusively) more pointedly directed at people with impairments less culturally legitimate. The underlying impulse of such questions that call upon disabled people to name their efforts to solve the problem of disability also belies the individualized nature of medicalization (that it is the individual's responsibility to get better), as well as the compulsory nature of able-bodiedness that insists those who do not meet an able-bodied standard account for their efforts to reach that standard. Such a seemingly simple, if pervasive, question illuminates the dominance of medicalization as a framework for understanding disability.

Dilemmas, Debates, and Unresolved Questions

Many scholars writing about medicalization specify that it refers to aspects of human life previously not understood as problems of a medical nature or within the purview of medicine. For instance, Peter Conrad states, "'Medicalization' describes a process by which nonmedical problems become defined and treated as medical problems, usually in terms of illness and disorder" (2007, 4). This understanding draws a distinction between medical and nonmedical problems, implying that there are experiences that are properly medicalized and those that are not.

Though few within disability studies explicitly define medicalization, its use within the field reveals an understanding that incorporates the broader processes of using medical knowledge to understand experiences and human differences. As a field, we might also query whether medicalization is strictly a process that affects humans and engage with those in animal studies who seek to challenge distinctions between humans and nonhumans. Disability studies' more comprehensive scope of medicalization as a process that describes all application of medicalized knowledge lends itself well to challenging such distinctions, given its focus on the *process* of medicalization and not on the specific individual illness or disability being medicalized.

The tension between these positions rests, to some degree, on different understandings of the scope of medicalization as well as different analytical approaches to medicalization, and it can be seen more fully in how the concept has been applied and discussed. Approaches that focus on medicalization as a process by which nonmedical experiences become medical tend to outline the construction of specific disease entities or disorders and detail the ways in which the associated experiences, states, or behaviors become a medical problem. These approaches retain the specific experiences or behaviors as the objects of analysis, leaving the processes of medicalization examined *only* within the context of the specific disease entity. To be clear, this approach reveals important insights about medicalization. However, it can lead to implications (or, in some instances, explicit arguments) that the disease entity or disorder has been wrongly or overly medicalized, implying that there are proper objects of medicalization. Scholars who approach medicalization in this way often draw a distinction between pathologies discovered and pathologies created.

A more comprehensive analysis of medicalization, one that takes the process of medicalization itself as the primary object of analysis, offers more systemic critiques. Disability studies approaches to medicalization also apply analytical frameworks that recognize disability as an experience situated within and framed by contexts. Such approaches do not draw hard distinctions between discovery and creation but instead argue for understanding *all* pathological designations as created, in the sense that their identification, naming, and treatment are part of broader cultural, social, historical, political, and economic processes. These processes, then, become the focus of analysis. In short, this view understands medicalization as describing the application of and authority embedded within medical knowledge without drawing distinctions between proper and improper objects of medicalization.

The Future of Medicalization

Much of the work on medicalization within disability studies outlines the devastating impact that the medicalization of disability has had on disabled people's lives. This work is key to mapping the processes that frame and perpetuate disability oppression. However, recent work has begun to also recognize that, within the current social, political, economic, historical, and cultural contexts, medicalization also provides access to care, supports, and legitimacy of experiences, however precarious, that those whose experiences are not recognized by medical knowledge do not have access to. Anna Mollow (2014) has recently argued for the importance of recognizing and centralizing what she calls "undocumented disabilities," or those experiences that medical knowledge has not authorized as legitimate.

Critical work within disability studies (and other disciplines) must also recognize such experiences as part of the effects of medicalization—which uses medical knowledge and authority to separate experiences into legitimate problems (which mobilizes resources) and illegitimate experiences seen as not really problems (for which resources will not be distributed). The material needs of those whose experiences have been delegitimized by these processes of medicalization have, at times, mobilized to advocate for greater research into their embodied experiences to produce the medical knowledge necessary to authorize those experiences as legitimate to access needed material resources.

Jeremy Greene points out, "The medicalization critique is typically a top-down approach which accuses a powerful and interested organization—most frequently the medical profession, the state, or the pharmaceutical industry—of manufacturing a disease and producing populations of patients to consolidate control over power and resources" (2012, 209). However, such a critique fails to acknowledge the degree to which many people or groups trying to access care, services, or recognition of experiential differences actively seek the authorization that medicalization can provide. This returns us to the question of who motivates medicalization. This top-down critique, as Greene reveals, has importantly identified the roles that the medical profession, state, and industry play in animating the processes of medicalization.

However, this understanding does not fully account for the active role that advocacy groups can play in the processes of medicalization. Future research on medicalization needs to recognize that people actively pursue medicalization *because of* medicalization. The fact that resources are so closely tied to medicalization makes people have to argue for and invest in these processes, perpetuating the authority of medical knowledge. However, if we recognize that medicalization is not only the authority of medicine and medical knowledge but also the permeation of that knowledge into other spheres, we can continue to target our interventions into these permeations. We might ask, then, how and what it would look like for medical knowledge to exist in the absence of medicalization.

Conclusion

We have recognized that medicalization is a process shaped by historical, political, cultural, social, and economic factors that impact people differently depending on race, class, gender, sexuality, ethnicity, age, and disability. In an effort to more explicitly call up the historical context and colonial legacy of medicine, Susan Burch (2015) explicitly includes "Western" as a designation before "medicine" to speak of Western medicine. This move calls attention to the dominance of (and colonial legacy within) Western medicine by drawing limits on what we mean when we say "medicine." It also recognizes that other ways of relating to bodyminds exist alongside Western medicine: indigenous, local, alternative, and Ayurvedic knowledges. Excavating and honoring these knowledges and finding affinities between them and critical disability or crip knowledges can help counter the devastating effects of medicalization.

Alyson Patsavas

See also: Business of Disability; Disability Studies; Medical Education; Medical Paternalism; Social Model of Disability

Further Reading

Burch, Susan. 2015. "Disorderly States: Institutionalization and American Indian Histories, 1900–1960s." Society for Disability Studies 28th Annual Conference. Hyatt Regency, Atlanta, GA. June 13.

Conrad, Peter. 2007. *The Medicalization of Society: On the Transformation of Human Conditions into Treatable Disorders.* Baltimore: Johns Hopkins University Press.

Greene, Jeremy, and Elizabeth Watkins, eds. 2012. *Prescribed: Writing, Filling, Using, and Abusing the Prescription in Modern America.* Baltimore: Johns Hopkins University Press.

Mollow, Anna. 2014. "Criphystemologies: What Disability Theory Needs to Know about Hysteria." *Journal of Literary and Cultural Disability Studies* 8, no. 2: 185–202.

Price, Margaret. 2015. "The Bodymind Problem and the Possibilities of Pain." *Hypatia* 30, no. 1: 1527–2001.

Mental Health and Developmental Disabilities

This entry discusses the issue of mental health concerns among people with developmental disabilities (DD). "Dual diagnosis" is a term applied to the coexistence of both DD and a mental health diagnosis (also referred to as psychiatric disabilities or mental illnesses). Some common examples are anxiety, depression, schizophrenia, attention deficit hyperactivity disorder (ADHD), and substance abuse disorders. This entry will discuss the history, prevalence, and current dilemmas and debates.

Background and History

For many years, mental health concerns among people with DD were largely ignored by researchers and clinicians. In general, it was believed that people with DD lacked the cognitive capacity to develop mental illness. This belief was strongly connected to the Freudian view, in which mental illness was the result of an imbalance between primitive urges and societal rules. Since people with DD were assumed to lack the cognitive skills to experience this conflict, it followed that they could not develop mental illness in the same way as people without disabilities. Later views held that people with DD could develop schizophrenia, as evidenced by aggressive or self-injurious behavior, but not other forms of mental illness. As the focus of psychology shifted away from a Freudian perspective and onto cognitive and biological models of mental health, the question of whether people with DD could experience mental illness was reexamined. In the early 1980s, researchers began to examine more closely case reports of people with DD and argue that poor mental health was not dependent on intellectual functioning.

Today, research shows that people with DD experience the same range of mental health concerns as people without disabilities. In fact, most research suggests that people with DD are *more* likely to develop mental illness than people without DD. That is not surprising given this population's high incidence of risk factors for developing mental illness, such as a history of abuse, high risk of living in poverty, high levels of stress, and lack of positive supports, friends, and intimate relationships. While there is no longer a debate over whether or not people with DD can experience mental illness, the focus has now shifted to how best to diagnose and treat mental illness within this population.

Important Points to Know about Mental Health and Developmental Disabilities

For many years, people with DD who lived outside of the family home lived in large, usually state-run, institutions. Medical and psychological care was provided in-house, and people with DD did not generally seek care in the community. With the recent movement toward *deinstitutionalization*, there has been a flood of people with DD seeking mental health care from community providers. However, there are considerable barriers for people with DD who need timely and accurate mental health care.

Barriers to Receiving a Diagnosis. One barrier to mental health care access for people with DD is related to funding. People with DD often rely on Medicaid or Medicare as their primary form of insurance; this may limit their choice of providers and the amount of care they can receive. Additionally, many mental health providers feel ill equipped to care for people with DD and have not received training for working with this population. One common issue has been referred to as "diagnostic overshadowing." This term refers to care providers missing symptoms or signs of secondary conditions because they mistake these symptoms as a part of the person's disability. A second area of concern is the lack of validated and reliable instruments for assessing mental health symptoms in people with DD. Some strides have been made in this area, including the *Diagnostic Manual-Intellectual Disability* (DM-ID), a desk reference book designed to aid clinicians in arriving at accurate diagnoses in people with DD. However, there remains much work to be done.

Barriers to Receiving Care. After receiving a diagnosis of a mental illness, people with DD may still not receive appropriate care. They may struggle to find a care provider who feels capable of providing care and may face insurance restrictions. There is a very high rate of psychotropic medication use among people with DD. People with DD are one of the most heavily medicated populations, despite the lack of adequate research on the long-term impact of these medications. Moreover, people with

DD are less likely to receive other forms of treatment, such as psychotherapy. People with DD are unlikely to be included in new medication or psychotherapy trials, and so they may miss out on new and effective forms of treatment. These barriers mean that many people with DD who have mental health concerns may not receive the care that they need.

Dilemmas, Debates, and Unresolved Questions

Approximately 50 percent of people with DD also show some level of behavioral concern, such as property destruction, self-harm, or harm to others. A significant number of people with DD are heavily medicated, are restricted from their community, and make frequent visits to the emergency room as a result of behavioral concerns. Researchers and clinicians have struggled with how to determine if behavioral concerns are a symptom of poor mental health, if poor mental health causes behavioral concerns, if they are entirely separate, or to what degree they overlap. This ambiguity is a concern for clinicians trying to provide appropriate diagnoses and treatment, as well as for care providers trying to manage behavioral concerns. A better grasp of how these two issues are related would help to provide appropriate care for all people with DD.

Conclusion

People with DD are likely to experience poor mental health. Yet, there is still much work to be done to effectively diagnose and treat mental illness in this population. Future initiatives should focus on training providers of mental health services to work with people who have DD, developing strong instruments to evaluate mental health concerns, and researching better methods for providing mental health support to people with DD. Policy changes, such as expanding insurance coverage for mental health care and support for research that captures the perspectives of people with DD, may also improve mental health care for people with DD.

Haleigh M. Scott

See also: Deinstitutionalization; Mental Health Self-Help and Support Groups; Race and Mental Health; *Primary Documents:* Excerpt from the President's Panel on Mental Retardation, Report of the Task Force on Law (1963); Declaration of Objectives from the Older Americans Act (1965)

Further Reading

Cooper, Sally-Ann, Elita Smiley, Jillian Morrison, Andrew Williamson, and Linda Allan. 2007. "Mental Ill-Health in Adults with Intellectual Disabilities: Prevalence and Associated Factors." *British Journal of Psychiatry* 190, no. 1: 27–35.

Fletcher, Robert Jonathan, Earl Loschen, and Chrissoula Stavrakaki. 2007. *DM-ID: Diagnostic Manual-Intellectual Disability: A Textbook of Diagnosis of Mental Disorders in Persons with Intellectual Disability.* New York: National Association for the Dually Diagnosed.

Krahn, Gloria L., Laura Hammond, and Anne Turner. 2006. "A Cascade of Disparities: Health and Health Care Access for People with Intellectual Disabilities." *Developmental Disabilities Research Reviews* 12, no. 1: 70–82.

Schalock, Robert L., Sharon A. Borthwick-Duffy, Valerie J. Bradley, Wil H. E. Buntinx, David L. Coulter, Ellis M. Craig, Sharon C. Gomez, et al. 2012. *Intellectual Disability: Definition, Classification, and Systems of Supports.* 11th ed. Washington, DC: American Association on Intellectual and Developmental Disabilities.

Mental Health Narratives

Mental health narratives are broadly defined as first-person narratives by people who identify as having a mental health disability. Mental health disabilities addressed in these narratives often include mood disorders (such as bipolar disorder or depression), schizophrenia, obsessive-compulsive disorder, and personality disorders (such as borderline personality disorder).

Characteristics of Mental Health Narratives

Narrative Structure. Mental health narratives comprise a broad range of topics and formats. The most typical narrative format used is linear, in which authors describe their life and experience from early childhood to the present. Examples of this format include Kay Redfield Jamison's *An Unquiet Mind: A Memoir of Moods and Madness*, in which the author relates her experiences of bipolar disorder; Elyn Saks's *The Center Cannot Hold: My Journey through Madness*, in which the author explores her experiences of schizophrenia; and Meri Nana-Ama Danquah's *Willow Weep for Me: A Black Woman's Journey through Depression*, in which the author relates the unique experiences of a black woman grappling with depression.

Some authors take a less linear approach, focusing on a specific period of time in their lives. An example of this format includes Kate Millett's *Loony-Bin Trip*, in which the author narrates her experience of living with bipolar disorder while trying to establish a woman's commune and avoiding medication and hospitalization, despite pressures from her partner. Another example is Susanna Kaysen's *Girl, Interrupted*, in which the author explores her experience of hospitalization for borderline personality disorder in the 1970s. Merri Lisa Johnson also explores her experience of borderline personality in her memoir *Girl in Need of a Tourniquet*, but her narrative structure moves back and forth in time, from her childhood to the present, focusing more on experience than on a cohesive narrative beginning with her childhood. In his memoir *Tranquil Prisons: Chemical Incarceration under Community Treatment Orders*, Erick Fabris situates his experience of hospitalization within the broader context of community treatment orders in Canada, orders that require people diagnosed with mental illness to adhere to a medication regimen if they wish to leave the psychiatric hospital. He terms this "chemical incarceration." Throughout the memoir, the author explores the broader issue of the dismissal and silencing of people diagnosed with mental illness.

Rhetorical Strategies. "Rhetorical strategy" refers to the way the authors position themselves in relation to the topic of disability and their readers (Couser 1997, 33). The authors try to convey to their readers something specific regarding their experience of disability. They rely on certain narrative strategies to do this. Many first-person narratives, including those about the experience of mental illness, use a variety of rhetorical devices.

The *rhetoric of triumph* is the one readers are most familiar with, and it composes narratives of individuals overcoming the limitations of their disabilities and framing themselves as inspirational. The rhetoric of horror, or the *gothic rhetoric*, narrates the experience of disability as a "dreadful" condition that should be avoided at all costs. This rhetoric is usually used by those who have experienced temporary disability and

are now effectively cured and can look back on their experience as a horrific thing of the past (34). Because mental illness can never be cured, only treated and managed, one might assume that the gothic rhetoric would not be used in mental health narratives. However, many authors of these narratives highlight the most horrific aspects of their experiences with mental illness, and subsequent treatments, before they find the road to recovery, so the narratives typically combine the rhetoric of horror and the rhetoric of triumph. Counterhegemonic, *postcolonial rhetoric* is aligned with disability studies as the narratives mainly focus on the physical, social, and cultural barriers that oppress people with disabilities, rather than on the disabling conditions themselves. There are elements of this rhetoric in many mental health narratives as well. Many of the authors highlight the judgment they have experienced from others, including colleagues and medical professionals, when they have disclosed their diagnoses.

Historical Overview

One of the first published memoirs narrating the experience of mental illness, titled *Memoirs of My Nervous Illness*, was authored by Daniel Paul Schreber in 1903. Schreber was diagnosed with what was then known as "dementia praecox." Today, the diagnosis is known as paranoid schizophrenia. Schreber's memoir was actively studied by famous psychoanalysts Sigmund Freud and Carl Jung and thus remained widely popular. In 1946, Mary Jane Ward published her semiautobiographical novel *The Snake Pit*, about her experiences in a mental institution. The novel was made into an Academy Award–winning film in 1948. Both the novel and film are credited with instigating dialogue and eventual reform of state mental institutions. In 1963, Sylvia Plath, using a pseudonym, published her autobiographical novel *The Bell Jar*, in which she relates her experiences of extreme depression, a suicide attempt, and hospitalization. The autobiographical novel is considered a classic and is regularly studied in high school and college English courses. In 1964, Joanne Greenberg published her semiautobiographical novel, *I Never Promised You a Rose Garden*, about her diagnosis with schizophrenia and hospitalization. Another noteworthy autobiographical novel about mental illness is *A Question of Power*, by Bessie Head, published in 1974. In the novel, Head, a South African woman, explores her experience of what is vaguely termed a mental breakdown while living in poverty as a refugee in Botswana.

Despite these sporadic publications throughout the century, the mental health memoir as a narrative format did not gain ground until the 1990s, with the publication of William Styron's *Darkness Visible: A Memoir of Madness*. Published in 1990, it is a narrative of the author's experience with severe depression. This book was followed by Elizabeth Wurtzel's *Prozac Nation*, published in 1994, in which the author explores her experience with depression and treatments with a variety of antidepressants.

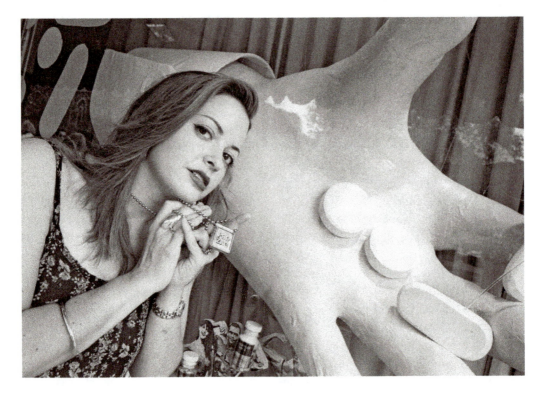

Elizabeth Wurtzel, author of the memoir *Prozac Nation*, holds up a locket with the word "Prozac" on it and poses for a portrait in front of a window display of a hand holding pills. The written narratives of people who identify as having a mental health disability can be extremely diverse and wide-ranging in their topics and formats. (Catherine McGann/Getty Images)

Narrative Control

People with mental illness experience a great deal of stigma and shame. Common misperceptions about people with mental illness include stereotypes of them as homicidal maniacs who should be feared, as irresponsible and incapable of taking care of themselves or making proper decisions, and as being childlike and in need of care. People with mental illness are also often thought to be at fault for their own struggles (Rüsch, Angermeyer, and Corrigan 2005). Such stigma leads to social isolation, fear of seeking treatment, and lack of employment opportunities.

Mental health narratives are commonly thought to help reduce the stigma of mental illness because they potentially generate new narratives that combat the common stereotypes and fears associated with having a mental health condition. It is important to note that the memoirs may often be more powerful because the authors—rather than psychiatrists, therapists, or any other medical professionals associated with treatment—become the authorities of their experience. While many mental health memoirs are inspirational in nature, namely stories of triumph and success after a lengthy and difficult battle, the authors are asserting control over how they are represented to their readers. They are dictating their own stories. For a population that has historically been highly discredited, this is a very empowering step. This attention to the voices of disabled people and the ways in which disabled people claim power over their own representation in these narratives is an important development in disability studies (Couser 1997).

Dilemmas, Debates, and Unresolved Questions

Many have pointed out that the majority of mental health narratives are written by white men and women, with very few by women and men of color. With a small number of exceptions, African Americans do not have the prestigious publication record of mental health narratives as do white men and women. Some have attributed this gap to greater stigma among the African American community concerning mental illness, citing the prevalent myth of the strong African American woman in particular (Bolden 2016). Similarly, few Latinx, indigenous/Native American people, and gender nonconforming individuals have published mental health narratives.

Another concern is access to treatment. For example, in Latinx communities, it can be difficult for people to find a culturally competent provider who can communicate in Spanish. Further, many times a mental health condition is misdiagnosed as a physical health condition. Despite the fact that "depression, substance abuse, and suicide represent the areas of greatest need with regard to the mental health of indigenous peoples," there remains relatively little research in this area. One memoir, *My Body Is a Book of Rules*, by Elissa Washuta, a woman from the Cowlitz Indian Tribe, explores her experiences with bipolar disorder and sexual assault as related to her native identity. Despite the important works of various women of color, the lack of first-person mental health narratives by nonwhite authors remains an issue of concern. This has the potential to contribute to the illusion that mental illness is a white person's disability (Bolden 2016).

Conclusion

Whether labeled as a genre or a subgenre, mental health narratives comprise a large number of the life writings by people with disabilities. These narratives continue to be released regularly. A potential future direction for disability studies is to explore the complex position of a physically disabled person who also has a mental health condition. Oftentimes, people with physical disabilities struggle with mental health issues, but symptoms are attributed to their physical disability rather than a separate condition. As mental health narratives stretch their boundaries, one can expect there to be more written by this population, as well as by people of color, who face a variety of different constraints in regard to stigma and access to treatment.

Meghann O'Leary

See also: Disability and Performance in Everyday Life; Life Writing; Madness, Mad Studies, and Psychiatric Survivors Stigma

Further Reading

Bolden, Christina. 2016. "Mental Illness Is Not Just a 'White Person's Disease.'" *Huffington Post*, June 8. http://www.huffingtonpost.com/christina-bolden/mental-illness-is-not-a-white-persons-disease_b_10309790.html.

Cohen, Alex. 1999. "The Mental Health of Indigenous Peoples: An International Overview." *Cultural Survival Quarterly Magazine* 23, no. 2 (June).

Corrigan, Patrick W., Beth Angell, Larry Davidson, Steven C. Marcus, Mark S. Salzer, Petra Kottsieper, Jonathon E. Larson, Colleen A. Mahoney, Maria J. O'Connell, and Victoria Stanhope. 2012. "From Adherence to Self-Determination: Evolution of a Treatment Paradigm for People with Serious Mental Illness." *Psychiatric Services* 63, no. 2: 169–173.

Couser, Thomas G. 1997. *Recovering Bodies: Illness, Disability and Life-Writing*. Madison: University of Wisconsin Press.

Pryal, Katie Guest. 2011. "The Genre of the Mood Memoir and the Ethos of Psychiatric Disability." *Rhetoric Society Quarterly* 40, no. 5: 479–501.

Rüsch, Nicolas, Matthias C. Angermeyer, and Patrick W. Corrigan. 2005. "Mental Illness Stigma: Concepts, Consequences and Initiatives to Reduce Stigma." *European Psychiatry* 20, no. 8: 529–539.

Wang, Amanda. 2017. "NAMI Latino Multicultural Action Center." https://www.nami.org/Find-Support/Diverse-Communities/Latino-Mental-Health.

Mental Health Self-Help and Support Groups

Mental health self-help and support groups and organizations are designed for people who have experience living with psychiatric disability. Self-help and support groups are often made up of people who identify with a psychiatric diagnosis, although many groups are geared specifically toward family members and some are open to both. People participate because they want to talk with other people who have the same experiences. They also want to learn new ways to cope with their illness, and they often want to help others. In addition to personal support, many self-help and support organizations focus on bringing about social change.

What Are Self-Help and Support Groups?

Although all the groups that fall under the category of self-help and support share the same overarching goals, they go about achieving those goals in different ways. The differences vary based on the concerns of the members or the beliefs of those who lead the groups. Sometimes the differences have more to do with the places the group meets. Many organizations create the support and self-help groups and provide the meeting spaces and through that process will often define how the groups are to function.

For example, sometimes a group will be formed by and will meet in a hospital setting where there is a strong focus on treating psychiatric disorders as a medical issue, as opposed to a community mental health center where there is a more holistic approach. It is important to first clarify the difference, and identify the overlap, between self-help groups and support groups.

Self-Help Groups. Self-help groups, sometimes referred to as mutual-help groups or organizations, are always led by *peers.* A peer in this case is defined as a person who shares the same diagnosis or problem as those attending the group meeting. Self-help groups can range from a few people getting together over a cup of coffee to large recovery programs such as Alcoholics Anonymous (AA). AA is a self-help group program for people who believe they are addicted to alcohol and want to stop drinking. People who wish to attend self-help groups can do so whenever they want and for as long as they want. Although some groups ask for donations to cover the cost of providing coffee, renting space, or providing materials for the group, there is generally little or no cost to attend. Many self-help groups are only available for people who identify with the problem being addressed. Not allowing others to attend can help group members feel comfortable enough to share their experiences and ask for support. Some self-help programs have a structured agenda and will offer "open" groups, often with expert speakers on identified topics of interest.

Support Groups. Support groups can include self-help groups, but the term also refers to groups that are led by people who provide professional mental health services. This difference in meaning can create confusion. Despite the fact that peer-led self-help groups fall under the category of a support group, professionally led groups are *never* considered self-help or mutual help. Some professionally led groups are open to anyone and have no attendance commitments or monetary requirements. On the other hand, many support groups that are led by professionals have a specific agenda that may be considered educational or therapeutic. When they do, participation in the support groups typically requires members to formally commit to attending and participating in the group process.

Purpose of Self-Help and Support Groups. Self-help and support groups are intentionally developed to meet the needs of a specific group of people who share a common experience. Some groups are developed for people addicted to drugs or alcohol; others are for people who identify with depression or bipolar disorder or psychotic disorders. Some groups are specifically designed to meet the needs of parents, spouses, or other family members. The National Alliance on Mental Illness (NAMI), an organization that provides education and support programs related to mental illness, was originally developed by and for family members of people who identify with psychotic disorders. Although they now offer a variety of different groups, they still have a strong family support component and as an organization continue to advocate for government policies that are most important to family members.

In all these cases, self-help support groups serve a basic purpose, which is to bring together people who are experiencing something they perceive as difficult and to help them relate and accept each other and their experiences, share coping strategies, establish social networks, and engage in advocacy.

Background and History

The history of mental health self-help and support groups is complicated. Still, it can help clarify the divide that exists in mental health support services today. According to Katz and Bender (2009, 280), mutual aid groups can be traced back to before the Middle Ages. Yet, many consider the beginning of the modern self-help movement to be the creation of Alcoholics Anonymous in 1935. During that year, two men, Bill W. and Dr. Bob S., developed a partnership based on the belief that alcoholism was a disease rather than the result of poor moral character. Both men had severe addiction to alcohol and believed that talking to other alcoholics would support their efforts to stay sober. Al-Anon, a program for family members, developed because Bill's wife, Lois, discovered that many wives of the men meeting in her living room were also in need of support and coping strategies.

Psychiatric Survivors and Consumer Groups. Later on, during the late 1960s, small groups of people, most of whom had been residents in state institutions for psychiatric disabilities, began to get together in small consciousness-raising groups, where they agreed that being held in an institution had done them more harm than good. Leaders of this movement called themselves *psychiatric survivors* and began to organize, taking to the streets to engage in acts of civil disobedience. Despite not having any money, groups of survivors started meeting together in churches and basements around the country. At one point, several of these groups worked together to hold a conference where people gathered to discuss the survivor movement and other issues affecting their daily lives. Over time, this gathering of people formed two different groups with very different ideas about how to live their lives. *Survivor groups,* such as the National Association for Rights Protection and Advocacy (NARPA), focused on fighting for the civil rights of people with

psychiatric disabilities. They fought against forcing people to accept treatment, such as going into an institution and taking medications, without their permission. They began to call out the negative effects that people experienced because of these actions forced on them. NARPA continues to work toward civil rights today, still without any federal support. *Consumer groups* consisting of many family members, such as NAMI, put most of their efforts into supporting research on medications and preventive services and continue to support policies that allow for forcing people to accept treatment against their will when it is believed that they lack the ability to make their own decisions.

In 1977, the National Institute of Mental Health (NIMH), a federal organization dedicated to the treatment of psychiatric disabilities, created the Community Support Project (CSP). The primary goal of the CSP was to come up with ways to improve services for people who had been discharged from institutions without the support they needed to live in the community. NIMH required CSP to include people with psychiatric disabilities in the discussion groups, which had never been done before. In 1984, CSP held the first national Alternatives Conference meant to bring survivors' ideas into the discussion regarding treatment and daily life. However, conference presentations were mostly about medicine and other forms of medical treatment, likely because the drug companies helped sponsor the conference. Thus, survivors felt their message was lost. The divide between the survivors and the consumer groups widened because of this conference. Despite sharing the belief that people with psychiatric disabilities can achieve a satisfactory life, these groups remain opposed as to how to reach that goal. Today NARPA remains a largely unrecognized and unfunded organization of survivors focused on advocating for self-determination and choice for people with psychiatric disabilities, while NAMI has become a very powerful parent/consumer voice, advocating for policies that lean more toward making sure people get treatment.

Important Points to Understand about Self-Help and Support Groups

Benefits of Self-Help and Support Groups. Throughout the history of self-help and support groups, the general mission has not changed: bring people together to share common experiences and decrease the fear and loneliness that accompanies a psychiatric diagnosis. People gain a number of benefits when they participate in self-help and support groups. Some studies indicate that people with psychiatric disabilities who participate in self-help and support groups feel they have better life management skills, have better self-esteem, and are more effective in their daily life. Other studies indicate that after participation people feel they have better coping skills, better relationship skills, and a better sense of well-being. Almost all participants state that the groups provide a sense of community, leaving them feeling less isolated and more empowered in their lives. One important and often overlooked benefit is that many people find that helping others helps them feel better about themselves.

Peer Support Specialists. Self-help groups are mainly run by peers who are not paid for their services and are not providing professional counseling. A separate and relatively new movement in mental health includes paid peer support staff in hospital mental health units and in community-based mental health service teams. People who serve in peer support positions, where they help people begin their recovery

process, identify as having a psychiatric disability and have received training as recovery specialists. *Peer support specialist* positions have been established for some of the same reasons as self-help and support groups: to give people a model of recovery, to help them experience decreased loneliness, and to allow them to connect with others who have a similar story. However, specialists' role on the treatment team is typically geared toward supporting the team's intervention plan instead of toward providing daily support.

Dilemmas, Debates, and Unresolved Questions

The debate between the survivor movement (focused on having the ability to make their own decisions in their lives and in their services) and the provider/consumer movement (focused on managing medications, symptoms, and daily function) is likely to continue for some time, especially given the social stigma that falsely labels people with psychiatric disabilities as dangerous. An important question that remains unresolved and unresearched revolves around the civic role of large support or advocacy organizations. NAMI, NARPA, the Depression and Bipolar Support Alliance (DBSA), and other large support organizations typically have teams of people who plan advocacy campaigns that support government and social policies consistent with their beliefs. One question these advocacy campaigns raise is how much influence these support organizations' advocacy efforts have on the beliefs of their members or on the way society understands psychiatric disability. Do such organizations form their advocacy goals after talking to their members, or do they intentionally (or unintentionally) encourage members to take on the organization's beliefs (Chaudhary, Avis, and Munn-Giddings 2013)? This question is important because if, for example, an organization advocates for forcing treatment on people because "they may be dangerous if they are not treated," then that organization is encouraging society to reject people out of fear. Such a stance could also cause people with psychiatric disabilities to internalize these attitudes and live in fear of hurting others, when, in reality, only a tiny fraction of people with mental illness are dangerous to others—about the same number as in the general population of people without these disorders.

The Future of Self-Help and Support Groups

The psychiatric survivors' movement focused on highlighting and demanding the civil and human rights of those with psychiatric disabilities. Disability studies programs are increasingly including important discussions about psychiatric disability, arguing that psychiatric disability is more the result of a society that does not understand these impairments and, as result, rejects people who think or do things differently. Longitudinal research indicates that people experience different levels of recovery from psychiatric illness, refuting long-held medical beliefs about the expected progressive and debilitating impact on daily life. Given these trends, the demand for peer-led services is likely to continue to grow.

Conclusion

People interested in attending or participating in self-help or support groups can call their local mental health service providers or go online and search for groups related to their concerns. Many of the groups meet in person at local civic organizations, private homes, churches, or health centers such as hospitals or county health departments.

Other groups meet virtually in online chat rooms or discussion boards. Large organizations, such as NAMI, DBSA, or Mental Health America (MHA), have lists of groups including the topic, the dates and times, and the contact numbers for people who can answer questions.

Lisa Mahaffey

See also: Community Living and Community Integration; Madness, Mad Studies, and Psychiatric Survivors; Self-Advocacy and Health Literacy; Self-Determination, Concept and Policy

Further Reading

Chaudhary, Sarah, Mark Avis, and Carol Munn-Giddings. 2013. "Beyond the Therapeutic: A Habermasian View of Self-Help Groups' Place in the Public Sphere." *Social Theory & Health* 11, no. 1: 59–80.

Davidson, Larry, and Thomas H. McGlashan. 1997. "The Varied Outcomes of Schizophrenia: Time to Author a New Story." *Canadian Journal of Psychiatry* 42, no. 1: 34–43.

Katz, Alfred, and Eugene Bender. 2009. "Self-Help Groups in Western Society: History and Prospects." *The Journal of Applied Behavioral Science* 12, no. 3: 265–282.

Kelly, John, and Julie Yeterian. 2011. "The Role of Mutual-Help Groups in Extending the Framework of Treatment." *Alcohol Research & Health* 33, no. 4: 350–355.

Pistrang, Nancy, Chris Barker, and Keith Humphreys. 2008. "Mutual Help Groups for Mental Health Problems: A Review of Effectiveness Studies." *American Journal of Community Psychology* 43: 110–121.

Seebohm, Patience, Sarah Chaudhary, Melanie Boyce, Ruth Elkan, Mark Avis, and Carol Munn-Giddings. 2013. "The Contribution of Self-Help/Mutual Aid Groups to Mental Health Well-Being." *Health and Social Care in the Community* 21, no. 4: 391–401.

Tomes, Nancy. 2006. "The Patient as a Policy Factor: A Historical Case Study of the Consumer/Survivor Movement in Mental Health." *Health Affairs* 25, no. 3: 720–729.

Microaggressions. See Discrimination and Microaggressions

Minority-Owned Businesses, Partnerships with

Given the changing demographics of people in the United States, it is apparent that job seekers of minority descent will become increasingly important to the country's economic and social well-being. To tackle the employment inequity problem, minority-owned and managed businesses located in highly populated immigrant neighborhoods—especially those in Latinx, African American, Asian American, and other immigrant or refugee communities— could help to provide culturally sensitive employment opportunities for skilled minorities who have disabilities.

Background

Problem of Disability Employment. Estimates report that the labor force participation rate for Americans with disabilities is at about 19.5 percent, compared with 68.5 percent for job seekers without disabilities. The issue of unemployment or underemployment for many working-aged individuals with disabilities remains problematic, especially for those who are also minorities, immigrants, or refugees. Compared to nondisabled workers, multicultural workers with disabilities experience higher rates of unemployment, higher rates of poverty-level income, limited access to

employee benefits and career options, disproportionate representation in low-skilled jobs, and higher rates of discrimination (Tsang et al. 2007).

Hiring Power of Minority-Owned Businesses. As American communities become more diverse, minority-owned businesses are having a noticeable impact on the nation's economy and workforce. According to the Department of Labor's Office of Disability Employment Policy (ODEP 2012), the current buying power of minority groups is estimated at $1 trillion. This figure is expected to increase substantially over the next 50 years as minority populations continue to grow. ODEP reports that immigrant and refugee populations have a strong history of creating businesses, which range from small, family-run operations to large-scale enterprises. Moreover, employment policies and programs, including vocational rehabilitation (VR), have the potential to increase the employment of people with disabilities by partnering with minority-owned businesses. Such innovative ventures could result in effective, sustainable partnerships that improve employment outcomes for qualified job seekers with disabilities from multicultural backgrounds.

Facts and Figures Relevant to Minority-Owned Businesses

According to the U.S. Department of Commerce's Minority Business Development Agency (2015), there are 5.8 million minority-owned businesses, compared to 20.1 nonminority-owned businesses. Minority-owned organizations consist of 1.9 million firms owned by African Americans; 237,000 owned by American Indians and Alaska Natives; 1.5 million owned by Asian Americans; 2.3 million owned by Hispanic Americans; and 38,000 owned by Native Hawaiians and Pacific Islanders.

Minority-owned firms contribute $1 trillion to U.S. economic output and create 5.8 million jobs annually. These firms average eight workers per business and $1 million in annual receipts. In spite of this economic power, minorities with disabilities remain unemployed in large numbers. However, through strategic public-private partnerships and awareness campaigns targeted to minority business owners, more minorities with disabilities could become part of the workforce through this sector.

The Minority Business Development Agency's Small Business Associations (MBDA 2010) reported the following figures:

- **Asian American–owned** firms grew 41 percent, to 1.5 million, from 2002 to 2007. They have continued to generate the highest annual gross receipts of any minority-owned businesses, at $506 billion in 2007, increasing 56 percent from 2002.
- The number of **Hispanic-owned** businesses totaled 2.3 million in 2007, up 44 percent from 2002. Receipts for Hispanic firms increased 55 percent, to $350.7 billion.
- **African American–owned** businesses grew to 1.9 million firms in 2007, up 61 percent from 2002—the largest increase among all minority-owned companies—and generated $135.7 billion in gross receipts, up 53 percent from 2002.

Despite the growing impact of minority businesses, the disability and employment sector continues to underuse them to advance employment opportunities for workers who come from these ethnically, racially, and linguistically diverse backgrounds. As a practical next step, it is critical that vocational rehabilitation (VR) employment specialists start building connections with minority-owned businesses that are loyal and dedicated to their communities, as a means to improve employment outcomes for members of the disability community.

Reaching Out to Minority-Owned Businesses

The outreach strategies that follow can help educate minority-owned businesses in the community about the benefits of hiring and retaining people with disabilities as employees. Building strategic partnerships among the state VR system, community-based organizations, and the local business community ensures that people with disabilities fully participate in their community and contribute to the local economy. Strategies to engage minority businesses in hiring people with disabilities include the following:

- working with minority and mainstream employers to demolish myths and reduce fears about hiring people with disabilities;
- helping to incorporate awareness of people with disabilities into overall hiring and general business practices;
- helping businesses actively identify and recruit people with disabilities from family networks and communities;
- helping businesses create job advertisements that encourage people with disabilities to apply;
- offering ADA-related and new disability rights regulation workshops in minority communities;
- diversifying the state VR agency's current pool of employers so that minority-owned businesses become part of the disability employment network;

- developing partnerships with agencies such as chambers of commerce in various ethnic communities;
- utilizing available benefits (such as supported employment or tax incentives), which are often underutilized when hiring people with disabilities;
- initiating partnerships with minority-owned businesses to provide holistic disability supports and resources that maximize individuals' full participation in their own communities;
- shifting attitudes toward people with disabilities by creating employment opportunities in various industries, including self-employment and entrepreneurship.

Conclusion

The important economic role of ethnic groups clearly indicates the need for innovative public-private partnerships to address the employment disparities facing immigrants and other minorities with disabilities. This entry attempts to encourage disability advocates and researchers to work with minority-owned businesses that want to recruit, hire, and retain employees with disabilities. It also provides resources and exemplary practices that can help disability providers engage with underserved and unserved multicultural communities.

Currently, workers with disabilities of all cultures tend to be hired by mainstream, nonminority businesses and rarely by employers of the same cultural background based on project field experiences. Although some nonprofit groups are addressing this problem, the for-profit minority business sector has gotten little attention. Outreach efforts that highlight success stories of employee-employer relationships in these communities can help shift negative attitudes associated with hiring a person with a disability.

Rooshey Hasnain

See also: Cultural Competence and Employment; Employer Attitudes; Employment, Barriers to

Further Reading

Hernandez, B., S. McCullough, F. Balcazar, and C. Keys. 2008. "Accessibility of Public Accommodations in Three Ethnic Minority Communities." *Journal of Disability Policy Studies* 19, no. 2: 80–85.

Ju, S., E. Roberts, and D. Zhang. 2013. "Employer Attitudes toward Workers with Disabilities: A Review of Research in the Past Decade." *Journal of Vocational Rehabilitation* 38: 113–123.

Kitching, J. 2006. "Can Small Businesses Help Reduce Employment?" *Environment and Planning Government and Policy* 24: 869–884.

Le, C. N. 2000. "Asian Small Businesses: Why Do So Many Asians Own Their Own Businesses?" *Asian Nation*. http://www.asian-nation.org/small-business.shtml.

Minority Business Development Association. 2010. "Number of Minority-Owned Businesses Increases but Economic Parity Remains Elusive." Washington, DC: U.S. Department of Commerce. Categories: Press Releases. http://www.mbda.gov/pressroom/press-releases/number-minority-owned-businesses-increases-economic-parity-remains-elusive.

Nota, L., S. Santilli, C. M. Ginevra, and S. Soresi. 2014. "Employer Attitudes towards the Work Inclusion of People with Disability." *Journal of Applied Research in Intellectual Disabilities* 27, no. 6 (November): 511–520.

Office of Disability Employment. 2012. "Business Strategies That Work: A Framework for Disability Inclusion." Washington, DC: Department of Labor.

Rao, D., R. A. Horton, H. W. H. Tsang, K. Shi, and P. W. Corrigan. 2010. "Does Individualism Help Explain Differences in Employers' Stigmatizing Attitudes toward Disability across Chinese and American Cities?" *Rehabilitation Psychology* 55, no. 4: 351–359.

Robb, M. A., and W. R. Fairlie. 2009. "Determinants of Business: An Examination of Asian-Owned Business in the USA." *Journal of Population Economics* 22: 827–858.

Tsang, W. H., B. Angell, W. P. Corrigan, Yueh-Ting Lee, K. Shi, S. C. Lam, S. Jin, and M. T. K. Fung. 2007. "A Cross-Cultural Study of Employers' Concerns about Hiring People with Psychotic Disorder: Implications for Recovery." *Social Psychiatry and Psychiatric Epidemiology* 42: 723–733.

U.S. Department of Commerce. Minority Business Development Agency. 2015. Fact sheet: U.S. Minority-Owned Firms. https://www.mbda.gov/sites/mbda.gov/files/migrated/files-attachments/052914 FactSheets.pdf.

Mobile Technology

Mobile technology (MT) refers to portable technologies that allow users to complete a variety of tasks through wireless Internet connectivity using cellular communications. Examples of MT include tablets, smartphones, electronic (e) readers, tablet-PCs, portable gaming devices, and MP3 players. MT has revolutionized the way we access and use the Internet. In doing so, it has transformed how we gather and disseminate information and communicate with one another. MT connects individuals to a world of digital information while on the go. It uses various apps to quickly access Web sites and services. Through MT, people are able to connect by phone, e-mail, and text messages; participate in social networking sites such as Facebook and Twitter; manage finances, appointments, schedules, and health care; and participate in various forms of entertainment, such as music, videos, photography, and games.

MT has become ubiquitous within the United States and other developed countries (Goggin 2015, 1). While it is unclear as to how many people around the world have access to and use MT, it has been argued that the impact and adaptation of MT has been rapid and widespread (Shane et al. 2012, 8). For example, in 2015, as many as 68 percent of American adults reported using smartphones, a number that was up from 35 percent just four years prior in 2011. Moreover, American adult tablet ownership (e.g., iPads and other tablet devices) rose from only 3 percent in 2010 to 45 percent in 2015 (Anderson 2015, 3). Little is known about MT usage in low-income countries or with differing populations. The use of and experience with mobile technology takes on different forms across different groups, places, and countries (Goggin 2015, 1).

Impact on the Disability Community

MT connects users and provides access to education, commerce, employment, and entertainment through wireless Internet connectivity (Foley and Ferri 2012, 192). Persons with disabilities have historically been less likely to report using the Internet and having access to information and communication technologies (ICTs) when compared to those without disabilities (Shane et al. 2012, 6). This gap in reported use can be due to a variety of factors, including barriers associated with income, education, employment, and accessibility. It has resulted in what is commonly referred to as the *digital divide* (Shane et al. 2012, 6), or the gap between those who have access to

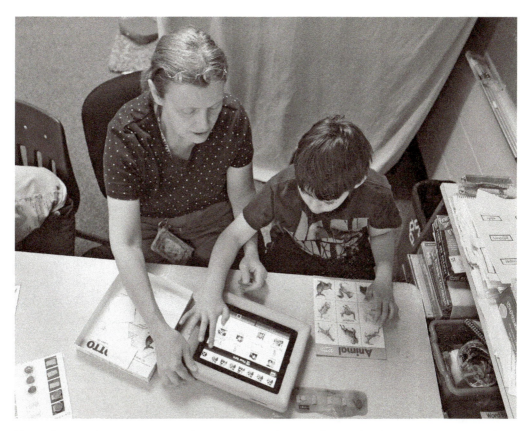

Karen Lajmoraki, an instructional assistant, works with Steven Moshuris, an autistic student who uses an iPad as a communication device, at Belle View Elementary School in Alexandria, Virginia. (Jahi Chikwendiu/The Washington Post via Getty Images)

ICTs and the Internet and those who do not have access.

Because of its affordability, portability, and omnipresence in today's society, MT carries with it the potential to increase access for people with disabilities. In doing so, MT can expand these individuals' participation in society (Shane et al. 2012, 8). MT can provide a gateway to information, socialization, education, employment, entertainment, health and safety, public services, and various tools to support daily activities (Shane et al. 2012, 8). As access to these mainstream technologies increases, so does the ability to challenge societal attitudes and media representations of disability. For some, mobile technology has become a means to access new forums for disability activism by using social networking sites or personal blogs (Foley and Ferri 2012, 194).

MT offers a variety of technological supports related to disability-specific needs. It has revolutionized the field of assistive technology, as such supports can be more affordable and socially desirable when compared to disability-specific assistive technology devices (Shane et al. 2012, 8). MT promotes access to necessary technology and may decrease stigmatization that can occur from the use of disability-specific assistive technology.

Persons with a variety of sensory, intellectual, physical, and communication disabilities have used MT to increase their participation in an assortment of desired daily activities. For example, MT can support access to print and digital information, communication, independence with daily activities, maintenance of safety, and ability to self-monitor or self-regulate. A full review of the many ways in which persons with disabilities have used MT is beyond the scope of this entry and would be quickly outdated because of the current rapid changes within the field of technology. However, some examples will be discussed to underscore this point.

Persons with intellectual or sensory disabilities may use specific apps for MT to aid in their ability to self-regulate, self-prompt, and self-monitor through video modeling or other visual supports (e.g., checklists and timers). Persons who are blind or have low vision, or those with intellectual or linguistic disabilities, may use MT to access print information through the use of built-in screen reading accessibility features or specialized screen reader and Braille apps. Those with various sensory or intellectual disabilities can use transportation and Global Positioning System (GPS) features built into MT to support their safety and community navigation. Finally, MT has arguably enhanced the communication opportunities for persons with complex communication needs with the addition of speech-generating applications. These applications generate speech to facilitate face-to-face and audio telephone communications for persons with communication disabilities.

Debates, Concerns, and Ongoing Considerations

Despite the many benefits that MT has brought to persons with disabilities, some ongoing debates and concerns must be considered. The first revolves around the issue of accessibility. MT can be inaccessible to persons with disabilities for a variety of reasons, ranging from financial barriers to educational barriers. In addition, because many mobile technologies and Internet Web sites are not universally accessible, physical, intellectual, or sensory disabilities may make using the devices and accessing desired applications nearly impossible.

Key Concepts

- Many would argue that MT provides persons with disabilities with many benefits, including the expansion of Internet access. This has increased connectivity and access to communication, services, and information for this population.
- MT has revolutionized assistive technology by incorporating specialized technologies into mainstream devices that are more affordable and socially desirable.
- Despite its many benefits, scholars express concerns regarding MT in terms of disability. Issues of accessibility and the impact of inaccessibility may lead to the creation of new forms of disability and social exclusion.
- Many argue the need for policies and procedures to ensure access to mobile technology for all individuals, regardless of disability.

Conclusions

MT has revolutionized the way modern society communicates, gathers and disseminates information, and conducts various educational, commercial, and economic activities. It has certainly had a substantial influence on members of the disability community by increasing access to the Internet and moving certain assistive technologies to the mainstream. There are concerns, however, regarding MT as it relates to disability. The inaccessibility of MT for many with disabilities can create areas of exclusion.

As MT becomes increasingly more popular and pervasive in today's society, we must ensure that policies are put in place and upheld to support equal access to MT for persons with disabilities, such as the Federal Communications Commission (FCC 2016, 11) policy ensuring the rights of people with disabilities to accessible ICT. Manufacturers and developers should consider ways in which their technology can be accessible to all of their consumers. One recommendation from those within the field of disability studies is to incorporate those with disabilities in the design and production of technologies (Foley and Ferri 2012, 196).

Stephanie Bay

See also: Alternative and Augmentative Communication; Assistive Technology, Use of in Minority Communities; Online Social and Professional Networks and Work

Further Reading

Anderson, Monica. 2015. "Technology Device Ownership." Pew Research Center. http://www.pewinternet.org/2015/10/29/technology-device-ownership-2015/pi_2015-10-29_device-ownership_0-01/.

Ellcessor, Elizabeth. 2016. *Restricted Access: Media, Disability, and the Politics of Participation.* New York: New York University Press.

Federal Communications Commission. 2016. "White Paper: Individuals with Cognitive Disabilities: Barriers to and Solutions for Accessible Information and Communication Technologies." https://apps.fcc.gov/edocs_public/attachmatch/DOC-341628A1.pdf.

Foley, Alan, and Beth A. Ferri. 2012. "Technology for People, Not Disabilities: Ensuring Access and Inclusion." *Journal of Research in Special Education Needs* 12, no. 4: 192–200.

Goggin, Gerard. 2015. "Disability and Mobile Internet." *First Monday* 20, no. 9.

Shane, Howard C., Sarah Blackstone, Gregg Vanderheiden, Michael Williams, and Frank Deruyter. 2012. "Using AAC Technology to Access the World." *Assistive Technology* 24, no. 1: 3–13.

Modernism

Modernism encompasses literary and cultural production that uses experimental techniques, such as flashbacks, fragmented narratives, and stream of consciousness, to respond to the conditions of modern life from the turn of the century to the mid-1940s. These conditions include World War I and World War II, a growing skepticism toward religion, increased migration, a sense of cultural decline, the decreasing importance of familial structures, and the increasing pace of life due to industrialization.

Important Issues to Know about Disability and Modernism

Cultural Production. By using modernism as a lens through which to read cultural production in the early 20th century, we are able to learn more about disabled life during this time. The antidisability tendencies in many modernist texts have led scholars such as Donald J. Childs to critique Anglo-American modernism's disciplining of the atypical bodymind. Virginia Woolf infamously stated that the mentally disabled "certainly should be killed" (Woolf 1979, 13). D. H. Lawrence asserted that "hopeless life should be put to sleep, the idiots and the hopeless sick and the true criminal" (Woolf 1979, 24). Scholarship on T. S. Eliot and Ezra Pound's conservatism highlighted modernism's fear of cultural degeneration and the masses. This conservatism cast modernism as unethical. Studies of transnational high modernism stress its valuations of opacity, genius, and highbrow difficulty which further amplifies the unattractive coupling of Anglo-American modernism and eugenics. *Eugenics* is an ideology that supports selective breeding to generate a population with the most desirable inherited traits. In the early and mid-20th century, this involved efforts to prevent the continuation of inherited disability conditions in the U.S. population.

Veterans and Early Government Initiatives. While modernism's relationship with eugenics was often tied to the persecution of those perceived as having congenital or inherited disabilities, veterans returning from World War I and World War II with psychiatric and physical disabilities generated a cultural crisis. Modernism strove to register this crisis in instances such as Ernest Hemingway's *The Sun Also Rises* or Dalton Trumbo's 1938 *Johnny Got His Gun.* In the early-20th-century United States, governmental initiatives (now recognized as predecessors to the ADA) created certain possibilities for disabled veterans and civilians but also foreclosed them. Laws such as the 1918 Soldiers Rehabilitation Act and the 1920 Smith-Fess Act focused on veterans to the exclusion of civilians and people with congenital disabilities but did not necessarily shield veterans from stigma and economic difficulties. Conversely, even as policies intended for veterans actively excluded other people with disabilities, especially women, people of color, and those considered "severely" disabled, these acts laid the groundwork for future social and economic inclusions that are still far from realization. Modernism also registered these exclusions in texts such as Nathanael West's novella *Miss Lonelyhearts*, wherein the main character returns to Depression-era New York City and encounters "crowds of people" who "moved through the street with a dream-like violence" with "their broken hands and torn mouths" (West 2009, 39).

Contestation of Normality. As modernist studies scholar Janet Lyon writes, "modernist aesthetics, with its emphasis on disproportion, fracture, and incompleteness, shares with disability theory a foundational contestation of the category of 'the normal'" (2011, 552). While modernist texts showcase a manifold cast of disabled characters, disability itself is also a site of formal possibility. For example, William Faulkner's 1929 novel *The Sound and the Fury,* a multiperspectival narrative of the decline of the Southern family, provides a sympathetic portrayal of Benjy Compson, a cognitively disabled man who was subjected to enforced sterilization; it was also groundbreaking in using stream of consciousness to narrate an intellectually disabled protagonist's perspective. Similarly, British modernist Virginia Woolf uses fragmented narratives and flashbacks to render Septimus Smith, a World War I veteran experiencing post-traumatic stress, in her 1929 novel, *Mrs. Dalloway.* As with Woolf's exploration of psychiatric disability throughout her work, James Joyce's inclusion of manifold disabled characters in *Ulysses* was, also in part, a reflection of his own experiences with disability.

Summary

In sum, modernism has a complex relationship with disability. While it confirms disability as crucial to artistic production, it can also promote cultural justifications for mistreating people with disabilities. However, modernist form was available to not only canonical writers but also disabled authors themselves, such as memoirist Katharine

Butler Hathaway or fiction writer Mary Jane Ward, author of the 1946 anti-institutionalization novel *The Snake Pit.*

Future Directions in Disability and Literary Modernism

More knowledge is needed about the relationship between modernist literature and disabled life, activism, and policies. Furthermore, modernist studies often exclude authors of color. For example, as I have argued elsewhere, by incorporating Afro-modernist artistic production into a wider notion of modernism, we also learn more about the politics of disability and illness during this time period. For example, some Afro-modernists, such as W. E. B. Du Bois, strategically embraced eugenic thinking to assert the supremacy of the black upper class. Others, such as Langston Hughes, Wallace Thurman, and Zora Neale Hurston, protested eugenic thought and medical segregation, which can be seen as a nascent form of disability rights protest (Waggoner 2017). In this way, we begin to see disability in modernism not merely as the presence of physical or psychiatric disability but also as critical engagements with such mechanisms of modernity as medical abuse, eugenic discourses, and the public health surveillance of racialized people.

Jess Waggoner

See also: Individualism and Independence; Life Writing; Medicalization

Further Reading

Childs, Donald J. 2001. *Modernism and Eugenics: Woolf, Eliot, Yeats, and the Culture of Degeneration.* New York: Cambridge University Press.

Lyon, Janet. 2011. "On the Asylum Road with Woolf and Mew." *Modernism/modernity* 18, no. 3: 551–574.

Lawrence, David Herbert. 2004. *Late Essays and Articles.* Edited by James T. Boulton. Cambridge: Cambridge University Press.

Waggoner, Jess. 2017. "'My Most Humiliating Jim Crow Experience': Afro-Modernist Critiques of Eugenics and Medical Segregation." *Modernism/modernity* 24, no. 3: 507–525.

West, Nathanael. 2009. *Miss Lonelyhearts & The Day of the Locust.* New York: New Directions.

Woolf, Virginia. 1979. *The Diary of Virginia Woolf.* Vol. 1: 1915–1919. New York: Mariner.

Mothers with Disabilities

An estimated 6.2 percent of parents in the United States who are currently caring for children under the age of 18 have disabilities (National Council on Disability 2012). What's more, women with disabilities are found to devote as much time to caregiving as nondisabled women (Shandra and Penner 2017). While much has been written about nondisabled mothers who care for disabled children, surprisingly little has been written about mothers with disabilities. This pattern both reflects and reinforces the binary of care, the pervasive assumption that disabled and nondisabled people can be neatly divided between those who receive care and those who provide it.

Background: Discrimination against Mothers with Disabilities

While most nondisabled women are expected to have children, women with disabilities experience an *imperative of childlessness.* Because Deaf and disabled women are often regarded as childlike and incompetent themselves, they are frequently met with disbelief and even hostility when they assume the role of mother. Furthermore, owing to the legacy of the eugenics movement, there remains a pervasive belief that disability could be eradicated if only those with genetic disorders would stop having children. Finally, Deaf and disabled women who mother confront stereotypes that women with disabilities are either asexual or hypersexual. These cultural values manifest in the many interactions that mothers with disabilities have with neighbors, medical and social service professionals, and even members of their own families.

Paradox of Visibility. Mothers with disabilities often experience a "paradox of visibility" (Frederick 2017a). On the one hand, they often feel as if they are living in a fish bowl. They feel hypervisible as they endure and expect intense scrutiny from medical professionals, the public, and even friends and family. Women with disabilities frequently report pervasive staring and reactions of shock, as well as unwarranted social service intervention, when they are out with their children. On the other hand, the issues with inaccessibility and a lack of representation in the mothering self-help industry all simultaneously render these women's identities, needs, and experiences invisible (Kuttai 2010).

Antidiscrimination Legislation. Title II of the Americans with Disabilities Act prohibits discrimination against parents and prospective parents with disabilities solely on the basis of their disability. Title II of the ADA also requires that public agencies in the child welfare system provide equal opportunities for disabled parents to maintain or regain custody of their children, which include providing appropriate accommodations so that parents may access services offered in the system.

Important Points to Understand about Mothers with Disabilities

Who Are the Experts? Much of the discrimination mothers with disabilities experience results from nondisabled people, who have little knowledge of disability communities, performing "imagination work" (Frederick 2014). These individuals imagine a range of scenarios, some of them highly unlikely, that a mother with a particular disability might face. As a result, with little knowledge of a particular impairment, they frequently arrive at the conclusion that, were they in the disabled mother's shoes, the outcome would be disastrous. Thus, it is critical to ask, "Who is the expert on disabled mothering?"

Cultural Norms. Disability communities have their own cultures, and individuals in these communities share strategies about how to routinely accomplish tasks that nondisabled people might think impossible. Disability communities also have shared cultural norms of acceptable and unacceptable actions that can differ from those of nondisabled communities. For example, blind parents often use a child leash to keep track of their young toddlers. While this might be off-putting to nondisabled observers, it is an accepted strategy in this community. Furthermore, when legitimate concerns are raised about child maltreatment perpetrated by a disabled mother, members of that disability community have the knowledge and resources to offer techniques or assessments that might not be imagined by nondisabled people who lack such expertise.

The Agency of Deaf and Disabled Mothers. Contrary to pervasive stereotypes that paint Deaf and disabled individuals as passive and childlike, women with disabilities are found to exercise a tremendous amount of agency and perform a heavy amount of labor to negotiate motherhood. First, Deaf and disabled mothers often must engage in more work to adapt equipment, to develop effective strategies for parenting, and to manage their own self-care in ways that do not diminish their role as mothers (Frederick 2017a; Malacrida 2009). Mothers with disabilities also perform a great deal of emotion work to combat deeply held cultural beliefs that describe them as unsuitable for motherhood. They work to interpret dominant values of motherhood so that they cultivate the confidence and belief in themselves that defy these cultural values (Kuttai 2010). They also often work to pass a social justice framing of disability to their children.

Resistance Strategies. Finally, mothers with disabilities engage in a great deal of work to resist the prejudice and discrimination surrounding them (Frederick 2017b). Some engage in *visibility politics*, assuming a highly visible role as educator and advocate. Some engage in *respectability politics*, paying great attention to their self-presentation in order to gain respect from the nondisabled majority. Finally, others practice *disengagement*, at times, restraining their movements, and sometimes their anger, to avoid the consequences of discrimination. Because these mothers' resistance strategies are often interwoven into daily interactions, the agency they exercise can often go unrecognized by the nondisabled majority.

Conclusion

The experiences of Deaf and disabled mothers include high levels of prejudice and discrimination, which often place their right to parent in jeopardy. Yet, these mothers also exhibit high levels of ingenuity as they develop adaptations to perform motherhood, as they guard against social judgments of others, and as they find new ways of interpreting motherhood that allow for their own confidence and success.

Angela Frederick

See also: Ableism; Self-Advocacy and Health Literacy; Sexuality Education for People with Intellectual Disabilities

Further Reading

Frederick, Angela. 2014. "Mothering While Disabled." *Contexts Magazine* 13, no. 4: 30–35.

Frederick, Angela. 2017a. "Risky Mothers and the Normalcy Project: Mothers with Disabilities Negotiate Scientific Motherhood." *Gender & Society* 31, no. 1: 74–95.

Frederick, Angela. 2017b. "Visibility, Respectability, and Disengagement: The Everyday Resistance of Mothers with Disabilities." *Social Science & Medicine* 181: 131–138.

Kuttai, Heather. 2010. *Maternity Rolls: Pregnancy, Childbirth, and Disability.* Halifax, Nova Scotia: Fernwood Publishing.

Malacrida, Claudia. 2009. "Performing Motherhood in a Disabling World: Dilemmas of Motherhood, Femininity and Disability." *International Journal of Qualitative Studies in Education* 22, no. 1: 99–117.

National Council on Disability. 2012. "Rocking the Cradle: Ensuring the Rights of Parents with Disabilities and Their Children." https://www.ncd.gov/publications/2012/Sep272012.

Shandra, Carrie, and Anna Penner. 2017. "Benefactors and Beneficiaries? Disability and Care to Others." *Journal of Marriage & Family* 79, no. 4: 1160–1185.

Museums

Museums play an important role in cultures around the world. Museums are publicly and privately funded institutions of any scale and are most commonly located in cities. They care for and maintain artifacts and document archives for the purpose of preserving objects of historical, cultural, artistic, and scientific significance. Museums also preserve material objects in digital archives, which have the potential to make the objects more *accessible* to audiences around the world.

What Is the Role of Museums?

Museums serve the important purpose of providing spaces where individuals can collectively reflect on the past, consider the contemporary moment, and think about the future. With the important role museums play in bringing people together to learn and reflect on the world, it is equally essential that museums be accessible to everyone, including people with disabilities.

Access and Education. Museums are dedicated to giving the public access to the artifacts they house and to education, such as historical and cultural context, and they provide important opportunities for the public to learn about other cultures, parts of the world, and time periods. This education can help promote understanding and equity across time and place. Museums have a responsibility not only to record history and represent culture as we commonly understand it but also to uncover stories of marginalized and oppressed people that may have been elided by dominant narratives, to represent multiple perspectives, and to ensure that their exhibits and educational programming are inclusive and accessible to everyone. The communities, peoples, and populations selected to be represented in museum exhibitions send a message about who is deemed valuable within the larger social culture and collective history. For these reasons, it is important to the disability rights movement and the achievement of disability justice that people with disabilities and representations of disability histories, arts, cultures, and perspectives be included in museum archives. This inclusion sends a powerful message that the

history and experiences of people with disabilities are important to understanding our past, present, and future.

Representations of Disability in Museums and Culture

Disability studies scholar Rosemarie Garland-Thomson writes, "The history of disabled people in the Western world is, in part, the history of being on display, of being visually conspicuous while politically and socially erased" (2002, 56). Historically and still today, although less frequently, people with disabilities have been socially disappeared through practices of *institutionalization*, which sent people with disabilities to live in such institutions as asylums, hospitals, boarding schools, and residential schools; as well as *discriminatory legislation,* such as the "ugly laws," which prohibited people with disabilities from being seen in public space throughout the 19th century (Schweik 2010, 1–2). At the same time, people with disabilities were put on display for profit in carnivals and freak shows from the 1850s to the 1980s in the United States (Gerber 1996, 43).

Through these cultural practices, people with disabilities were usually not considered to be valuable members of society. One way to correct exclusion of people with disabilities is to include them in the stories that museums tell. Disability is an intersectional identity, and the history of disability is woven throughout all regional, religious, ethno-racial, and civil rights histories, as well as others. As such, people with disabilities should be deliberately included in the ways that museums represent these histories and cultures.

Disability histories, cultures, and politics are represented in many museums across the United States. The Museum of disABILITY History in Buffalo, New York, offers permanent, temporary, touring, and virtual exhibitions that explore such topics as institutions' development as places to house people with disabilities, the rise of eugenics and its impact on people with disabilities, the rise of the self-advocacy movement, and African Americans' experience of disability from colonial times to desegregation (Museum of disABILITY History, n.d.). The National Museum of American History in Washington, D.C., had a disability history exhibition in 2015 in celebration of the 25th anniversary of the Americans with Disabilities Act (ADA). Along with chronicling historical treatment of people with disabilities in the United States, this exhibit—which is now a virtual exhibition—tells the story of how the disability rights movement led to the establishment of the ADA. These exhibitions play an important role in marking the treatment and contributions of people with disabilities throughout history and ensuring that this history is entered into public knowledge.

How Museums Are Inclusive to People with Disabilities

Equally as important as making sure that people with disabilities and disability history, culture, and politics are properly represented in museums is the responsibility museums have to be accessible and inclusive.

The ADA "guarantees that people with disabilities have the same opportunities as everyone else to participate in the mainstream of American life" (ADA.gov 2010). Museum spaces and environments are covered under ADA policy. Making museums accessible to people with disabilities extends beyond the requirement to ensure that these spaces are barrier-free. For example, the Smithsonian Institution in Washington, D.C., published a comprehensive resource in its Smithsonian Guidelines for Accessible Exhibition Design. This resource provides guidelines for museum accessibility beyond what is minimally required by the ADA's standards for accessible design. Making exhibitions accessible is important, as people with disabilities are part of museums' diverse audience. However, because accessible exhibitions are designed with considerations for how people interact with space, language, information, arts, and artifacts, they benefit not just people with disabilities but all museum attendees.

Best Practices

The Smithsonian Guidelines for Accessible Design provide detailed instructions and explanations for how to curate, build, and maintain accessible exhibitions. Museum curators are beginning to take heed of these and other standards and best practices. These practices include writing exhibition content, such as exhibition statements, in plain language; creating audio description for all visual material; providing captioning for all auditory features (including tactical or touchable) components; hanging wall-mounted work and setting display tables at an accessible height; planning accessible circulation routes throughout the exhibition; using accessible lighting design, which may include brightly lit accessible paths and minimal flashing or strobe lighting; and creating accessible emergency evacuation plans. Museum programming can also be made accessible by the inclusion of relaxed museum hours for people who feel more comfortable when they can make noise and move about freely; tours featuring American Sign Language (ASL), audio description, and plain language interpretation; and touch tours.

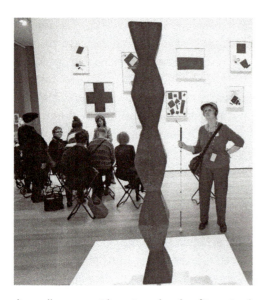

A small group with various levels of impaired vision tour *Inventing Abstraction*, an exhibit at the Museum of Modern Art in New York City. Museums must take numerous steps to ensure that exhibits are barrier-free and accessible to all patrons. (Don Emmert/AFP/Getty Images)

Creating a Culture of Inclusion

Following accessibility standards and best practices ensures that museums comply with ADA legislation, and it also allows them to uphold their commitment to be inclusive spaces wherein everyone, most especially people with disabilities, has access to the archives and education that they hold. Building and curating accessible exhibitions, as well as programming accessible events, sends a strong message that people with disabilities are anticipated and desired as museum visitors and important members of the community.

Future of Disability and Museums

People with disabilities must be meaningfully included in museums, both in educational displays and as audience members.

Museums offer the public access to a range of artifacts and history, giving us a collective sense of who we are and what we value as a culture. Therefore, including people with disabilities sends a powerful message that people with disabilities are a valuable part of society and culture.

Eliza Chandler

See also: Americans with Disabilities Act (ADA); Contemporary Art; Fine Arts

Further Reading

ADA.gov. 2010. "ADA Standards for Accessible Design." https://www.ada.gov/2010ADAstandards_index.htm.

Garland-Thomson, Rosemarie. 2002. "The Politics of Staring: Visual Rhetorics of Disability in Popular Photography." In *Disability Studies: Enabling the Humanities*, edited by Sharon Snyder, Brenda Brueggemann, and Rosemarie Garland-Thomson, 56–65. New York: Modern Language Association.

Gerber, David. 1996. "The 'Careers' of People Exhibited in Freak Shows: The Problem of Volition and Valorization." In *Freakery: Cultural Spectacles of the Extraordinary Body*, edited by Rosemarie Garland-Thomson, 38–54. New York: New York University Press.

Museum of disABILITY History. n.d. "Permanent Exhibits" and "Temporary Exhibits." http://museumofdisability.org/.

National Museum of American History. n.d. "Disability History." http://americanhistory.si.edu/ topics/disability-history.

Schweik, Susan. 2010. *The Ugly Laws: Disability in Public*. New York: New York University Press.

Smithsonian Institution. "Smithsonian Guidelines for Accessible Exhibition Design." n.d. http://accessible.si.edu/pdf/Smithsonian%20Guidelines%20for%20accessible%20design.pdf.

N

Natural Supports

Natural supports are relational features of an environment that provide accessibility, security, and a sense of belonging without unnecessary complications. In other words, natural supports are support systems people have as a result of relationships within their families and communities.

What Are Natural Supports?

Provided through unstructured, reciprocal relationships (Department of Developmental Services, n.d.), natural supports give assistance or benefit to individuals within nonspecialized settings. Usually, the term implies support given to someone who experiences disability.

While some view the exclusion of disabled people to be a necessary evil in particular settings, natural supports exemplify the strength, possibility, and viability of community sites that embrace inclusion instead. In schools and community centers, opponents of inclusion have claimed it is a difficult and unreasonable practice, often ignoring the practicality of natural supports. Within communities that provide support systems for one another, disabled individuals and others who might be marginalized by outside forces can ultimately thrive.

Background

Although the term "natural supports" was introduced first in 1988 (Project 10, 2016) to describe support that is not paid for, people have been benefitting from support systems developed through relationships for ages.

Families and neighbors have often relied on each other in interdependent relationships, acknowledging that everyone needs support of some kind and that giving it to each other is natural. However, the term itself is primarily used by professionals within special education and rehabilitation to assess how an individual's needs can be met.

Real-Life Examples

The following examples from one girl's experience illustrate what natural supports can look like:

- *Family belonging.* Maggie's earliest memories of belonging come from her family, where she was the third of six children. The family always planted a huge garden and expected the whole family to participate in tending to it. Although she could not walk through the rows of plants to pull weeds and pick vegetables, she still had to take part. When her siblings picked green beans, her mother gave her the job of snipping them, or pinching off the stems, which they didn't want to eat. When it was time to harvest corn, she worked alongside those who removed the husks. Her job was not always the same as her siblings' tasks, but it was seen as just as valuable.

  In a large extended family, belonging was never orchestrated or contrived when they gathered for family events. Spending time with four girl cousins close to her age helped form her expectations for friendship. Each of her cousins knew that she needed someone to lean on when they walked anywhere together; one or two of them were always by her side. She was never forgotten or left behind. At family reunions when meals were served buffet style, the girls shared plates of food and drinks, which two or three of them carried. As young children, they worked out these buddy systems that ensured they could be together, not isolated or excluded.

- *Community belonging.* Outside of her family, Maggie enjoyed ready access to her rural community, although it was not always perfect. Once when her classmate, Lori, welcomed friends to her 10th birthday party, Lori's mother noticed that Maggie had yet to arrive. She called Maggie's mother right away to invite the girl and apologize that her daughter had not extended an invitation. Maggie went to the party and enjoyed the time with her classmates. Regardless of why Maggie was not initially invited, one mother stepped in and made more than a symbolic gesture to ensure that she was not left out.

- *School belonging.* The schools Maggie attended were not completely accessible, yet in many situations, her peers made her feel as if she belonged. Attending a high school without an elevator, she worked hard to get from one class to another while using crutches and carrying books, until two boys suggested they take turns piggybacking her from art class to biology class every day. She agreed, and they were there for her, expecting only friendship in return.

One year, a surgery just before the school year began necessitated her use of a wheelchair. One of her classes was in a portable classroom that had no ramp. The teacher was unsure what to do when he saw her at the bottom of the steps. When two of her cousins showed up to take the same class, they simply stacked their books on her lap as one took the back of her wheelchair and one took the front; together, they lifted her up the three steps. Watching them, others learned to step in to offer a lift if the cousins were not there.

Dilemmas, Debates, and Unresolved Questions

The conception that disabled people need specialized help from professionals is pervasive in schools and communities. This idea often leads to segregation. Historically, the idea has been used as justification to institutionalize people, to send them to separate schools and classrooms, and to exclude them from various public services. Through segregation, individuals lose access to natural supports and the benefits that come with them. Further, fear develops about "unknown others," which serves to uphold this segregation.

The Future of Natural Supports

Within schools and communities, recognition of the value of natural supports can help stabilize the general welfare and health of disabled individuals and move communities to form more supportive relationships. Instead of continuing an overreliance on specialized services and professionals to meet the needs of individuals, further integration will allow for the growth of natural supports.

With natural supports, inclusion is not always lost in the language of idealized futures. It happens in families and intimate spaces. It happens without formal consensus or elaborate protocols, and it can yield experiences that can strengthen both disabled and nondisabled youth who engage in the experience from a desire to promote and profit from belonging.

Suzanne Stolz

See also: Inclusive Education; Inclusive Language as Advocacy; (In)Exclusion in Education; Self-Determination in Education

Further Reading

Department of Developmental Services, Services and Supports Section. n.d. "How to Develop Natural Supports." http://www.dds.ca.gov/Publications/docs/Natural_Supports.pdf.

Project 10. 2016. "Natural Supports." http://project10.info/DetailPage.php?MainPageID=106&PageCategory=A-Z%20Library%20or%20Terms&PageSubCategory=None.

Neoliberalism

"Neoliberalism" is used to describe a form of capitalism that has been dominant globally since the 1970s. Under neoliberalism, governments work to eliminate barriers that might impede the ability of capitalists to act freely in the market, generally by emphasizing the importance of private rather than public goods and services.

What Is Neoliberalism?

Neoliberalism is a political economy—that is, a form of economic organization that is implemented and sustained by national or international political entities (including governments; transnational organizations, such as the United Nations; or multinational corporations). Under a neoliberal form of governance, individual nation-states are at times described as "smaller," as advocates of neoliberalism often explicitly say they are against "big government." There is some truth to this description because government regulations of what capitalists can do have been loosened or eliminated and because many public services or agencies (including those focused on the needs of disabled citizens) have been trimmed or privatized. In another sense, however, neoliberalism continues to rely on a large, interventionist state. The role of the state has simply *shifted away from* providing for the public welfare and protecting citizens from the potential excesses of capitalism. National, government-run health care systems, for example, protect citizens from private insurance companies making a quick profit on illness, injury, or disability. The role of the state under neoliberalism has *shifted to* safeguarding the capacity of capitalists to accumulate rapidly massive profits, and to installing a neoliberal consensus in every corner of the globe. Neoliberal states generally have large and well-financed security operations (the police and the military) to carry out these functions.

Historical Overview

The writings of economist Milton Friedman and those trained by him at the University of Chicago in the 1960s and 1970s are often credited with providing the philosophical foundation for neoliberal thought. These ideas were not, initially, well received in Europe and North America, not least because they were perceived as eliminating a social safety net: unemployment protection, disability compensation, and free and accessible health care. Cultural commentator Naomi Klein, in fact, called neoliberalism "disaster capitalism" and argued that "shocks" of some sort (natural disasters such as earthquakes or human-made shocks such as war) are needed to push neoliberal ideas through (Klein 2007). The coup that ousted democratically elected President Salvador Allende of Chile on September 11, 1973, bringing to power the dictator Augusto Pinochet (and the neoliberal policies he implemented), is a prime example of disaster capitalism. Similar "shocks" ushered in neoliberal policies in other South American countries, preparing the way for neoliberalism's ascendency in the 1980s in the United States and the United Kingdom with the elections of Ronald Reagan and Margaret Thatcher. Since that time, Thatcher's idea that "There Is No Alternative" to neoliberalism has sedimented around the globe.

Levels of Neoliberalism

Neoliberalism is a form of capitalism that has cultural effects at both a systemic (or *macroeconomic*) level and at the level of everyday life (or *microlevel*). At the macroeconomic level, neoliberalism relies on "flexible" production that can be distinguished from the "mass" production of the previous era in the history of capitalism. This previous era is often termed "Fordist" because of its association with the factories and assembly lines of Henry Ford. The Fordist era was characterized by both mass production (often of such commodities as automobiles that were largely the same) and government checks on capital's ability to accumulate profit too rapidly. Fordism privileged capital accumulation over the long term and allowed for the construction of a "welfare state" to protect workers. The neoliberal era, in contrast, is characterized by flexible production (often of commodities targeted at smaller groups or niches). This production is often flexibly outsourced to locations where labor costs are cheapest. The state, in this context, works not to check capital's ability to accumulate profit rapidly but to facilitate it.

At the level of everyday life, Fordism required a certain conformity: mass production required mass consumption, which required a certain sameness from the population. Fordism thus relied on normalization, and those perceived as too different—including disabled people; lesbian, gay, bisexual, and transgender (LGBT) people; or racial minorities—were stigmatized or pathologized. Not surprisingly, the LGBT, disability, and civil rights movements resisted the normalization and stigmatization of Fordism. These movements demanded that certain identities (for example, disabled identity) be recognized and valued as such. Neoliberalism, at the level of everyday life, thus no longer necessarily requires conformity or normalization. Distinct identities are often celebrated rather than stigmatized. In relation to disability, neoliberalism has in this way generated deep paradoxes: disabled identity might be recognized and celebrated in some locations. The Paralympic Games, for instance, receive massive sponsorship from multinational corporations and are watched by millions around the globe. However, at the same time, the public services upon which many disabled people rely are cut or privatized.

Conclusion: The Future of Neoliberalism and Disability

Although some saw the global economic crisis of 2008 as the beginning of the end for neoliberalism, others understood it as allowing for harsher forms of neoliberalism to be imposed. Indeed, that has been the case as *austerity* has been pushed on countries such as Spain and Greece: harsh cuts to disability services and other benefits have been coupled with the accelerated privatization of national health care systems. In the UK under David Cameron, in particular, a harsh austerity regime has targeted virtually all disability benefits, including funds allowing disabled people to live independently or to access affordable housing. Resistance to such policies, however, has emerged around the world. Disabled people have engaged in occupations of public spaces and marches designed to draw attention to how neoliberalism has disproportionately affected people with disabilities. Disabled people and allies in some locations have experimented with "social medical centers" that attempt to provide community-based care separate from the inadequate services provided by the neoliberal state. Even if neoliberalism tolerates, or at times even celebrates, disability, disabled artists in many locations have generated performances, disseminated stories, and created installations highlighting how privatization and the shrinking of the public sphere make the lives of most disabled people increasingly precarious.

Robert McRuer

See also: Colonialism; Globalization; Poverty; Welfare to Work

Further Reading

Duggan, Lisa. 2003. *The Twilight of Equality? Neoliberalism, Cultural Politics, and the Attack on Democracy.* Boston: Beacon Press.

Floyd, Kevin. 2009. *The Reification of Desire: Toward a Queer Marxism.* Minneapolis: University of Minnesota Press.

Harvey, David. 2005. *A Brief History of Neoliberalism.* Oxford: Oxford University Press.

Klein, Naomi. 2007. *The Shock Doctrine: The Rise of Disaster Capitalism.* Toronto: A. A. Knopf Canada.

McRuer, Robert. 2018. *Crip Times: Disability, Globalization, and Resistance.* New York: New York University Press.

Seymour, Richard. 2014. *Against Austerity: How We Can Fix the Crisis They Made.* London: Pluto Press.

Normalization and Discipline

The concepts of normalization and discipline have received increasing attention in disability studies and philosophy of disability, due in large part to growing interest throughout the humanities and social sciences in the work of Michel Foucault. These theoretical debates are both complex and important for understanding disability. This entry offers some background of the term "normal" and its relation to normalization and discipline, provides an overview of Foucault's claims about normalization and discipline, and indicates some of the distinct ways that disability theorists have used the concept of normalization in disability theory.

Background

In a number of places, Foucault aimed to show that normalization and discipline are vital mechanisms of a relatively recent form of power that he called "biopower." Foucault described biopower in this way:

> By [biopower] I mean a number of phenomena that seem to me to be significant, namely, the set of mechanisms through which the basic biological features of the human species became the object of a political strategy, of a general strategy of power, or, in other words, how, starting from the eighteenth century, modern Western societies took on board the fundamental biological fact that human beings are a species. (2007, 1)

Foucault argued that the consolidation of the modern concept of *normal* legitimized and occurred in tandem with the new statistical knowledge and other techniques of population management that stemmed from biopower. The norm accomplished this expansion of power in two ways: (1) by enabling discipline to develop from a simple set of constraints into a mechanism; and (2) by transforming the negative restraints of the juridical into the more positive controls of normalization. Foucault regarded normalization as a central—if not *the* central—strategy of biopower's management of life. Foucault claimed that, since the 18th century, the power of the normal has combined with other powers such as the law and tradition, imposing new limits upon them. The normal, he explained, was established as a principle of coercion through the introduction of standardized education; through the organization of national medical professions and hospital systems that could circulate general norms of health; and through the standardization of industrial processes and products and manufacturing techniques.

Ian Hacking (1990) has noted that the first meaning of "normal" that any current English dictionary provides is something like "usual, regular, common, typical." According to the *Oxford English Dictionary*, this usage became current after 1840, with the first citation of "normal, or typical" appearing in 1828. Hacking has noted that the modern sense of the word "normal" was not, however, furnished by education or cloistered study but rather by the study of life (161–62). Hacking explained that the word "normal" became indispensable because it provided a way to be objective about human beings, especially given the inseparability of the notion of normal from its opposite, namely, the pathological. The word "normal," he wrote, "uses a power as old as Aristotle to bridge the fact/value distinction, whispering in your ear that what is normal is also all right" (160). Hacking has also pointed out that although the normal stands "indifferently for what is typical, the unenthusiastic objective average, it also stands for what has been, good health, and what shall be, our chosen destiny" (169). It is especially noteworthy for disability

studies that, as Hacking noted, our modern usage of the word "normal" evolved in a medical context.

In the late 1700s, there was a significant reconfiguration of the concept of the pathological and its relation to the normal. Disease came to be regarded as an attribute of individual organs, rather than as a characteristic of the entire body. Pathology, likewise, became the study of unhealthy organs, rather than the study of sick or diseased bodies. Unhealthy organs could be investigated, in part, by the chemistry of fluids, such as urine or mucus, that actual living beings secreted. The concept of the normal came into being as the inverse of this concept of pathology: a given state of affairs or process of the body was normal if it was not associated with a pathological organ. The pathological became defined as deviation from the normal, and all variation became characterized as variation from the normal state. Pathology was no longer conceived as different in kind from the normal but rather as continuous with, and as a deviation from, the normal (164). This new understanding of the normal and the pathological that emerged in the late 1700s is one, but only one, component of what Shelley Tremain has referred to as "the diagnostic style of reasoning" (Tremain 2010, 2015), which is a style of reasoning that has enabled the consolidation and expansion of biopower.

Overview of Foucault's Claims

Foucault (1977) argued that normalization thus became one of the great instruments of power at the close of the classical age; that is, the power that the norm harnessed was shaped through the disciplines that began to emerge at this historical moment (184). From the end of the eighteenth century, the indicators of social status, privilege, and group affiliation have been increasingly supplemented, if not replaced, by a range of degrees of normality that simultaneously indicate membership in a homogeneous social body (viz. a population) and serve to distinguish between subjects, divide them from each other, classify them, categorize them in a number of ways, and rank them in a host of hierarchies. In *Discipline and Punish* (1977), Foucault noted that normalization initially emerged in the eighteenth-century military school, orphanages, and boarding schools as an effective form of punishment. In Foucault's terms, discipline is neither an institution, nor an apparatus, but rather a particular type of power and a modality for its exercise, comprising a whole set of instruments, techniques, procedures, levels of application, and targets. Discipline is an "anatomy" of power, a technology of power that may be assumed by (1) particular institutions—such as, schools or hospitals—to achieve a certain end; or (2) authorities that use it as a means to reinforce and reorganize their established means of power; or (3) apparatuses that use it as their mode of functioning; or (4) state apparatuses whose primary function is to assure that discipline reigns over society in general—that is, the police (215–216). As a technology that facilitated the expansion of biopower, disciplinary normalization aims to make the body more efficient and calculated in its acts, movements, gesture, and expression, to produce a body that is "docile," that is, a body that can be subjected, used, transformed, and improved. Modern discipline can be summed up thus: it enables subjects to act to constrain them.

Foucault (1977) claimed that disciplinary "punishment"—that is, normalization—has brought into play five distinct normalizing operations: first, individual actions are referred to a totality that is simultaneously a field of comparison, a space of differentiation, and a rule to be followed; second, individuals are in turn differentiated from each other in relation to this rule, which functions as a minimal threshold, as an average, or as an optimal outcome toward which individuals must move; third, the natures, grades and levels, and abilities of individuals are hierarchized and quantified; fourth, these quantifying and hierarchizing measures introduce the constraint of a conformity that must be achieved; fifth, the limit of difference, the far side of "the abnormal" that will define difference per se in relation to all other specific differences, is codified and enforced by penalty (correction, segregation, and so on). The five elemental modes of normalization are thus: comparison, differentiation, hierarchy, homogeneity, exclusion. The punitive impulse that regulates normalization compares, differentiates, hierarchizes, and excludes individuals to homogenize a population that, by virtue of its homogeneity, can be more effectively utilized and modified. In short, the disciplinary power of the norm relies upon coercion rather than open repression or violence (215–20).

Disability Theorists and Normalization

Because of its inescapable historical association with pathologization and coercive correction, the idea of normalization has a checkered past in disability theory and research. In the last decades of the 20th century, some disability theorists and researchers promoted the idea of normalization as emancipatory, both individually and socially, and as a sign of both personal and social progress. Most notably, Wolf Wolfensberger gave birth to a social movement, grounded in the "normalization principle," that denounced the forced institutionalization of "cognitively impaired people." The "normalization movement" aimed to integrate these people into the wider community by enhancing their self-perceptions and abilities to advocate for themselves and transforming their appearances to make them more socially accepted (Yates 2015). Michael Oliver explained the principle upon which the normalization movement relied, in this way: "Normalization theory offers disabled people the opportunity to be given valued social roles in an unequal society which values some roles more than others" (in Drinkwater 2015, 233). The normalization principle was eventually renamed "social role valorization" to stress the *normativity* of normalization. Chris Drinkwater (2015) has argued, however, that although normalization theory was renamed "social role valorization," the power-knowledge regime that is productive of a "normal life" remained unexamined. As Drinkwater explained it, the motivational assumption that underlies these normalizing strategies is that certain people find it difficult to learn how to behave "appropriately"—that is, normally. Drinkwater argues that a more tacit assumption that underlies social role valorization is that these people *ought* to learn normal (valued) behaviors to acquire normal (that is, valued) lifestyles (233).

Conclusion and Future Directions

In Foucault's 1978–79 lecture course at the Collège de France (later published in English as *The Birth of Biopolitics*), he linked his claims about the historical emergence of biopower and its objects with his approach to the theme of government (2008). Recall that, for Foucault, modern power is productive rather than merely repressive: it produces objects and induces effects. Foucault argued that power is more a question of "government"—that is, the direction of conduct—than it is a question of confrontation between adversaries. Foucault used the term "government" in this 16th-century sense to refer to the art of government—that is, any form of activity that aims to shape, guide, or affect the conduct of oneself or someone else—proposing that the term be defined, in general, to mean "the conduct of conduct" (1982).

In an important 1982 interview, Foucault explained that he adopted this earlier, broad meaning of the term "government" because it encompasses both calculated modes of action that structure the field of possible action of oneself or other people and legitimately constituted forms of political and economic subjection. Analyses of force relations that construe power as government (that is, as the direction of conduct) take into consideration innumerable practices that have previously been assumed to fall outside the scope of power. These considerations include technologies of normalization that act as mechanisms for the systematic objectivization of subjects as (for instance) deaf, criminal, and mad, and techniques of self-improvement and self-transformation (technologies of the self), such as weight-loss programs and fitness regimes, assertiveness training, Botox injections, breast implants, psychotherapy, and rehabilitation—in addition to recognizably power-laden procedures and practices such as state-generated prohibitions and punishments and global networks of social, economic, and political stratification, the deleterious effects of which congeal disproportionately along disabling, racialized, and gendered lines. Foucault maintained that although power appears to be merely repressive, the most effective exercise of power consists in guiding the possibilities of conduct and putting in order the possible outcomes. Thus, Foucault's work on normalization and government instructs disability theorists and activists to develop new ways to resist and subvert the increasingly novel strategies and mechanisms that power produces, as well as to move beyond the confines of social models of disability that rely upon outdated and parochial notions of power as fundamentally repressive.

Shelley Tremain

See also: Criminal Justice System and Incarceration; Medicalization

Further Reading

Drinkwater, Chris. 2015. "Supported Living and the Production of Individuals." In *Foucault and the Government of Disability*, edited by Shelley Tremain, 229–44. Ann Arbor: University of Michigan Press.

Ewald, François. 1991. "Norms, Discipline, and the Law." In *Law and the Order of Culture*, edited by Robert Post, 138–161. Berkeley: University of California Press.

Foucault, Michel. 1977. *Discipline and Punish: The Birth of the Prison*. Translated by Alan Sheridan. New York: Vintage Books.

Foucault, Michel. 1982. *Michel Foucault: Beyond Structuralism and Hermeneutics*. Edited by Hubert L. Dreyfus and Paul Rabinow. Chicago: University of Chicago Press.

Foucault, Michel. 2007. *Security, Territory, Population: Lectures at Collège de France, 1977–1978*. Translated by Graham Burchell. New York: Palgrave Macmillan.

Foucault, Michel. 2008. *The Birth of Biopolitics: Lectures at the Collège de France, 1978–1979*. Edited by Michael Senellart. New York: Palgrave Macmillan.

Hacking, Ian. 1990. *The Taming of Chance*. Cambridge: Cambridge University Press.

Tremain, Shelley. 2015. "This Is What a Historicist and Relativist Feminist Philosophy of Disability Looks Like." *Foucault Studies*, June 19. http://rauli.cbs.dk/index.php/foucault-studies/article/view/4822/5268.

Tremain, Shelley. 2010. "Biopower, Styles of Reasoning, and What's Still Missing from the Stem Cell Debates." *Hypatia: A Journal of Feminist Philosophy* 25, no. 3: 577–609.

Williams, Lindsey, and Melanie Nind. 1999. "Insiders or Outsiders: Normalisation and Women with Learning Difficulties." *Disability & Society* 14, no. 5: 659–672.

Yates, Scott. 2015. "Truth, Power, and Ethics in Care Services for People with Learning Difficulties." In *Foucault and the Government of Disability*, edited by Shelley Tremain, 65–77. Ann Arbor: University of Michigan Press.

"Nothing about Us without Us"

The expression "Nothing about Us without Us" is widely used by political activists with disabilities around the world as a slogan emphasizing political empowerment. The slogan's power derives from its opposition to the long-experienced exclusion and degradation of people with disabilities. The slogan emphasizes the central role disabled persons want to play regarding the issues, services, policies, and programs directly affecting them. The slogan emphasizes control and voice. As Ed Roberts, one of the leading figures of the international disability rights movement, has said, "If we have learned one thing from the civil rights movement in the U.S., it's that when others speak for you, you lose" (Driedger 1989, 28).

What Is "Nothing about Us without Us"?

Nothing about Us without Us resonates with the philosophy and history of the disability rights movement, an international movement that has embarked on a mission parallel to those of other social movements. The politics and philosophy of the disability rights movement have evolved out of an emerging consciousness of political activists worldwide. The politics and philosophy of the disability rights movement incorporate the interconnected principles of empowerment and human rights, integration and independence, self-help and self-determination. The meaning of these concepts and the places they programmatically lead can be different and have different strategic importance depending on the time and place they are embraced and the divergent politics of the movement's activists.

The disability rights movement's demand for control has universal appeal because the needs of people with disabilities and the potential for meeting those needs are everywhere conditioned by a dependency born of powerlessness, poverty, degradation, and institutionalization. This condition of dependency is presently typical for hundreds of millions of people throughout the world.

Historical Overview

Only in the past 40 years has the condition of disability and disabled persons begun to change. It has been during this period that we have witnessed the increasing use of the slogan "Nothing about Us without Us," which was first used among disability rights activists in South Africa. Although little noticed and affecting only a small percentage of people with disabilities, this transformation has been profound. For the first time in history, politically active people with disabilities are beginning to proclaim that they know what is best for themselves and their community.

Important Points to Know about the Topic

The disability rights movement is not unlike other new and important social movements demanding self-representation and control over the resources needed to live a decent life.

People with disabilities have formed a wide array of organizations to respond to political and personal needs. Each organization has its own motivation and agenda, lines of communication and leadership, and expectations and scope. These range from small political action and self-help groups, social clubs, and income-generating initiatives to large national and regional federations or coalitions of disability-related groups. These organizations, given their specific circumstances and histories, have developed strategies and patterns of organization that in a very short time have advanced the overall progress of their communities. They have promoted an increased identification with others who have disabilities and an interest in what many have come to call "disability culture." The slogan "Nothing about Us without Us" captures the essence of these developments. To understand anything about people with disabilities or the disability rights movement, one must recognize their individual and collective necessities. "Nothing about Us without Us" forces people to think about the broad implications of "nothing" in various political-economic and cultural contexts. Further, a growing number of people with disabilities have developed a consciousness that transforms the notion and concept of disability from a medical condition to a political and social condition.

"Nothing about Us without Us" requires people with disabilities to recognize their need to control and take responsibility for their own lives. It also forces institutions and systems to incorporate people with disabilities into the decision-making process and to recognize that the experiential knowledge of these people is pivotal in making decisions that affect their lives. While the number of people affected is relatively small, a movement has emerged. The disability rights movement has developed its own ideology and politics. The slogan "Nothing about Us without Us" is a demand for self-determination, independence and integration, empowerment and human rights, and self-help and self-determination. The demand "Nothing about Us without Us" affirms the essence of these principles.

Dilemmas, Debates, and Unresolved Questions

Self-determination requires people with disabilities to control all aspects of their collective experience. It means that we are able to take responsibility for our own lives, and we do not need or want you to manage our affairs; that we best understand what is best for us; and that we demand control of our own organizations and programs and influence on the government funding, public policy, and economic enterprises that directly affect us. The demand for self-determination provocatively and intuitively attacks the ideology of paternalism; the existing political elite and power structure; social institutions like family, school, the medical establishment, social agencies, and charities; and the political, economic, and social dependency people have been forced into. This principle is not without risk as it tends to promote a go-it-alone approach that would require people to actually take control of their lives, an endeavor many people with disabilities are not prepared for. Analogies of failed efforts at deinstitutionalization of people with mental illness come to mind. As a practical matter, self-help and self-determination are illusory short-term goals but extremely important and powerful demands.

There are further challenges, two of which stand out. One is how to successfully resolve the contradiction between the individual and the collective. The question of how individuals long isolated by political, economic, and social marginalization can find each other and unite around their common experiences of oppression while accommodating each other's profound differences has an often perplexing history. The contradiction between the individual and the collective is particularly complex among people with disabilities because of our isolation, stigmatization, and fragmentation into categories (physical disability, intellectual disability, cognitive disability, deaf and hard of hearing, blind and visually impaired, and so on). Add to this the wide spectrum of experiences that exist among people with disabilities and that are filtered by class, gender, and race, and a future politics based on "Nothing about Us without Us" is hard to predict.

Conclusion and Future Directions

A remarkable and unprecedented paradigm shift has recently occurred, representing a historic break with the traditional perception of disability as a sick, abnormal, and pathetic condition. This shift poses a fundamental challenge to the ideological oppression of people with disabilities, for it sees disability as normal, not inferior, and demands self-determination over the resources people with disabilities need. This new perspective unfolds out of a changing world where a relatively few political activists with disabilities are challenging the old ways of thinking about and treating disability. The stories of these people provide compelling evidence for the basis and direction of this paradigm shift.

Jim Charlton

See also: Disability Protests; Disability Rights Movement (DRM); Self-Advocacy Movement; Self-Determination, Concept and Policy

Further Reading

Abberley, Paul. 1987. "The Concept of Oppression and the Development of a

Social Theory of Disability." *Disability, Handicap and Society* 2, no. 1: 5–19.

Charlton, James I. 1998. *Nothing about Us without Us: Disability Oppression and Empowerment.* Berkeley: University of California Press.

Driedger, Diane. 1989. *The Last Civil Rights Movement: Disabled People's International.* New York: St. Martin's Press.

Erevelles, Nirmala. 2011. *Disability and Difference in Global Contexts: Enabling a Transformative Body Politic.* New York: Palgrave McMillan.

O

Occupational Therapy

Occupational therapy (OT) is a health and rehabilitation profession that works with people—often who have experienced disease, injury, impairment, or disability—throughout the lifespan to maximize their ability to participate in meaningful activities or occupations.

Background and History

While the consideration of health as a factor of occupational engagement has been a part of various cultures and societies since antiquity, the "professionalization of Occupational Therapy" (Frank and Zemke 2009, 144) began in the late 19th and early 20th centuries in the United States and United Kingdom. The emergence of standardized training programs and professional organizations, such as the American Occupational Therapy Association, were linked to increasing industrialization occurring in the Western world and to the progressive political movements that emerged at this time to address the social and public health issues often linked to this changing economic and cultural environment. Early OT services focused heavily on reform for conditions for people labeled with mental illness and on the use of occupational engagement as an intervention to address mental health issues.

After World War I and World War II, the field shifted focus to working with wounded veterans and began to embrace the rehabilitation model of medicine, which also emerged as a result of the wars. During this time, the profession also allied itself more with the medical fields, moving away from its alignment with social work and transformative models of service and care (Frank and Zemke 2009). The body of OT literature became dominated by the voices of physicians and quests for scientific understandings of how occupations affected individuals and individual body structures or functions. While early figures in OT in the United States were instrumental in passing laws related to social reform, the field increasingly became regulated by vocational rehabilitation regulations that arose out of World War I, causing a shift in practices and theoretical foundations.

The field in the United States has continued to be influenced by political and social forces in the last century, such as the creation of social security programs, the rise of the for-profit health insurance industry, and the worldwide influence of neoliberalism on public policy and services from the 1980s onward (Frank and Zemke 2009). This model of OT, with its heavy rehabilitative focus, has heavily influenced the proliferation and development of OT around the world. While the profession has become increasingly international, with notable expansion in Asia and South America at the end of the 20th century and beginning of the 21st century, it remains dominated by the United States and Europe, particularly regarding practitioner membership in national organizations and knowledge generation through widely disseminated English-language publications.

In recent decades, there have been increasing calls for OT to acknowledge its progressive roots and adopt a social transformation model of practice. In 2004, the World Federation of Occupational Therapists issued a position paper on community-based rehabilitation, which recognized the large worldwide population of people with disabilities, a majority of whom live in "developing countries," who are consistently denied access to occupational engagement and the opportunities to participate in meaningful roles and their communities (Frank and Zemke 2009). This acknowledgement of community-based services and the connections between the profession and the disability community at large has been influential in more current debates within the field.

What Is Occupational Therapy?

OT services can be provided in a wide variety of settings or environments, but in the United States, they are most frequently provided in hospitals, long-term care or skilled nursing facilities, and schools (American Occupational Therapy Association 2015). Services can be provided by occupational therapists, who currently require a master's degree for entry-level practice, and OT assistants, who are supervised by occupational therapists and have an associate's degree. Practitioners must complete educational and certification requirements that are standardized and monitored by various national regulatory bodies and that often have additional continuing education requirements to maintain certification and licensure, which can vary by state and practice setting.

Practice Frameworks. As outlined in the American Occupational Therapy Association's (2014) "Practice Frameworks," which serves as a guiding document that provides standardized definitions and conceptualizations of commonly used terminology in the field, OT services center around the collaboration between the practitioner and receiver

of services, typically referred to as "clients," in a process often referred to as "client-centered practice." The process includes three stages:

1. Evaluation and analysis of occupational performance.
2. Identification of targeted service outcomes.
3. Development and implementation of an intervention plan.

While services typically follow the order detailed above, it is acknowledged that these three aspects of the process inform each other and that adjustments can be and are made continuously throughout service provision.

Interventions. There are five main approaches to interventions in OT: (1) the use of *occupations or activities* chosen based on activity demands, client factors, goal, and environments; (2) the use of *preparatory methods and tasks*, such as physical modalities, orthotics, assistive technology, wheeled mobility, or environmental modifications, to prepare for occupational engagement; (3) *education and training* related to occupational performance; (4) *advocacy* undertaken by either the practitioner or the client; and (5) *group-based services* (American Occupational Therapy Association 2014). Within these approaches, the foci of interventions in OT center on *health promotion*; *skill acquisition* or development; *restoration* of abilities after injury, illness, or functional decline; *maintenance* of performance; environmental and activity *modifications* or adaptations; and *prevention*.

Outcomes. Outcomes for OT services can be broken down into eight categories:

1. Improvement or enhancement in occupational performance

2. Prevention of unhealthy conditions, risk factors, diseases, or injuries
3. Health and wellness
4. Quality of life
5. Participation
6. Role competence
7. Well-being
8. Occupational justice

In the United States, the services OT practitioners provide are influenced by *state regulations and practice-setting policies*, which are often heavily influenced by *health care insurance reimbursement*. Another influential factor in service provision is *evidence-based practice*, or guidelines and decision making based on the use of research and other scientific knowledge.

Important Points to Know about Occupational Therapy

Occupation and Engagement. Within the field, occupations are defined as any activities that people regard as purposeful and meaningful to engage in throughout their daily routines. They are seen as essential elements of people's identity and role engagement and unique to the individual's wants, needs, and expectations. In this framework, occupations are categorized as *activities of daily living (ADLs)*, which encompass personal bodily care activities often essential to basic survival and well-being, such as bathing, dressing, hygiene, and eating tasks; *instrumental activities of daily living (IADLs)*, which are often more complex than ADLs but still support daily life routines, including care of others, shopping, home maintenance, personal financial management, health management, community mobility, and safety maintenance; *rest and sleep*; and any activities related to exploration or participation in *education, work, play, leisure,* and *social* interactions.

Engagement in occupations is viewed as an interaction between *client factors*, including individual characteristics such as values, beliefs, body structures, and body functions; *performance skills*, which are the ways client factors come together as actions, such as motor skills, process skills, and social interaction skills; and *performance patterns*, which are the habits, routines, rituals, and roles composing performance skills. The cultural, personal, physical, social, temporal, and virtual *contexts* or *environments* affect all of these aspects (American Occupational Therapy Association 2014). The relationships between client factors, performance skills, performance patterns, occupations, and the environment are seen as transactional rather than hierarchical.

Rehabilitation. The field of rehabilitation medicine and science focuses on the improvement of physical, cognitive, and sensory functions for people who have experienced losses or impairments in these areas because of injury, illness, or other mechanisms. Services and care under this framework are primarily focused on restoring function to the maximum extent possible and increasing a client's ability to independently participate and complete activities or occupations, with adaptations and use of equipment or devices as needed (Magasi 2008). In addition to OT, other professions typically, but not exclusively, involved in rehabilitation services include physiatrists or physical medicine and rehabilitation physicians, rehabilitation nurses, physical therapists, speech and language therapists, recreational therapists, and registered dietitians.

Occupational Justice. Occupational justice, a relatively new concept discussed in the OT literature, views participation in occupation as a human right. These rights are further developed and described as the right to

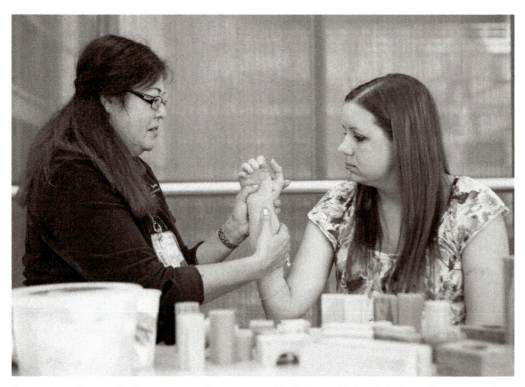

Occupational therapist Renee Portenier massages Emily Fennell's hand during a therapy session, at the Ronald Reagan UCLA Medical Center, in Los Angeles, California. Fennell was UCLA's first hand-transplant recipient. Occupational therapists work with individuals on the activities that they consider purposeful and meaningful to their lives. (Ann Johansson/Corbis via Getty Images)

experience *meaningful* occupations, the right to participate in a *variety* of occupations that support inclusion, the right to make *choices* related to occupations, and the right to *equal* opportunities for occupational participation. From an occupational justice lens, practitioners and services should focus on the recognition of the importance of social policies, beliefs, political forces, and power dynamics that can either enable or restrict participation.

Critical Occupational Therapy. "Critical occupational therapy" refers to an increasing number of scholars in the field who are challenging long-held foundations of the profession, such as definitions of participation (Mirza, Magasi, and Hammel 2016), constructions of disability and evidence-based practice (Phelan 2011), client-centered

practice (Whalley Hammell 2015), and the role of OT in politics (Frank and Zemke 2009). This paradigm is influenced by other critical fields of study, including disability studies, in reflexively examining how OT as a profession and its individual practitioners position themselves in relation to people with disabilities and how the profession examines attitudes, power, and identity related to disability.

Dilemmas, Debates, and Unresolved Questions

Challenging Views on Participation. The previously discussed shifts in the field of OT, and the emergence of critical narratives within its body of research, suggest increased recognition of the importance of rights, advocacy, and social consciousness. For example, while participation is heavily emphasized as a focus of OT services and addressing participation disparities in a variety of environments is viewed as a distinct contribution that the field makes in health care, there have been some critical examinations of how the profession views participation and how these conceptualizations affect the lives of people with disabilities and other recipients of OT services. Other research is challenging traditional rehabilitation and medical conceptualizations of participation that attempt to quantify this construct and make standardized measurements of what constitutes desirable or undesirable levels of participation. Mirza, Magasi, and Hammel (2016) argue that traditional understandings of participation fail to capture the complex experiences of people with disabilities related to their navigation within their communities. Knowledge about the unique meanings and experiences of participation may help guide practices that support engagement in occupations and contribute to an evidence base that increasingly acknowledges that participation for people with disabilities is not just a matter for medical or rehabilitation services but a matter of rights. However, the connections between participation and social justice or occupational justice are also criticized for being underdeveloped at this point (Mirza, Magasi, and Hammel 2016).

Challenging Positivism. Evidence-based practice has also been critiqued for its overwhelmingly positivist approach. This approach minimizes the importance of qualitative research and strengthens OT's ties to medicine instead of highlighting knowledge created by and with people with disabilities and other client groups. Positivism in OT relies on normed assessments to evaluate client needs and plan interventions that aim to meet those norms. Phelan (2011) asserts that such evidence-based practice may be perpetuating ideologies that continue to marginalize people with disabilities and that practitioners need to carefully consider their intentions with these actions. Similarly, Whalley Hammell (2015) argues that current conceptualizations of client-centered practice fail to recognize or encourage practitioners to recognize their privilege and power over their clients with disabilities, and this omission can lead to assumptions that reinforce inequalities and limited opportunities.

Partners in Advocacy. In addition to recognizing and addressing power imbalances in rehabilitation services, Magasi (2008) urges practitioners to advocate for policy change that directly affects the resources and services available to people with disabilities. Practitioners should also partner with disability organizations within communities as a valuable source of knowledge and peer support. While OT as a profession is concerned with improving people's lives at its core, failures to critically examine ongoing practices are seen as threats to undermine this mission. There appears to be limited research that moves beyond a description of how and why disability studies can be incorporated into OT and how it actually operates within day-to-day practices of practitioners, particularly within current economic and political climates.

The Future of OT and Disability

If these two fields are to be better integrated with the goal of providing services more in line with what the disability community wants and needs, understanding how practitioners view and use elements of disability studies in their practice is essential to making practical and implementable recommendations for the field. Another area of future study is in educational practices, at both entry and continuing education levels. Investigators should study how OT affects attitudes toward disability and the incorporation of disability studies in OT services. How are practitioners and students asking themselves about their attitudes and beliefs about disability, their privilege, and their power, and how do these attitudes affect their practices and interactions on a regular basis? To what extent does OT consider how to include a wider variety of voices in the dialogue and knowledge creation about best practices, and how do these actions challenge or perpetuate stereotypes? As the field of OT in the United States enters its second centennial, considerations of its place within the health care and rehabilitation fields and its connections to the disability community are paramount to shaping its future directions.

Alisa Sheth Jordan

See also: Activities of Daily Living (ADLs); Community Living and Community Integration; Health Care Provider Activism; Therapist, Role in Activities of Daily Living (ADLs)

Further Reading

American Occupational Therapy Association. 2014. "Occupational Therapy Practice Framework: Domain and Process." *American Journal of Occupational Therapy* 68, Supplement 1: S1–48.

American Occupational Therapy Association. 2015. "2015 AOTA Salary & Workforce Survey Executive Summary." https://www.aota.org/Education-Careers/Advance-Career/Salary-Workforce-Survey.aspx.

Frank, Gelya, and Ruth Zemke. 2009. *A Political Practice of Occupational Therapy.* London: Churchill Livingstone.

Magasi, Susan. 2008. "Infusing Disability Studies into the Rehabilitation Sciences." *Topics in Stroke Rehabilitation* 15, no. 3: 283–287.

Mirza, Mansha, Susan Magasi, and Joy Hammel. 2016. *Occupying Disability: Critical Approaches to Community, Justice, and Decolonizing Disability.* New York: Springer.

Phelan, Shanon K. 2011. "Constructions of Disability: A Call for Critical Reflexivity in Occupational Therapy." *Canadian Journal of Occupational Therapy* 78, no. 3: 164–172.

Whalley Hammell, Karen R. 2015. "Client-Centred Occupational Therapy: The Importance of Critical Perspectives." *Scandinavian Journal of Occupational Therapy* 22, no. 4: 237–243.

Olmstead v. L. C. (1999)

On June 22, 1999, the Supreme Court of the United States issued a landmark "decision" that called for the community integration of people with disabilities and ruled that unnecessary isolation was disability discrimination. *Olmstead v. L. C.* 527 U.S. 581 (1999) would have wide-reaching policy implications for dismantling thousands of institutions in the United States. The "Olmstead decision," as it became known, challenged the paradigm that institutional settings that segregate individuals from the general community best served people with significant disabilities. *Olmstead* stood for the proposition that people with disabilities are worthy of participating in community living. The implementation of *Olmstead* continues today as people with disabilities and their advocates work toward integration into the most inclusive settings possible.

Background

Title II of the Americans with Disabilities Act of 1990 (ADA) set the legal framework for community integration. Title II is the public services portion of the ADA. It requires that "no qualified individual with a disability shall, by reason of such disability, be excluded from participation in or be denied the benefits of the services, programs, or activities of a public entity, or be subjected to discrimination by any such entity" (42 U.S.C. §12132). Congress also instructed the U.S. attorney general to issue regulations defining forms of discrimination under Title II. The "integration regulation," commonly known as the "integration mandate," thus states: "A public entity shall administer services, programs, and activities in the most integrated setting appropriate to the needs of qualified individuals with disabilities" (28 CFR Section 35.130(d) [1998]).

What Is *Olmstead*?

In *Olmstead v. L. C.* (1999), two women, with intellectual disability and mental illness, argued that Title II's integration mandate meant they should be released from a state psychiatric hospital. Civil rights attorneys from the Atlanta Legal Aid Society chose these women, Lois Curtis and Elaine Wilson (L. C. and E. W.), to serve as representatives for thousands of individuals in similar situations. L. C. and E. W. were both voluntarily admitted to state hospitals for psychiatric treatment. After several years, both women remained institutionalized after their treating medical teams concluded that their needs could be met in community-based settings. This hospital "seal of approval" that both women could live in the community made it unlikely that defendants, Georgia's Department of Human Resources, could successfully argue that the plaintiffs required further institutional care. Instead, it focused the attention on the problem of the state's long *waiting lists* to receive community care—a problem pervasive throughout the United States.

Important Points to Understand About *Olmstead*

Supreme Court Decision. Justice Ruth Bader Ginsburg, delivering the opinion of the court, upheld the ADA's integration mandate, ruling that defendants could not segregate L. C. and E. W. in a state hospital long after their medical teams had recommended their transfer to community care.

The Supreme Court declared that "unjustified isolation . . . is properly regarded as discrimination based on disability" (*Olmstead* 1999, 597). The court held that, to reach the goal of integration, states would have to make reasonable modifications to their programs, services, and activities to include individuals with disabilities. However, the court also held that states do not have to make fundamental alterations to provide community-based care. Under the "fundamental-alteration" defense, states may consider their resources (such as cost and range of services available) when determining whether they have made a reasonable modification. In this way, some individuals with disabilities might be "properly" confined in a facility for care and treatment when there cannot be a more integrated setting appropriate to their needs.

Impact of Olmstead. The *Olmstead* decision led to the mass deinstitutionalization, or the release, of individuals with disabilities from state mental hospitals, nursing homes, and intermediate health care facilities. Since *Olmstead v. L. C.*, communities have made considerable changes to provide its citizens with disabilities with meaningful engagement. In this way, the courts, federal agencies, and policy makers have developed different areas of *Olmstead* enforcement.

However, today millions of individuals with disabilities remain in segregated settings away from the community. Though *Olmstead* prompted deinstitutionalization efforts, the Supreme Court held that a state could keep some individuals with disabilities institutionalized *and* establish compliance with the ADA if it demonstrates that it has:

A comprehensive, effectively working plan for placing qualified persons with [disabilities] in less restrictive settings, and a waiting list that moved at a reasonable pace not controlled by the State's endeavors to keep its institutions fully populated. (*Olmstead* 1999, 584)

States thus have created their respective "*Olmstead* plans" to comply with this mandate. *Olmstead* continues to be applied as legal precedent for individuals with disabilities who wish to further challenge unnecessary segregation and demand community services. These cases are often referred to as "*Olmstead* litigation."

Various decisions, such as in *Makin v. Hawaii* 114 F.Supp.2d 1017 (D.Haw. 1999), have ruled that *Olmstead* applies to individuals living outside of institutions on waiting lists to receive community services. Courts have concluded that individuals who are at risk of institutionalization because of a lack of appropriate community services also fall under *Olmstead*'s protection. (*See also Fisher v. Oklahoma Healthcare Authority*, 335 F.3d 1321 [10th Cir. 2003].) Several cases have been filed on behalf of residents in nursing facilities arguing that these facilities fall under segregated institutions not appropriate under *Olmstead*. Courts, in cases such as *Rolland v. Cellucci* 52 F.Supp.2d 231 (D.Mass. 1999) and *Olesky v. Michigan* (2000) have held that residents of nursing facilities may bring *Olmstead* cases. The Tenth Circuit held that Oklahoma's fiscal problem, by itself, does not lead to an automatic conclusion that providing community services would be a fundamental alteration. Newer litigations have questioned whether *Olmstead* mandates mental health services in the most integrative settings and whether group homes, sheltered workshops, and other day programs for individuals with disabilities comply with *Olmstead*.

The U.S. Department of Health and Human Services, Office of Civil Rights, is the federal agency charged with ensuring *Olmstead* compliance. They have conducted enforcement activities, such as developing settlement agreements with the states, to ensure that individuals with disabilities receive services in the least restrictive environments.

Conclusion

Olmstead remains an important court decision for individuals with disabilities as they navigate not only their treatment and care in the most integrated settings but also full inclusion into mainstream society. *Olmstead*-type policies and cases may continue to include other aspects of social inclusion—for example, in the area of employment, where staggering numbers of individuals with disabilities are unemployed. Employment is a fundamental aspect of U.S. society that brings its citizens into mainstream life. Thus, attorneys might argue that bridging the gap of employment of individuals with disabilities responds to the heart of *Olmstead*. The mandates of *Olmstead* are not complete, and individuals with disabilities will continue to fight for inclusion.

Katherine Perez

See also: Americans with Disabilities Act (ADA); Community Living and Community Integration; Deinstitutionalization; *Primary Documents:* Excerpt from the U.S. Supreme Court Decision in *Olmstead v. L. C.* (1999)

Further Reading

ADA.gov. n.d. "Olmstead: Community Integration for Everyone." https://www.ada.gov/olmstead/olmstead_enforcement.htm.

National Disability Rights Network. 2004. "Q&A about *Olmstead* Interpretations." http://www.ndrn.org/public-policy/community-integration/346-qaa-about-olmstead-interpretations.html.

Ng, Terence, Alice Wong, and Charlene Harrington. 2011. "Home and Community-Based Services: Introduction to *Olmstead* Lawsuits and *Olmstead* Plans 11." *Community Living Policy Center.* http://www.pascenter.org/olmstead/downloads/Olmstead_report_2011.pdf.

Online Social and Professional Networks and Work

Over the past 20 years, online social networking sites (SNS) have become an integral part of many people's daily routines as entertainment, a source of news, a marketplace to buy and sell, a platform for community organizing, and a resource for looking for employment.

What Are Online Social and Professional Networks and Work?

Conventional wisdom has long considered networking and "who you know" the most effective source of finding employment. Networking remains an important part of the job-seeking process in an increasingly online world. Job seekers and recruiters are increasingly supplementing in-person networking with online connections (Garg and Rahul 2017). Online personal and professional networks minimize the effort required to maintain connections to close friends and acquaintances, who may be able to offer job-seeking support.

Background and History

Disability communities have found different advantages to communicating through social media. Adolescents and adults with cerebral palsy who use alternative and augmentative communication (AAC) devices have reported that social networking sites allow them to communicate more easily, more effectively, and at a pace they can control (Caron and Light 2016). Instant messaging on social media creates a platform for people who are Deaf or hard of hearing to contact businesses, public figures, and friends. Deaf SNS users can communicate in real time with hearing and Deaf peers. Autistic people have used SNS such as Twitter and Tumblr using the hashtag #ActuallyAutistic to create an online community that is intended to be an autistic-only space to network with other autistic people. Activists from all disability groups created an ongoing conversation on Twitter using the hashtag #CripTheVote, to discuss and organize around disability-related policies and draw attention to the disability voting bloc. Through tags like these, disability communities build relationships, critique policy and media, and articulate priorities for change.

Important Points to Know about the Topic

Widespread use of social and professional networking sites has cemented their importance in job-seeking, organizing, and community-building efforts by people with disabilities. SNS are an essential part of community organizing in disability communities, as they are used to share information about proposed policy changes, candidate platforms, and meet-ups, marches, and boycotts. People with disabilities who cannot attend events use SNS to follow along through live streaming, sharing photos, and live tweeting.

SNS offer a niche community connection that was not previously available. Disability communities share more casual in-group knowledge about work opportunities and offer advice on job seeking and disability disclosure. SNS are a platform for people with and without disabilities to promote workplace alternatives, including freelance work and different forms of self-employment (e.g., blogging, creative work, and individual sales within network).

Dilemmas, Debates, and Unresolved Questions

Internet access and SNS accessibility affect which groups can gain the potential benefits of SNS use and which groups continue to experience barriers to use. The term "digital divide" refers to the rift between groups of people who have access to tech devices and the Internet and those who do not. People with disabilities are more likely to be older adults and more likely to live in poverty, with additional factors contributing to lack of Internet access at home (Anderson and Perrin 2017).

Accessibility of Web sites themselves is another potential barrier to online participation for people with disabilities. Online accessibility was not directly addressed in the original text of the Americans with Disabilities Act (ADA) when it passed in 1990. As a result, online accessibility has been addressed in small pieces through case law and regulations. The Justice Department has since acknowledged that the promise of the ADA will not be fulfilled until businesses and municipalities make their Web sites accessible.

While SNS have some accessibility features built into their structure, the sites share responsibility for access with

businesses and the general public who produce the content for the platform. Some social media content requires a certain level of literacy to fully engage, which may keep some people with disabilities from fully accessing the benefits of SNS for connecting with employers and disability communities. Additionally, SNS structures are often not set up with appropriate section labels or image and link descriptive text for convenient use by people with blindness and low vision (National Council on Disability 2011). When new accessibility features are developed for apps and Web sites, companies are often ineffective at communicating about the existence and use of the features.

While SNS have opened up additional opportunities for people with disabilities to find employment, they also open up a risk that job seekers with disabilities will face discrimination in the hiring process if potential employers see that individuals have disabilities on their social media profiles. Most employers report that they use social media for recruitment and background checks. Use of SNS as part of the hiring process is not prohibited by current Equal Employment Opportunity laws; however, the discrimination based on text or photos with observable characteristics that may identify a potential employee as having a disability is prohibited.

The Future of Online Social and Professional Networks, Work, and Disability and Conclusions

This topic will grow and change as the cycle of new technologies leads to shifts away from certain platforms to others. For example, some younger social networking users have fully transitioned from Facebook, Twitter, and LinkedIn to newer platforms like Instagram and Snapchat. With each new platform that is developed and used, there will be new issues with accessibility and privacy for job seekers with disabilities. While there is potential for community building and empowerment on SNS platforms, this potential is balanced by the fact that accessibility is retrofitted, the inability to avoid harassment and trolling, and the potential for employment discrimination. Social networking has shown potential to be both an enabling and disabling force in the lives and work of people with disabilities, and continued consideration of SNS application to disabled people is necessary to hold SNS companies accountable for their practices.

Amy Heider

See also: Communication; Employment, Barriers to; Social Capital; Youth with Disabilities, Employment of

Further Reading

Anderson, Monica, and Andrew Perrin. 2017. "Disabled Americans Are Less Likely to Use Technology." Pew Research Center. http://www.pewresearch.org/fact-tank/2017/04/07/disabled-americans-are-less-likely-to-use-technology/.

Brown, Victoria R., and E. Daly Vaughn. 2011. "The Writing on the (Facebook) Wall: The Use of Social Networking Sites in Hiring Decisions." *Journal of Business and Psychology* 26, no. 2: 219–225.

Caron, Jessica, and Janice Light. 2016. "Social Media Has Opened a World of 'Open Communication': Experiences of Adults with Cerebral Palsy Who Use Augmentative and Alternative Communication and Social Media." *Augmentative and Alternative Communication* 32, no. 1: 25–40.

Department of Justice. 2015. "Nondiscrimination on the Basis of Disability: Accessibility of Web Information and Services of Public Accommodations." The Department of Justice. https://www.reginfo.gov/public/do/eAgendaViewRule?pubId=201504&RIN=1190-AA61.

Garg, Rajiv, and Rahul Telang. 2017. "To Be or Not to Be Linked: Online Social Networks and Job Search by Unemployed Workforce." *Management Science, Articles in Advance.* 1–16.

Lee, Sang M., Soon-Goo Hong, Dong-Han An, and Hyun-Mi Lee. 2014. "Disability Users' Evaluation of the Web Accessibility of SNS." *Service Business* 8, no. 4: 517–540.

National Council on Disability. 2011. *The Power of Digital Inclusion: Technology's Impact on Employment and Opportunities for People with Disabilities.* https://ncd.gov/publications/2011/Oct042011#toc1.

Wong, Alice, Andrew Pulrang, and Gregg Beratan. 2018. #Cripthevote. http://cripthevote.blogspot.com/.

P

Paralympics

The Paralympic Games, the second largest multisport event in the world, is elite-level competition for athletes with disabilities (Brittain 2012). Further, it is the largest multisport event for people with disabilities. The number of countries participating in international disability sport has grown over time, as the 2016 Summer Games in Rio de Janeiro welcomed 4,316 athletes from 158 countries, competing in 22 different sporting events (International Paralympic Committee 2016).

Background and History

Dr. Ludwig Guttmann, the founder of the Paralympic Movement, encouraged sport participation by wounded war veterans at Stoke Mandeville Hospital in the United Kingdom. Stoke Mandeville believed sport participation to be a valuable part of the

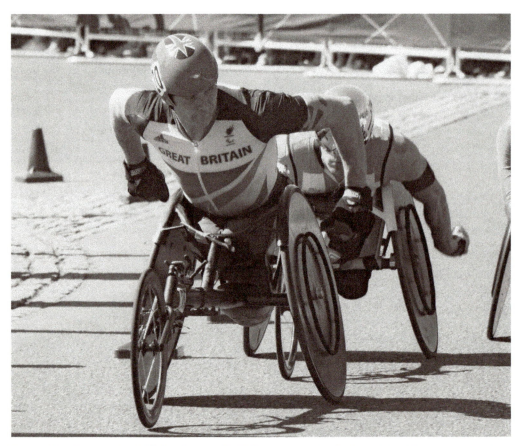

David Weir leading the 2012 Paralympic T54 Marathon in the final straight. His victory resulted in his fourth gold medal of the 2012 Summer Paralympics. (Rkaphotography/Dreamstime.com)

rehabilitation process. As this belief caught on in other rehabilitation centers, patients began to come together for a national competition each year. This annual gathering eventually became what was the first Paralympic Games. In 1948, coinciding with the timing of the Olympic Games, the Stoke Mandeville Games occurred, marking an important milestone in terms of competition for athletes with disabilities. Those games later evolved into the Paralympic Games, which were first held in Rome, Italy, in 1960, with 400 athletes from 23 countries. For a comprehensive history of the Paralympic Games, refer to *From Stoke Mandeville to Stratford: A History of the Summer Paralympic Games*, by Ian Brittain (2012).

"Paralympic" derives from the Greek preposition "para," meaning beside or alongside. The significance of the name is the intention that the Paralympics are parallel to the Olympics, and the name illustrates that the two movements were intended to exist side by side (International Paralympic Committee 2016). Since the Summer Games of Seoul, Korea, in 1988 and the Winter Games in Albertville, France, in 1992, the Paralympics have taken part in the same cities and venues as the Olympics because of an agreement that cities who place an Olympic bid are also bidding on the Paralympic Games.

Important Points to Understand about the Paralympics

Governance Structure. The International Paralympic Committee (IPC), founded in 1989, is the global governing body of the Paralympic Movement, which oversees and organizes the Summer and Winter Paralympic Games. The IPC is also the international federation (IF) for ten sports, meaning that they oversee the governance process, rules, and policies for those sports. The ten sports that are governed by the IPC are world para alpine skiing, world para athletics, world para biathlon, world para cross-country skiing, world para ice hockey, world para powerlifting, world shooting para sport, world para snowboard, world para swimming, and world para dance sport. For these sports, the IPC also coordinates world championships.

There are independent IFs who oversee other sports for athletes with, and in some cases without, disabilities. For example, the International Table Tennis Federation (ITTF) is the governing body for athletes with and without disabilities who compete in table tennis. Alternatively, the International Wheelchair Rugby Federation oversees wheelchair rugby, but it is not connected to the World Rugby Federation. Overall, the IPC membership comprises 179 national Paralympic committees (NPC), 4 international organizations of sports for the disabled (IOSD), 16 international sport federations, and 4 regional organizations (International Paralympic Committee 2016).

Unlike most other nations, the United States does not have a sports ministry. The U.S. Olympic Committee (USOC) serves as both the National Olympic Committee and the National Paralympic Committee for the country. The NOC and NPC are the bodies within a country that organize and represent the Olympic and Paralympic athletes of that nation. There are few other countries where the Olympic and Paralympic athletes are governed by the same entity. U.S. Paralympics is a division formed in 2001 within the nonprofit structure of the USOC. Nationally, U.S. Paralympics operates as the national governing body or high-performance management organization for six sports: alpine skiing, cycling, Nordic skiing (biathlon and cross-country skiing), snowboarding, swimming, and track and field.

Paralympians. Paralympians are athletes with disabilities who have competed in a Paralympic Games. While athletes may be named to national teams for world championships or other elite-level international competitions, the term "Paralympians" is only for those who were on a national team that competed at the Paralympic Games. For example, being an athlete with a disability who competes as part of a member of a Paralympic sport club or at nationals does not equate to being a Paralympian. Athletes may also be a member of a national team, such as one that competes at world championships but not the Paralympics.

Classification. Athletes with disabilities are classified based on the sport they are competing in and the nature and level of their disability. Classification provides a structure for competition. Athletes competing in para sports have an impairment that leads to a competitive disadvantage in comparison to athletes without disabilities. Consequently, a system is in place to minimize the impact of impairments on sport performance and to ensure that the success of an athlete is determined by skill, fitness, power, endurance, tactical ability, and mental focus. This system is called classification. Since different sports require different abilities, each sport logically requires its own classification system.

Eligibility. The Paralympic Movement offers sport opportunities for athletes who have at least one of ten eligible impairments outlined by the IPC: impaired muscle power, impaired passive range of movement, limb deficiency, leg length difference, short stature, hypertonia, ataxia, athetosis, visual impairment, and intellectual impairment. The Paralympic Movement adopted the definitions for the eligible impairment types as

described in the World Health Organization International Classification of Functioning, Disability, and Health (ICF). Each Paralympic sport decides for which impairment groups they provide sporting opportunities in their classification rules. While some sports (such as athletics or swimming) include athletes of all impairment types, other sports, (such as goalball, a sport designed specifically for visually impaired athletes) are specific to one impairment type and still others (such as equestrian or cycling) are specific to a selection of impairment types.

Dilemmas, Debates, and Unresolved Questions

Doping. As with any elite sport, the integrity of Paralympic competition is maintained through doping control and organizations such as the U.S. Anti-Doping Agency (USADA) and World Anti-Doping Agency (WADA). There are a few unique elements to consider in Paralympic sport. The classification structure, briefly described above, and policies are constantly changing. Therefore, it is important to consider performance doping, whereby athletes may fake it in classification, such as downplaying their limitations to gain assignment to a different classification and potentially an advantage in competition. In Paralympic sport, mechanical doping is also an important phenomenon, whereby some types of equipment and technology that mediate participation could be deemed an unfair advantage (e.g., a type of prosthetic).

Media Representation. Paralympic athletes, particularly in the United States, are trying to earn more equitable media representation. Historically, the Paralympic Games get less airtime and viewership on network television in the United States, whereas other countries air footage constantly on public or private television stations. However, if the Paralympics are not on television and are not given similar media opportunities, then it makes it harder to generate ticket sales for the Paralympic Games and corporate interest for sponsorship to support televising.

Financial Support. Corporate sponsorship opportunities and backing of Paralympic athletes are not equitable with those of Olympic athletes. The monthly stipends (direct athlete support) and medal bonuses are not equitable in the United States either, making it challenging for Paralympians to be full-time athletes. For example, for the 2016 Rio Paralympic Games, U.S. Paralympians received only $5,000 from the USOC for winning gold. U.S. Olympians received $25,000 for their gold medals. In other countries, there is greater monetary support of Paralympians. Complicating matters further, even within the United States, there are differences in the direct athlete support funding based on the type of sport and governance structure.

The Integration Debate. There is some debate on whether or not the Paralympic Games should (or could) ever be integrated into the Olympic Games. Proponents of this idea put inclusion at the heart of the argument, believing that integration of elite athletes with disabilities with elite athletes without disabilities is fundamental. One of the arguments against integration is the enormous increase in size of the event. So far, events that have tried to integrate athletes with and without disabilities (such as the Commonwealth Games) have had to make major cuts to the schedule, thereby limiting available events to allow athletes to complete the competition in the available time.

Summary

- The Paralympic Games provide elite, high-level competition with rigorous competition standards for athletes with disabilities. The Paralympic Games are not the same as Special Olympics, and Paralympians are not the same as Special Olympians. Special Olympics provides sport opportunities targeted for children and adults with intellectual disabilities and encourages participation of all.
- Paralympians are athletes who have competed at the Paralympic Games representing their respective country. Paralympians are not the same as Olympians. Olympians are athletes who have competed at the Olympic Games. However, Paralympians train as hard as Olympians, and many are full-time athletes who make a living competing and obtaining sponsorship endorsements.
- Athlete classification in the Paralympic Movement is a key feature. Classification systems are unique to each para sport and perform two critical functions: (1) define who is eligible to compete in para sports, and (2) group athletes into sport classes. Classification aims to minimize the impact of impairment and allow for fair competition.
- The Paralympic Movement, bigger than just the games, has gained momentum and further reach to demonstrate the power and role sport plays in the promotion of disability rights, accessibility, inclusion, and health (Blauwet and Willick 2012; Forber-Pratt 2015).

Future of Paralympians and the Paralympics

The growth of the Paralympic Movement over the last several decades has allowed for an increase in the number of available sports, participating athletes, and media support. The United States traditionally has a strong presence at the Paralympic Games, in the number of both athletes and medals won, and this presence is expected to continue to grow with the continued support from sponsors and institutional resources. The overall growth of the Paralympic Movement has made the need for increased awareness and education about the Paralympics and Paralympians even more vital. In particular, there is an increased need for coaching development and for involvement and integration with school-based sport systems, which can serve as a direct pipeline for athlete identification and recruitment. Additionally, continued engagement with academic researchers and innovators to further the knowledge base of physiological, psychological, and social factors of Paralympic sport and the Paralympic Movement remains important for the continued success of technological and equipment advancements. Finally, the classification system remains a highly debated topic in Paralympic sport, and continued research needs to be conducted to further inform the classification process and protocols that work to maintain the integrity of sport.

Anjali Forber-Pratt and K. M. LeFevour

See also: Body Enhancement; Health and Fitness, Access to; Identity; *Primary Documents*: Table of the Medals Won in the Atlanta Paralympics (1996)

Further Reading

Blauwet, Cheri, and Stuart E. Willick. 2012. "The Paralympic Movement: Using Sports to Promote Health, Disability Rights, and Social Integration for Athletes with Disabilities." *PM&R* 4, no. 11: 851–856.

Brittain, Ian. 2012. *From Stoke Mandeville to Stratford: A History of the Summer Paralympic Games.* Champaign, IL: Common Ground Publishers.

Brittain, Ian, and Aaron Beacom. 2018. *The Palgrave Handbook of Paralympic Studies.* Basingstoke, UK: Palgrave Macmillan.

Forber-Pratt, Anjali. 2015. "Paralympic Sport as a Vehicle for Social Change in Bermuda and Ghana." *Journal of Sport for Development* 3, no. 5: 35–49.

International Paralympic Committee. 2016. "International Paralympic Committee." https://www.paralympic.org/.

Paraprofessionals

Paraprofessionals work in schools under the supervision of certified or licensed teachers. They support teaching and learning in many areas (e.g., instruction and education, employment, and independent living skills). They most often support students with disabilities. They may also support classrooms with high enrollment, intensive support needs, or an early-childhood emphasis.

What Is a Paraprofessional?

"Paraprofessional" is a title; paraprofessionals are people hired to assist teachers and students across instructional environments. They are most frequently used as supports for special educators and their students. They also support students in schools that implement multitiered programs, such as multitier system of supports (MTSS) or response to intervention (RTI) and Positive Behavioral Intervention & Supports (PBIS). Although their specific roles vary by district, school, teacher, and environment, they generally support students' access to quality instruction, environments, and experiences. If a student has more intensive needs related to behavior or independent functioning, the individualized education program (IEP) team may suggest the use of a one-on-one paraprofessional to provide additional support.

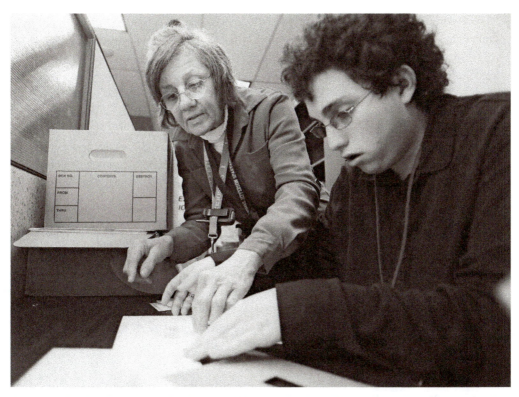

A paraprofessional works with a 2I-year-old high school student with autism. Paraprofessionals work primarily in schools and are most frequently utilized to support special educators and their students. (Helen H. Richardson/The Denver Post via Getty Images)

The use of paraprofessionals as supports for students with disabilities is not without controversy. Research has identified several concerns that need to be considered by stakeholders. These will be addressed in more detail in the following sections, along with iterance to the importance of the topic to disability studies.

The term "paraprofessional" refers to school employees in a school setting. Paraprofessionals are not synonymous with personal care attendants, home care assistants, and personal assistants in adult-living or independent living settings, nor are they school employees. Instead, they are the employees of people with disabilities (consumers) receiving the service or support to live self-directed lives. A similarity in the roles may occur in some types of tasks or funding.

Background/History

According to the Council for Exceptional Children, paraprofessionals have assisted special educators for over 50 years. In this section, research regarding paraprofessionals, including a comprehensive literature review, was compiled by the work of Zanton (2015), and it demonstrated (a) an increase in the use and need of paraprofessionals, (b) the changing role and tasks, (c) and varied expectations and qualifications. Specifically, over the past 30 years, the number of paraprofessionals supporting classroom education in U.S. schools has increased dramatically. Specifically, in 1986, approximately

150,000 paraprofessionals were employed nationwide; then in 2010, there were 1,233,400 paraprofessionals. By 2022, that number is expected to have risen by an additional 105,000 jobs. Paraprofessionals are employed in 91 percent of public schools. This number indicates a high likelihood of students' exposure to paraprofessionals.

Important Points to Know about the Topic

A Role Changes. Once primarily a clerical position that supported the teacher by performing noninstructional tasks (e.g., copying, collating), the role of the paraprofessional has become increasingly one of hands-on work with students. "Typical responsibilities are adapting materials, assisting with group activities, facilitating peer interactions, providing one-on-one instruction, participating on Individualized Education Program (IEP) implementing team member, other school team member, assisting with personal care, and providing behavioral supports" (Zanton 2015, 1).

Paraprofessionals increasingly serve as the primary instructors for students with disabilities (especially those with more significant disabilities); however, relying on paraprofessionals is quite controversial (Downing, Ryndak, and Clark 2000). Suter and Giangreco asserted that there is "no sound conceptual or theoretical rationale supporting the notion that students with disabilities should receive primary or extensive instruction from the least trained, lowest paid staff" (2009, 82). Some researchers question whether, even with ongoing training, paraprofessionals can provide a free appropriate public education, as mandated by the Individuals with Disabilities Education Act. In the area of academics, typically yet not systematically, paraprofessionals are specified to be used to provide maintenance instruction on already acquired skills so that the student can practice and become fluent in the skill to mastery. However, the research findings vary on paraprofessionals as purely for maintenance of skills.

Federal Criteria. Each state must follow federal criteria for paraprofessionals under the No Child Left Behind Act (NCLB 2002) and the Every Student Succeeds Act (ESSA 2016): "Specifically, each State and its LEAs must continue to ensure that each paraprofessional . . . has a secondary school diploma or its recognized equivalent and has completed at least two years of study at an institution of higher education, obtained an associate's or higher degree, or met a rigorous standard of quality and can demonstrate, through a formal State or local academic assessment, knowledge of, and the ability to assist in instructing, reading, writing, and mathematics" (U.S. Department of Education 2016, 21).

Paraprofessionals as Catalysts of Inclusive Practices. Paraprofessionals are particularly common in various special education services. Many stakeholders (e.g., teachers, parents, and administrators) view inclusion as more manageable or acceptable with a paraprofessional (Zanton 2015). The assumption may be that paraprofessionals are likely to know and use a continuum of supports, starting with natural supports, as a catalyst for inclusive practices. Even if a paraprofessional has obtained a teaching degree, if employed as a paraprofessional, that individual is expected to comply with the standards and their duties, not the duties of a hired certified or licensed educator.

Dilemmas, Debates, and Unresolved Questions

Training. Given this level of instructional responsibility, paraprofessional training should naturally be a high priority for school districts; however, it is often ineffective, inadequate, and at times nonexistent. This lack of quality leaves paraprofessionals unprepared and often reliant on observation, on-the-job experience, and self-instruction to learn the key skills needed in classroom settings (Downing, Ryndak, and Clark 2000). Without proper training, paraprofessionals may not know appropriate strategies to support children's intellectual, behavioral, social-emotional, and motor development. Paraprofessionals themselves have reported receiving insufficient training.

Dependency versus Self-Determination. According to the deficit model of disability, our society often views people with disabilities as helpless or less than their peers without disabilities because they may need additional support in daily activities (Stolz 2010). Hence, paraprofessionals often serve to closely supervise and assist students with disabilities in school environments and, later, in vocational and community settings. Concerns have been raised over the informal practice of *hovering*, in which staff provide too much or unnecessarily intensive supports rather than encouraging independence and using natural supports. Hovering inhibits learning and social opportunities, increases the likelihood of dependency on adult support, and reinforces conceptualizations of students with disabilities as deficient and thus as requiring an adult.

Adults with disabilities who rely on the support of others are less likely to live in the community, be employed, and have social opportunities with friends, and as children, those who require high levels of adult support remain dependent on others if they are not systematically taught otherwise (Zanton 2015). Paraprofessionals are rarely taught to use systematic instructional procedures,

including cueing responses, allowing sufficient response time before intervening, using individualized prompting levels, and correcting errors. These procedures are essential for promoting independence, which is the primary educational focus for many children with intellectual disabilities. Given the importance of independence skills, it is crucial for paraprofessionals to receive sufficient training.

It is important that those with disabilities be included in the discussion of paraprofessional support. Obstacles, areas for improvement, gaps, and successes are often learned from student voices. In a 2007 study by Broer, Doyle, and Giangreco, former students felt protected by paraprofessionals from bullying but also felt that they were not important enough for the teacher's attention. Other potential negative impacts include reinforcing the deficit model approaches, isolating students with disabilities from teachers and peers, and providing possibly inadequate instruction.

The Future of Paraprofessionals and Conclusions

Paraprofessionals have become an integral part of the special education team and of some general education settings. The concerns discussed previously should continue to be studied, particularly as the need is projected to increase dramatically. For example, research has shown that paraprofessionals can benefit from training focused specifically on the skills used with their students (Zanton 2015). Paraprofessionals can learn instructional and behavioral strategies that facilitate skill development and self-determination. Such training may be an appropriate practical focus for teachers and administrators while researchers continue to study new possibilities.

Jessica Zanton

See also: Every Student Succeeds Act (ESSA); Free Appropriate Public Education; Natural Supports; Schoolwide Systems of Supports; Self-Determination in Education; Special Education

Further Reading

Broer, Stephen, Mary Beth Doyle, and Michael Giangreco. 2007. "Perspectives of Students with Intellectual Disabilities about their Experiences with Paraprofessional Support." http://www.advocacyinstitute.org/advocacyinaction/Student_Perspectives_Paraprofessionals.shtml.

Downing, June E., Diane L. Ryndak, and Denise Clark. 2000. "Paraeducators in Inclusive Classrooms: Their Own Perspectives." *Rural Special Education Quarterly* 26, no. 3: 3–15.

National Center on Educational Statistics. "Description and Employment Criteria of Instructional Paraprofessionals." https://nces.ed.gov/pubsearch/pubsinfo.asp?pubid=2007008.

Stolz, Suzanne. 2010. "Disability Trajectories: Disabled Youths' Identity Development, Negotiation of Experience and Expectation, and Sense of Agency during Transition." Unpublished doctoral dissertation. San Diego: University of California San Diego.

Suter, Jesse C., and Michael F. Giangreco. 2009. "Numbers That Count: Exploring Special Education and Paraprofessional Service Delivery in Inclusion-Oriented Schools." *Journal of Special Education* 43, no. 2: 81–93.

U.S. Department of Education. 2016. "Transitioning to the Every Student Succeeds Act (ESSA)." https://www2.ed.gov/policy/elsec/leg/essa/essafaqstransition62916.pdf.

Zanton, Jessica. 2015. *Evaluating the Effect of a Staff Training Package for Paraprofessionals to Teach Communicative Behavior to Students with Special Needs.* Unpublished doctoral dissertation. Urbana: University of Illinois.

Performance of Everyday Life. See Disability and the Performance of Everyday Life

Personal Care Attendant Services

Personal care attendant (PCA) services provide individuals with the chance to live and work independently, allowing them the chance to be a part of their community. Living and working independently means that the individual has choice and control. For many people with disabilities, their attendants can be an extension of themselves. This is true given all the tasks that a personal care attendant is responsible for. In 2000, the World Institute on Disability (2000, 18–19) created a list of the six components that PCA services entail. These components are as follows:

1. Attendant services that encompass personal services, paramedic services, and household tasks
2. Communication services
3. Cognitive and emotional support services
4. Management of services
5. Transportation services
6. Work-related services

The job of a personal care attendant is that not only of an assistant but also of a nurse, housekeeper, chauffeur, etc. Therefore, these services are invaluable to people who need them. In this entry, you will learn a brief background of PCA services, some limitations or restrictions that make it difficult for people to receive these services, and some pieces of legislation that set out to rectify these issues.

Background and History

Until the latter half of the 20th century, people in need of personal care services in the United States relied solely upon family, friends, and institutions to get their needs met. In the 1950s, PCA programs were created by Rancho Los Amigos Hospital in Los Angeles, California, and the National Foundation for Infantile Paralysis (March of Dimes), who established their respective programs as a more cost-effective way to assist polio survivors (Glazier 2001). However, by 1960, these programs ceased to exist. It was not until 1981 that the home and community-based services (HCBS) waiver authority was established (Smith et al. 2000). The HCBS waiver authority allowed states for the first time to provide services within the home in order to meet the needs of people with disabilities.

Optional State Programs

Medicaid, which is the primary funding source for most government-funded PCA programs, is a state and federally funded program. The only home and community-based program that the state is required to fund is Home-Health (Grossman et al. 2007). This program does not meet the needs of many people with disabilities. The two programs serving those with more extensive needs are optional for states.

One optional program, the *State Plan*, offers less flexibility when it comes to service packages and income criteria, but functional, or level of need, eligibility is less restrictive (LeBlanc, Tonner, and Harrington 2001). Financial and need criteria for services provided under the optional State Plan are determined using each state's

standards and left to the discretion of each state (LeBlanc, Tonner, and Harrington 2001).

HCBS waiver programs, on the other hand, offer a wider range of services. However, under HCBS waivers, states do not have to include all categories of people with disabilities or medically needy individuals; financial criteria must meet federal standards; and there must be a limit set by each state on the number of people served (LeBlanc, Tonner, and Harrington 2001). In many states, there are waiting lists for HCBS services. In 2011, average waiting lists for HCBS services were more than two years long, and waiting lists had increased by 19 percent from the previous year (Ng et al. 2014).

In 2009, HCBS services under both State Plans and HCBS waiver programs composed 45 percent of Medicaid spending on long-term care, and funding increased from $17 billion in 1999 to $52 billion in 2009 (Ng et al. 2014). The expansion of Medicaid HCBS services has promoted the prevalence of people with disabilities living in the community. Having an increased number of people with disabilities living in the community is a step in the right direction, though many people still do not get the services they need. In 2010, 10.9 million people needed services, and 1.8 million people resided in nursing homes (Ng et al. 2014) because they could not get the services that they needed in order to reside in the community. As such, family and friends are still primary and vital sources of care and assistance for people with disabilities. For instance, 92 percent of people with disabilities living in the community receive some form of unpaid help (Kaye, Harrington, and LaPlante 2010).

Each state has different eligibility criteria for receiving Medicaid benefits.

Additionally, each state provides different levels of services. For example, Louisiana has a supportive independent program that provides 24-hour PCA services, in the home as well as out in the community, to people with disabilities (Louisiana Department of Health and Hospitals 2011), although this program has had some major budget cuts and has an estimated 14-year waiting list. On the other hand, Illinois's program does not provide such an extensive amount of services.

Eligibility Criteria

Along with the differences in the amount and types of services being provided among states, there are also criteria that must be met in order to qualify for government-funded PCA programs. Two of the major criteria are disability and income. Although every state claims to serve a variety of disabilities, few programs provide services for visual, hearing, and cognitive impairments. One must also provide some form of documentation that gives a detailed description of the person's functional limitations. These limitations are then rated through an assessment process (World Institute on Disability 2000). However, because assessments often are not individualized to a given person, one's needs may be left out of the assessment. Since these assessments are not individualized, the individual's needs often get left in the hands of those in power (such as medical professionals or family members). The assessment of disability and the scope of disabilities that are actually provided for, therefore, leave many people with disabilities dependent and isolated.

Income is another factor in determining eligibility that leaves people with disabilities who are in need of PCA services dependent and isolated. Half of the U.S. PCA programs limit eligibility to people whose incomes fall well below the poverty level (World Institute on Disability 2000). For example, in Louisiana, to qualify for services one must qualify for Medicaid. In order to qualify for Medicaid, one cannot make more than three times Social Security Income (SSI) before taxes are taken into account (Louisiana Department of Health and Hospitals 2011). Current SSI is $733 per month; therefore, three times that amount would be $2,199 before taxes. However, if a person requires an extensive amount of services in order to complete activities of daily living, this amount would not even begin to cover the needed care. There are only a few state programs that actually encourage employment. For example, Ohio allows an individual to earn up to 600 percent of the federal poverty level (Ohio Rehabilitation Services Commission 2011). As of January 2012, the federal income poverty level is $11,770 (Medicaid 2015). The income criteria in most states trap those in need of care in a state of dependency where they must continue to rely upon public benefits.

This dependency is a far cry from what PCA services are meant to achieve, which is independence. Not only do income restrictions impose penalties on individual employment, but there are also penalties put on those who choose to get married. "Marriage penalties" occur when a service user's spouse's income is counted toward determining eligibility for services. For example, an individual can have up to $2,000 in resources per month, whereas a married couple can only have $3,000 (New Opportunities Fact Sheet 2011). Therefore, many people have to choose between opting out of marriage in order to get the care that they need and having to often go without services, leaving them dependent on their spouse or family for personal care support.

Model Comparison

According to the World Institute on Disability (2000), there are three models guiding PCA services: the medical model (provider direction), family model (family direction), and independent living model (user direction). Under the medical model, the individual's needs and wants are assessed by a medical professional and controlled through a provider agency, whereas, in the family model, the consumer's needs and wants are directed by a family member. In both cases, those in need of care have little or no control when it comes to the management and direction of their own care. However, the independent living model puts users in control of directing and managing their own services. Recent studies have shown that access to and control over their own care has a positive impact on those in need of services (Clark, Hagglund, and Sherman 2008; Jurkowski, Jovanovic, and Rowitz 2002). However, for many people with disabilities, being in control of their own care is not an option. For instance, among PCA services consumers living in the community, 79 percent use volunteer or unpaid personal assistance by family or friends (World Institute on Disability 2000). In order to change PCA services on the basis of a medical or a family model that leaves those with disabilities dependent, we must view these services in an independent living and social justice model that views all people as interdependent on one another, puts people who need care in control, and treats all people with dignity.

Legislation

The landmark court case *Olmstead vs. L. C.* (1999), involved two women with developmental disabilities in Georgia who remained institutionalized after medical professionals recommended home and community-based services. As a result, states are now mandated to ensure that people with disabilities are in the most integrated setting, and each state must have a comprehensive plan for providing care within the community setting (Center for an Accessible Society 2012). Following this case, two pieces of legislation have been brought before Congress that would have helped to make home and community-based services a requirement in every state. Those pieces of legislation are the Medicaid Community Attendant Services and Supports Act and the Community Choice Act. Both pieces of legislation would require that funds be allocated to PCA programs (Center for an Accessible Society 2012). These acts would also create a national program of home and community-based services (ADAPT 2012). The Community Choice Act would also allow services regardless of age or disability and would also have an option to serve individuals with incomes above the current institutional income limitation in order to promote employment (ADAPT 2012). Although these acts have been presented to Congress numerous times, they have yet to be passed (Center for an Accessible Society 2012; ADAPT 2012).

Conclusions

In the United States, PCA services have come a long way from their early beginnings in the 1950s. Yet, there is still a long way to go. The first step in this process would be to have a national policy across states making PCA services a requirement and not just an option, as proposed by the Medicaid Community Attendants and Supports Act (Center for an Accessible Society 2012). Along with a national policy, income limits need to be raised or a sliding scale based on income needs to be implemented in order for the United States to live up to its goal to "assure equality of opportunity, full participation, independent living, and economic self-sufficiency" (Kittay 2011, 50). To achieve these goals, there should be a deliberate move away from the medical model and the "sick role," toward a social justice model of interdependence and dignity for all when it comes to care.

Ashley Volion

See also: Caregivers and Care Recipients; Direct Service Workforce; Ethics of Care; Medicaid

Further Reading

ADAPT. 2012. "Community Choice Act." http://www.adapt.org/cca.

Center for an Accessible Society. 2012. "MiCassa." http://www.accessiblesociety.org/topics/persasst/micassa01.htm.

Clark, Mary J., Kristofer J. Hagglund, and Ashley K. Sherman. 2008. "A Longitudinal Comparison of Consumer-Directed and Agency-Directed Personal Assistance Service Programmes among Persons with Physical Disabilities." *Disability and Rehabilitation* 30, no. 9: 689–695.

Glazier, Raymond. 2001. "The 'Re-Invention' of Personal Assistance Services." *Disability Studies Quarterly* 21, no. 2.

Grossman, Brian R., Martin Kitchener, Joseph T. Mullan, and Charlene Harrington. 2007. "Paid Personal Assistance Services: An Exploratory Study of Working Age Consumers' Perspectives." *Journal of Aging & Social Policy* 19, no. 3: 27–45.

Jurkowski, Elaine, Borko Jovanovic, and Louis Rowitz. 2002. "Leadership/Citizen Participation: Perceived Impact of Advocacy Activities by People with Physical Disabilities on Access to Health Care, Attendant Care and Social Services." *Journal of Health & Social Policy* 14, no. 4: 49–61.

Kaye, H. Stephen, Charlene Harrington, and Mitchell LaPlante. 2010. "Long-Term Care: Who Gets It, Who Provides It, and How Much?" *Health Affairs* 29, no. 1: 11–21.

Kittay, Eva F. 2011. "The Ethics of Care, Dependency, and Disability." *Ratio Juris* 28, no. 1: 49–58.

LaCAN. 2014. "End the Wait and Fill the Slots. http://www.laddc.org/files/Waiver FactSheet102213.pdf.

LeBlanc, Allen, M. Christine Tonner, and Charlene Harrington. 2001. "State Programs Offering Personal Care Services." *Health Care Financing Review* 22, no. 4: 155–171.

Legal Information Institute. 1999. "Olmstead v. L.C." http://www.law.cornell.edu/supct/html/98-536.ZO.html.

Louisiana Department of Health and Hospitals. 2011. "Department of Health and Hospitals Office for Citizens with Developmental Disabilities (OCDD) Waiver Supports and Services." http://new.dhh.louisiana.gov/assets/docs/OCDD/waiver/NOW/NOW_FactSheet-2011.pdf.

New Opportunities Fact Sheet. 2011. U.S. Equal Employment Opportunity Commission. https://www.eeoc.gov/laws/regulations/adaaa_fact_sheet.cfm.

Ng, Terence, Charlene Harrington, Mary-Beth Musumeci, and Erica Reaves. 2014. "Medicaid Home and Community-Based Services Programs: 2010 Data Update." Kaiser Family Foundation. http://kff.org/medicaid/report/medicaid-home-and-community-basedservice-programs/.

Ohio Rehabilitation Services Commission. 2011. Opportunities for Ohioans with Disabilities Personal Care Assistance Program. http://ood.ohio.gov/Portals/0/RSC-4007%20FINANCIAL%20STATEMENT.pdf.

Smith, Gary, Janet O'Keeffe, Letty Carpenter, Pamela Doty, Gavin Kennedy, Brian Burwell, and Loretta Williams. 2000. "Understanding Medicaid Home and Community Services: A Primer." U.S. Department of Health and Human Services.

http://aspe.hhs.gov/daltcp/reports/primer.htm.

World Institute on Disability. 2000. "PAS Fundamentals History, Structure, Utilization and Adequacy of Existing PAS Systems." http://wid.org/publications/downloads/PAS%20Fundamentals.pdf.

Physical Therapy

Physical therapists are health care professionals with extensive training in human anatomy and physiology, movement science, pathology, and therapeutic modalities, including exercise and functional task training. Physical therapy is just one specialty within the broader field of rehabilitation medicine, which focuses on improving *health-related quality of life* for individuals across the lifespan (American Physical Therapy Association 2016). People seek out, or are referred to, physical therapists for many different reasons, some of which include acute or chronic musculoskeletal injury, new-onset neurological conditions (such as stroke or spinal cord injury), or impairments that are present at birth (such as cerebral palsy or spina bifida). There is a complex relationship between disability and physical therapy. This might seem surprising, considering that one of the primary roles of a physical therapist is to assist persons who have been injured, have had an illness, or have a disability, in augmenting or improving aspects of their physical performance and everyday function (American Physical Therapy Association 2016).

What Is Physical Therapy?

Physical therapy treatment can take place in the home, a hospital, an outpatient clinic, or a school, and treatment is *individualized* to address the concerns and goals of the people, their family, and often their medical team. For one person, physical therapy might consist of wheelchair mobility skills and assistive technology training, while for another it might focus on postural exercises and breathing strategies for pain relief, and for another still, it might focus on high-intensity strengthening to return to a sport. Regardless of mode, physical therapy aims to maximize function in whatever way is most meaningful for the person receiving services.

Background and History

The profession of physical therapy, as a sector of the larger rehabilitation industry, has its roots within governmental and charitable programs that were established following the return home of disabled veterans from World War I and II (Albrecht 1992). While initial goals focused on reintegration of veterans back into the workforce, growth into a multidisciplinary sector of overall health care provision resulted. This growth focused on preventive or restorative treatment interventions to improve function to the greatest extent possible, either through remediation or compensation. This period was also a major turning point in the early recognition of the rights of disabled people to access service programs and *assistive technology* (Albrecht 1992).

The Medical Model View. The field of rehabilitation historically has been influenced by a *medical model* view of disability, whereby disability is defined as an undesirable deficit residing in an individual and intervention is recommended to remediate or normalize such deficit as best as possible (Kielhofner 2005). Although there have been challenges to this view of disability from within the field, resulting in a slow philosophical shift within some professional

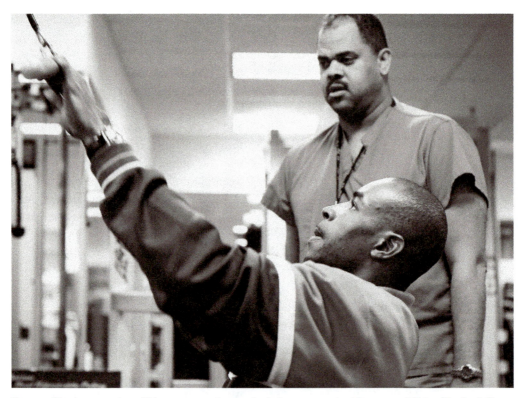

Eugene Simpson, an Iraq War veteran, in physical therapy at the Veterans Affairs Medical Center in Washington, D.C. Physical therapists receive extensive training in human anatomy but are also educated to recognize and address other complex social factors that impact rehabilitation services. (Jeff Hutchens/Getty Images)

circles, evidence of the medical model perspective remains pervasive in physical therapy practice (Gibson et al. 2009). For example, wording in the American Physical Therapy Association's (2016) *Guide to Physical Therapist Practice* notes that one of the primary roles of the physical therapist is to "prevent the onset, symptoms, and progression of impairments, functional limitations, and disabilities that may result from diseases, disorders, conditions, or injuries." Other scholars have pushed for a shift in the profession, away from "disability prevention" toward the promotion of health, wellness, and participation for disabled people (Rimmer 1999).

The ICF Model View. Physical therapy practice, as with most professional practices

within the broader rehabilitation field in the United States, uses the World Health Organization's International Classification of Functioning, Disability, and Health (ICF) as a model to categorize various domains of health and function that have an overall impact on an individual's participation in meaningful life activities. Physical therapists often use the ICF model as a framework to identify areas of strength and limitation in an individual's daily function and to structure treatment interventions in those areas to maximize function and improve participation.

The ICF model is a biopsychosocial framework, which includes domains of (1) body structures/functions; (2) activities/activity restrictions; (3) participation/

participation restrictions; (4) personal factors; and (5) environmental factors as intersecting components of a person's health experiences (Imrie 2004). These domains are not linear or meant to imply causal relationships. However, each domain can influence, or be influenced by, each other domain as it may relate to meaningful aspects of a person's life, such as employment, community life, and education. The ICF model was adopted in part as a result of criticisms from disability communities that previous health models had reduced the concept of disability to focus only on medical conceptualizations, highlighting individual physical or intellectual limitations rather than social or environmental causes of disability. Many people believe the ICF represents a more holistic view of health and disability that considers social and environmental contexts in research, practice, and policy making; however, ongoing discussions of the meanings and utilizations of the ICF model mimic historical criticisms of its focus and meaning for disabled people (Imrie 2004).

Benefits of Physical Therapy

Physical therapy has been shown in scientific research to significantly improve function and participation persons who have experienced an illness or injury or who have lifelong or new-onset impairments. Participants in physical therapy research have reported significant improvements in pain, functional mobility with and without assistive devices or technology, and participation in instrumental activities of daily living as well as recreational and social activities (Magasi 2008). Most physical therapy research is conducted in the positivist research tradition, which utilizes scientific inquiry to quantify outcomes, often using standardized tests, measures, and evaluation tools that are overwhelmingly focused on the body structures/function domain and the activity/activity limitation domain of the ICF. In practice, translation of research findings facilitates a primary focus on treatments to and for the body or adaptations or compensations meant to remediate impairment (Gibson et al. 2009).

Dilemmas, Debates, and Unresolved Questions

Internalized Ableism. Despite the benefits that may be associated with physical therapy treatment, there remain significant dilemmas and debates surrounding the mechanisms of physical therapy practice, and the underlying implications these practices have for disabled people. In fact, the field of disability studies has been steadfast in its criticism of medicine and rehabilitation in general. Although scholars recognize the "well-intentioned" application of therapeutic interventions by rehabilitation professionals, they contend that there are several unintended consequences of remediating impairment, in that disabled people may internalize messages that disability and impairment are inherently negative, thus devaluing their bodies and identities as tragic or "less-than" (Abberley 1995). Further, scholars in disability studies suggest that rehabilitation focuses solely on the individual, while negating the social, environmental, and economic factors that contribute to disability.

Impact of Normalization. The field of disability studies notes that another consequence of rehabilitation, resulting from the dominance of the medical model viewpoint, lies in the assumption that impairments are deficits that should be "fixed" or "normalized," which assumes that a comparatively normalized state is more desirable than a disabled one. Scholars argue that this view has the potential to undermine the self-worth of an individual and the disability pride and culture within a community. A second consequence that arises from medical model thinking is the assumption that rehabilitation professionals are experts because of their training, rather than disabled people being experts in their own lives and disabilities. Despite a trend toward *person-centered* care, where individuals collaborate with their health care providers to codirect their treatments and medically related decision making, the rehabilitation processes, and the balance of decision-making power, still reside with rehabilitation professionals (Magasi 2008).

Bodily Impairment and Experience. Disability studies scholarship has offered alternative models in conceptualizing disability. The social model, for example, claims that, while bodily impairment exists, it is a value-neutral way of being in the world and that disability is a constructed phenomenon—a combination of social, political, and environmental barriers—resulting in the persistent oppression of people with impairments. However, critiques of this model have recognized that for many disabled people, bodily experiences of impairment do matter and are as important in defining disability as the social and environmental discriminations faced. If both bodily experiences of impairment and social discriminations are legitimate and important in a person's experience of disability, then there is a likely place for such rehabilitative services as physical therapy in the lives of disabled people, but only if enacted on their own terms.

The Future of Disability and Physical Therapy

Physical therapy intervention may greatly assist in alleviating pain, restoring or maintaining functional mobility, or enhancing a person's accessibility to different environments. As a result, it can actually play a role in helping to prevent marginalization, empowering individuals in their health care decision making, and enhancing social participation (Ripat and Woodgate 2011). However, given the complex history of how physical therapy practice has been conceptualized and actualized, what might this shift look like? What strategies can physical therapists and other rehabilitation professionals use in responding to critiques from within disability studies?

One possible solution is for physical therapy education curriculums to elevate their practices to incorporate multiple understandings of disability or to incorporate more disabled people into the professional fold, as instructors or students. Another possible future direction is to explore how clinical practice can shift toward incorporating a greater emphasis on the domains of the ICF that pertain to participation, personal factors, and environmental factors. Further, physical therapists have an opportunity to explore advocacy and policy work that deals with inaccessible spaces in the built environment and the promotion of user-centered design, as well as to combat discrimination in its many forms. Finally, physical therapists must reexamine professional power relationships and embrace disabled people's expertise in their own lives and abilities to be the primary decision makers in their own health care needs and goals.

Heather Feldner

See also: Disability Studies; International Classification of Functioning, Disability, and Health (ICF); Therapeutic Recreation; Therapist, Role in Activities of Daily Living (ADLs)

Further Reading

Abberley, Paul. 1995. "Disabling Ideology in Health and Welfare: The Case of

Occupational Therapy." *Disability & Society* 10, no. 2: 221–232.

Albrecht, Gary L. 1992. *The Disability Business: Rehabilitation in America*. Newbury Park, CA: Sage Publications.

American Physical Therapy Association. 2016. "Role of a Physical Therapist." http://www.apta.org/PTCareers/RoleofaPT/.

Gibson, Barbara E., Johanna Darrah, Deb Cameron, Goli Hashemi, Shauna Kingsnorth, Céline Lepage, Rose Martini, Angela Mandich, and Dolly Menna-Dack. 2009. "Revisiting Therapy Assumptions in Children's Rehabilitation: Clinical and Research Implications." *Disability and Rehabilitation* 31, no. 17: 1446–1453.

Imrie, Rob. 2004. "Demystifying Disability: A Review of the International Classification of Functioning, Disability and Health." *Sociology of Health & Illness* 26, no. 3: 287–305.

Kielhofner, Gary. 2005. "Rethinking Disability and What to Do about It: Disability Studies and Its Implications for Occupational Therapy." *American Journal of Occupational Therapy* 59, no. 5: 487–496.

Magasi, Susan. 2008. "Infusing Disability Studies into the Rehabilitation Sciences." *Topics in Stroke Rehabilitation* 15, no. 3: 283–287.

Rimmer, James H. 1999. "Health Promotion for People with Disabilities: The Emerging Paradigm Shift from Disability Prevention to Prevention of Secondary Conditions." *Physical Therapy* 79, no. 5: 495–502.

Ripat, Jacquie D., and Roberta L. Woodgate. 2011. "Locating Assistive Technology within an Emancipatory Disability Research Framework." *Technology and Disability* 23, no. 2: 87–92.

Poetry

"Disability poetry" refers to poems that spring from the lived experience of moving through the world with a disability. While not limited in subject matter to disability in any of its facets, disability poetry often seeks to explore and validate the lives and perceptions of disabled people in an ableist world.

What Is Disability Poetry?

Sometimes referred to as crip poetry, disability poetry is informed by and contributes to disability culture. Disability poetry recognizes and rejects the ableism that permeates contemporary culture. Like the rest of the disability arts movement, crip poetry repudiates views of disability as a shameful, pitiable, tragic, and individual phenomenon. This viewpoint is not a denial of the pain and functional limitations that may come with impairment; in fact, disability poetry is often informed by a heightened awareness of those aspects of impairment. But crip poetry is also sharply aware that a major part of the impact disabilities have on lives results from the ways those human differences are interpreted culturally and responded to by society, so often with prejudice, marginalization, and discrimination. Lynn Manning's poem "The Magic Wand" explicitly addresses this point by describing the transformation the persona undergoes, from black man to blind man, through the simple act of unfolding his white cane.

The Magic Wand
by Lynn Manning

Quick-change artist extraordinaire,
I whip out my folded cane
and change from black man to blind man
with a flick of my wrist.
It is a profound metamorphosis—
From God gifted wizard of roundball
dominating backboards across America,
To God-gifted idiot savant

pounding out chart-busters on a cock-
eyed whim;
From sociopathic gang-banger with
death for eyes
To all seeing soul with saintly spirit;
From rape deranged misogynist
to poor motherless child;
From welfare-rich pimp
to disability-rich gimp;
And from 'White man's burden'
to every man's burden.

It is always a profound metamorphosis.
Whether from cursed by man to
cursed by God
or from scripture condemned to God
ordained,
my final form is never of my choosing.
I only wield the wand;
You are the magician.

Manning's poem displays several characteristics common to crip poetry: a challenge
to stereotypes and an insistence on self-
definition; foregrounding of the perspective
of people with disabilities; an emphasis on
embodiment, especially atypical embodiment; and alternative techniques and poetics.

It is important to note that the range of
human circumstances that today we call *disability* has been part of human experience
since there have been humans. Since the earliest days, the verbal art of poetry has been created by those who today would be considered
disabled, among other people. Too, since disability has been part of the human experience
from the beginnings of the species, disability
has been a topic of poetry since early on.

But whether famous poems of the past
could be considered disability poetry is
open to debate. The description of disability
poetry, with its emphasis on disability culture and a rejection of ableism, might seem
to be limited to poems from the latter part of
the 20th century on. For example, whether
John Milton's "On His Blindness," a poem
from the 17th century, could be considered
disability poetry is a rich question to explore.

One of the major impulses of crip poetry
is to resist stereotyping and the limits of
the socially imposed handicapped identity
through an insistence on defining oneself.
Disability poetry often explicitly rejects social
pressure to pursue a forever-elusive normality
and instead finds value and strength within
disability experience, not *in spite of* impairments but *because of* and *through* them. This
is portrayed in Cheryl Marie Wade's "I Am
Not One of The," in which the persona force-
fully rejects the labels that are applied to her.

I Am Not One of The
by Cheryl Marie Wade

I am not one of the physically
challenged—

I'm a sock in the eye with gnarled fist
I'm a French kiss with cleft tongue
I'm orthopedic shoes sewn on a last of
your fears

I am not one of the differently abled—

I'm an epitaph for million imperfect
babies left untreated
I'm an ikon carved from ones in a
mass grave at Tiergarten, Germany
I'm withered legs hidden with a
blanket

I am not one of the able disabled—

I'm a black panther with green eyes
and scars like a picket fence
I'm pink lace panties teasing a stub of
milk white thigh
I'm the Evil Eye

I'm the first cell divided
I'm mud that talks
I'm Eve I'm Kali
I'm The Mountain That Never Moves
I've been forever I'll be here forever
I'm the Gimp
I'm the Cripple
I'm the Crazy Lady

I'm The Woman With Juice

Credit: "I Am Not One of The," Cheryl Marie Wade Papers, Bancroft Manuscripts Number 2017/262, Carton 2, The Bancroft Library, University of California, Berkeley.

The speaker of this poem rejects the euphemistic labels applied to her by a world that would prefer to not discuss disability and rather to simply stereotype her. Instead, she articulates an identity for herself. She claims a kinship with disabled people through history, including those hidden away, left to die, even executed for their disabilities. Each time she rejects the euphemism, she replaces it with images that confound common expectations for people with disabilities—images of strength, of action, of sexual attraction and pleasure. The poem situates people with disabilities not in the margins but in the center of human experience ("I'm the first cell divided . . . I've been forever I'll be here forever"). By the end of the poem, she has claimed negative terminology ("gimp," "cripple," "crazy") for her own, transforming the terms with the final, triumphant assertion: "I'm the Woman with Juice."

Important Points to Understand about Disability Poetry

Disability has typically been described by nondisabled people. Another characteristic of disability poetry is that not only is it situated within the lived experience of disabled people but it specifically comes from the perspective of people whose bodies and minds have been deemed abnormal. Whether from wheelchair height or through impaired eyes or ears, crip poetry foregrounds an alternative perspective. Sometimes that alternative perspective is specifically addressed in the poem, as in "Harvest" by Stephen Kuusisto, when the speaker seeks to "admire the white moon of the morning, / even if my eyes tell me there are two moons."

Embodiment. Embodiment is another characteristic of disability poetry. Crip poetry demonstrates a powerful awareness of and sensitivity to nonstandard bodies. With its attention to alternative ways of being in the world, crip poetry seeks to redefine what it means to have and be a body in the world.

In Mark O'Brien's poem "The Man in the Iron Lung," the speaker describes his dream life in "the body electric" that inserts itself in "the map of my body." As it whooshes beautiful lies of invulnerability, it forces its way not just into his lungs but into his sense of who he is. Eli Clare describes a far different anomalous embodiment in "Learning to Speak": "I practiced the sounds *th, sh, sl* / for years, a pianist playing endless / hours of scales. I had to learn / the muscle of my tongue."

Because of this emphasis on exploding the limits of acceptable bodies in the world, embodying poems through performance is an important part of disability poetry. Disability is centrally about bodies, how they look and act, and how they are construed, so this embodiment is a crucial strategy. People with disabilities are often told to disregard their flawed, unsatisfactory bodies; paying the attention that poems evoke and reward is a powerful antidote, one that is intensified and multiplied through performance. And, as with other disability arts, events that include the performance of crip poetry are an important site for the continuing development of disability culture.

Alternative Poetics. Alternative poetics can be found in disability poetry as well. Anomalous ways of moving through the world can lead to formal differences in poems; for example, using a respirator to breathe has significant potential to influence rhythms and use of the line. Cerebral palsy had a significant impact on the poetry of Larry Eigner, including on the length of his poems—it was difficult for him to put a new piece of paper in his typewriter—and his distinctive use of space on the page. It is important to note that alternative embodiment, cognition, and rationality do not guarantee alternative poetics, but anomalous ways of encountering the world seem likely to influence a disabled writer's poetry.

Conclusion

Since the disability movements going back to the early 20th century have sought full access and equal opportunity for people with disabilities, a prominent question for disability poetry is how to integrate disability insights into a poetry that is about more than the experience of disability in an ableist world. People with disabilities are far more than merely carriers of that difference; their poetry should find ways to focus on the particular while reaching for the stars. A second direction for disability poetry may be to engage more profoundly with poetry that emerges with other minority experiences. The oppression that disabled people experience is not separate from the oppression that members of other minority groups experience; these related experiences can help to drive a poetry that not only reflects but contributes to a more inclusive world.

Disability poetry springs from the lived experience of moving through the world with a disability, but the poetry continues to evolve, reflecting not only those experiences but also the imaginations of poets with a wide variety of ways of moving through the world.

Jim Ferris

See also: Contemporary Art; Crip and Crip Culture; Disability and Performance in Everyday Life; Embodiment; Fine Arts; Life Writing; *Primary Documents*: Cheryl Marie Wade's "Disability Culture Rap" (1994); Laura Hershey's Poem "You Get Proud by Practicing"

Further Reading

Bartlett, Jennifer, Sheila Black, and Michael Northen. 2011. *Beauty Is a Verb: The New Poetry of Disability*. El Paso, TX: Cinco Puntos.

Fries, Kenny. 1997. *Staring Back: The Disability Experience from the Inside Out*. New York: Plume.

Wordgathering: An Online Journal of Disability Poetry and Literature. 2017. "Index." http://www.wordgathering.com/index.html.

Poverty

Poverty and disability are linked in many ways, with the result being that Americans with disabilities are more likely to be living in poverty compared to persons without disabilities, regardless of the definition of poverty being used.

Channels Linking Disability and Income Poverty

Using a traditional definition of poverty as "low income," poverty is linked to disability in many and complex ways. First, there could be factors, such as violence, that independently lead to both disability and poverty. It is more commonly noted that disability and poverty reinforce each other as part of a vicious cycle known as the "cycle of poverty."

Linking Poverty to Disability and Disability to Poverty

Poverty may lead to disability through hunger and malnutrition, a lack of access to health care, or poor living conditions. For instance, malnutrition in infants and young children may lead to developmental delays or physical impairments.

Conversely, the onset of disability may lead to lower living standards, poverty, and hunger through adverse impact on education, employment, earnings, and increased expenditures related to one's impairment. Disability may prevent school attendance of children and youth with disabilities, restricting their ability to gain the education necessary to succeed as part of the workforce. For those who become disabled as adults, disability may prevent work or constrain the kind and amount of work a person can do, lowering income for the individual and the household and potentially resulting in poverty and hunger. Barriers to social participation, whether physical or social, contribute to poverty because of discrimination in the labor market or in the school system.

Additional Costs of Disability

Disability may require additional expenditures for the individual and the household, which can also lead to poverty. Such additional expenditures arise in relation to mainstream services (like health care) or disability-specific services (like assistive devices or personal care) and may be made worse by a barrier-filled environment. For instance, a public transportation system that is not wheelchair accessible will leave wheelchair users in situations where they are more likely to become isolated from economic opportunities or to incur higher transportation costs.

These complex links are a reminder that the policy issue cannot simply be one of "disability prevention" but must include awareness that for those who are born with or who become disabled, poverty is a potential concern throughout the lifespan.

The Poverty Status of Persons with Disabilities in the United States

Persons with disabilities have higher rates of poverty using the traditional poverty measure employed by the U.S. government, which compares available family-level financial resources to required expenditures to maintain a particular standard of living. The official poverty line in the United States takes into consideration family pretax income relative to estimated food expenditures in the 1960s, adjusted for inflation and family structure. The official poverty measure not only is used to identify the proportion of federal, state, and local populations that are *income poor* but also serves as the basis for determining eligibility for participation in many public programs designed to assist low-income families. In determining eligibility for program participation, many programs set family resource thresholds relative to the official poverty line (for example, 135 percent or 185 percent of poverty).

Considering a Disability-Adjusted Poverty Standard. The official poverty measure, however, does not account for the value of noncash benefits, including publicly provided health insurance; housing; nutrition assistance; variations in costs of living across the country; or disability status. This official poverty measure is problematic as there are additional costs associated with disability that can affect standards of living and subtract from available financial resources within households that include a person with a disability. For example, imagine two households just above the *poverty threshold*. If one of these two households contains a member with a disability, medical and transportation expenses could be higher for that household, forcing a lower standard of living. Put another way, the household with disabilities may technically fall above the poverty threshold but may maintain a standard of living that is more similar to households without disabilities that are identified below the poverty threshold.

Supplemental Poverty Measure. The recent Supplemental Poverty Measure (SPM) developed by the U.S. government is an alternative that addresses some of these concerns. It broadens the definition of resources to include after-tax income and noncash benefits and adjusts for child care, medical and transportation costs, and geographic cost-of-living differences. These resources are compared to estimated expenditure thresholds including food, clothing, shelter, and utilities. Both official poverty and the SPM are routinely reported by the federal government, providing a way to identify the population that falls above or below the established thresholds as "nonpoor" or "poor." Given these modifications, official poverty and the SPM to some extent identify different populations. Again, however, using SPM, persons with disabilities are more likely to be poor than the rest of the population.

Resources and Poverty. Sufficient resources are certainly key to acquiring essential commodities. However, as the saying goes, "money cannot buy happiness." Individuals may have adequate income yet lack personal health, social relationships, access to health care, education, employment, and political voice. If one intrinsically values these other components as part of overall well-being, then an individual who has been disadvantaged in one of these dimensions can also be considered "poor" in that dimension.

Multidimensional Poverty Measures. Multidimensional poverty measures emerged in light of this criticism. These measures extend beyond low income or expenditures and capture the extent to which individuals experience deprivations in several aspects of well-being, such as health, education, social connectedness, and material well-being. Such measures have been used more frequently on the international stage than they have in the United States. The Multidimensional Poverty Index, for example, measures economic development in terms of assets/living conditions, health, and education. Multidimensional poverty measures tend to capture individuals who are deprived in several important aspects of well-being but who are not necessarily deprived in terms of income or expenditures.

Americans with disabilities consistently face high rates of multidimensional poverty. Americans with disabilities have been found to be more likely to experience multiple deprivations when deprivations are measured in terms of income, health, education, employment, political participation, and social connectedness.

Not all persons with disabilities are poor, whatever the definition of poverty. In addition, not all persons with disabilities face the same rates of poverty. Consistently, research identifies a range of negative outcomes based on the type, severity, and duration of a particular condition. Short-term and less-severe conditions tend to have less negative impacts and consequently lower rates of poverty.

Conclusion

In the United States, persons with disability experience higher rates of poverty than other persons, whether poverty is defined in terms of low income or multiple deprivations. The strength of the association between disability and poverty varies depending on the type, duration, and severity of a disability. However, most persons with disabilities in the United States are not poor.

The association and the many channels that link disability and poverty are a reminder that this is a policy issue that is not simply about *disability prevention*; it is also a cross-cutting issue of *disability inclusion* in employment, education, health care, social and political participation, and economic opportunities throughout the lifespan.

Katie Jajtner, Debra Brucker,
and Sophie Mitra

See also: Disability Demography; Neoliberalism; Social Capital

Further Reading

Brucker, Debra L., and Andrew J. Houtenville. 2014. "Living on the Edge: Assessing the Economic Impacts of Potential Disability Benefit Reductions for Social Security Disability Beneficiaries." *Journal of Vocational Rehabilitation* 41, no. 3: 209–223.

Brucker, Debra L., Sophie Mitra, Navena Chaitoo, and Joseph Mauro. 2015. "More Likely to Be Poor Whatever the Measure: Working Age Persons with Disabilities in the United States." *Social Science Quarterly* 96, no. 1: 273–296.

Mitra, Sophie, Patricia A. Findley, and Usha Sambamoorthi. 2009. "Health Care Expenditures of Living with a Disability: Total Expenditures, Out-of-Pocket Expenses, and Burden, 1996 to 2004." *Archives of Physical Medicine and Rehabilitation* 90, no. 9: 1532–1540.

She, Peiyun, and Gina A. Livermore. 2007. "Material Hardship, Poverty, and Disability among Working Age Adults." *Social Science Quarterly* 88, no. 4: 970–989.

United Nations. 2013. *The State of the World's Children 2013: Children with Disabilities.* New York: UNICEF.

United Nations Development Programme. 2010. *Human Development Report 2010: The Real Wealth of Nations—Pathways to Human Development.* New York: United Nations.

Prenatal Testing/Selective Abortion

Prenatal testing for disability looks for the presence of certain genetic conditions that lead to impairment or disability. While a number of conditions can be tested for, the most commonly discussed genetic condition is Down syndrome. This entry will focus on the debates around the uses of prenatal testing for Down syndrome specifically because of the commonly held belief that a prenatal diagnosis of Down syndrome should result in aborting that fetus. More than a belief, the importance of the controversy around prenatal genetic testing and selective abortion is indicated by the estimated 68 percent to 72 percent (Natoli et al. 2012) termination of Down syndrome fetuses in the United States. Disability rights activists and scholars have critiqued the availability and uses of prenatal genetic testing because of the high selective abortion rates, arguing that *both* the availability and use of prenatal testing reveal significant bias against disability (Parens and Asch 2000). In order to understand the disability scholars' critiques of prenatal testing, one needs to know how prenatal testing works.

Prenatal Genetic Screening and Testing Technologies

Prenatal genetic testing involves a series of screening and diagnostic testing technologies and practices. *Screening* is a way of examining the probability that a fetus has a condition, and it cannot provide definitive answers. Common methods of screening use ultrasound images and measure certain protein levels in the mother's blood to detect the likelihood that certain chromosomal conditions are present in the fetus. These blood serum screenings are known as first-trimester, sequential, triple, or quad screens, depending on the particular combination and timing of each serum screening test. They are performed between 11 and 15 weeks of pregnancy. These screens have been in use since the 1980s. Any screening tests with results that indicate a higher than average likelihood of the presence of a chromosomal condition are flagged, and it is suggested that the parents undergo amniocentesis or chorionic villus sampling (CVS) to determine whether the fetus actually has that genetic condition. Both amniocentesis and CVS are *diagnostic* tests, which means that they can determine with 99.99 percent certainty whether or not the fetus actually has the condition. Amniocentesis and CVS are both considered invasive tests because their methods involve extracting a sample of fetal tissue through a needle through the abdominal wall (amniocentesis) or vaginally using a catheter (CVS). Both diagnostic tests have about a 1 percent risk of miscarriage associated with them. The risk of miscarriage has played a large role in how expectant parents make decisions about whether to have the testing done or not. The profession of *genetic counseling*, while not limited only to amniocentesis and CVS, has developed out of the circumstances surrounding prenatal genetic testing and its

implications for what disability signals for expectant parents. Initially established as a gatekeeper to keep parents from having children with disabilities, the profession is currently much more inclusive and positive about genetic disability diagnosis and life with a disability.

Noninvasive Prenatal Genetic Screening and Its Implications

However, a recent technological development in screening has important implications for how prenatal genetic testing is used and, thus, how disability is understood. In 2011, a technology known as *cell-free placental DNA screening* was implemented in clinical practice. This technology uses a maternal blood sample, very similarly to the serum screens mentioned above, but instead of measuring the presence of proteins in the mother's blood, the technology extracts fragments of "cell-free" placental fetal DNA to examine whether the fetus has a chromosomal condition. As of this writing, cell-free placental DNA screening most commonly looks for three chromosomal conditions: Edwards' syndrome, Patau syndrome, and Down syndrome. While commercially branded tests, including MaterniT21, Panorama, Verifi, and Harmony, are still considered screening tests and not diagnostic tests, the reported specificity and sensitivity rates of these tests are both very high, particularly for Down syndrome. High specificity and sensitivity mean that the probabilities are very high that the screening tests are identifying positives when the condition is actually there and identifying negative results when the condition is not there. As a result, cell-free placental DNA screening tests are blurring the lines between screening and diagnostic testing models. Cell-free placental DNA screening tests are currently only recommended for "high-risk" pregnancies, but commercial laboratories continue to urge for use in the general population. Such companies have also begun expanding the conditions to include sex chromosome–linked conditions, including Klinefelter's and Turner's syndromes, and also provide fetal sex if patients desire

Disability Activist/Scholar Critiques of Prenatal Genetic Testing

Disability activists and scholars have been vocal about their concerns with the increasing availability, uptake, and popularity of prenatal genetic testing because of the impact of decisions about selective abortion on both currently existing disabled people and potential disabled people-to-be. As with much disability studies scholarship, the disability rights and scholarly work critiquing prenatal genetic testing and selective abortion has largely developed as a response to certain social values and assumptions about disability itself. These assumptions include an understanding of disability as an individual problem or lack and as something to be avoided if possible. The critiques described below view the technologies and practices of prenatal genetic testing as *eugenic* practices that seek to eliminate disability wherever possible. Some of the most thoughtful and well-articulated critiques have emerged from legal and moral philosophy scholars, including Adrienne Asch, Erik Parens, and Rosemarie Garland-Thomson, as well as social scientists, including Carol Gill, Marsha Saxton, and Adam Hedgecoe. The "expressivist" argument (Parens and Asch 2000; Saxton 1997; Gonter 2004) claims that prenatal genetic testing expresses rejection toward all disabled people. These theorists state that prenatal testing, in conjunction with the decision to terminate a

fetus on the basis of disability, is ethically problematic first because it is harmful to current disabled people by perpetuating discriminatory ideas about disability. Many disabled people view the idea that expectant parents would choose to not have a child with a genetic condition as discriminatory not only toward the fetus in question but toward all those who share the genetic condition or, more generally, status as a disabled person. Second, these theorists have identified that the decision to abort on the basis of disability is often based on misinformation or lack of information about disabled embodiment. The *disability paradox* (Albrecht and Devlieger 1999) has been invoked to describe the phenomenon of disabled people reporting higher quality of life than might be expected. This argument removes the justification for selective abortion that assumes that life with a disability is not worth living. The importance of communicating the experience of life with a disability, then, is a key recommendation to change perceptions of what disability means. A third component of the disability activist/scholarly critique is that selective abortion on the basis of disability is an act of *synecdoche*, or mistaking the part for a whole (Parens and Asch 2000). This critique is also connected to parental expectations about who and what their child will become and is perhaps the particular critique that most directly attends to parental hopes and fears about their children. This strand of critiques is pulled together by the underlying assumption that prenatal genetic testing and selective abortion are two linked practices—that prenatal genetic diagnosis always leads to at least the possibility or consideration of selective abortion.

However, the emergence of cell-free placental DNA screening tests requires rethinking the necessity of placing prenatal genetic diagnosis and selective abortion side by side. Cell-free placental DNA screening tests are increasingly used in place of diagnostic testing, as many patients view them as noninvasive alternatives to amniocentesis or CVS. This places screening, as a phenomenon that attempts certainty and deals in risk and probability, at the center of this debate. In light of the rise of cell-free placental DNA screening tests, Scott Woodcock's (2009) argument helps shift the debates around prenatal testing and selective abortion. Woodcock has argued for maintaining human diversity because it offers social and mutual benefits to everyone, instead of only focusing on preventing harm against certain individuals. Woodcock views the expressivist argument as "all or nothing" because if expressivists did not claim that harm was done to existing persons with disabilities through prenatal testing, then they would not be against prenatal testing at all (2009).

Legislation and Education

There have been several attempts to legislate selective abortion and several attempts to provide more comprehensive education about life with genetic disability. In 2008, Congress passed the Prenatally and Postnatally Diagnosed Conditions Awareness Act, also known as the Kennedy-Brownback Act. The act calls for the collection and dispersal of information about outcomes for individuals living with chronic illness or disability. At least two states have used this act as a template; Massachusetts' version (HB 3825) and Ohio's law (HB 552) provision the same access to information about the conditions, services, and supports. The act also can be seen as attempting to cross the congressional aisle, as it enjoys bipartisan support, but

it remains unfunded and unregulated. The Kennedy-Brownback Act's underlying thesis is that information can influence policy and practice. This idea is supported by Kelly's (2009) findings that a majority of parents of children with disabilities either "choose not to choose" by abstaining from having more children or choose against prenatal screening for subsequent pregnancies. In contrast, Ormond et al. (2003) explored how medical trainees, including genetic counseling students, view genetic disabilities. Quality of life was perceived largely in terms of functional or medical aspects of disability instead of more subjective aspects. These two studies reveal the gap between families' experiences of disability and perceptions of disability within medical trainee settings, and they demonstrate the need for further research regarding these disparate understandings of disability.

At the state level, several attempts have been made to ban selective abortion. North Dakota passed a ban (HB 1305) on disability- and sex-selective abortion in 2013, the same day as it passed a ban on abortions after a fetal heartbeat is detected. Indiana (SB 334) has also passed a bill to ban disability-selective abortions.

Disability activists and scholars can continue to refine critiques of prenatal genetic screening and testing by delinking the practices of testing from the outcome of selective abortion. This move may help develop policies that emphasize how disability is a way of life for many individuals and families, instead of only focusing on the isolated act of selective abortion. Moving toward information-related legislation could, in turn, help cultivate state and federal policies that provide long-term services and supports for individuals with disabilities and their families.

Conclusion

Prenatal genetic screening and testing will continue to expand in both their technological capabilities and clinical uptake. As technology expands, it will become increasingly difficult for disability activists and scholars to engage with the issue of defending the personhood of people with disabilities without an understanding of how disability operates as a set of social meanings, how these meanings are embodied by people, and how medical technologies and practices interact with these meanings and bodies. Future areas for research include studying how the current usage and understanding of various screening and diagnostic tests are affecting the process and outcomes of prenatal clinical care, as well as continuing to understand better how to maximize true social inclusion of people with disabilities.

Aleksa Owen

See also: Bioethics; Ethics; Eugenics; Genetic Screening; Medical Paternalism; Medicalization

Further Reading

Albrecht, Gary L., and Patrick J. Devlieger. 1999. "The Disability Paradox: High Quality of Life Against All Odds." *Social Science & Medicine* 48, no. 8: 977–988.

Gonter, Carolyn. 2004. "The Expressivist Argument, Prenatal Diagnosis, and Selective Abortion: An Appeal to the Social Construction of Disability." *Macalester Journal of Philosophy* 13, no. 1: Article 3.

Kelly, Susan E. 2009. "Choosing Not to Choose: Reproductive Responses of Parents with Children with Genetic Conditions or Impairments." *Sociology of Health & Illness* 31 no. 1: 81–97.

Natoli, Jamie, Deborah L. Ackerman, Suzanne McDermott, and Janice G. Edwards. 2012. "Prenatal Diagnosis of Down Syndrome: A Systematic Review of Termination Rates 1995–2011." *Prenatal Diagnosis* 32, no. 2: 142–153.

Ormond, K. E., C. J. Gill, P. Semik, and K. L. Kirschner. 2003. "Attitudes of Healthcare Trainees about Genetics and Disability: Issues of Access, Health Care Communication and Decision Making." *Journal of Genetic Counseling* 12, no. 4: 333–349.

Parens, Erik, and Adrienne Asch. 2000. *Prenatal Testing and Disability Rights.* Washington, DC: Georgetown University Press.

Saxton, Marsha. 1997. "Disability Rights and Selective Abortion." In *Abortion Wars: A Half Century of Struggle, 1950–2000*, edited by Rickie Solinger, 374–395. Berkeley: University of California Press.

Woodcock, Scott. 2009. "Disability, Diversity, and the Elimination of Human Kinds." *Social Theory and Practice* 35, no. 2: 251–278.

Preventive Health Care

Preventive care includes a wide variety of health services designed to prevent illness or to diagnose it at an early stage of development. Prevention and early diagnosis are critical for saving money and time, as well as for improving overall health and well-being.

The seven main areas of preventive health care and screening services include the following:

1. Diabetes, blood pressure, and cholesterol testing
2. Sexually transmitted disease (STD) screening
3. Cancer screening
4. Regular visits to a physician
5. Prenatal care
6. Behavioral interventions for risky behavior
7. Vaccinations

Approaches to Prevention

A wide range of health care services are considered preventive care, ranging from general physicals and routine blood tests to very specific screening services for cancer or mental health concerns. In other words, preventive health care should incorporate the entire body. Prevention services can be categorized into three main groups: primary, secondary, and tertiary prevention.

- *Primary prevention.* The provision of care before there is evidence of disease.
- *Secondary prevention.* Care services provided after disease has begun but before symptoms are evident.
- *Tertiary prevention.* Health care interventions implemented after disease is evident to resolve the condition or to prevent further progression.

The Centers for Disease Control and Prevention (CDC) estimated that 100,000 lives could be saved in the United States if everyone received the recommended clinical preventive care. In addition, preventive health care has many economic benefits, both in the form of cost savings in the health care system and in improvements in well-being and quality of life. The costs of treating a small tumor in the early stages, for example, are much less than the costs of extensive surgery and chemotherapy in later-stage cancers. Similarly, with smoking prevention and cessation programs, primary or secondary prevention costs are less than tertiary care costs linked to morbidities caused by smoking. It is a well-known fact that the United States spends more on health care than any other developed nation yet has some of the worst health outcomes of any developed nation.

Access to Preventive Health Care

By utilizing preventive health services and screenings, we can improve health outcomes for all Americans. However, having access to preventive care is especially important for persons with disabilities, who typically have inequitable access to services. We know that an individual with a disability is at a higher risk for poor health than an individual without a disability. The CDC (2016) reports that individuals with disabilities are more likely to have poorer overall health, less access to adequate health care, and a greater likelihood of engaging in risky health behaviors. Adding to the critical need to incorporate high-quality preventive health care services for persons with disabilities is the higher rate of largely preventable secondary conditions in this population.

Past and Future Trends in Preventive Health

Preventive medicine has a long history in the United States. The use of vaccinations is perhaps the best-known example of preventive medicine. Vaccinations are usually safe, are widely implemented, and protect individuals from infectious agents that otherwise could result in serious illnesses or death.

A key historical development in preventive medicine was the advancement of laboratory technology. This trend has allowed the development of ever more sophisticated tests capable of detecting diseases much earlier in their progression. Today's testing innovations continue to push this trend forward by using genetic testing to identify genetic predispositions for specific diseases and conditions. The application of genetic screening to unborn children is controversial, and it raises a number of critical ethical issues, discussed in greater depth elsewhere in this volume.

The Affordable Care Act (ACA) has elevated the role of preventive health services, mandating insurance coverage for a wide range of such services, from sexually transmitted disease (STD) testing to type 2 diabetes screening. The ACA provisions represent critical recognition of the importance of preventive care by making screening and services more accessible to all Americans, especially pregnant women seeking prenatal care. Access to prenatal care is extremely important for identification of potential problems in both maternal and child health.

Recent initiatives in primary prevention for Americans with disabilities emphasize the importance of being physically active and having a nutritious diet—that is, the importance of lifestyle choices. Given the role of inactivity and poor diet in elevated obesity rates among those with disabilities in the U.S. population generally, and the comorbidities associated with obesity, encouraging and facilitating the role of healthy lifestyle choices is an emerging and potentially critical form of preventive health care.

Tina Schuh

See also: Genetic Screening; Health Determinants; Health Disparities; Health-Related Quality of Life; Wellness and Health Promotion

Further Reading

Association of State and Territorial Health Officials (ASTHO). 2013. "Access to Preventative Healthcare Services for Women with Disabilities." http://www.astho.org /Access-to-Preventive-Healthcare-Ser vices-for-Women-with-Disabilities-Fact -Sheet/.

Ervin, David, Brian Hennen, Joav Merrick, and Mohammed Morad. 2014. "Healthcare for Persons with Intellectual and Developmental Disability in the Community." *Frontiers in Public Health* 2, no. 83: 108.

Ervin, David, and Joav Merrick. 2014. "Intellectual and Developmental Disability: Healthcare Financing." *Frontiers in Public Health* 2, no. 160: 1–3.

Peacock, Georgina, Lisa Iezzoni, and Thomas Harkin. 2015. "Healthcare for Americans with Disabilities: 25 Years after the ADA." *The New England Journal of Medicine* 373, no. 10: 892–893.

World Health Organization. "Disability and Health: Fact Sheet." http://www.who.int /mediacentre/factsheets/fs352/en/.

Primary Care, Barriers to

A primary care provider (PCP) provides routine primary care and can be a source of usual care for most nonurgent health care needs. PCPs are often the gateway to services people with disabilities need to maintain health and live independently. Barriers to primary care can arise when a person with a disability is trying to find care, pay for care, or gain physical access to a provider's office. Barriers also arise with interpersonal communications or interactions with office staff.

Many people with disabilities report that they do not have a usual source of health care—a particular doctor's office, clinic, health center, or other care setting where they seek care and medical advice. In part, this is due to barriers to primary care. For that reason, awareness and elimination of barriers for people with disabling conditions become extremely important.

Most people with disabilities are in good health and see the doctor no more frequently than others. They are not "sick" and do not want to be cured. They seek primary care services that provide the same quality and access to care as their nondisabled counterparts, but their impairments and functional limitations often make them more vulnerable to certain health problems. They experience health conditions, such as heart failure or pneumonia, that they share with the nondisabled population, as well as conditions, such as urinary tract infections or pressure sores, more likely to appear among people with certain physical disabilities (DeJong et al. 2002). Although most research focuses on barriers to care for people with physical and sensory disabilities, people with intellectual and psychiatric disabilities also face barriers to care.

Finding Care

People with disabilities and significant health care needs must consider many factors in choosing a primary care provider. Three factors especially unique to disability are provider knowledge of disability, the costs of accommodations, and transportation.

Knowledge of Disability. Most primary care physicians are not prepared to address the unique health care needs of people with disabilities, partly because they see so few patients with any one disabling condition. They may see more patients with common conditions, such as intermittent low-back pain or diabetes, but relatively few patients with less common conditions. When asked, patients with disabilities wished that clinicians had some basic familiarity with their condition, listened to the patient's descriptions of issues, and knew when to make a referral to a specialist (DeJong et al. 2002).

Health care professionals and medical students say they are often unsure how to interact with and treat people with significant disabilities. A study revealed that medical students admitted knowing little about people with disabilities but were open to changing their views (Iezzoni and O'Day 2006). The students also confessed to having discriminatory attitudes toward

morbidly obese people, who may be considered disabled because of limited mobility. Further, they reported not knowing whether it was appropriate to talk to their patients about the disability and having little knowledge about disabilities in general. Students had much more difficulty in both interpersonal skills and physical examination skills when the patient had a disability, indicating a need for more training in this area (Brown et al. 2010). Health care professionals also described specific educational needs, such as how to (1) access disability resources, (2) coordinate care and adapt health checkups to the disability, (3) address sexuality and contraception with patients, (4) order durable medical equipment, (5) complete forms for disability status and home care, and (6) plan for hospital discharge (Morrison, George, and Mosquedo 2008).

Compared with the general population, people with certain disabilities are at greater risk for other common health conditions, and they often experience these conditions differently. They may require a somewhat different or extended treatment that takes into account both their disability and the resulting functional limitations. For example, people with mobility impairments may be at greater risk of coronary heart disease, renal failure, or earlier onset of diabetes and may need a longer recovery period or a different exercise regimen to address these conditions (DeJong et al. 2002).

People with congenital conditions—that is, disabilities that are present from birth or early childhood, such as cerebral palsy and spina bifida—face special barriers to finding willing and knowledgeable physicians. As children, people with congenital conditions typically receive health care from pediatricians, often within specialized clinics for children with disabilities. But few primary care physicians trained in adult medicine learn about caring for people with congenital conditions, and these patients have trouble finding a provider as they get older. As a result, many continue to see their pediatrician well into adulthood, even though the pediatrician may be ill equipped to handle adult medical issues, such as family planning, pregnancy, or substance abuse.

Cost of Accommodation. Any patients, whether they have a disability or not, may find it difficult to find a provider who takes their insurance. People with disabilities often must find a practice that accepts public health insurance, such as Medicare or Medicaid. Some practitioners will not accept patients with these insurance plans because, compared to private plans, Medicare and Medicaid do not pay providers as much for their services. Given that many people with disabilities depend on public health insurance, this is a significant challenge to finding a provider.

Even if a provider does accept public health insurance, the payments from the insurance plan may be inadequate. Basic services, like routine office visits, can cost more for people with disabilities because of additional time, personnel, testing, or equipment required. Insurance plans have a certain set fee for each service a provider offers, and these fees do not take into account whether patients have special health care needs or require extra help to receive a service. If the payments do not cover the cost of the services, clinicians either have to absorb the extra costs or refuse to accept these patients.

The reimbursement that providers receive for routine primary care is insufficient for many people with disabilities, particularly for those with chronic conditions, as care for these patients usually takes more time (particularly when several conditions need to be addressed). Any additional costs of serving people with disabilities, such as providing a sign language interpreter, are generally not covered by insurance. Finding a medical practice that will absorb any extra costs, if needed, is crucial for many people with disabilities.

Transportation. Finally, some people with disabilities may face barriers in getting to a provider's office. People who do not drive must find a practice that is close to home or near public transportation. People who cannot use regular mass transit must rely on paratransit services—specialized door-to-door services for people with disabilities. Paratransit services must be scheduled in advance and often require long wait times for the vehicle to arrive, meaning that a trip to a doctor's office can take most of a day or that the patient may be late for the appointment. People in rural areas where public transportation is lacking must find alternatives, such as friends or volunteers, to take them to doctor's appointments, and they often have to travel to a larger city to find a practitioner who provides the specialized care they need.

Paying for Care

People with disabilities often lack sufficient insurance, making it difficult to afford care. Many are not employed and, as a result, rely on public health insurance or lack insurance altogether. Others may have once been employed but developed a disability that stopped them from working; these individuals may apply for Social Security Disability Insurance (SSDI) and will eventually become eligible for Medicare, but they must wait 29 months for coverage, leaving many without insurance at a particularly vulnerable time.

Uninsured people with disabilities face many more barriers to accessing care than do nondisabled people without health insurance, and people with certain types of disabilities, such as intellectual or mental health problems, may be at an even greater disadvantage. People without insurance may forego preventive and primary care, which can lead to more care in emergency rooms or higher health care costs down the road, or they have to pay high out-of-pocket costs.

People with disabilities who do have insurance may still have to pay out of pocket for services that their insurance will not cover. Generally, for an item or service to be covered by Medicare or private insurance, it must be deemed "medically necessary." Most definitions of medical necessity include surgery or other services to treat an acute condition but do not consider the ongoing health and functional maintenance needs of people with disabilities who want to live independently in the community. These needs may include physical or occupational therapy to maintain their functional ability, durable medical equipment such as wheelchairs, or personal assistance in the home. Medicaid generally covers personal assistance or durable medical equipment, but people must keep their earnings low to qualify for the program. If they lose their coverage, they must pay high out-of-pocket costs or go without the service or equipment entirely.

Gaining Physical Access to the Health Care Office

The Americans with Disabilities Act (ADA) requires health care facilities to be physically accessible to people with disabilities, but this requirement only applies to new construction or to major changes made to existing buildings. Many health facilities were built before the passage of the ADA or similar state laws, and making these facilities accessible is only required if it is "readily achievable"—in other words, if it can be done without "significant difficulty or expense." Physical access can still be a challenge for people with physical disabilities, including wheelchair users. Barriers may include doors that are too narrow, do not have automatic openers, or have cumbersome hardware (knobs rather than levers); cramped spaces and narrow corridors; inaccessible restrooms; and elevators that are small, hard to operate, or nonexistent. Blind or low-vision patients may find it challenging to navigate a facility once inside if there is no Braille or raised print on the room signs.

Inaccessible medical equipment, such as exam tables, radiography machines, and scales, pose other barriers for people with physical disabilities. Exam tables that do not raise and lower can be a major problem for wheelchair users, but they also can pose problems for people with less severe mobility impairments who may have trouble climbing up on them. To have a complete medical exam, wheelchair users must be lifted onto the exam table, which can be dangerous for the staff person and the patient. Patients report receiving inadequate pelvic exams or other routine care while sitting in the wheelchair rather than on the exam table, which contributes to the lower rates of Pap smears and mammograms for women with disabilities than for other women. Patients also report inadequate monitoring of body weight, in part because of inaccessible scales. Specially designed exam tables, weight scales, and mammography equipment can make the exam more comfortable and thorough, but practice staff who buy this equipment often do not know about these types of medical equipment. Administrators need more education not only about the availability of accessible equipment but also about the importance of this equipment for patients with disabilities and their physicians.

Communicating with the Provider

Good communication, including respect for and responsiveness to each patient's preferences, needs, and values, is essential. However, negative attitudes and mistaken beliefs surrounding disability can make it difficult for patients and providers to have effective and meaningful interactions. Disability can dominate the conversation in overt and subtle ways. Ineffective communication reinforces the patient's belief that the provider is not interested in or sensitive to the particular needs of patients with disabilities. This belief has significant consequences for patients, who may be less likely to seek care or to follow up on clinician recommendations.

In studies of patient experiences with health care, people with disabilities stress the importance of placing the person, *not* the disability, first. They want clinicians to treat them as adults, communicate with respect in an appropriate pace and tone of voice, listen to their needs, and refrain from making assumptions about the quality of their lives. Patients with disabilities do not expect to be cured, but they would like to receive health care that allows them to make autonomous decisions about their care and to be treated with the same respect given to patients without disabilities. Many people with disabilities rate their quality of life much higher than their medical providers do. In fact, their perceived quality of life is similar to the self-perceived quality of life of people without disabilities. Many people with disabilities bring a wealth of knowledge about their health and needs based on their life experience. Clinicians can tap into this experience through open, respectful communication with patients. Active

listening and good communication will engender mutual respect and trust between the provider and patient.

Clinicians sometimes assume that the patient is seeing them for a problem related to his or her disability, when in fact the problem may be unrelated. Such physicians are treating the disability first instead of the person—for example, asking questions about a visual or mental impairment when the medical issue the patient sought care for was related to chest pain. This focus on the disability can be a barrier to care because it could cause the provider to overlook the main problem, delay care, or make the patient feel that the provider isn't listening. The chief complaint should be evaluated without consideration of the disability unless the situation or type of treatment warrants it. The patient should be offered the same types of treatment that would be offered to patients with a similar diagnosis without a disability.

Another issue is providers' reluctance to talk with patients with disabilities about sensitive subjects, such as sexuality, smoking, or substance use. Although providers often avoid these topics even with patients without disabilities, fewer women and men with disabilities are asked about reproduction, birth control, or sexually transmitted diseases or about smoking and substance use (Iezzoni 2011). Clinicians may believe that people with disabilities are uninterested or unable to engage in sexual activity or that smoking or substance abuse helps patients deal with difficulties in their lives. People with disabilities use drugs and alcohol at least as often as others but are asked about it less often. Furthermore, they may use pain medication that has been prescribed for their disability, which in combination with alcohol or other drugs could have severe medical consequences. These topics should be addressed during a primary care visit.

People who are deaf or hard of hearing may face unique challenges in obtaining care, as these patients may request a sign language interpreter (someone who translates spoken words into sign language). Some clinicians believe that writing notes or lip reading are adequate substitutes for interpreters. However, writing notes is slow and cumbersome, and notes may not include complete information. People who are deaf or hard of hearing report difficulties understanding words when lip reading, especially when physicians speak quickly, turn away, bow their heads, speak in an accent, or have beards or masks. Even in the best circumstances, lip reading is generally inadequate because many English sounds are not clearly visible on the lips. However, even when a person does have a sign language interpreter, communication barriers can arise when clinicians speak to the interpreters rather than to the patients themselves. Similarly, clinicians may speak to the family member or personal assistant, bypassing the patient. The same principles for communication with patients using sign language interpreters or personal assistants apply as for oral foreign language interpreters: keep eye contact with the patients and speak directly to them, not to interpreters or assistants. Unless clinicians talk directly to patients, they might not benefit from the patients' knowledge of their own conditions or treatment regimens. Without providers' recognition of how to fully engage these populations in respectful, open communication, the quality of care or the patient's ability to follow instructions may suffer.

Interacting with Office Staff

Each member of the medical office staff plays a role in creating a welcoming environment for people with disabilities. This environment includes reception staff, intake nurses, physician's assistants, and supporting staff in the lab or other areas. The receptionist, who is often the first contact with the patient, can be welcoming and friendly or can cause distress. For example, deaf patients may miss an appointment because they did not hear the receptionist call their name. Blind patients encounter embarrassing situations when staff help them complete forms with sensitive information in a lobby or public area. Making sure a deaf person knows his or her name has been called, or helping a blind patient complete forms in a private room, will address these problems.

Some patients need assistance getting to the examination room. Wheelchair users report being pushed without their permission, and blind patients report being grabbed rather than being asked what type of help they need. Asking the patient first and making sure the office is accessible, with unobstructed hallways and appropriate signage, can address these issues.

Once in the examination room, clinicians should recognize how important assistive devices, such as a cane or wheelchair, are to the patient. Clinicians should ensure that the equipment is nearby and that the patient can readily access it. Clinicians should also respect the patient's decision about whether a family member or personal assistant is in the room during the exam. Some patients may want the person with them to help them get on the exam table or talk to the clinician. Others may want to discuss sensitive, private information, such as abuse in the home, with the clinician without the presence of the assistant. Telling patients when something unpleasant is about to happen, such as warning a person who is blind about a needle stick, can also make the exam less stressful.

Summary and Conclusion

Barriers to primary care make it difficult for people with disabilities to get the same quality of care that other people receive, which affects their well-being. Although breaking down these barriers may seem onerous, many can be overcome with common courtesy and effective communication, which will let patients know they are respected and valued. The more satisfied patients are with their health care and the more comfortable they are with practitioners, the more likely they are to keep their appointments and follow doctors' advice.

Bonnie O'Day and Holly Matulewicz

See also: Health Care, Barriers to for Minorities; Health Disparities; Health Insurance; Preventive Health Care; Self-Advocacy and Health Literacy

Further Reading

Brown, Rachel S., Catherine Leigh Graham, Nancy Richeson, Junlong Wu, and Suzanne McDermott. 2010. "Evaluation of Medical Student Performance on Objective Structured Clinical Exams with Standardized Patients with and without Disabilities." *Academic Medicine* 85: 1766–1771.

DeJong, Gerben, Susan E. Palsbo, Phillip W. Beatty, Gwen C. Jones, Thilo Kroll, and Melinda T. Nari. 2002. "The Organization and Financing of Health Services for Persons with Disabilities." *The Milbank Quarterly* 80, no. 2: 261–301.

Iezzoni, Lisa I. 2011. "Eliminating Health and Health Care Disparities among the Growing Population of People with Disabilities." *Health Affairs* 30: 1947–1956.

Iezzoni, Lisa I., and Bonnie L. O'Day. 2006. *More Than Ramps: A Guide to Improving Health Care Quality and Access for People with Disabilities.* Bethesda, MD: Oxford University Press.

Morrison, Elizabeth H., Valerie George, and Laura Mosquedo. 2008. "Primary Care for Adults with Physical Disabilities." *Clinical Research and Methods* 49, no. 9: 645–651.

Protests, Disability Rights Movement. See Disability Protests

Public Health

Public health is a discipline that focuses on the promotion of health and the prevention of disease at the population level. Public health workers seek to address societal and structural barriers that make it difficult for people to access health care by working to increase health equity across population groups, and by doing so, they build healthy communities. The needs of people with disabilities have often gone overlooked in public health initiatives, but the discipline is beginning to include people with disabilities in their thinking about health and the ways in which they are interacting with the broader environment.

Public health provides the means for identifying individuals who need access to services, and issues of access are important concerns for the disability community. Public health practitioners emphasize policy and focus their work on increasing access to care. Given the emphasis on promoting health and making health care available to entire communities, the population of people with disabilities is a good fit for targeting public health initiatives.

Community health assessments, which describe the health of entire communities via data collection, are some of the most powerful tools in public health. Data drives policy and informs practice. A great deal of the data collection surrounding issues of disability comes from public health initiatives focused on developing a better understanding of the health needs of this population.

Essential Public Health Frameworks

To gain a deeper understanding of the way in which public health and disabilities fit together, it is important to have a basic knowledge of some of the main themes and frameworks that influence public health practice. These include understanding social determinants of health, the life course model, and the social-ecological model.

An examination of individual risk factors for a disease does not give a full picture of a person's health status. Public health practitioners work to address health inequity that is related to the social determinants of health, which are features of the environment where people live and work. For example, an individual with limited mobility is more likely to be obese when compared to nondisabled counterparts. The social determinants of health help to explain why this is the case. Social determinants of health can include such factors as the number of grocery stores in a neighborhood, the accessibility level of parks or green spaces, lead exposure, access to clean water, and other conditions of the physical environment in which the person lives. Considering these contextual determinants of health as opposed to focusing only on biological markers, such as body mass index (BMI), allows us to have a fuller understanding of the causes of poor health and the reasons that differences exist between groups. The social determinants of health are particularly useful for identifying factors that may exacerbate the negative impact that an impairment has on an individual's health.

The life course model is an additional public health framework that is helpful in describing how the social determinants can affect an individual over time. The approach highlights the outcome of negative influences in terms of the compounding effects of time through length of exposure. The key themes that are used to frame the way the model affects health are timing, environment, and equity. That is, today's experiences and the things one is exposed to now will influence tomorrow's health. Health trajectories are particularly affected during critical or sensitive periods (timing). Also, the broader community environment strongly affects the capacity to be healthy (environment). Finally, while genetic makeup offers both protective and risk factors for disease conditions, health disparities reflect more than just genetics and personal choice (equity). The last point emphasizes social inequality and the role of the environment in the health of persons with disabilities. The focus of this model is on promoting the reduction in the number of risk factors and adverse exposure variables that one encounters throughout one's lifetime in an effort to improve overall health.

A third important public health framework is the socio-ecological model, which organizes the social determinants of health and connects them to health outcomes. This model is often described along dimensions that move from individual level, which explores the biological and personal factors, to the very macro level, which reflects broader factors at play across society and culture. Different models employ varying schemes and levels of effect.

Healthy People 2020

Healthy People 2020 is the consensus statement about the nation's health promotion and prevention priorities. The Healthy

People 2020 goals require that public health departments across the country actively engage the disability community in order to improve the overall health of the population. These goals strive to do the following:

- increase the number of population-based data systems that include in their core a standardized set of questions that identify people with disabilities
- increase the number of health promotion programs for people with disabilities and caregivers
- reduce the proportion of adults with disabilities who are aged 18 years and older who experience delays in receiving primary and periodic preventive care due to access barriers
- increase the proportion of youth with special health care needs whose health care provider has discussed the transition from pediatric to adult health care
- reduce unemployment among people with disabilities and increase employment levels
- increase the proportion of children with disabilities, birth through age 2, who receive early intervention services in home or community-based settings

Moving Forward

Maintaining and improving the health of individuals with disabilities is a public health issue that will continue to persist as our population ages. People with disabilities who are living in low resource areas and have been exposed to health risks over time have unique concerns that must be addressed. Innovative solutions are needed to provide the necessary supports that can allow for effective care of people with disabilities. With its interdisciplinary and systems-level approach to addressing health issues, public health is positioned as a field

foundational to improving health outcomes of people with disabilities.

Sarah Agamah

See also: Health Determinants; Health Disparities; Primary Care, Barriers to; Wellness and Health Promotion

Further Reading

McMenamin, Terence M., Thomas W. Hale, Douglas Kruse, and Haejin Kim. 2005. "Designing Questions to Identify People with Disabilities in Labor Force Surveys: The Effort to Measure the Employment Level of Adults with Disabilities in the CPS." Bureau of Labor Statistics. http://www.bls.gov/ore/pdf/st050190.pdf.

Office of Disease Prevention and Health Promotion. 2014. "Disability and Health." https://www.healthypeople.gov/2020/topics-objectives/topic/disability-and-health/objectives.

Office of Disease Prevention and Health Promotion. 2014. "Rethinking MCH: The Life Course Model as an Organizing Framework." https://www.healthypeople.gov/2020/topics-objectives/topic/disability-and-health.

Talley, Ronda C., and John E. Crews. 2006. "Framing the Public Health of Caregiving." *American Journal of Public Health* 97, no. 2: 224–28.

U.S. Department of Health and Human Services Health Resources and Services Administration Maternal and Child Health Bureau. 2010. "Rethinking MCH: The Life Course Model as an Organizing Framework." Health Resources and Services Administration. http://www.hrsa.gov/ourstories/mchb75th/images/rethinkingmch.pdf.

Public Transportation

Accessible, affordable transportation provides people with disabilities access to opportunities in employment, education, recreation, health care, and independent community living. There are many different forms of transportation that people with disabilities have access to, depending on where they live. Public transportation modes include buses and trains (for travel within metropolitan areas and across regions), air travel, taxis, and door-to-door programs.

Background and History

Prior to any of the disability rights laws, there were no policies that required transportation providers to build and maintain accessible vehicles or transit stations for people with disabilities. Often transportation infrastructure was built on elevated lines or subway lines without consideration for whether all people could access those stations. Similarly, buses, motor vehicles, and trains were not built for people with disabilities to use them independently. Because much of the transportation infrastructure in the United States was built before the 1970s, many barriers continue today.

Policies on Accessible Transportation. Several laws helped shape transportation systems in the United States to become more accessible for people with disabilities. The Rehabilitation Act of 1973 was the first major law that prohibited discrimination against people with disabilities on transportation receiving federal financial assistance. In 1990, Title II of the Americans with Disabilities Act (ADA) set forth specific aspects of public transportation that have to be in place for the transportation to be considered accessible to people with disabilities. Newly built and remodeled transit stations must be accessible according to the architectural guidelines known as the Americans with Disabilities Act Accessibility Guidelines (ADAAG). These guidelines are standards for newly built and altered facilities, and they are enforceable under the ADA. Additionally, Title II requires new vehicles purchased by public transit agencies to be accessible, which includes bus boarding, movement within the bus, and the presence of securement for wheelchairs. Communication on public transit vehicles and at stations also must be accessible to people who have sensory disabilities, such as hearing or visual impairments.

With the passage of the ADA, areas with transit systems became required to provide an alternative service for people who could not use local buses and trains. However, this requirement only applied to areas that are within three-quarters of a mile of a transit route. The main alternative is *paratransit*, which is a door-to-door demand/response service from a person's home to a destination. Users pay per ride, and the cost can only be twice as much as what is paid on buses and trains.

Important Points to Know about Public Transportation and Disability

Despite shifts in federal policy and class action lawsuits, results of a large national survey conducted by the National Organization on Disability and the Kessler Foundation indicate that inadequate transportation is a problem for more than one in three people with disabilities. Many people with disabilities use their own cars or rely on family or friends instead of taking public transit, which can be very limiting to independent community travel.

Municipal Transit Systems. Local buses and trains are part of what is known as a "fixed-route system," which has predetermined routes and stops in a community and is run by a local transit agency. Municipal transit accessibility is complicated because access for one group is not necessarily access for all. For example, people with mobility disabilities benefit from lifts, ramps, and wheelchair securement, whereas people with sensory disabilities benefit from stop announcements, and people with cognitive disabilities benefit from assistance provided by vehicle drivers.

According to the 2013 National Transit Database, 84 percent of all vehicles used by public transit agencies and 79 percent of transit stations were compliant with ADA standards. These figures are reported by transit agencies. Many of the stations in larger metropolitan cities with older infrastructure have much lower rates of ADA compliant stations, as low as 21 percent in New York City. Areas in rural parts of the country have additional problems in accessing transportation. Rural towns often do not

have access to any fixed-route system. As a result, there is no requirement that any form of paratransit be provided. This can leave people with disabilities in rural areas highly dependent on friends and family and with a feeling of isolation. Some special transportation services, such as local shuttles and van pools, are provided in rural areas, but they are typically limited in their trip frequency.

Where there are fixed-route systems, there is a common problem with schedules and the fixed-route transit not running often enough for people to count on it. People with disabilities often face many barriers in the pedestrian environment that prevent getting to or from transit stops, such as lack of sidewalks, uneven or cracked sidewalks, steep sidewalks, and missing curb ramps to

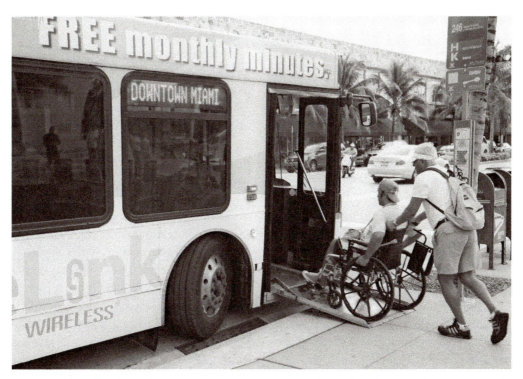

A man uses a wheelchair ramp to board a bus in Miami, Florida. Access to public transportation is an integral aspect of community living for many people with disabilites. (Jeffrey Greenberg/ UIG via Getty Images)

transition from the sidewalk to the street at intersections. While many buses are now equipped with ramps or lifts, automatic audio announcements, and visual stop displays, maintenance issues often make the bus inaccessible, which may result in people being stranded at a bus stop or completely missing their stop.

Greyhound and Amtrak. Buses and trains that travel between cities are known as "intercity public transportation." Amtrak, the largest U.S. intercity train system, is run by the federal government and provides train service between U.S. cities in 46 states. All Amtrak stations were supposed to be completely accessible by 2010. However, studies by the National Disability Rights Network and Amtrak's Office of the Inspector General showed that many stations were still not ADA compliant. Several lawsuits were filed, and in 2015, the U.S. Department of Justice found that Amtrak was in violation and was discriminating against people with disabilities. It outlined what Amtrak was required to do to come into compliance.

Over-the-road buses provide low-cost bus service between U.S. cities. Greyhound, the largest intercity bus company in the United States, provides transportation to nearly 18 million passengers. Greyhound was a target of many ADA protests because of its lack of accessibility in the late 1980s and 1990s. The Over-the-Road Bus Transportation Accessibility Act, signed in 2007, provided the requirements for these companies, which often don't have set stations but rather pick up people at designated locations on the road. As a result of this law, it is unlawful for over-the-road bus companies to deny passage to people with disabilities.

Paratransit. Users of paratransit often have issues with the quality and timeliness of paratransit services, which affects whether people really consider the services reliable or not. This can affect individuals in getting to medical appointments, employment, and other important community activities. There has been criticism from transit providers that the cost of providing paratransit is exceedingly high and is continually growing with increased demand. Transit agencies are pushing to move people away from paratransit and toward fixed-route systems, even if only for some of their local trips. Disability advocates respond by saying that the claim of an increased demand is overblown. A recent report by the Transportation Cooperative Research Program (TCRP) indicates that for every person with a disability riding paratransit, there are between one and five people with disabilities who ride a fixed-route system.

Mobility Management. Mobility management is a growing transit industry practice that involves managing the transportation of a local area, coordinating services, and ensuring efficiency in the transit system as a whole. Trained mobility managers help to coordinate transportation for people with disabilities across the various transportation modes available in a given area. *Travel training* is an important component of mobility management. Travel trainers help individuals with disabilities plan out routes to their most visited locations and become oriented to the whole travel experience. This service can be especially helpful for people with cognitive disabilities, who may need to develop skills in time management, literacy, attention, and problem solving to be able to navigate a transit system independently.

Taxis. Taxicabs can be a vital resource for people with disabilities, but often taxis are not designed to accommodate individuals who have wheelchairs or other mobility devices. According to the ADA, taxicab operators cannot discriminate against people with disabilities or charge them higher fees. However, there are no requirements about taxi fleets and the accessibility of their vehicles. In several cities, there have been large efforts to work with taxicab associations on providing more accessible fleets, comprising vehicles that allow wheelchair users to roll into the cab and that have straps to secure a wheelchair during the drive. After an outcry from disability advocates about the lack of accessible taxis, the Freedom Taxi Company now provides an accessible fleet of taxis in Philadelphia, Pennsylvania. In 2013, a group of disability advocates filed a class action lawsuit against the city of New York for having so few accessible cabs. The city settled the lawsuit and agreed on a mandate to make 50 percent of taxis accessible by 2020.

Air Travel. For many years, people with disabilities had substantial difficulty accessing air travel in the United States, as policies varied from airline to airline. Airlines imposed various restrictions or requirements, such as flying with a companion, for people with disabilities. Following various lawsuits, Congress signed the Air Carrier Access Act of 1986, which set out to ensure equal access to air travel. According to the act, airlines cannot refuse air travel to anyone, regardless of disability, or charge higher rates to people with disabilities. Further, airlines must provide accommodations on flights, and they must transport any kind of wheelchair onboard the aircraft. New aircrafts are required to be built using accessibility standards for entry, seating, and lavatories. Airport facilities are also required to be accessible and to meet the standards for independent use as set forth by the ADA.

Future Directions. New technology aids people with disabilities in using public transportation. In many cities, apps that alert when buses or trains are coming help to plan out local travel and make using transit more efficient and reliable. In some cities, developers have made apps that track when parts of the transit system are not working. For example, an app will alert a user if there is an issue with a station elevator. This information can be communicated to travelers with disabilities ahead of time to allow them to plan an alternate route instead of getting stuck on a train platform. For individuals who are blind or have low vision, some apps and other assistive devices provide audio instructions that can be followed to move around a transit station independently. Such apps, which use GPS signals and other technologies, can let people with cognitive disabilities know when to get off and on buses or trains.

Conclusion

The laws and policies that transportation agencies must follow reshaped public transportation, making it a realistic possibility for people with disabilities. However, several challenges remain, and much improvement is needed before people with disabilities can feel that public transportation is a truly accessible and reliable form of travel. Lack of transportation in general continues to be an ongoing obstacle. Financial challenges often force transit agencies to make difficult decisions, such as cutting service in certain areas with less usage.

Yochai Eisenberg

See also: Americans with Disabilities Act (ADA); Community Living and Community Integration; Employment, Barriers to; Independent Living

Further Reading

Federal Transit Administration. 2017. "American Disabilities Act." http://www.fta.dot.gov/civilrights/12325.html.

National Aging and Disability Transportation Center. "Project Action Transportation." http://www.projectaction.org/.

National Transit Database. 2018. https://www.transit.dot.gov/ntd.

NCD Report. n.d. http://www.who.int/chp/ncd_global_status_report/en/.

Rosenbloom, Sandra. 2007. *The Future of Disability in America*. Washington, DC: National Academies Press.

TCRP Report. 2016. "Strategy Guide to Enable and Promote the Use of Fixed-Route Transit by People with Disabilities." http://www.trb.org/Publications/Blurbs/170626.aspx.

U.S. Department of Transportation. 2015. "Air Carriers Access Act." http://www.transportation.gov/airconsumer/passengers-disabilities.

Q

Quality of Life

The concept of quality of life (QOL) is not new, as a discussion of what constitutes personal well-being dates back to Plato and Aristotle. To appreciate fully the importance of this concept, it is necessary to understand its semantic meaning. "Quality" makes us think of the excellence or "exquisite standard" associated with human characteristics and positive values such as happiness and satisfaction; "of life" indicates that the concept concerns the very essence or essential aspects of human existence. Although this semantic meaning has remained the same over time, since the 1980s there has been significant progress in how the QOL concept is conceptualized, measured, and applied to persons with disabilities.

A common definition of individual quality of life is that it *is a multidimensional phenomenon composed of core domains that constitute personal well-being.* These domains are influenced by both personal characteristics and environmental factors. One's quality of life is the product of these characteristics and factors and can be influenced positively through public policy, quality enhancement strategies, quality thinking, and outcomes evaluation.

QOL is conceptualized as being composed of core domains and domain indicators. *QOL domains* are the set of factors that constitute personal well-being and represent the range over which the QOL concept extends and thus defines a life of quality. *QOL indicators* are QOL-related perceptions, behaviors, and conditions that give an indication of the person's well-being and are used as the basis for QOL assessment. Although there are numerous QOL conceptual models, the present article focuses on the one developed and validated by Schalock and Verdugo (Schalock et al. 2016). The model encompasses the eight core domains and exemplary indicators summarized in table 1.

Approach to Disability

Historically, disability was viewed as a defect, and the cause of the deficit was thought to be centered within the person. Current conceptualizations of disability are closely related to social-ecological models that view human function as the result of a person's condition interacting with environmental factors that can either hinder or facilitate the person's functional level and, especially, quality of life. Chief among the environmental factors that facilitate or enhance are attitudes stressing that disability exists in the environment rather than the person. Supports reduce the discrepancy between the person's capabilities and the environmental demands and, hence, enhance the person's functioning level and opportunity for involvement and participation. Each of these actions is directly related to the core QOL principles of inclusion, self-determination, equity, and empowerment.

Measurement

How one measures QOL is a long-standing debate in the field. Current practices include the following: (1) use a measurement framework that incorporates core QOL domains

Table 1: Quality of Life Domains and Exemplary Indicators

Domain	Exemplary Indicator
Personal Development	Education status Personal competence (cognitive, social, practical)
Self-Determination	Autonomy/personal control Goals and personal values Choices
Interpersonal Relations	Interactions (e.g., social networks) Relationships (family, friends)
Social Inclusion	Community integration Community roles
Rights	Human (respect, dignity, equality) Legal (citizenship, access, due process)
Emotional Well-Being	Contentment (satisfaction, enjoyment) Lack of stress (predictability and control)
Physical Well-Being	Health status Activities of daily living (self-care, mobility)
Material Well-Being	Employment status Possessions

Source: Schalock, Robert L., Miguel-Angel Verdugo, Laura E. Gomez, and Hans S. Reinders. 2016. "Moving Us Toward a Theory of Individual Quality of Life." *American Journal on Intellectual and Developmental Disabilities* 121, no. 1: 1–12.

such as those listed in table 1; (2) employ domain-referenced indicators such as those listed in table 1 as the actual items assessed; (3) employ four to six items per domain; (4) use a three-to-six-point Likert rating scale as the metric to assess each item; (5) provide two versions of the assessment scale that contain the same items, but use one for self-report and the second (involving more objective indicators) for the report of others; and (6) establish the reliability and validity of the assessment instrument.

Quality of life assessment information can be used for multiple purposes at the level of the individual, organization, and system. *The guiding principle is that QOL information is* not *used to compare persons.*

- At the individual level, the information can be used as (1) the basis for a dialogue regarding what is important to the person, thus providing a *communication platform*; (2) a way to provide a holistic view of the person and those domains associated with a life of quality; and (3) feedback to the individual, family members, and organization personnel regarding whether the services and supports provided to the person are influencing one or more QOL domains. This latter use requires that QOL domains are used as a *framework for either providing supports or for developing individual education or support plans* that align individualized supports to personal goals, assessed support needs, specific QOL domain-referenced enhancement strategies, and QOL-related outcomes.
- At the organization level, QOL assessment information is typically aggregated across individuals and used for reporting, benchmarking, and quality improvement.
- At the systems level, QOL assessment information is typically aggregated across organizations within the service delivery system and used for developing provider profiles and systems-wide quality improvement.

Research

Research has played a significant role in both validating the concept of QOL and determining the role that both personal and environmental variables play in QOL-related outcomes. For example, the eight QOL domains listed in table 1 have been shown in cross-cultural research studies to have etic (or universal) properties, whereas QOL domain-referenced indicators have emic (or culture-bound) properties. Since the mid-1980s, and concomitant with the emergence of the approach to disability and organization transformation and systems change described earlier, research studies have also demonstrated that individualized supports and less restrictive, more inclusive environments are associated with positive outcomes across the eight QOL domains. Participatory action research, which involves persons with disabilities in partnership roles in the conduct of research, widely uses QOL-related outcomes as the "evidence" in the development of evidence-based practices.

Implications

Today, most students with disabilities are educated in regular classrooms, and most adults with disabilities live in the community and participate in employment, recreation, and community activities (Braddock et al. 2015; U.S. Department of Education 2014). This has not always been the case, since historically individuals (and especially those with significant limitations in intellectual functioning, adaptive behavior, and behavioral health) were relegated to large, segregated facilities. As a sensitizing notion, and an overriding principle for supports delivery, the concept of quality of life can significantly affect how organizations and service delivery systems approach persons with disabilities. The goal is to have organizations and systems transformed into entities that (1) emphasize QOL-related supports and evaluate QOL outcomes; (2)

implement supports in partnership with persons with disabilities; (3) provide critically needed professional education and support provider development; (4) engage in continuous quality improvement based on the needs of organizations and systems to be both effective and efficient; and (5) are creative in developing programs that are of value to the individual, the person's family, and society (Schalock and Verdugo 2013).

The actions of both professionals and support providers have high stakes for individuals and their quality of life. Thus, it is essential that both groups incorporate into their thinking and daily activities four essential concepts that when implemented enhance the quality of the support recipient's life: (1) an appreciation for the capacity of the individual; (2) a QOL-related language of thought and action; (3) the supports paradigm; and (4) a sensitivity to QOL-related behavioral indicators.

The Supports Paradigm

The supports paradigm began influencing the field of disabilities in the mid-1980s and augments the social-ecological model of disability. Supports are intended to bridge the gap between the individual's functioning and participation opportunities and the requirements of the person's social and physical environment. Minimizing this gap enhances individual functioning and increases meaningful participation. The net result is an improvement in one's quality of life. An overview of the specific components of a system of supports and their intended consequences is presented in table 2.

Conclusion

In conclusion, for each of us, the quest for a life of quality is a journey. We have come a long way in our understanding of what

Table 2: A System of Supports Components, Exemplary Strategies, and Potential Outcomes

Potential Outcomes	System Component	Exemplary Strategy
Natural supports	Support networks (e.g., family, friends, colleagues, generic agencies)	Increased social inclusion, interpersonal relations, social-emotional well-being
Technology based	Assistive and information technology	Increased cognitive functioning, control, and life-long learning
Education and training	Universal design for learning	Enhanced adaptive behavior and personal functioning
Environmental accommodation	Smart homes, modified transportation, job accommodation	Enhanced personal development, community living, and integrated employment
Incentives	Involvement, recognition, personal goal setting	Increased motivation and achievement
Personal strengths	Incorporating interests, skills and knowledge, and positive attitudes into support plans	Increased self-regulation, autonomy, and self-determination
Professional services	Access to allied health services	Increased personal development, physical and behavioral health, interpersonal relations, and emotional well-being

quality of life is, how it can be assessed, and how the QOL concept can become a language of thought and be applied to enhance personal development, self-determination, interpersonal relations, social inclusion, rights, and emotional, physical, and material well-being.

In the end, it is the journey that makes our effort worthwhile. Thus, we try always to improve the quality of life for all people, understanding that there is no end, no stopping point—and that we are always striving for improvement. Thus, quality of life is not an end but simply the meaning of the experience, the process of life. Maybe, in the words of the old Chinese proverb, "the journey is the reward."

Robert L. Schalock

See also: Health-Related Quality of Life; International Classification of Functioning, Disability, and Health (ICF); Life Expectancy

Further Reading

Braddock, David, Richard Hemp, Mary C. Rizzolo, E. Shea Tanis, Laura Haffer, and Jiang Wu. 2015. *State of the States in Developmental Disabilities*. Washington, DC: American Association on Intellectual and Developmental Disabilities.

Brown, Ivan, Chris Hatton, and Eric Emerson. 2013. "Quality of Life Indicators for Individuals with Intellectual Disabilities: Extending Current Practices." *Intellectual and Developmental Disabilities* 51: 316–322.

Keith, Kenneth D., and Robert L. Schalock. 2018. *Cross-Cultural Quality of Life: Enhancing the Lives of Persons with Intellectual Disability*. Washington, DC: American Association on Intellectual and Developmental Disabilities.

Nussbaum, Martha C. 2011. *Creating Capabilities: The Human Development Approach*. Cambridge, MA: Belknap Press of Harvard University Press.

Reinders, Hans S., and Robert L. Schalock. 2014. "How Organizations Can Enhance the Quality of Life of Their Clients and Assess Their Results: The Concept of QOL Enhancement." *American Journal of Intellectual and Developmental Disabilities* 119: 291–302.

Schalock, Robert L., and Miguel-Angel Verdugo. 2012. *A Leadership Guide for Today's Disabilities Organizations: Overcoming Challenges and Making Change Happen.* Baltimore: Brookes.

Schalock, Robert L., and Miguel-Angel Verdugo. 2013. "The Transformation of Disability Organizations." *Intellectual and Developmental Disabilities* 51, no. 4: 273–286.

Schalock, Robert L., Miguel-Angel Verdugo, Laura E. Gomez, and Hans S. Reinders. 2016. "Moving Us Toward a Theory of Individual Quality of Life." *American Journal on Intellectual and Developmental Disabilities* 121, no. 1: 1–12.

Thompson, James R., Robert L. Schalock, John Agosta, Lilia Teninty, and Jon Fortune. 2014. "How the Supports Paradigm Is Transforming Service Systems for Persons with Intellectual Disability and Related Developmental Disabilities." *Inclusion* 2: 86–99.

U.S. Department of Education. 2014. "38th Annual Report to Congress on the Implementation of the Individuals with Disabilities Education Act." https://www2.ed.gov /about/reports/annual/osep/2016/parts-b -c/38th-arc-for-idea.pdf.

Queer Identity and Politics

The intersection of queerness and disability is a rich area of study for research, activism, and art. There are similarities in theories about queerness and disability, as well as similar lived experiences between queer and disabled people. There is also a subgroup of queer, disabled people who have unique experiences at the intersection of both identities.

In this entry, "queer" is defined as an umbrella term that includes the entire lesbian, gay, bisexual, and transgender (LGBT) community. Likewise, disability is defined broadly, including physical, mental, emotional, and sensory disabilities. One should note that the word "queer" often has a political meaning in the LGBT community, similar to the word "crip" in the disability community.

Queer-Disability Intersections

There are many intersections between the queer and disability communities. Both communities have similar shared experiences of medicalization (having their identities viewed as medical conditions), lack of access to health care, and criminalization (having their identities viewed as legal or criminal problems). Many queer and disabled people also have similar experiences of growing up in nondisabled or nonqueer community and developing identity, coming out, and finding community later in life (sometimes called "chosen family"). Because both disabled people and queer people are often told by medical or legal officials what to think of their identities, self-determination (the freedom to choose one's own life path) and self-definition (the freedom to define one's own identity) are important in both disability and queer communities.

There are myths about disability, sexuality, and queerness in the media. These myths have real effects for disabled and queer people in society. Myths that disabled people are not sexual or are sexual only in ways that are not considered normal, can affect disabled people who want to be proud of their queer identity. Some of these myths lead people to assume that disabled people cannot be queer.

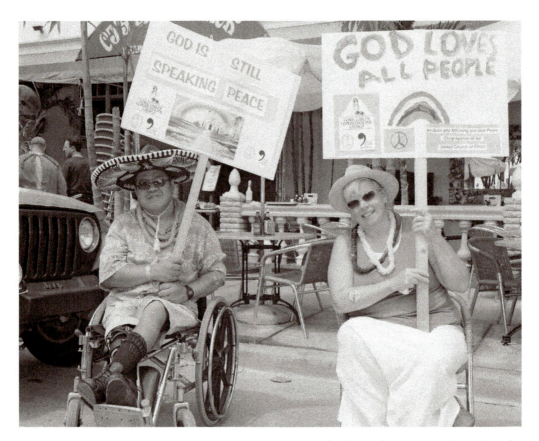

A disabled man and woman in wheelchairs hold signs at a Gay Pride Day event in Miami Beach, Florida. There are similar theories about queer and disability identities, as well as many activists who identify as both queer and disabled. (Jeff Greenberg/UIG via Getty Images)

Although there are many similarities between queer and disabled identities, there are some differences between these experiences. There are also people who have different experiences because they are both queer and disabled. Queer and disability intersections include both ideas (queer theory and disability theory) and people (queer and/or disabled people).

Background and History

Identities of both queer and disabled communities have a history of being viewed as individual medical problems by physicians and scientists. Starting in the 19th century, queerness was seen as a mental illness in much of the world. Psychiatrists researched the causes of queerness and tried to find "cures." Many queer people were subjected to harsh medical interventions, including electroshock therapy and lobotomy, in an attempt to "cure" them (Cruz 1998). Attempts to cure queerness continued from the 20th century into the 21st in the form of "reparative therapy" or "gender orientation conversion therapy." While conversion therapy is banned in some U.S. states, it continues today. The modern queer rights movement has fought hard for the medical community to stop viewing queerness as a mental illness. Homosexuality was removed from the DSM in 1973, although other diagnoses that apply to transgender and queer people, like gender identity disorder and later gender dysphoria, stayed in the DSM. Many Americans now believe that people are born queer. Fewer Americans view queerness as a disease.

Similarly, disability is frequently considered a personal medical problem in need of pity and cure. The medical model view of disability is common, and physicians and scientists spend a lot of time and money trying to prevent or cure disability. The disability movement has not yet been as successful as the queer movement in changing public opinion to view disability as a social identity instead of a medical problem. Disabled people are still institutionalized (put into nursing homes, hospitals, or institutions) at high rates and face continued struggles to claim their right to live with or without medical treatment.

Queer people are overrepresented in prison (Meyer et al. 2017). Disabled people—specifically those with mental illness, intellectual disabilities, and learning disabilities—are also overrepresented in prison, making up more than half of the prison population in some studies (Smith 2005). Both queer and disabled people face harsh medical and social treatments because of their identities. This treatment may be particularly intense for those people who are both queer and disabled. Both queer and disabled persons have been deeply affected by scientific and social views about their identities.

Related Policy

Several policies are relevant to both queer and disability communities and politics. The Americans with Disabilities Act (ADA), a defining policy for disability rights in the United States, also protects persons with HIV/AIDS (a health condition that disproportionately affects queer people) against discrimination.

Although the ADA has created many protections against employment discrimination because of disability, discrimination and inaccessibility remain large problems. Employment discrimination is also a major issue for queer people; discrimination because of sexual orientation and gender identity is legal in most U.S. states (Human Rights Campaign [HRC] 2017). Similarly, housing discrimination and accessibility are major issues for both queer and disabled people. Housing discrimination because of sexual orientation and gender identity is legal in most U.S. states (HRC 2017).

Throughout history, immigration policies have excluded both queer and disabled migrants from entering the United States. HIV-positive immigrants were banned from entering the United States from 1993 until 2010.

As of June 2015, same-sex marriage (marriage equality) became legal in the United States. This legalization of same-sex marriage had important legal effects for queer disabled people as well, because same-sex partners could more easily share health care coverage.

Key Concepts

Queer scholars played an important role in disability studies. In 2000, disabled queer people worked together to host an international Queer Disability Conference in San Francisco. There have also been queer and disabled working groups at conferences. Queer theory has been used to develop disability studies theory. Scholars have used the intersection of disability and queerness to unite on shared experiences. Scholars have also created theory about the ways that queerness and disability inform each other, as seen in Carrie Sandahl's "Queering the

Crip or Cripping the Queer" (2003), Robert McRuer's *Crip Theory* (2006), and Alison Kafer's *Feminist, Queer, Crip* (2013).

Performance artists and visual artists have also explored the intersections of queerness and disability by including activism in their art. One example is Sins Invalid, a queer, disabled, people of color–led performance art group based in Oakland, California. This group also works with intersectional issues of police brutality, institutionalization, and criminalization. Designers and visual artists like Sky Cubacub, creator of Rebirth Garments in Chicago, embrace the intersection of queerness, disability, and other marginalized identities by creating custom-made clothing as a point of affirmation, pride, and community building. Petra Kuppers, director of The Olimpias performance project in Ann Arbor, Michigan, also uses queer and disabled social justice initiatives. These groups also overlap with communities of color and the fat/body positive community.

Queer and disabled scholars and activists have often also seen disability and queerness as a site for memoir and storytelling, such as in Eli Clare's *Exile and Pride: Disability, Queerness, and Liberation*; Corbett O'Toole's *Fading Scars: My Queer Disability History*; and Terry Galloway's *Mean Little Deaf Queer*. Queer and disabled people also have a strong presence in Internet and blog communities, such as in the NeuroQueer blog, a blog celebrating queer, neurodiverse work. The related independent publishing house, Autonomous Press, publishes the work of queer, disabled, and other marginalized writers. There are also disability categories in other social justice blogs, such as The Body Is Not an Apology and Autostraddle.

Dilemmas, Debates, and Unresolved Questions

Although there are many intersections of queerness and disability in culture and scholarship, it is important to note that discrimination against queer and transgender people in disability community has limited coalition and activism. Likewise, inaccessibility in queer spaces has limited disability inclusion in the queer community. Queer community events often take place in inaccessible spaces, and many queer organizations fail to include disabled community members in their leadership and planning. In the past, Centers for Independent Living refused to serve some people living with HIV/AIDS, creating further divides and limiting access (O'Toole 2015).

How can we break down barriers between queer and disability communities that keep us from supporting each other? Are disabled and queer communities working more closely than before, or have the issues simply shifted and evolved? These questions remain complex and unanswered, but they are useful in examining the landscape.

Conclusion: The Future of Queer-Disability Intersectionality

There is great potential for coalitional organizing across and within queer and disability communities around issues affecting both groups. Queer and disability communities could collaborate in advocacy for inclusive sexual education, improved bathroom accessibility (see the work of People in Search of Safe and Accessible Restrooms [PISSAR]), and improved mental health care for queer and disabled people. Queer and disability communities could also stand together against employment and housing discrimination, police brutality, institutionalization, incarceration, and conversion therapy. Within the academy, future work is needed to theorize queer and disability intersections and to increase representation of queer and disabled people's perspectives in research.

Elizabeth Adare Harrison and Alison Kopit

See also: Crip and Crip Culture; Critical Disability Studies; Intersectionality of Race, Gender, and Disability; Medicalization

Further Reading

Clare, Eli. 1999. *Exile and Pride: Disability, Queerness, and Liberation.* Cambridge: SouthEnd Press.

Cruz, David. 1998. "Controlling Desires: Sexual Orientation Conversion and the Limits of Knowledge and Law." *Southern California Law Review* 72, no. 5: 1297.

Human Rights Campaign (HRC). 2017. "State Maps of Laws and Policies." https://www.hrc.org/state-maps/housing.

Kafer, Alison. 2013. *Feminist, Queer, Crip.* Bloomington: Indiana University Press.

McRuer, Robert. 2006. *Crip Theory: Cultural Signs of Queerness and Disability.* New York: New York University Press.

Meyer, Ilan, Andrew Flores, Lara Stemple, Adam Romero, Bianca Wilson, and Jody Herman. 2017. "Incarceration Rates and Traits of Sexual Minorities in the United States: National Inmate Survey, 2011–2012." *American Journal of Public Health* 107, no. 2: 267–273.

O'Toole, Corbett. 2015. *Fading Scars: My Queer Disability History.* Fort Worth, TX: Autonomous Press.

Sandahl, Carrie. 2003. "Queering the Crip or Cripping the Queer: Intersections of Queer and Crip Identities in Solo Autobiographical Performance." Special issue of *GLQ: A Journal of Lesbian and Gay Studies* 9, no. 1–2: 25–56.

Smith, Phil. 2005. "'There Is No Treatment Here': Disability and Health Needs in a State Prison System." *Disability Studies Quarterly* 25, no. 3.

R

Race and Mental Health

Racial discrimination is a source of perceived stress. For the majority of nonwhite and multiracial individuals, discrimination is accompanied by stress, which in turn has a negative effect on both physical and mental health. As a result, it can be argued, race indirectly affects mental health by means of experienced discrimination.

How Does Race Affect Mental Health?

Knowing the impacts of stress from perceived racial discrimination and the consequences for the mental health of nonwhite populations is significant. For example, the health of African Americans has been steadily declining; not all of the decline may be traced to inequalities in other areas, such as socioeconomic status. Stress is a normal part of life, and individuals will experience differences in how vulnerable they are to the effects of stress. The body has neurological systems that protect other systems in the body from the negative impacts of stress. However, if these protective processes are activated too frequently, "overactivation" can occur and lead to physical or mental health problems.

There are serious implications of overactivation, or excess stress. The negative symptoms due to repeatedly adapting to stress are called "allostatic load." People who are black have been found to have higher allostatic loads compared to people who are white and are of the same age. Higher-income individuals who are black also have a greater probability of having a larger allostatic load than economically disadvantaged people who are white. These racial disparities suggest that the health of black Americans may be affected, to some degree, by race.

Acknowledgment of these racial disparities is important to disability studies because the field seeks to express the perspectives of persons who are disabled and, therefore, marginalized. People who are black and multirace individuals are already marginalized groups. These groups are further marginalized given the impact of race on mental health and related disability.

Background and History

In 1997, David R. Williams, a sociology and public health professor at the University of Michigan, and his colleagues investigated how racial differences in socioeconomic status, social class, perceived discrimination, and other types of stress influenced the differences in the physical and mental health outcomes between people who are black and people who are white. The researchers felt that previous studies conducted in the area of racial health disparity were racist. Earlier research studies assumed results showing health declines for minority groups meant that race was the cause of inherent biological differences between people. Breaking from this trend, Professor Williams and his team defined race as a social construction. In other words, the meaning of race in society is the product of beliefs about race and not a result of race creating biological differences. Williams and his colleagues did not believe that races were distinct from one another; they argued that the decline in the health status of black Americans is better understood by studying differences in income and wealth between white and nonwhite people in the United States. In 2003, Professor Williams, along with other researchers, concluded that health may be negatively influenced by the stress of racial discrimination, with mental health being particularly affected. Environmental stressors like urban noise, air pollution, and overcrowding should also be considered stressors related to race, as these too may result from underlying discrimination.

The work of Professor Williams and his team has been extended by the work of Professor Arline Geronimus, also at the University of Michigan. In 2006, Geronimus examined whether black Americans experience more health deterioration than white people of the same age. Professor Geronimus found that African Americans have a higher allostatic load than people who are white. She states that these differences are due to our race-conscious society. Her work aims to prove that stress is the cause of physical and mental problems in nonwhite populations. Professor Geronimus coined the term "allostatic load."

Race, Mental Health, and Disability

Differences in race are accompanied by differences in mental health status. This correlation is partly because of greater exposure to perceived discrimination potentially resulting in differences in vulnerability to stress. Often, minority populations are assumed to have poor coping methods when faced with a major stressor. It is important to consider that these individuals may be coping with the secondary stress of perceived discrimination as well.

The 2001 *Supplement to the Surgeon General's Report of 1999* was an important document about race and mental health. The supplement addressed how culture, race, and ethnicity influence the way mental health services are used and delivered. The report expressed concerns regarding disparities for minorities in the prevention and treatment of mental illness. When Professor David Williams studied the decline of minority health outcomes, he found the decline to be most prominent in the area of mental health. Racial and ethnic discrimination was associated with more chronic health problems, depressive symptoms, and diagnosed depression, as well as reduced life satisfaction.

The supplement pointed out that many of the disparities due to the racism in society are on the levels of both individual and society. Thus, it is significant that nonwhite individuals and families are more likely to be of lower socioeconomic status compared to white people. Multiracial people experience among the highest levels of psychological distress (Bratter and Eschbach 2005). Nonwhite individuals are also more likely to have a disability, including serious mental illness. Because of the disadvantages that result from being poor or having a disability, minority populations may have less access to doctors, medication, general care, and other medical necessities. This lack of access to appropriate care and services can make mental health conditions worsen. Thus, the negative consequences of untreated mental health issues will disproportionately affect people of color, who are more likely to have lower income, limited opportunities, and less access to care.

Dilemmas, Debates, and Unresolved Questions

A dilemma for racial and ethnic minorities is their mistrust of the mental health system. Many researchers mention this mistrust as a barrier to receiving treatment. Hispanic American people tend to under-use mental health services. This problem is compounded within the mental health system; many providers do not understand the importance of involving extended family members when treating people of Hispanic origin. This lack of understanding dis-suades Hispanic people from fully utilizing mental health treatment options.

Stigma is a major obstacle for minorities seeking mental health treatment. Some research has found that African American people with major depressive disorder do not seek professional mental health treatment because of fears of being hospitalized or institutionalized. People who are Asian American have been found to delay mental health treatment until symptoms are severe. They may experience cultural barriers, such as language barriers, lack of insurance, and unfamiliarity with available mental health resources. However, though Asian Americans delay treatment until symptoms become too difficult for them to deal with alone, once the symptoms have reached a point of severity, they seek mental health services at a rate greater than the general population does.

Native Americans and Alaska Natives are disadvantaged in terms of the mental health care they receive. Native Americans and Alaska Natives have the most access to culturally appropriate health care in their own native communities, where they are served by the Indian Health Service. However, they are increasingly moving from their reservation communities into urban settings. This change often affects access to health care. In their own communities, the federal government funds their health care services (though the amount of money is very limited).

More Native Americans and Alaska Natives have disabilities when compared to people who are white. They also experience persistent mental illness at a greater rate than the general population. Native American men experience alcoholism, suicide, and depression at much higher rates than the general population. Many mental health providers who provide services to Native people do not provide culturally appropriate services. In addition, there are also few providers of services for Native Americans and Alaska Natives.

Conclusion: The Future of Race, Mental Health, and Disability

International perspectives have expanded our understanding of mental health disability. In the United States, hearing voices and having hallucinations are considered to be forms of mental illness. However, in some small minority cultures in Africa and South America, for example, those who hear voices or have hallucinations are considered holy or divinely gifted. There are now social movements in Western cultures to consider such symptoms as extrasensory events and not abnormal.

Psychiatry is experimenting with treating serious mental health conditions without medication. For example, in Finland, a treatment known as open dialogue involves a person experiencing severe symptoms being surrounded by mental health professionals, friends, and family. The individual receives support through their relationships, and without medication. This treatment has proved to have long-term mental health benefits. The future of alternative mental health treatment continues to evolve.

Andrea Cooke

See also: Criminal Justice System and Incarceration; Intersectionality of Race, Gender, and Disability; Mental Health and Developmental Disabilities; Mental Health

Self-Help and Support Groups; *Primary Documents*: Article on "Drapetomania" in Dr. Cartwright's *Diseases and Peculiarities of the Negro Race* (1851)

Further Reading

Ben-Moshe, Liat, and Sandy Magnana. 2014. "An Introduction to Race, Gender, and Disability Studies, and Families of Color." *Women, Gender, and Families of Color* 2, no. 2: 105–114.

Bratter, Jennifer L., and Karl Eschbach. 2005. "Race/Ethnic Differences in Nonspecific Psychological Distress: Evidence from the National Health Survey." *Social Science Quarterly* 86, no. 3: 620–644.

Geronimus, Arline T., Margaret Hicken, Danya Keene, and John Bond. 2006. "'Weathering' and Age Patterns of Allostatic Load Scores among Blacks and Whites in the United States." *American Journal of Public Health* 96, no. 5: 792–797.

U.S. Department of Health and Human Services. 2001. *Culture, Race and Ethnicity—A Supplement to Mental Health: A Report of the Surgeon General.* Rockville, MD: U.S. Department of Health and Human Services, Substance Abuse and Mental Health Services Administration, Center for Mental Health Services.

Williams, David R., Yan Yu, James S. Jackson, and Norman B. Anderson. 1997. "Racial Ethnic Differences in Physical and Mental Health: Socio-economic Status, Stress and Discrimination." *Journal of Health Psychology* 2, no. 3: 335–351.

Refugees. See Immigrants and Refugees

S

Schoolwide Systems of Supports

Schoolwide systems of supports for people with disabilities are prevention-oriented frameworks or approaches that assist school personnel in (1) adopting and organizing educational practices based on research evidence (i.e., evidence-based practices); (2) implementing those practices effectively; and (3) maximizing academic, social, emotional, and behavioral outcomes for all students in a school, including students with disabilities (Sugai and Horner 2002). Schoolwide systems of supports for people with disabilities are systematic and effective approaches for improving academic and social behavior outcomes for all children and youth in schools.

Schoolwide Systems of Supports Frameworks

Schools use different types of supports frameworks. A multi-tiered system of supports (MTSS) is a multilevel, prevention-oriented framework for organizing a school's resources to address each individual student's academic and nonacademic needs. A MTSS is preventive in that it allows for early identification of academic and nonacademic needs and for timely intervention for students who are at risk for poor learning outcomes. A MTSS is organized by tiers of interventions that vary in intensity and are accessed by students on the basis of student need. The tiers, sometimes referred to as levels of prevention, are described as tier 1, primary/universal supports with a focus on prevention; tier 2, secondary/targeted supports with a focus on early intervention; and tier 3, tertiary/individualized supports with a focus on intensive intervention. Positive behavioral interventions and supports (PBIS) and response to intervention (RTI) are examples of multilevel, schoolwide prevention frameworks for improving academic and social behavior outcomes for all students. PBIS and RTI frameworks share core features: School-based teams use data-informed decision making. Regular screening allows for early identification of student academic and nonacademic needs so timely, evidence-based interventions may be used for students who are at risk for poor learning outcomes. Student progress is continuously monitored. Students access a tiered continuum of interventions with adjustments in intensity and nature of supports based on a student's responsiveness. In a MTSS framework such as PBIS and RTI, there is priority emphasis on high-quality implementation of interventions to ensure students receive full benefit. Schoolwide systems of supports frameworks like PBIS and RTI have been used as an approach to change the way school personnel think about and plan quality instruction and inclusion of persons with disabilities in schools.

Background/History

People with Disabilities and Inclusion. American social movements, such as the women's rights movement, the civil rights movement, the disability rights movement, and the independent living movement, that evolved during the 1970s and 1980s are examples of the ongoing importance of extending individual rights to formally disenfranchised groups, facilitating the inclusion of those groups into the mainstream of society (Carr et al. 2002). The inclusion movement for people with disabilities continues in education with a trend toward supporting students with disabilities in general education settings and away from the historically default practices of segregation in special education facilities based on disability. MTSS supports inclusive practices as opposed to the long-established exclusion approach.

Children with Disabilities and the Law. A significant step toward expanding inclusive educational opportunities for children with disabilities was the Education for All Handicapped Children Act (Public Law (PL) 94-142). Congress enacted PL 94-142 in 1975 to support states and localities in protecting the rights of, meeting the individual needs of, and improving the results for children with disabilities and their families. This landmark law is currently enacted as the Individuals with Disabilities Education Act (IDEA), as amended in 1997 (U.S. Department of Education 2017). In the IDEA, Congress stated:

> Disability is a natural part of the human experience and in no way, diminishes the right of individuals to participate in or contribute to society. Improving educational results for children with disabilities is an essential element of our national policy of ensuring equality of opportunity, full participation, independent living, and economic self-sufficiency for individuals with disabilities.

With P.L. 94-142, Congress responded to concern for the more than 1 million children with disabilities who had been excluded entirely from the education system and those who had only limited access to the education system, denying them an appropriate education. The latter group comprised more than half of all children with disabilities who were living in the United States in the early 1970s. Families, educators, and researchers focused on improved access to educational opportunities for children with disabilities over the last quarter of the 20th century (U.S. Department of Education 2017).

The goals of improving educational results for children with disabilities are expressed in PBIS and RTI connections to the IDEA. In amending the IDEA both in 1997 and in 2004, Congress recognized the potential of PBIS to prevent exclusion and improve educational results (PBIS 2017). Congress's reasons for encouraging the use of PBIS stem from the historic exclusion of individuals with emotional and behavioral disabilities from educational opportunities.

In the IDEA 2004 amendments, states are allowed, but not required, the use of a process based on the child's "response to scientific, research-based intervention" (i.e., RTI) as part of their criteria for determining whether a child has a specific learning disability (Individuals with Disabilities Education Act 2004). Additionally, over time, different models of RTI have emerged (e.g., the problem-solving model) for supporting the academic and social behavior needs of all students in both general and special education environments.

Important Points to Know

Real-Life Example: Ben's Story. Ben is a person with disabilities who attended a middle school with a PBIS schoolwide system of supports in place. Ben needed a communication board (a device that enables a person with disabilities to communicate through pictures) to help him succeed in school. Ben's middle school leadership team met and looked at schoolwide behavior data regularly. The team found that some students were receiving discipline referrals for problems they were having in the hallways during transitions between classes. Ben was one of those students. The team decided that the students needed extra support in learning behavior expectations for moving through the hallways during transition times. The intervention was reteaching the expectations to those students, giving them opportunities to practice transitioning between classes correctly, and acknowledging their successes. Once the intervention began, the team checked on the progress of the students regularly and found that all the students were improving except for Ben. They realized that he needed even more support to be successful. Ben's teacher suggested that additional pictures be added to his communication board to assist him in understanding the behavior expectations and in learning the behavior skills for transitioning between classes in the hallways. Along with new communication board pictures, Ben was given more reteaching of the expectations, opportunities to practice transitioning between classes correctly, and acknowledgement of his successes. The team continued to check Ben's progress and found that over time Ben was no longer receiving discipline referrals.

Ben's story is an example of a schoolwide system of structures and procedures enabling adults to support a student with disabilities to successfully remain fully included in his school. This is possible when:

- adults and students share common vision, values, language, and experience;
- school personnel consider how environment affects student learning, moving away from a medical model approach that assumes an intraindividual (i.e.,

within the student) source of learning problems; and
- school personnel select and effectively use evidence-based practices to benefit students.

Dilemmas, Debates, and Unresolved Questions

Multilevel schoolwide systems of supports offer a promise of improving educational outcomes for all students. Some propose that more school-district demonstrations of implementing these systems across all schools, for all academic and social behavior skills, at all three intervention levels, for all students, are needed to understand the impact schoolwide systems of supports have on improving outcomes for all students, especially children and youth with disabilities. Schoolwide systems of supports require school personnel to have the knowledge and skills to be able to implement frameworks like PBIS and RTI and sustain them over time. Critics and supporters of schoolwide systems of supports both argue that educational agencies need adequate access to, including funding for, training for school personnel in methods and approaches of schoolwide systems of supports to ensure those methods and approaches will be effective. If, as Congress stated, "disability is a natural part of the human experience" and we move away from, as Ware (2004) described, the "hunt for disability" in order to "fix" or prevent difference, what role might a sustained schoolwide learner-centered approach have in transforming the marginalization and stigma of disability?

Future Directions for Schoolwide Systems of Supports for People with Disabilities

Conversations continue about ways for school personnel to choose and design evidence-based interventions, partner with families, address the needs of students with disabilities who are also English-language learners, and include the perspectives of students with disabilities within schoolwide systems of supports frameworks. Families, educators, and researchers continue to study and discuss the impact schoolwide systems of supports have had on producing measurable and significant outcomes for all students, including students with disabilities in schools.

Susan Sarno Gasber

See also: Inclusive Education; Inclusive Language as Advocacy; (In)Exclusion; Natural Supports; Paraprofessionals; Transitional Experiences of Students with Disabilities

Further Reading

Carr, Edward G., Glen Dunlap, Robert H. Horner, Robert L. Koegel, Ann P. Turnbull, Wayne Sailor, Jacki Andersen, Richard W. Albin, Lynn K. Koegel, and Lise Fox. 2002. "Positive Behavior Support: Evolution of an Applied Science." *Journal of Positive Behavior Interventions* 2, no. 3: 131–143.

Individuals with Disabilities Education Act, 34 CFR §300.307(a)(2). 2004.

Positive Behavior Interventions and Supports. 2017. "PBIS and the Law." http://www.pbis.org/.

Sugai, George, and Robert H. Horner. 2002. "The Evolution of Discipline Practices: School-wide Positive Behavior Supports." In *Behavior Psychology in the Schools: Innovations in Evaluation, Support, and Consultation*, edited by James K. Luiselli and Charles Diament, 23–50. New York: Haworth Press.

U.S. Department of Education. 2017. "History: Twenty-Five Years of Progress in Educating Children with Disabilities through IDEA." https://www2.ed.gov/policy/speced/leg/idea/history.html.

Ware, Linda. 2004. *Ideology and the Politics of In(Exclusion)*. New York: Peter Lang Publishers.

Section 504 of the Rehabilitation Act

Section 504 of the Rehabilitation Act of 1973 provided protection from exclusion for people with disabilities in the United Sates. While short and concise, Section 504 has implications for secondary schools, postsecondary educational institutions, and employment sites, making it invaluable for the protection of people with disabilities.

What Is Section 504 of the Rehabilitation Act of 1973?

The Rehabilitation Act was passed in 1973 as a continuation of the Smith-Fess Act of 1920, which started vocational rehabilitation (VR) services for the civilian population in the United States. The purpose of the Rehabilitation Act of 1973 was to increase funding of the VR programs in each state and offer more services (Scotch 2001). The Rehabilitation Act of 1973 includes the following seven titles (U.S. Department of Education 2010, 3):

1. VR Services
2. Research and Training
3. Professional Development and Special Projects and Demonstrations
4. National Council on Disability
5. Rights and Advocacy
6. Employment Opportunities for Individuals with Disabilities
7. Independent Living Services and Centers for Independent Living

Several agencies are responsible for carrying out the seven titles, including the

Department of Education (specifically the Office of Special Education and Rehabilitative Services [OSERS] and the Rehabilitation Services Administration [RSA]); the Departments of Labor and Justice; the Equal Employment Opportunity Commission (EEOC); the Architectural and Transportation Barriers Compliance Board; and the National Council on Disability (NCD). In the original Rehabilitation Act of 1973, section 504 stated:

No otherwise qualified individual with a disability in the United States, as defined in section 705 (20) of this title, shall, solely by reason of his or her disability, be excluded from the participation in, be denied the benefits of, or be subjected to discrimination under any program or activity receiving Federal financial assistance or under any program or activity conducted by any Executive agency or by the United States Postal Service. (29 U.S.C. §701)

This sentence on antidiscrimination for agencies receiving federal funding is the entirety of section 504 and was developed based on Title VI of the Civil Rights Act of 1964. However, while the Civil Rights Act refers to race and ethnicity, Section 504 refers to disability (Scotch 2001). This language was originally used in an attempt to amend the Civil Rights Act of 1964 in 1972, subsequently resulting in the language's inclusion in the 1973 Rehabilitation Act as section 504 (Scotch 2001). Section 504 of the Rehabilitation Act was not discussed during its passage. Scotch (2001) notes that it is unclear why the legislators did not discuss the statement.

The inclusion of Section 504 in the Rehabilitation Act of 1973 was critical for people with disabilities. The passage of the Civil Rights Act of 1964 brought about protections for some people, but not those with disabilities. People with disabilities needed protection in a world that was exclusionary, and Section 504 was able to accomplish that.

Important Points to Understand about Section 504

Section 504 and Secondary Students with Disabilities. Section 504 affects students with disabilities in all levels of their education. While in secondary school, some students do not receive special education services but instead qualify for services and protection under Section 504. When they become adults, if attending postsecondary education, they are covered by the ADA and Section 504. Typically, these are students with learning disabilities that require classroom accommodations, such as extended time for exams. Section 504 indicates that students must have physical access to education, as well as to needed accommodations and modifications to participate fully (U.S. Department of Education 2010).

Some students with disabilities may not be entitled to services under Individuals with Disabilities Education Improvement Act (IDEIA), but they may qualify for services under Section 504. There are different requirements for students receiving services under Section 504. Unlike the IDEIA, the school system is not required to initiate services; rather, the student or the family must identify the need for services to the school (Stodden, Jones, and Chang 2002). Students receiving services under Section 504 are not required to have an *individualized education program* (IEP) (National Center for Learning Disabilities 2014) because these students do not need the same level or types of supports and services necessary for students with disabilities covered under the IDEIA. However, students with disabilities found eligible under Section 504 will receive a *504 plan* that serves as a guide to the supports and services needed to attain successful education outcomes (National Center for Learning Disabilities 2014).

Transition to Postsecondary Education. The main laws that protect students with disabilities in postsecondary education are the Americans with Disabilities Act of 1990 (ADA) and Section 504 of the Rehabilitation Act of 1973. The ADA protects students in publicly funded or privately funded institutions, while Section 504 of the Rehabilitation Act of 1973 protects students with disabilities in institutions receiving any public funding (Thomas 2000). Because of this difference, policy discrepancies surface for students with disabilities as they transition from protection under IDEIA to the ADA and Section 504.

Overall, both the ADA and Section 504 state that postsecondary institutions cannot deny admission or otherwise discriminate against students with disabilities (Thomas 2000). Postsecondary institutions may not have the same resources as secondary schools, but they still must make every effort to provide reasonable or alternative accommodations (Thomas 2000). Further, students with disabilities are no longer entitled to the services included under the IDEIA and now must meet the eligibility requirements of the ADA and Section 504. Namely, students with disabilities must self-identify as having a disability and pay for and provide the necessary documentation (Shaw 2006; Stodden, Jones, and Chang 2002). This change often causes confusion as many students and families discover that having an IEP or a Section 504 plan does not guarantee services in postsecondary education.

Section 504 and Employment. Students transitioning to employment are covered under the ADA but may also be covered under Section 504. The ADA is widely acknowledged as the main legislation protecting people with disabilities in employment, as it covers both publicly and privately funded organizations. However, people with disabilities are also covered under Section 504 if employed by an organization receiving public funding (Office of Civil Rights 2006).

Conclusion

Section 504 of the Rehabilitation Act of 1973 came about during an era of exclusion and oppression for people with disabilities. The act led to the provision of protection for people with disabilities across education and employment settings. While the goal of the Rehabilitation Act was to increase funding to the Vocational Rehabilitation program, Section 504 has provided much more than could have ever been imagined, particularly in the area of postsecondary education.

Jessica Awsumb

See also: Americans with Disabilities Act (ADA); Individuals with Disabilities Education Improvement Act (IDEIA); Vocational Rehabilitation; *Primary Documents*: Excerpt from the Rehabilitation Act (1973); Kitty Cone's "Short History of the 504 Sit In" for the Twentieth Anniversary of the Sit In (1997)

Further Reading

Americans with Disabilities Act of 1990, as Amended, Pub. L. No. 110-325, §2, 104 Stat. 328. 2008.

National Center for Learning Disabilities. 2014. "Section 504 of the Rehabilitation Act of 1973." http://www.ncld.org /disability-advocacy/learn-ld-laws/adaaa -section-504/section-504-idea-comparison -chart.

Office of Civil Rights. 2006. "Your Rights under Section 504 of the Rehabilitation Act." http://www.hhs.gov/ocr/504.html.

Section 504 of the Rehabilitation Act of 1973. 1973. Pub. L. No. 93-112, §87 Stat. 394.

Scotch, Richard. 2001. *From Good Will to Civil Rights: Transforming Federal Disability Policy.* Philadelphia: Temple University Press.

Shaw, Stan. 2006. "Legal and Policy Perspectives on Transition Assessment and Documentation." *Career Development for Exceptional Individuals* 29, no. 2: 108–113.

Stodden, Robert A., Megan A. Jones, and Kelly B. T. Chang. 2002. "Services, Supports and Accommodations for Individuals with Disabilities: An Analysis across Secondary Education, Postsecondary Education and Employment." *Postoutcomes Network of the National Center on Secondary Education and Transition.* http://www.ncset.hawaii.edu/publications/pdf/services_supports.pdf.

Thomas, Stephen B. 2000. "College Students and Disability Law." *Journal of Special Education* 33, no. 4: 248–257.

U.S. Department of Education. 2010. "Annual Report Fiscal Year 2010: Report on Federal Activities under the Rehabilitation Act of 1973, as Amended." http://www2.ed.gov/about/reports/annual/rsa/2010/rsa-2010-annual-report.pdf.

Selective Abortion. See Prenatal Testing/Selective Abortion

Self-Advocacy and Health Literacy

"Self-advocacy" is defined as "being independent, defending one's rights, asserting oneself, and taking responsibility for one's self" (Aspis 2002). It is also a campaign to promote efforts to challenge and change barriers to full participation of people with disabilities in all aspects of society—including health management and access to quality health care. "Health literacy" is defined as "the degree to which individuals have the capacity to obtain, process, and understand basic health information and services needed to make appropriate health decisions" (White 2008). Having the combined abilities to self-advocate *and* skills in health literacy is important for any person in accessing, navigating, and managing the day-to-day activities that help maintain and optimize health.

What Is Health Literacy?

Much of the research on health literacy focuses on a person's basic skills, such as the ability to read medical instructions like prescriptions, fill out insurance forms, or understand what a doctor is saying during an appointment and why. However, some experts argue that understanding a person's health literacy requires looking at many other factors beyond a person's ability to read, write, and do math calculations. New definitions of health literacy include *functional health literacy*, which is the combination of a person's abilities and the challenges and demands of the task at hand, and *critical health literacy*, which is the ability to analyze information to then use it to gain greater personal control over health care decisions and health management (Nutbeam 2008). These new definitions suggest that health literacy is more about a balance among the individual's abilities, the demands of the task, and the processes or strategies a person uses when interacting or performing health-related activities.

Barriers in Health Literacy. If providers fail to consider this combination between a person's abilities and the multiple demands of any given task, they neglect to understand what is needed to help support successful health literacy and capacity for individual health management. For people with disabilities, the work experienced during interactions with health care professionals often includes addressing intersecting barriers of physical access, access and use of necessary health information, and confronting stigmas of disability that providers may hold. Many of these barriers can typically be removed when health care environments have accommodations for people with disabilities as part of their everyday standards of practice. An example of this would be providing large-print presurgical instructions for a person with low vision, Braille instructions for a person who is blind, or ensuring a referred diagnostic clinic has a ramp and accessible equipment for a person who uses a wheelchair.

Need for Self-Advocacy. People with disabilities face multiple barriers to health care yet often have greater demands for health care and access to services. These barriers and demands come in many forms, including barriers to physical access to providers for basic care and prevention programs, complicated medical insurance programs for people with disabilities, and attitudinal barriers from providers who view people with disabilities and their health only from a *medical model* perspective. These barriers are very often avoidable when health care systems account for the needs of people with disabilities. However, often, these needs are not considered, placing the work to overcome them on top of the primary health concerns the person has. To gain access, a person with a disability very often must self-advocate for the right to an accommodation to receive equitable care. For many people with disability, basic health literacy requires both understanding these barriers and having strategies of self-advocacy to make a request for an accommodation to receive health care services.

Background and History

Lack of access due to barriers in primary and preventive health care services is a leading cause of limited use of basic health care services for people with disabilities. In the United States, laws exist to eliminate access barriers and support full participation of people with disabilities in all aspects of society—including health care. Section 504 of the Rehabilitation Act of 1973 is a federal civil rights bill that prohibits discrimination on the basis of disability by government agencies, schools and universities, health facilities, and programs (Scotch 2001). The Americans with Disabilities Act (ADA), a groundbreaking civil rights law passed in 1990, provides people with disabilities the right to make reasonable requests to health care providers for accommodations to access care. Despite these laws, many health care facilities and much medical equipment (such as accessible scales and exam tables, medical information, and health promotion programs) continue to be inaccessible. Requests for accommodations by people with disabilities are often ignored or denied because of a failure of government or medical agencies to enforce these laws. As a result, the responsibility falls back on people with disabilities to advocate for access to health care, requiring that they understand when and how to request an accommodation to receive the necessary care. This requirement substantially increases the demand on a person's basic, functional, and critical health literacy.

Eliminating Health Disparities

Improved health literacy is a major agenda across state and national health organizations. The primary goal of this agenda is to reduce health disparities among the U.S. population. Part of Healthy People 2020, a public health campaign, focuses on improving the health literacy of the U.S. population by simplifying the language and approaches providers use to communicate health information. *Plain language* (simplifying the language used) and *teach-back* (clients repeat in their own words what they have been told) approaches by providers are some of the campaigns and strategies being used to ensure clear information exchange occurs during client-provider interactions. These approaches, however, which address more of the basic health literacy of reading, writing, and math, fail to consider many of the barriers that people with disabilities (PWD) experience. The barriers often prohibiting access to care for PWD are better understood when thinking about skills of *functional* and *critical* health literacy.

Recognition of the health literacy needs for different minority groups has led to specific programs that focus on reducing health disparities stemming from the different demands on a group's health literacy (e.g., foreign language translation accommodations for non-English speaking populations). People with disabilities experience significant disparities in health compared to their nondisabled peers, but no health literacy programs exist that focus on understanding the health literacy demands of this large minority group. Using the extended definitions of functional and critical health literacy, policy makers and providers might have an increased awareness of the demands and obstacles faced by PWD. An example of the health literacy demands of some PWD is knowing the recommended height of an examination table for ease in transferring for a person who uses a wheelchair. This simple bit of information can remove the ambiguity of "accessible exam table"

to make it more straightforward and easier to understand for both providers and PWD when planning an appointment. Consideration of technical specifications on accessibility may open the door for providers and policy makers to recognize how medical equipment specifications and accommodations in health care might also be part of the U.S. health literacy campaign.

Dilemmas, Debates, and Unresolved Questions

The National Assessment of Adult Literacy was a survey conducted in 2003 to document the literacy level of the U.S. population. It found that only 12 percent of Americans had enough health literacy skill to understand the basic medical information that is communicated in a doctor's visit (White 2008). Since this survey, low health literacy remains a major concern for U.S. public health programs. Yet, the way health literacy is defined and assessed determines the focus of interventions. Policy makers consistently refer back to the U.S. Department of Health and Human Services definition of health literacy (White 2008) and focus on individual *capacity* in reading and math skills as the primary contributor to overall health literacy. Policy changes then lead to interventions intended to simplify written instructions or provide supplemental literature, such as photos or diagrams. However, some policy makers and providers are beginning to use definitions of functional and critical health literacy, focusing on the balance between the person and task demand, as well as the person's ability to critically analyze information. These efforts are targeting standardizing practices of inclusion of accommodations, universal design, and training in disability awareness. Approaches that focus on functional and critical health literacy when considering accommodation needs might also be termed "disability health literacy," as awareness of the social barriers to health and the ways they contribute to disparities in health outcomes for people with disabilities is vital to understanding how to improve access to health care.

Enforcing Accessible Health Care

The Affordable Care Act (ACA) includes language that would provide for increased Department of Justice enforcement capability on accessibility standards for health care facilities. The ACA also directs the U.S. Access Board to develop and issue regulatory standards for medical diagnostic equipment for accessible entry, use of, and exit for people with disabilities. In January of 2017, the Medical Diagnostic Equipment Accessibility Standards Advisory Committee issued standards for diagnostic equipment for use by providers to make health care more accessible for PWD. These standards are not mandatory, and the U.S. Department of Justice has yet to adopt them. The laws to equal access are there, but the current system, structure, and attitudes of many providers and policy makers fail to acknowledge that lack of accommodations places undue obstacles and demands on accessing health care for the disability community. As a result, barriers persist, and strategies and tools in self-advocacy remain a critical component of disability health literacy.

Future Directions: Self-Advocacy as Part of Health Literacy

Self-advocacy skills intersect with health literacy skills for people with disabilities because of the need to address barriers to access to primary and preventive health care. As long as U.S. civil rights laws that promise access to health care facilities, equipment, and services are not enforced, people with disabilities will have to obtain the knowledge and skills to self-advocate for care. If, however, health literacy intervention approaches shift to embrace more of the functional and critical definitions, the intersections of personal and environmental factors would be more often considered. If so, people with disabilities may see a reduction in many of the barriers they face in access to health care. In the meantime, self-advocacy as part of *disability health literacy* will continue to be important for accessing, processing, understanding, and using medical information and medical services in health care management for PWD.

Laura VanPuymbrouck

See also: Primary Care, Barriers to; Public Health; Self-Advocacy Movement; Self-Determination, Concept and Policy

Further Reading

Aspis, Simone. 2002. "Self-Advocacy: Vested Interests and Misunderstandings." *British Journal of Learning Disabilities* 30, no. 1: 3–7.

Longmore, Paul K., and Lauri Umansky. 2001. *The New Disability History: American Perspectives.* New York: New York University Press.

Nutbeam, Don. 2008. "The Evolving Concept of Health Literacy." *Social Science & Medicine* 67, no. 12: 2072–2078.

Scotch, Richard. 2001. "American Disability Policy in the Twentieth Century. In *The New Disability History: American Perspectives*, edited by Paul K. Longmore and Lauri Umansky, 375–392. New York: New York University Press.

Shakespeare, Tom. 2012. "Still a Health Issue." *Disability and Health Journal* 5, no. 3: 129–131.

White, Sheida. 2008. *Assessing the Nation's Health Literacy: Key Concepts and*

Findings of the National Assessment of Adult Literacy (NAAL). Chicago: American Medical Association Press.

Self-Advocacy Movement

Self-advocacy is a movement where people with disabilities speak up for their rights and make decisions about their own lives. It is a constant process where self-advocates learn from others about how best to advocate for themselves. Many self-advocates belong to groups that are run by people with disabilities with the supports that they choose and the understanding that everybody needs to respect one another's roles, even during disagreements. In these groups, self-advocates learn to support each other, make friendships, and help create change in the world to make it better for people with disabilities and others. The term "self-advocate" does not mean that people only advocate for themselves, but it means that people with disabilities are able to speak up for themselves and express what is important to them personally, and do not need others to speak for them.

History

The self-advocacy movement in the United States is a human rights movement of and by people with disabilities, usually intellectual and developmental disabilities (IDD). Although origins of the movement date earlier, in the United States, self-advocacy grew significantly during the 1970s and 1980s (Caldwell 2010). According to Self Advocates Becoming Empowered (SABE), the largest self-advocacy organization in the United States, self-advocacy involves people with disabilities working together to take charge of their lives, fight discrimination, and advocate for justice (SABE 1991).

SABE was formed in September 1990 at a meeting in Colorado, where a steering committee for the organization was developed. Two representatives from each region of the United States were elected to be on a committee to help formalize the organization. In 1994, SABE held a board meeting in Knoxville, Tennessee, where SABE developed its bylaws and logo. Its next few meetings were focused on learning to work together as a team and getting to know one another, while developing a set of goals that the national organization would address as a group.

Current Landscape

While SABE is one of the more well-known self-advocacy organizations, since the early 1990s, several self-advocacy organizations have been developed; these organizations have built a network of supports for individuals with IDD entering the self-advocacy movement. People involved in self-advocacy learned to advocate for themselves by creating a system of supports and gaining the confidence to speak up for their rights. Individuals with IDD have learned self-advocacy skills and exercised them in various areas of their lives, such as the workplace, school, housing, transportation, and other places where they have experienced discrimination because of their disabilities. Self-advocates who have been a part of this movement for over a decade are seeking more opportunities to expand their reach and to grow as leaders.

Increasingly, self-advocates have been important parts of state and national efforts toward the inclusion of people with IDD in all aspects of society. In particular, self-advocacy has been an important part of University Centers on Excellence in Developmental Disabilities (UCEDD), of which there is at least one in each state that is focused on research, training, information dissemination, and other services related to people with IDD. UCEDDs are required to have self-advocates as part of their advisory committees to provide feedback and direction to the centers and the work they do. In addition, many UCEDDs have hired self-advocates and involve them in research projects. The Administration on Intellectual and Developmental Disabilities (AIDD), the federal body that funds UCEDDs, includes self-advocates on review and monitoring teams that evaluate the agencies that it funds, including state DD councils and protection and advocacy groups. Importantly, Leadership Education in Neurodevelopmental and Related Disabilities (LEND) programs that provide long-term, graduate-level interdisciplinary training to a variety of clinical disciplines have recently begun to include self-advocates in the training. This trend was started by the LEND program in Illinois in 2010.

State DD councils are also funded by AIDD, and they are important for self-advocacy programs in individual states. Many DD councils fund self-advocacy summits and conferences to bring self-advocates together to continue to learn from one another and work together toward a common goal. Many of the programs offer scholarships for self-advocates to attend these summits and other events around the state to practice their advocacy. DD councils are also required to ensure that at least half of the council is composed of persons with IDD.

Some other resources that are important to self-advocates include the following:

- National Youth Leadership Network (NYLN), which was created to teach youth with disabilities about self-advocacy
- National Gateway to Self-Determination

- Employment First, a policy that promotes employment for self-advocates

Support for Self-Advocacy

A key aspect of self-advocacy is self-determination. Although self-determination can hold multiple meanings, a consistent theme is that self-determination is about people directing their own lives in positive ways (Nonnemacher and Bambera 2011). The self-determination of people with IDD is viewed as the right of individuals to direct their own services to improve their quality of life. As other facets of people's lives are properly established and people are gaining access to meaningful employment, self-advocates can now be supported to move up in the hierarchal structure and take on leadership roles.

When developing supports and working with a support person, there are a couple of things to keep in mind: have more than one person supporting you in your life, and know that your support will not be there forever.

People providing supports should also keep a few rules in mind: make sure that the support you provide is individualized and specific to each person that you support; ask the person what kind of supports they need (make sure that they have proper support at home, adequate transportation, and stable housing); and make sure you work as a team.

Organizations that include people who receive support should also do the following:

- clearly outline the job responsibilities
- if the person will need to work out of the office, go over the responsibilities (e.g., times and dates, costs of traveling, the necessity of a support staff during travel)
- understand what supports the person will need day to day to complete tasks

- provide training if the person feels less comfortable about a particular responsibility
- provide a clear line of communication so the person with a disability feels comfortable going to someone if any questions or issues arise
- build a trusting environment for the person with a disability to explore, learn, and make mistakes without consequences while still feeling supported in attempts to grow

Conclusion

The important thing to remember about self-advocacy is that it takes self-advocates working together with supports to be successful. Self-advocacy is about an individual's life, so it is extremely important. People who are self-advocates want to express self-determination, and sometimes they need support to do this, but it is important that the support does not take over. Self-efficacy is an interdependent relationship, and it is okay for self-advocates and their supports to disagree with one another, as long as there is respect between self-advocates and between self-advocates and their support. Working together, self-advocates and their supports can make the world a better place.

Tia Nelis

See also: Disability Rights Movement (DRM); Disability Rights Movement (DRM), History and Development of; Self-Determination, Concept and Policy; Sexuality Education for People with Intellectual Disabilities

Further Reading

Caldwell, Joe. 2010. "Leadership Development of Individuals with Developmental Disabilities in the Self-Advocacy Movement." *Journal of Intellectual Disability Research* 54, no. 2: 1010–1014.

Nonnemacher, Stacy L., and Linda M. Bambara. 2011. "'I'm Supposed to Be in Charge': Self-Advocates' Perspectives on Their Self-Determination Support Needs." *Intellectual and Developmental Disabilities* 49, no. 5: 327–340.

Self Advocates Becoming Empowered. 1991. "Mission Statement." http://www.sabeusa.org.

Self-Determination, Concept and Policy

Self-determination is the level of control individuals have over the direction of their life and the extent to which they are the ones deciding on and making changes to improve their quality of life. A self-determined individual recognizes a need for a change, decides to take action, and acts in accordance with attaining said goal.

What Is Self-Determination?

For a person's actions to be considered "self-determined," the behaviors must be self-regulated, self-realizing, psychologically empowering, and done autonomously (Wehmeyer and Field 2007). *Self-regulated* people can use different strategies and make various plans of action depending on the circumstances, as well as make changes as needed to achieve their goals. The *self-realization* piece refers to the knowledge people have about their own beliefs, abilities, and goals. Self-determined people know who they are and what they want. *Psychological empowerment* is the confidence that allows people to make changes to improve their life. Without that empowerment, it is unlikely people would attempt to do so. Lastly, to act *autonomously*, people must make the changes based on their own desires and complete the process with only the support that is necessary. It is not enough for people to act in a manner that results in change. Those people must have decided to act in a certain way to produce the changes that they specifically desired for the purpose of improving their quality of life.

Important Points to Understand about Self-Determination

The level to which persons with disabilities become self-determined is affected by their cognitive and social abilities; their educational, personal, and community living experiences and opportunities; and their perception of themselves as well others' perceptions of them. Although much of the literature on self-determination is in the field of special education and disability, it is an important concept throughout the lifecourse. Most people develop an adequate level of self-determination without explicit instruction or assistance. Specifically for those individuals with disabilities who need that *support*, self-determination also depends on the level and quality of the assistance received and the opportunities available.

Perception of Control. Self-determination is based in part on the perception of control that individuals have over relevant aspects of their environment. It is characterized by how individuals perceive their level of control over the current situation and future outcomes. Perceptions of control affect the ways individuals interact with the world around them, as well as the level of desire for these interactions. Individuals who exhibit decreased levels of self-determination, or who perceive limited control over their world, often struggle with seeking out opportunities, setting goals, and achieving desired outcomes. With regards to students with disabilities, their degree of

self-determination has been associated with higher academic success; better engagement with schoolwork; greater participation in IEPs, transition planning, and goal setting; more postsecondary success; and more positive postsecondary quality of life. More self-determined students are also more readily able to solve problems and obtain what they want, leading to fewer negative behaviors.

Active Engagement. Self-determination is attained through active engagement in planning one's own future or being provided with opportunities to participate in such planning. Instruction should include learning to set appropriate and attainable goals and practicing self-advocacy, self-management, self-awareness, and problem-solving strategies. Methods for increasing the level of self-determination for students with disabilities include direct instruction in topics like goal setting; stage setting, such as having students plan their IEPs; person-centered planning (PCP); self-management practice; and student-generated assignments and activities. As often as possible, these strategies should be incorporated into natural settings, such as vocational tasks and community-based instruction. Resources can be found on the National Secondary Transition Technical Assistance Center Web site and on the Intervention Central Web site.

Debates, Unresolved Questions, and Future Directions

The primary methods for assessing self-determination levels include the *Arc's self-determination scale* (Wehmeyer 1995) and the *American Institutes for Research (AIR) self-determination scale* (Wolman et al. 1994). Both scales analyze teacher, student, and parent perceptions of self-determination levels to give a more balanced perspective on the individual's level of self-determination. Shogren et al. (2008) compared the two scales and found that each of the measures of self-determination focused on a different aspect of the self-determination construct. They concluded that it appears educators are providing objective ratings of their independent perceptions of students' capacity and opportunity for self-determination, while students' ratings are influenced by the strong relationship they see between their capacity and opportunity for self-determination. While further research is needed to verify these findings, they suggest that teachers do not perceive a strong relationship between students' capacity for self-determination and the opportunities they are provided.

Michael Wehmeyer, a leading researcher of self-determination, and his colleagues created the *self-determination learning model of instruction (SDLMI)* (2000). It is a supplement to existing curricula to help increase the emphasis on self-determination in students' school days, specifically in the areas of goal setting, choice making, and problem solving. Embedding self-determination skills into the school day instead of having a separate time to teach self-determination skills helps students learn to use them and see their importance. Wehmeyer and other researchers continue to look for better ways to teach students self-determination skills and make sure they generalize those skills to their lives to achieve better postsecondary outcomes. The existing research has focused on how to assess a student's level of self-determination, how to teach the skills to individual students, and what impact self-determination skills have on postsecondary outcomes. The newest directions of research have involved looking more specifically at the state of self-determination of students of color; the degree that self-determination is incorporated into academic instruction is linked to

the Common Core Standards for teaching English language, arts, and mathematics; and the effectiveness of behavior intervention plans. Additionally, there is a need for assessing the impact of large-scale self-determination interventions. Another shift in focus has been the process of starting the instruction with younger students.

Samantha Walte and Robert Maddalozzo

See also: Individualized Education Program (IEP); Natural Supports; "Nothing about Us without Us"; Self-Determination in Education

Further Reading

Shogren, K. A., M. L. Wehmeyer, S. B. Palmer, J. H. Soukup, T. D. Little, N. Garner, and M. Lawrence. 2008. "Understanding the Construct of Self-Determination: Examining the Relationship between the Arc's Self-Determination Scale and the American Institutes for Research Self-Determination Scale." *Assessment for Effective Intervention* 33: 94–107.

Wehmeyer, M. L. 1995. *The ARC's Self-Determination Scale: Procedural Guidelines.* Arlington, TX: ARC.

Wehmeyer, M. L., and S. L. Field. 2007. *Self-Determination: Instructional and Assessment Strategies.* Thousand Oaks, CA: Corwin Press.

Wehmeyer, M. L., S. B. Palmer, M. Agran, D. Mithaug, D. Martin, and J. Martin. 2000. Promoting Causal Agency: The Self-Determined Learning Model of Instruction. *Exceptional Children* 66: 439–453.

Wolman, J. P., P. Campeau, P. Dubois, D. Mithaug, and V. Stolarski. 1994. *AIR Self-Determination Scale and User Guide.* Palo Alto, CA: American Institute for Research.

Self-Determination in Education

Self-determination is referred to as the capability to steer one's own life in a valued direction and ways that are personally meaningful (Wehmeyer 2014). Depending on the environment in which self-determination occurs, is taught, or is valued, there may be various perspectives on delineating autonomy, self-agency, and self-determination. Promoting, modeling, teaching, and measuring self-determination among youth with and without disabilities is understood as meaningful, but specific to youth and adults with disabilities, self-determination is often interpreted in multiple and complex ways (Stolz 2010).

What Is Self-Determination in Youth with Disabilities?

Empirical evidence illustrates that self-determination can directly influence the success of youth with disabilities (Wehmeyer 2014; Shogren et al. 2013). The significance of self-determination has been highlighted by policy, legislature, and funding. According to Shogren and colleagues (2013), enhanced self-determination plays an important role in improving student outcomes, employment status, postsecondary participation, autonomy, and quality of life. Consequently, the promotion of students' self-determination now constitutes a significant component of best practices in the education and lives of youth with disabilities. Prominent scholars in the field have concluded that youth with disabilities benefit from instruction and support given to hone their self-determination skills (Chou et al. 2016; Cowley and Bacon 2013; Izzo and Horne 2016). Educator preparation guidelines now specify instruction of self-determination.

The *Education Teacher Performance Assessment* (edTPA), a policy mandate in many states in the United States, identifies self-determination as a best practice in special education instruction (Cowley and Bacon 2013). There is a need for all individuals to live a self-determined life. However, the instruction in self-determination may vary relative to the district, school, teacher, environment, or demographic details, such as identity, experience, race, religion, perceived gender roles, age, or definition of disability and intensity of access supports (of the student and the educator). Therefore, it is necessary to understand that there are multiple perspectives about the concept of self-determination and people with disabilities. Although self-determination occurs across the lifespan, in schools with youth with and without disabilities, it is a common expectation that students are often assessed on their level of skill and knowledge regarding self-determination—whether as a social-emotional competency or as a life skill. For example, in individualized education programs (IEPs), transition planning starts in early high school, and self-determination is typically measured in independent living, postsecondary education, and employment goals. These skills may affect inclusion or exclusion in future opportunities across all of life's setting (e.g., employment, housing, transportation, relationships, and learning).

Background and History

Cowley and Bacon stated that "the roots of self-determination in the U.S. can be traced back to Jeffersonian democracy" (2013, 465). They explained how the concept of self-determination has evolved and has been gradually appropriated by the government and adopted in the medical field. Although multiple definitions exist, a significant step forward is acknowledging and defining self-determination at state and federal levels in the United States. An evolution from a solely medical perspective includes the perspective of people with disabilities and experts in issues of self-advocacy, self-agency, and self-determination. Although not interchangeable, these terms are related because they affect issues of equity, influence, choice, dignity, and self-efficacy.

Self-determination is an essential component for all individuals, including people with disabilities. The skills leading to improved self-determination, such as problem solving, goal setting, and decision making, allow youth to assume greater control, direction, and responsibility. Furthermore, when young people with disabilities show that they can get things done and take responsibility for decision making and planning, others may change how they perceive them and what they expect from them (Wehmeyer 2014). Youth with disabilities have insisted that having control over their lives, instead of relying on someone to direct them, is important to their self-esteem and self-worth (Izzo and Horne 2016). Additionally, "testimonials show how self-determination and a positive self-concept are fostered and reinforced by mentors. Mentoring helps students who often feel alone in connecting to a larger community of people who lend support to students through critical junctures and transitions" (Izzo and Horne 2016, 12). Mentoring by a person with a disability is valuable, and it greatly influences the self-determination and self-agency of the student with the disability (Stolz 2010).

Important Points to Know about Self-Determination and Youth with Disabilities

Outcomes and Supports. Overall, self-determination consists of specific skills, including choice making, problem solving, goal setting, attainment, autonomy, self-observation, self-advocacy, and self-awareness (Cowley and Bacon 2013). Shogren

and colleagues (2013) explained that after graduating, youth with disabilities who are self-determined have a better chance of getting jobs that offer benefits, such as health coverage and leisure, and were more likely to be living independently. Stolz (2010) recommended that schools provide opportunities for students to identify their own needs and solutions, provide room for error to reduce students' fear of risk, and provide natural opportunities for students to lead and share their perspectives, thus enhancing the feeling that disabled students are capable and valued.

Although the promotion of self-determination is gaining prominence in such areas as policy initiatives, best practice suggestions, and assessment tools (e.g., Supports Intensity Scale) (Thompson 2004, 2008), relatively little is known about the different perspectives regarding how self-determination is addressed for youth with disabilities. The perspectives of students, parents, and educators on self-determination and the adoption of instruction to promote the self-determination of youth with disabilities vary. These perspectives related to self-determination can be compared by evaluating individual perspectives, attitudes about disability, "environmental context, and socio-cultural experiences" (Stolz 2010, 50).

Dilemmas, Debates, and Unresolved Questions

The topic of self-determination has accrued a reasonable amount of attention from scholars, parents, and special educators. A number of issues have come up concerning the multiple perspectives of self-determination and youth with disabilities. One of the key issues is the common misunderstanding that self-determination is evidenced as binary, or in absolutes of yes or no, for many youth with disabilities but that, for nondisabled peers or adults, the matter of self-determination can be relative; therefore, messages regarding the expectation or mastery of self-determination can be inconsistent (Stolz 2010).

In addition, youth with disabilities who lack expected self-determination skills may have increased potential to be segregated from peers, not obtain admittance into or continuance of postsecondary supports, or reduced choices. One notable controversy is that even though the topic of self-determination is thought to be relevant, many teachers have little knowledge of implementation, mainstream approaches, or alternate approaches (Wehmeyer 2014). Moreover, students with varying disabilities and levels of support may receive mixed messages due to lack of training for educators, community members, families, students, and school administrators (Izzo and Horne 2016; Shogren et al. 2013; Stolz 2010).

Self-determination is often misidentified as a largely internal or intrinsic characteristic. This potential misconception is problematic for people with disabilities, as they may require supports and interdependence as a right, regardless of their level of self-determination skills (Cowley and Bacon 2013). Disability is diverse, and the attempt to neatly fit the important skills of self-determination across political, social, cultural, learning, employment, living, identity, and environmental aspects provides a venue for questions about the existing structures that define what it means to lead a self-determined life. Stolz (2010) researched further how students with disabilities are often taught to comply in schools and how as a result their voices are not authentically participating in decision making, are absent, or are even discredited: "Not offending others has been particularly important for disabled youth who have often felt dependent on having good relationships with those around them" (22).

The Future of Self-Determination and Conclusions

Considerable efforts have been directed toward understanding self-determination in youth with disabilities. However, there remains much to be accomplished, especially in seeking and understanding the different perspectives and in implementation of self-determination related to youth with disabilities (Stolz 2010). The inclusion and leadership of learners, researchers, and scholars with disabilities in studies about topics related to self-determination may contribute to a broader and more authentic perspective related to topics affecting people with disabilities so that these important skills can be equitably valued, taught, and applied.

Ameen Alhaznawi

See also: Individualized Education Program (IEP); (In)Exclusion; Natural Supports; Transition from High School; Transitional Experiences of Students with Disabilities

Further Reading

Chou, Yu-Chi, Michael Wehmeyer, Susan Palmer, and Jaehoon Lee. 2016. "Comparisons of Self-Determination Among Students with Autism, Intellectual Disability, and Learning Disabilities: A Multivariate Analysis." *Focus on Autism and Other Developmental Disabilities* 32, no. 2: 124–132.

Cowley, Danielle, and Jessica Bacon. 2013. *Self-Determination in Schools: Reconstructing the Concept through a Disability Studies Framework*. Montclair, NJ: Montclair State University.

Izzo, Margo, and LeDerick Horne. 2016. *Empowering Students with Hidden*

Disabilities: A Path to Pride and Success. Baltimore: Brookes Publishing.

Shogren, Karrie, Michael Wehmeyer, Susan Palmer, Graham Rifenbark, and Todd Little. 2013. "Relationships between Self-Determination and Postschool Outcomes for Youth with Disabilities." *The Journal of Special Education* 48, no. 4: 256–267.

Stolz, Suzanne. 2010. *Disability Trajectories: Disabled Youths' Identity Development, Negotiation of Experience and Expectation, and Sense of Agency during Transition.* Unpublished doctoral dissertation, University of California, San Diego.

Thompson, James. 2004. *Supports Intensity Scale.* Washington, DC: American Association on Intellectual and Developmental Disabilities.

Wehmeyer, Michael. 2014. "Framing the Future." *Remedial and Special Education* 36, no. 1: 20–23.

Self-Identification and Self-Diagnosis for Autism

Autism spectrum disorder (ASD) is a lifelong state of being that influences an individual's social interaction and communication styles. The medical diagnosis also requires repetitive behaviors, unusual reactions to sensory stimuli, or strong interests in specific topics. There are vast efforts to develop and disseminate methods to identify autism at earlier and earlier ages; currently, children can be reliably and stably diagnosed as early as their toddler years. Meanwhile, there is little effort put into developing reliable and accessible methods to diagnose adults. This situation has led to efforts by some in the adult autistic community to self-diagnose.

Background

Rise of Self-Diagnosis. In the disability community, self-identification and self-diagnosis involve issues among autistic self-advocates related to *disability authenticity*; *biocertification* (or medical, educational, and institutional verification); and *self-understanding.* The phenomenon of self-diagnosis is somewhat unique to autism among psychiatric conditions. People with schizophrenia, for instance, often do not recognize the presence of or need for a diagnosis. While people may self-diagnosis with conditions like depression and anxiety, these labels are not often associated with the levels of identity formation, community connection, or sociocultural mobilization seen in autism.

Diagnosis in Adulthood. There are many reasons an adult may not have an autism diagnosis despite meeting criteria. Some adults were diagnosed in childhood but were never made aware of their diagnosis or have lost records of their diagnosis. Other individuals are unable to access a diagnostician familiar with diagnosing adults because of geographic location (such as living far away from a qualified diagnostician) or few resources such as money, time, and energy. While insurance or schools usually cover diagnostic practices in the United States for children, such services are not often covered for adults. Obtaining an official diagnosis in adulthood can cost hundreds or even thousands of dollars as an out-of-pocket expense, making this practice financially inaccessible to many.

Unlike diagnosis in childhood, obtaining an autism diagnosis in adulthood has few, if any, formal rewards, particularly in the United States. In fact, an adult diagnosis can result in workplace, social, and educational discrimination. When a child is diagnosed with autism, a host of therapeutic and educational services become available. These services are often provided by the child's school system or are covered by insurance.

However, an autism diagnosis usually does not yield adults access to services outside of possibly pharmacological or psychological services, which can be accessed with a host of diagnoses that do not carry the stigma or cost of an autism diagnosis. Many adults learn to develop their own coping mechanisms for navigating the neurotypical world or access informal support on the Internet or through relationships (e.g., with a workplace mentor), social support groups, or, for some, programs in higher education (though the latter two may also be quite costly). Regardless, many self-advocates who are diagnosed in adulthood, either by a professional or through self-assessment, do find comfort and self-understanding as a result of having a diagnosis with which to identify. Additionally, there is a vibrant, supportive autistic community, particularly online, where one can find like-minded individuals. For these reasons, adults may want to seek out a diagnosis or begin to self-identify as autistic.

Important Points to Understand about Self-Diagnosis

Advantages and Disadvantages. There are various benefits and disadvantages of professional autism diagnoses for adults who have not previously been diagnosed. Autism or *neurodivergent* communities are emerging as unique and robust sites of *biocitizenship*, or groups that collect under a common biological profile to assert rights and support. Here, autistic self-advocates use the concept of neurodiversity to claim shared neurological states deserving of acceptance, accommodation, culture, and community. Whether a formal diagnosis results in these goals varies. Although diagnosis does provide a legal right to accommodations and protection against discrimination, further stigma and

mistreatment or misunderstanding may occur in practice after diagnosis. Yet even self-advocates who support the principles of neurodiversity and related concepts such as autistic expertise may support professional diagnoses to validate a self-diagnosis that other autistic people may have already endorsed.

Biocertification. Despite the fact that there are many children and adults who meet criteria for autism but lack a formal diagnosis, some self-advocates assert that to belong in the autistic community, one must access professional diagnoses. The process of biocertification, or obtaining official documents verifying one's state of being, firmly situates one in the autistic community. For many this is preferable despite distrust of and dislike for professional methods directed at autistic people and ways of talking about autism in general. Others extend this distrust and distaste to reject professional input in autism verification overall, preferring to rely on self-expertise instead. Deciding whether to use professional expertise to ensure one's autism status or eschew the entire process is a personal choice. Yet, this choice is also often shaped by institutionalized hierarchies, such as the common barriers to access adult diagnosis mentioned above, which prevent certain types of people from accessing the structures they need to be biocertified and, thus, the benefits of doing so.

Dilemmas, Debates, and Unsolved Questions in Self-Diagnosis

Autism and Authenticity. In the autistic self-advocacy and neurodiversity communities, there is a robust debate on the acceptability of self-diagnoses, primarily centered on whether people who self-diagnose should be accepted in the community. This tension reflects the need to create and sustain a welcoming space for autistic people to develop community where they can be themselves and to ensure that space is safe from outsiders, who can be stigmatizing or nonrepresentative. There are some general arguments for and against the inclusion of self-diagnosed autistic people in the autistic community. Some of the most prevalent arguments against include the need for professional training to accurately diagnose autism and issues related to authenticity. The former argument asserts that autism is a complex and complicated state of being that is difficult to identify without professional training. Some self-advocates assert that matching outside traits with internal experiences is problematic and, thus, negates the process of self-diagnosis. Further, some argue that if the traits were not identified in childhood, then they must reflect some other, less significant condition.

Inaccurate Advocacy. Arguments related to authenticity align with these points but focus on the people who can and cannot represent the autistic community and on the role of inaccurate advocacy and public representation in motivating self-diagnosis. Some self-advocates feel disconnected from individuals who have not been professionally diagnosed, noting a distinction between the experiences of carrying an autism diagnosis and suspecting oneself to be autistic. These differences can lead to different needs and values, and so many advocates believe that the right to represent the autistic community should lie with those officially diagnosed. Other self-advocates who are skeptical of self-diagnosis believe that those who self-diagnose are doing so to access the supportive autistic community, and they may feel concerned that those who self-diagnose add competition for scarce resources or increase the perception of autistic activists as

trivializing or denying disability. Similarly, autistic self-advocates who argue against acceptance of self-diagnosis assert that some self-identifiers became inspired by inaccurate media portrayals showing autistic adults as merely funny, quirky individuals, suggesting that being autistic is a fun or lighthearted experience. However, these representations fail to recognize the complexity of living as an autistic person, and most autistic adults do not relate to these representations.

Self-Knowledge and Expertise. On the other side of the debate are self-advocates who support self-diagnosis. Many of these individuals note a high level of misdiagnosis and a general distrust of the medical and scientific professions. This distrust is related to continuing psychiatric critique that identifies areas in which psychiatric diagnoses and practices serve to disempower certain types of people. Arguments in the realm of medical and psychiatric doubt rest on two primary premises: that professionals are not better at identifying autism than autistic people and that the high variability within autism ensures that many diagnoses are guesses. Building on the first premise, there is a notion of the autistic *self-expert*, working from direct experiences with an autistic mind and life, as a better source than a trained professional, who can only access external behavior and expressed thoughts or feelings. Self-advocates may also critique clinical judgment because of medical diagnoses' basis in a pathological framework that excludes neutral differences and strengths; some self-advocates may identify autism based on alternative criteria. Regarding the second premise of high variability in autism, many self-diagnosed people stem from groups with which professionals and assessments have less understanding, such as women, gender and sexual minorities, people of color, and adults. Factors such as culture and life experience may lead autistic people to present differently, such as when adults (perhaps especially women) learn to "mask" their autism or "pass" for neurotypical, through self- and social awareness that allows them to internalize neurotypical norms and suppress ongoing differences and struggles. Thus, a trust of self-knowledge often supersedes that of a diagnostician.

Navigating Challenges. Another argument in support of self-diagnosis applies a pragmatic approach in a field with a dominant focus on children. Professionals well-versed and interested in diagnosing adults can be difficult to locate or access by those living in remote areas or who may be un- or underemployed. Finally, many autistic adults who self-diagnose do so to avoid any workplace- or insurance-based discrimination that may come from obtaining an official diagnosis. While recognizing autism in oneself can alleviate long-felt alienation and misunderstanding, official diagnoses may bring about another set of issues. For some, self-diagnosis is a way to navigate these challenges.

Conclusion

The debate on self-diagnosis relates to wider issues of determining who belongs in an often tight-knit, supportive community and how to ensure that the community remains authentic and safe. This process is complicated when considering an identity like autism, which has shifted widely in diagnostic definition, social acceptance, and recognizability. And without specific physical or biological markers on which to rely for a definitive diagnosis, there is a level of subjectivity involved in interpreting certain behaviors and histories as autistic or neurotypical (i.e., normative), especially

for autism's social communication criteria, given that interpersonal behaviors vary by sociocultural context. It will be important and interesting to trace the debate on self-diagnosis in the autistic community, as it will provide important insights into neurocommunities and neurodiversity acceptance.

Jennifer C. Sarrett and Steven K. Kapp

See also: Community; Disclosure and Self-Identification; Self-Advocacy Movement; Self-Determination, Concept and Policy

Further Reading

Baggs, A. M., Phil Schwarz, Joel Smith, and Laura Tisonick. 2013. "Who Can Call Themselves Autistic?" Autistics.org. http://www.autistics.org/library/whois autistic.html.

Brownlow, Charlotte, and Lindsay O'Dell. 2013. "'Hard-wired from the Factory'? Autism as a Form of Biological Citizenship." In *Worlds of Autism: Across the Spectrum of Neurological Difference*, edited by Joyce Davidson and Michael Orsini, 97–114. Minneapolis: University of Minnesota Press.

Samuels, Ellen. 2014. *Fantasies of Identification: Disability, Gender, Race.* New York: New York University Press.

Sarrett, J. C. 2016. "Biocertification and Neurodiversity: The Role and Implications of Self-Diagnosis in Autistic Communities." *Neuroethics* 9, no. 10: 23–36.

Schaber, A. 2014. "ASD Paper Diagnosis vs. Self-Diagnosis: Pros and Cons." *Neurowonderful (Web log).* http://neurowonderful.tumblr.com/post/89986388881/asd-paper-diagnosis-vs-self-diagnosis-pros-and.

Walker, N. 2014. "Neurodiversity: Some Basic Terms and Definitions." *Neurocosmopolitanism (Web log).* http://neurocosmopolitanism.com/neurodiversity-some-basic-terms-definitions/.

Service Animals

A service animal is defined as a dog that is trained to perform tasks for a person with a disability (ADA Amendments Act 2008). To qualify as a service animal under the law, the tasks the dog performs must be specifically related to the individual's disability. The ADA also recognizes miniature horses as service animals in some circumstances.

What Do Service Animals Do?

Service animals can be trained to perform an array of tasks for people with a wide variety of impairments. The types of impairments animals may be trained to respond to include, but are not limited to, mobility impairments, vision impairments, and hearing impairments. Service animals enhance independence for people with disabilities, making them a valuable tool in the lives of

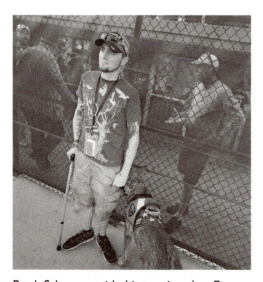

Brad Schwarz, with his service dog Panzer, attends a Chicago Cubs baseball game at Wrigley Field in Chicago, Illinois, with a group of veterans from the Wounded Warrior Project. Only dogs and miniature horses are recognized as service animals under the ADA. (Scott Olson/Getty Images)

many individuals. The training a service dog undergoes depends on the needs of the dog's eventual handler.

For Visual Impairments. Guide dogs are perhaps the most well-known category of service animals. These dogs are trained to guide individuals who are blind or have low vision through a variety of environments, like schools and work buildings, busy city streets, and public transportation. An important hallmark of a guide dog is "intelligent disobedience," which entails the dog disobeying the handler's command if complying would put the team in obvious danger, such as walking in front of an oncoming car. The miniature horses that are recognized as service animals most often perform guide work, similar to that of a guide dog.

For Mobility Impairments. For people with mobility impairments, dogs can be trained to do things like pick up dropped items, carry items, pull a manual wheelchair, push doors and drawers closed and open them with the use of tug straps, turn lights on and off, and tug off clothing. Commands can be chained together to enable the dog to perform a sequence of related commands, giving the opportunity for the dog and handler team to complete complex tasks such as retrieving a soda from the fridge, doing the laundry, or completing a purchase transaction at a store.

For Hearing Impairments. Service animals that assist individuals with hearing impairments will alert and orient their handler to different sounds by nudging the handler and going to the location of the sound. Hearing dogs can be taught to respond to numerous sounds, but some of the most common are the phone, smoke alarms, sirens, the person's name, and items falling or being dropped.

For Seizure and Diabetic Alerts. Dogs can also assist with alerting to seizures for handlers with conditions such as epilepsy, or alerting to changes in blood sugar for those living with diabetes. Diabetic alert dogs detect small changes in blood sugar through the scent of their handler. Dogs are often trained to respond to high and low blood sugar changes in different ways. For instance, dogs may be trained to sit in front of their handler when they detect high blood sugar or bow in response to low blood sugar; both actions would prompt the individuals to test their blood sugar.

Unlike the other categories of service dogs described above, dogs that can detect seizures are usually born with this ability, and training is used to help the dogs harness these skills. It remains unclear what triggers a seizure alert dog to warn their handlers of an oncoming seizure. It is possible that the dogs are responding to changes in biological functioning of the brain or to small scent changes that occur when seizure activity is about to begin. Training alone usually will not produce an effective seizure alert dog. There are also seizure response dogs that do not necessarily have the innate ability to predict seizures but are trained to perform tasks during and after a seizure. Although the tasks service dogs perform for their disabled handlers vary widely, the amount of independence they can bring to the individuals they work with is immeasurable.

Background and History

The first service dog team in the United States was recognized in 1928 and consisted of a German shepherd guide dog named Buddy and his handler, Morris Frank (The Seeing Eye, n.d.). Within a year, Frank went on to cofound The Seeing Eye with Buddy's trainer, Dorothy Harrison Eustis, in Morristown, New Jersey. The Seeing Eye remains the longest-running service dog organization in the United States. In the

past few decades, service dog organizations have become significantly more prevalent both in the United States and abroad, with hundreds of programs available worldwide. Many of these programs can be located through the database maintained by Assistance Dogs International (ADI), a coalition of service dog organizations that have passed ADI's accreditation standards.

Legislation and Service Animals. There are several pieces of legislation that define and outline provisions for the use of a service dog. The ADA is perhaps the most well-known piece of disability rights legislation that addresses it. This law mandates that businesses open to the public, employers of 15 or more employees, and entities receiving state and local government funding make reasonable accommodations for individuals with disabilities. The law requires that privately owned businesses and establishments open to the public modify their policies and procedures to permit the use of a service dog. Although the ADA does not specifically address the use of service animals in employment settings or state and local government establishments, the use of a service dog is typically considered a *reasonable accommodation* in these settings.

When it is unclear whether an animal qualifies as a service animal, entities covered under this law are only legally allowed to ask two questions to service animal handlers to make the determination: (1) "Is the service animal required because of a disability?" and (2) "What work or task has the animal been trained to perform?" Entities are not allowed to require an individual to demonstrate what the dog does for them or to ask for documentation. However, many service dog handlers and programs choose to have their dogs wear vests or other accessories in public that indicate they are working animals. A business owner or other entity covered under the ADA does have the right to ask a person to remove a dog from the premises if the dog is not under the control of the handler or if it is not housebroken.

In addition to the ADA, there are other pieces of legislation that permit the use of assistance animals. The Fair Housing Act (FHA) of 1968 and the Air Carrier Access Act (ACAA) of 1986 address the use of both service dogs and *emotional support animals* (animals whose primary purpose is to provide emotional comfort). The FHA was amended in 1988 to allow service dogs and emotional support animals to accompany their owners in rented dwellings that do not typically allow animals as a reasonable accommodation. In the case that a dwelling requires a pet deposit, these fees must be waived for individuals needing assistance animals. The ACAA allows passengers with disabilities to fly with an accompanying service dog or emotional support animal free of charge.

Unlike the ADA, the FHA and ACAA do allow landlords and airlines to ask for documentation of the need for an assistance animal. Landlords may not inquire about the specific nature of the person's disability under the FHA, but they can ask for documentation that the person has a disability and that the animal helps with the disability in some way. The landlord may also ask questions similar to those allowed under the ADA. According to the ACAA, airlines may ask for documentation, such as the animal's identification card, presence of a harness or vest, or verbal assurances. In the case of an emotional support animal or psychiatric service dog, documentation from a medical professional stating why the animal must travel with the person may be requested. As the use of assistance animals

continue to evolve, so too does the legislation that protects the rights of the animal-handler team.

Important Points to Understand About Service Animals

Although service animals, therapy animals, and emotional support animals (ESA) are often lumped into the category of "assistance animals," there are important distinctions to be made between them.

Service Animals versus Emotional Support Animals. Service animals are trained to do specific tasks to mitigate the handler's disability. On the other hand, emotional support animals (ESAs) are not task trained and are used primarily for emotional comfort and support. ESAs are typically dogs or cats but may be of varied species. While ESAs may accompany their owners in the cabin of an airplane and are allowed access to dwellings, they are not covered under the ADA and do not have the public access rights that service animals do.

For example, an individual diagnosed with a condition like post-traumatic stress disorder who acquires a dog primarily to provide emotional support with its presence alone would be considered an ESA. This dog would not be entitled to run errands with its owner in spaces where animals typically are not allowed. However, with documentation from a health care professional stating that the ESA is needed, this dog may accompany its owner on aircrafts and live in the housing their owner inhabits. Alternatively, in the case that this same individual acquires a dog *trained* to do specific tasks to mitigate the implications of the disability, this dog would then be considered a psychiatric service dog. Tasks the psychiatric service dog might perform include standing in front of its handler in crowded places to ease symptoms or entering a room before the handler to alert the individual of the presence of another person. Psychiatric service dogs are afforded the public access rights of service animals under the ADA.

Facility Dogs and Therapy Dogs. A more recent category of assistance animal is the facility dog. These dogs are paired with someone who works for an organization that serves individuals with disabilities or high-risk populations, such as juveniles in the criminal justice system or children and adults who have been victims of violent crime. Facility dogs are *task trained* to assist individuals with disabilities, as service dogs are. For instance, a facility dog may assist a patient undergoing physical therapy by retrieving a ball or holding a rope being used for resistance. Unlike therapy dogs, facility dogs do have public access rights under the ADA when they are accompanying and working for a person with a disability in public spaces.

Therapy animals typically visit hospitals, nursing homes, detention centers, schools, and communities in crisis, for the purpose of providing emotional comfort and support to many people. Although therapy dogs do not have to be formally certified, often facilities will require some type of certification for the animals to enter the facility and visit with occupants. Some of the most well-known certifying organizations include Therapy Dogs International and the American Kennel Club with their Canine Good Citizen test. Regardless of the category these animals fall under, they all provide a unique and essential function for the people they serve.

Dilemmas, Debates, and Unresolved Questions

Certification Concerns. The prevalence and use of assistance dogs has evolved tremendously over the past several decades, and with this evolution comes unresolved issues and dilemmas. One issue that has been a topic of much debate is the training and certification process of dogs being given public access rights. Many service dog organizations require a dog to undergo rigorous temperament testing, two years of training, and public access testing before graduating as a service dog. However, there is currently no national standard of training or accreditation process a dog must pass to work as a service dog. As long as it qualifies under the parameters set forth by the ADA, the dog is granted public access rights. Many people and service dog organizations have voiced concern that the lack of an official accreditation process is potentially hazardous to the public as well as to working dog teams. Also, dogs who are not properly trained but are being used as service dogs damage the reputations of legitimate service dogs, leaving open the possibility that business owners could begin to lobby to revoke the rights granted to service dogs.

Fraud Concerns. The presence of fraudulent service dogs has grown tremendously with the rise of the Internet. The Internet has made it increasingly easy to acquire official-looking service dog equipment, leading some to take advantage of the lack of accreditation required and pass their pet dogs off as working dogs. Along with that, some people have taken the opportunity to profit off of people's ignorance about the lack of accreditation required under the ADA. There are numerous Web sites that are charging large amounts of money for official-looking ID cards and superfluous "certifications" for their animals.

Profiteering. An instance of profiteering that has become a large problem within the service dog community is the existence of programs that charge thousands of dollars to consumers wishing to purchase service dogs and that subsequently do not provide a sufficiently trained dog as promised. That's not to say there aren't legitimate programs and organizations that charge money for service animals. Purchasing a service animal is often an appealing option to people who cannot or do not want to wait on a waitlist of a nonprofit organization that will provide a fully trained service dog free of charge. However, given there is the potential for fraud in the service dog industry, it is up to consumers to educate themselves thoroughly about the options available and make informed decisions that best meet their needs.

Standardized Accreditation. Although there are sound arguments in favor of the creation of a standardized certification process for all service dogs, there are also compelling reasons against it. One of the most prevalent arguments against a standardized accreditation process is that it will make it more difficult for people who wish to train their own service dogs and not go through an established program or work with a professional trainer. A process like this would also be very difficult to implement fairly and uniformly across the country. This remains an issue without any clear-cut solutions or answers.

Conclusion

New ways in which animals can help humans are continuing to be researched and discovered. As the relationships between animals and humans change, so too will the definition of service animals and the policies surrounding them. Regardless of changes to come, the bond between animals and people will remain significant, especially in the lives of people with disabilities.

Janie Meijas

See also: Americans with Disabilities Act (ADA); Animal-Assisted Therapy (AAT); Community Living and Community Integration; Independent Living

Further Reading

Assistance Dogs International. 2017. "Program Search." http://www.assistancedo gsinternational.org/members/programs -search/.

The Seeing Eye. 2015. "History." http://www .seeingeye.org/about-us/history.html.

U.S. Department of Justice. "Fair Housing Act." https://www.justice.gov/crt/fair-housing -act-2.

Sexual Violence

Sexual violence against people with disabilities is a serious problem that is growing larger. Both children and adults experience high rates of sexual violence, despite many efforts to protect them. The reasons for this are complex and many layered.

What Is Sexual Violence?

According to the U.S. Centers for Disease Control and Prevention (CDC), sexual violence can be defined as a sexual act committed against someone without that person's freely given consent (2015). This definition covers many types of nonconsensual sexual activities, including child sexual abuse, sexual assault, incest, intimate partner violence, and sexual harassment. Sexual violence can occur in many forms, including rape, attempted rape, other forced sexual activity, unwanted sexual touching, child pornography, other sexual activity in the presence of a minor, sex trafficking, and unwelcome sexual advances or verbal harassment of a sexual nature in the workplace or learning environment.

Background and History

Based on the data available, people with disabilities experience sexual violence at much higher rates than those without disabilities. One estimate from the U.S. Department of Justice states that people with disabilities over the age of 12 experienced rape or sexual assault at more than three times the rate of people without disabilities. The rate of serious violent victimization (rape, sexual assault, robbery, or aggravated assault) was highest for people with cognitive disabilities among all the disability types measured (U.S. Department of Justice 2015a). Research studies on the sexual abuse of children estimate that children with disabilities are also three times more likely to be sexually abused than children without disabilities. Children with intellectual disabilities are at especially high risk, almost five times more likely to be sexually abused than children without disabilities (Smith and Harrell 2013, 4). An intellectual disability is a type of disability that affects both the intellectual functioning and adaptive behavior of a person, with the disability occurring before the age of 18 years, according to the American Association on Intellectual and Developmental Disabilities (AAIDD 2013).

Important Factors about Sexual Violence and People with Disabilities

A number of factors contribute to these high rates of sexual violence against people with disabilities. While the vulnerability of people with disabilities is widely recognized, many people underestimate the high rates of sexual violence against them. One reason for this is the presence of attitudes in our society that devalue and isolate people with disabilities. People with disabilities become invisible to the dominant society, and their lived experiences are relatively unknown to most people. These attitudes contribute to the high level of vulnerability to abuse experienced by many people with disabilities. In addition, many people have difficulty viewing people with disabilities as sexual beings. For example, people with disabilities often receive little to no information about sexual education and sexual violence prevention. This lack of information can make it difficult for people with disabilities to assess their level of risk in dating and social relationships, leaving them more vulnerable to sexual violence.

Perpetrators and Reporting of Sexual Violence. Many people believe strangers represent the greatest danger of committing acts of sexual violence. This is a myth. Most sexual violence is committed by someone the victim knows. This is also true for people with disabilities. One of the reasons people with disabilities experience greater vulnerability to sexual violence from someone they know is because they may have more needs for support and personal care assistance than people without disabilities. Family members, intimate partners, personal care assistants, health care workers in institutions such as nursing homes or residential centers, and others who work in disability service agencies are among the people who have committed sexual violence against people with disabilities. There are also incidences where a person with a disability commits sexual violence against another person with a disability. Not knowing how to report sexual violence and not having access to a method to communicate what has happened can serve as barriers for people with disabilities who have experienced sexual violence. When they are able to report sexual violence, people with disabilities are often not believed. These are yet additional factors contributing to the vulnerability of people with disabilities, as well as contributing to the underreporting of the crime.

Disability-Specific Abuse. People with disabilities are also at higher risk of experiencing multiple types of abuse, including disability-specific abuse. Disability-specific abuse occurs when the abuser takes away access to the supports or communication aids that the person with a disability needs to get through the day. It may mean taking away a person's wheelchair, medications, computer, communication device, or other assistive technology supports. Disability-specific abuse can go on for long periods of time and may be combined with other forms of abuse, such as sexual violence. Violence, including abuse, directed at a person with a disability because of the offender's bias against people with disabilities is a hate crime.

Accessibility. Another barrier identified by sexual violence survivors with disabilities is the lack of accessibility in community resources and organizations that help people who have experienced sexual violence. A lack of accessibility may mean that the physical location of the rape crisis center or health center lacks a ramp or accessible exam rooms. It may also mean that the written materials, such as consent forms, informational pamphlets, and other resources, are not accessible to people with intellectual disabilities, for example. In addition, the staff working in these community organizations may have had no training on the specialized needs of people with disabilities, and they may feel unprepared or lack confidence on how to work effectively with this population.

Efforts to Address Sexual Violence and Future Directions

In an effort to address the alarming problem of sexual violence, the federal government passed the Violence Against Women Act in 1994 because women have been disproportionately affected by sexual violence. When the act was reauthorized in 2000, one of the newly designated priority areas of funding was "Training and Services to End Violence Against Women with Disabilities." The goals of this grant program were to establish and strengthen collaborative relationships and organizational capacity across the various disciplines and professions in order to better provide safe, accessible, and effective services to individuals with disabilities who experience sexual assault, domestic violence, dating violence, and stalking (U.S. Department of Justice 2015a). This is one important example of how policymakers are becoming increasingly aware of the problem and making it a priority to fund initiatives across the country to better address the problem.

Another important resource can help address the problem of sexual violence against people with disabilities: the advocacy efforts of people with disabilities themselves. People with disabilities want to know about healthy sexuality and ways to prevent sexual violence. Learning about and engaging in health sexuality has been called sexual self-advocacy. Encouraging and supporting the sexual self-advocacy of people with disabilities can help combat sexual violence. Providing sexuality education in accessible formats, promoting choice and support for healthy relationships, and understanding the sexual rights of people with disabilities are all important components of sexual self-advocacy (Friedman et al. 2014, 529). Holding offenders accountable and increasing the knowledge and training of providers on how to work with sexual violence survivors with disabilities should remain a priority until the abuse of people with disabilities is stopped.

Linda Sandman

See also: Abuse; Self-Advocacy Movement; Sexuality Education for People with Intellectual Disabilities

Further Reading

American Association on Intellectual and Developmental Disabilities. 2013. "Definition of Intellectual Disability." http://aaidd .org/intellectual-disability/definition #.VyZtLfkrLIU.

Barnard-Brak, Lucy, Marcelo Schmidt, Steven Chesnut, Tianlan Wei, and David Richman. 2014. "Predictors of Access to Sex Education for Children with Intellectual Disabilities in Public Schools." *Intellectual and Developmental Disabilities* 52, no. 2: 85–97.

CDC—Injury Prevention and Control: Division of Violence Prevention. 2015. "Sexual Violence: Definitions." Accessed November 28, 2015. http://www.cdc.gov/violencepre vention/sexualviolence/definitions.html.

Friedman, Carli, Catherine K. Arnold, Aleksa L. Owen, and Linda Sandman. 2014. "'Remember Our Voices Are Our Tools': Sexual Self-Advocacy as Defined by People with Intellectual and Developmental Disabilities." *Sexuality and Disability* 32, no. 4: 515–532.

Smith, Nancy, and Sandra Harrell. 2013. "Sexual Abuse of Children with Disabilities: A National Snapshot." *Vera Institute of Justice, Center on Victimization and Safety, Issue Brief*, March 2013. http://www.vera .org/sites/default/files/resources/down loads/sexual-abuse-of-children-with -disabilities-national-snapshot.pdf.

U.S. Department of Justice, Office of Justice Programs, Bureau of Justice Statistics. 2015a. "Crime Against Persons with Disabilities, 2009–2013—Statistical Tables." http://www.bjs.gov/content/pub/pdf/ capd0913st.pdf.

U.S. Department of Justice, Office of Violence Against Women, Grant Programs. 2015b. "Discretionary Grant Programs." http://www.justice.gov/ovw/grant-pro grams#thag.

Sexuality Education for People with Intellectual Disabilities

People with intellectual disabilities (ID) experience higher rates of sexual violence than people without disabilities. People with disabilities, family members, caregivers, professionals, educators, and support staff have expressed concerns about balancing the protection of people with ID and the sexual rights to relationships, privacy, marriage, and procreation. International entities like the World Health Organization and national organizations like the National Guardianship Association have affirmed the *sexual rights* of people with ID. While these policy standards exist, people with ID in community and institutional settings continue to be denied access to sexuality education and to self-determination in sexual expression.

Important Points to Know about Sexual Education for People with Intellectual Disabilities

National Sexuality Education Standards. There are national sexuality education standards for youth without disabilities, as well as curricula for students in special education. However, there is a lack of "evidence-based" standards and curricula for people with ID specifically. Educators have worked to bring a sexuality and disability focus to health programming under the term "sexual health." However, many people with ID continue to need a variety of sexuality education options, while having limited access to information and supports.

Need for Accessible Content. Content and program delivery can be made more accessible for people with ID through modifications like plain language, images such as photos and drawings, and body-part models. This accessible content emphasizes public versus private behaviors, as well as sexual boundaries with disability support staff. The experience, knowledge, and practical skills of educators and clinicians are critical for making sexuality education accessible for people with ID. While curriculum fidelity is important, sexuality education becomes accessible for people with ID when content is modified and tailored for individual learners.

Dilemmas around Sexual Consent Capacity. Clinicians often begin working with people with ID after sexual violence has already occurred, and they may be asked to establish "sexual consent capacity." Clinicians use various instruments and assessments to determine if an individual with ID is able to communicate "yes" or "no" to sexual activity. As with sexuality education, there are few standardized, evidence-based instruments for measuring sexual consent capacity. The use of sexual consent capacity assessments largely depends on the training, skill, and approach of individual clinicians or clinics. Establishing sexual consent capacity is especially difficult given the general lack of accessible sexuality education for people with ID. Even if a person with ID has consented to sexual activity, there may still be negative consequences if clinicians cannot establish sexual consent capacity. For example, people with ID may be denied access to romantic relationships of their choosing. Also, if sexual consent capacity cannot be established, someone abusing an individual may not be stopped, because the person with ID is not considered to have the capacity to be a witness in court.

Conclusion and Future Directions

Sexuality education, sexual violence prevention, and measurements of sexual consent capacity cannot be separated. Ongoing, comprehensive sexuality education throughout the lifespan helps to increase the sexual consent capacity of people with ID. People with ID who have access to sexuality education can increase their sexual consent capacity and are more likely to engage in healthy, chosen sexual relationships; recognize sexual violence; report incidents of violence; and seek help when needed. Many activists with ID refer to themselves as "sexual self-advocates." Sexual self-advocates work for their sexual rights, especially when it comes to obtaining sexuality education, increasing sexual consent capacity, and having chosen romantic and sexual relationships. Sexual self-advocates have demanded sexuality education with a focus on the "dignity of risk" and an emphasis on saying "yes" and "no" to sexual life on their own terms. Sexual self-advocates work to resist stereotypes about people with ID as being childlike, asexual, hypersexual, or automatically in need of sterilization. Sexual self-advocates are working to transform systems that normalize sexual violence (also known as "rape culture") and to resist the sexual oppression of disabled people.

Rebekah Moras

See also: Abuse; Developmental Disabilities Assistance and Bill of Rights Act; Eugenics; Inclusive Education; Sexual Violence

Further Reading

Association of University Centers on Disabilities. 2017. Sexual Health Special Interest Group. http://www.aucd.org/template/page.cfm?id=975.

Gill, M. 2015. *Already Doing It: Intellectual Disability and Sexual Agency.* Minneapolis: University of Minnesota Press.

Lyden, M. 2007. "Assessment of Sexual Consent Capacity." *Sexuality and Disability* 25, no. 1: 3–20.

Sandman, L., K. Arnold, L. Bolyanatz, C. Friedman, C. Saunders, and T. Wickey, directors. 2014. *In My Voice: Sexual Self-Advocacy*. Video/DVD. Chicago: University of Illinois at Chicago, Sexuality & Disability Consortium.

Ward, K., R. Windsor, and J. P. Atkinson. 2012. "A Process Evaluation of the Friendships and Dating Program for Adults with Developmental Disabilities: Measuring the Fidelity of Program Delivery." *Research in Developmental Disabilities* 33: 69–75.

Siblings

The term "sibling" is used to refer to people who have a brother or sister with a disability. Siblings can include sibling-like relationships beyond blood or genetic connections with a person with a disability.

Why Are Siblings Important?

Siblings often have the longest relationship of their lives with each other and have shared history and memories, especially when they have grown up together (Cicirelli 1995). Siblings teach each other skills that help them prepare for other relationships in life. For example, siblings can learn from each other how to fight and make up, as well as how to confide in and comfort one another. Siblings of people with disabilities may play a support, advocacy, or caregiving role, especially as they get older. The peer nature of the sibling relationship uniquely positions siblings to support each other to lead self-determined lives in many areas such as employment, voting, transportation, relationships and sexuality, health care, housing supports, and more.

Each sibling has a unique experience. Even each child within a family can have a very different perception. Yet, there are often similarities within that difference.

However, siblings of people with disabilities are often overlooked and sometimes even forgotten in terms of their experience, perspective, and needs. More awareness is needed about the sibling experience.

Important Points to Understand about Siblings

Experiences of Siblings of People with Disabilities. The experience of every person who is a sibling is unique. Although each person has a different situation, there are often common threads among siblings of people with disabilities. As children, siblings of people with disabilities experience the range of emotions similar to all sibling relationships. In addition, some siblings experience unique concerns and opportunities related to being the sibling of someone with disabilities. Concerns may include feeling embarrassed about the behavior of their siblings, guilt over any negative feelings they have, and resentment about the attention their sibling may receive. Additionally, some siblings may feel pressure to achieve or to be perfect since they do not want to add more stress for their parents.

Being a sibling of a person with disabilities also provides many opportunities. Some siblings are more accepting of difference, are more attune to other people's needs, and can be creative problem solvers for their disabled siblings. Siblings can learn to be advocates at a young age with and for their brothers and sisters with disabilities.

The sibling relationship changes over time in terms of emotional closeness. As adults, siblings are affected by their experience with their brothers and sisters with disabilities as well. Some siblings are influenced in their career path and vocation as a result of their sibling experience. Being a sibling of a person with a disability can become part of some people's identity. As adults, siblings often play support roles, which can include being advocates and caregivers.

Support Needs. The needs of siblings across the lifespan are often not addressed. The focus is typically on parents and the person with disabilities. However, the sibling experience needs more attention. Often when people think about sibling support, they think about children who are siblings. There are a few supports available for young siblings. For example, "Sibshops" are gatherings for siblings to obtain peer support and education within a recreational context. Regardless of age, *peer support* is important for siblings to be able to connect and network with other siblings of people with disabilities to learn from each other and validate each other's feelings.

There are a number of online support groups for siblings, including SibNet for adults, Sib20 for those in their twenties, and SibTeen for teenagers. Siblings also need information at different points of their lives to help them respond to questions from classmates about their sibling's disability, deal with bullying, learn how to navigate the system of disability supports and services, plan for the future as their parents age, learn how to advocate with and for their brothers and sisters with disabilities, and much more (Arnold, Heller, and Kramer 2012).

Planning for the Future. Depending on the needs of the person with disabilities, siblings often become the next generation of caregivers when parents are no longer able to fill the role. Siblings often juggle multiple caregiving responsibilities, such as caring for their aging parents, their own children, and their brothers and sisters with disabilities. As siblings become more involved in the care of their brother or sister with a disability, their own support needs increase. Therefore, it is critical to understand what supports siblings need from their viewpoint. Also, as siblings get the support they need, their brothers and sisters with disabilities will have better outcomes.

Even when siblings anticipate taking on a caregiving role in the future, siblings are often not involved in future planning discussions. Information is not always passed down from parents to siblings, and siblings have a very steep learning curve when they take on a greater support role in the life of their brother or sister with disabilities. Starting the difficult dialogue of planning for the future is challenging for families. Professionals can help support families to work through this future-planning process so everyone in the family has a voice in the process and a choice in future potential role.

Dilemmas, Debates, and Unsolved Questions about Siblings

Sibling Research. The research on the experiences of siblings of people with disabilities has changed over the years. Research has shifted from focusing on the negative impact on siblings to incorporating the positive aspects and becoming more balanced about the benefits and detriments of the sibling experience. For example, early research corroborated ideas of professionals that siblings would be negatively affected by interacting with a person with disabilities, and this research was used as a reason for institutionalizing children with disabilities. For this reason, many siblings did not grow up together, and some people were never even told they had a sibling with disabilities who was sent away to an institution. Numerous stories and films by siblings reuniting with their institutionalized siblings in adulthood shared the complex emotions and impact this separation had on people's lives. Additionally, the early research on siblings gathered information from the parents, particularly the mother, about their perception of the relationship between their children with and without disabilities.

More recently, the research literature about siblings has grown, and it shows a balance of positive and negative implications of the sibling experience for people who have a disabled brother or sister. Most of the research focuses on siblings of people with intellectual and developmental disabilities, with some research on siblings of people with mental health disabilities or on siblings of children with cancer. The current research is dominated by the perspective of white middle-class women who are fairly engaged in the lives of their brothers and sisters with disabilities. There is a need for more diverse sibling perspectives in the research, including the perspectives of people with disabilities about their sibling relationships.

Family Support Funding. Many of the people with intellectual and developmental disabilities in the United States have brothers and sisters. The majority of this population in the United States live with their families (Braddock et al. 2017). Moreover, parents are getting older while people with disabilities are living longer. As parents age and become less able to support their adult child with disabilities, sibling involvement becomes more necessary. Even though the majority of people with developmental disabilities are living with and receiving support from their family, only a small amount of funding goes to family support services in most states (Braddock et al. 2017). Hence there is a disparity between the reality of families as predominant caregivers for people with disabilities and the concomitant lack of financial support that the government invests to support families.

Policy and Advocacy. Siblings are often left out of policies intended for families.

For example, the Family and Medical Leave Act (FMLA) does not specifically include siblings in the law. Many families are also affected by state-specific Medicaid regulations that make it difficult for people with disabilities to move to a new state and maintain their Medicaid services and supports. These regulations can put families in a difficult position if they want or need to be more geographically mobile to pursue job or other opportunities. Does the person with disabilities and his or her family stay tied to a state because of essential and often life-saving Medicaid services that are needed? Or does the person with disabilities move to a new state and risk starting from square one when trying to get needed supports and services, which often have long waiting lists? Or do families split up geographically? These policies affect many siblings and influence the choices they make in terms of where they choose to live and which job opportunities they decide to pursue.

Future Directions in Sibling Leadership

It became evident that more support needed to be developed and focused on siblings, and a group of primarily adult siblings created the Sibling Leadership Network (SLN) in 2007. The SLN is working to get the sibling voice to the policy table so that issues that affect families take into consideration the sibling role. The SLN is a national nonprofit with state chapters dedicated to providing siblings of people with disabilities the information, support, and tools needed to advocate with their brothers and sisters and promote the issues important to them and their entire families (Heller et al. 2008). Siblings are an untapped constituency for advocacy efforts in the disability rights movement, and engaging siblings in causes can help increase power in numbers.

The SLN brings together siblings and people with disabilities from across the United States and engages them in the disability advocacy movement to effect greater change for people with disabilities and their families. Of course, there are times when the needs and perspectives of people with disabilities and siblings clash or conflict, and this dynamic plays out both in families and through state and national policy efforts.

Conclusion

Sibling relationships affect siblings of people with disabilities in many ways throughout their lives. While the sibling experience and perspective are often overlooked, siblings have support needs that when addressed provide better outcomes for their entire families. The research on siblings of people with disabilities is limited, though it is growing, and more is needed that incorporates diverse sibling perspectives and includes the voice of siblings with disabilities. There is an opportunity for siblings to engage in advocacy with their brothers and sisters with disabilities to influence issues that affect their families as well as other families.

Katie Arnold

See also: Family Caregivers and Health; Family Support Movements; Natural Supports; Special Education, Role of the Family in

Further Reading

Arnold, Catherine K., Tamar Heller, and John Kramer. 2012. "Support Needs of Siblings of People with Developmental Disabilities." *Intellectual and Developmental Disabilities* 50, no. 5: 373–382.

Braddock, David, Richard E. Hemp, Emily S. Tanis, Jiang Wu, and Laura Haffer. 2017. *The State of the States in Intellectual and Developmental Disabilities.* Washington, DC: American Association on Intellectual and Developmental Disabilities.

Cicirelli, Victor G. 1995. *Sibling Relationships Across the Lifespan.* New York: Plenum Press.

Heller, Tamar, Ann Kaiser, Don Meyer, Tom Fish, John Kramer, and Derrick Dufresne. 2008. "The Sibling Leadership Network: Recommendations for Research, Advocacy, and Supports Relating to Siblings of People with Developmental Disabilities." *The Rehabilitation Research and Training Center on Aging with Developmental Disabilities.* September 15. http://sibling leadership.org/wpcontent/uploads/2013/02 /SLN-White-PaperFinal-2.pdf.

Sign Language Interpreters

A sign language interpreter is someone who facilitates communication between d/Deaf (capitalization has cultural implications) and hearing language users. Interpreters provide communication services that run the gamut of life experiences, including education, employment, health care, and entertainment. Interpreters may perform these services in person or through a digital interface and are often considered to be allies to the historically oppressed Deaf community.

What Is Sign Language Interpreting?

In the United States, an interpreter is generally fluent in (at least) American Sign Language (ASL) and English as well as the respective cultures of those languages to produce accurate and culturally appropriate interpretations. Although there are many different types of interpreting (such as consecutive interpreting, translation, and sight translation), sign language interpreters predominantly provide communication services through *simultaneous interpretation*, requiring the interpreter to continually

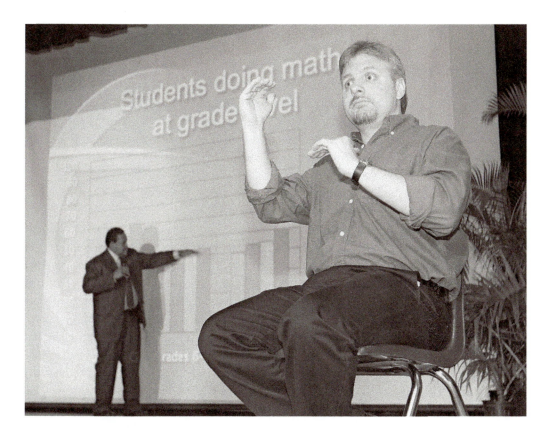

A sign language interpreter at work during a town hall meeting. There is a pressing need for more qualified interpreters across the United States. (Jeff Greenberg/UIG via Getty Images)

receive one language and quickly comprehend and express its meaning into another language within seconds while remaining neutral to the message and its users. This intense mental process often requires that interpreters work in teams to avoid mental fatigue and facilitate accurate interpretation.

Background and History

The earliest documentation of ASL interpreters records them to largely be siblings of children of Deaf people, clergy, and educators of deaf children (Humphrey and Alcorn 2007). Communication services provided up until that time were informal, infrequent, and unpaid (Ball 2013). This was because interpreter education programs were not established until the 1950s by funding made available through the passage of the Vocational Rehabilitation Amendments of 1954. Yet, ASL was not considered to be an actual language until nearly a decade later (Stokoe 1960).

Simultaneous Interpretation. The first occurrence of simultaneous interpretation is documented to have been at the Nuremberg Trials of 1945–1949 after World War II, in which the trial proceeded simultaneously in four languages (Gaiba 1998). The new technique was so efficient and effective when done well that it was quickly popularized and incorporated as the primary technique of interpreting in the United States.

Models of Interpretation. The "helper model" was the first model of interpreting, stemming from philosophies that d/Deaf people were deficient and incapable of handling their own affairs. Subsequently, the interpreter was conceptualized as a personal aide and caretaker in addition to communication facilitator for the d/Deaf individual. However, this approach is now considered paternalistic and oppressive to a d/Deaf person's *self-agency*. The next interpreting model went to the other extreme as a rigid communication "conduit" in which the interpreter functioned as a machine and did not prioritize cultural mediation but rather a verbatim interpretation between individual signs and words instead of complete concepts. This model resulted in confusing interpretations and little accountability of the interpreter's influence on interactions. The model that followed was known as the "bilingual/bicultural model," which situates cultural mediation at the core of linguistic interactions. This approach requires the interpreter to have the sociolinguistic fluency to represent messages and meaning accurately and appropriately between two language users.

The Importance of Sign Language Interpreters

Before the establishment of many disability rights laws, such as the Rehabilitation Act of 1973, the Americans with Disabilities Act (ADA), and the Individuals with Disabilities Education Act (IDEA), the majority of d/Deaf people were denied access to information in many important life events, such as education, employment, health care, and legal services. In addition, the historically poor quality of d/Deaf education established further barriers to communication through low English literacy levels. A readily accessible, visually based sign language is learned in conjunction with or often instead of English. Therefore, printed English is often just as inaccessible as spoken English but can be made accessible through the work of a sign language interpreter. Antidiscrimination legislation ensures that organizations and programs must provide sign language interpreters to ensure d/Deaf people have access to information and the opportunity to participate equally in mainstream society.

Dilemmas, Debates, and Unresolved Questions

Power and Authenticity. Although sign language interpreting education, training, and practice seems streamlined when compared to the field's beginning, interpreters still face many challenges in regard to negotiating power and authenticity within interpreted interactions. Some of these issues are related to the culture, language, and modality fluency as well as the need to maintain enough interpreters in the field to satisfy the demand for interpreters who represent the diverse identities of d/Deaf people and successfully navigate the role of the "neutral interpreter."

Formalization of the Field. Historically, sign language interpreters were family members of d/Deaf people or were otherwise heavily involved in the Deaf community, which promoted their exceptional fluency in Deaf culture and sign language. The formalization of interpreter education began attracting people from outside the community who have not had immersive learning opportunities, which could negatively affect the quality of interpretation.

Communication Modalities. Controversies around Deaf educational practices have invented a variety of communication modalities in addition to ASL, producing a community of diverse communication styles that interpreters are expected to know. A communication modality is not actual sign language but rather a manual representation of spoken language. Some of these modalities include Signed Exact English, Manually Coded English, Pidgin Signed English, Conceptually Accurate Signed English, Transliteration, and Cued Speech. Most interpreter training programs cover these modalities only superficially, if at all, which inadequately prepares new interpreters for the actual communication needs of the Deaf community.

Lack of Qualified Interpreters. The advent of legal protections for language access and increased awareness of Deaf rights has greatly increased the demand for sign language interpreters. However, the arduous training and credentialing involved to become a professional interpreter is a deterrent for many approaching the career, causing a great disparity between supply and demand. The lack of available interpreters often means that Deaf individuals must forego language access to an activity that they wish to attend.

Lack of Diversity. An additional concern is the lack of diversity in the interpreting profession, which does not reflect the diversity of the Deaf community. Sign language interpreters in the United States are predominantly heterosexual, white, college-educated females, while Deaf people reflect a general cross section of the lower socio-economic populations of the United States. Since sign language interpreters act as the voice for Deaf consumers, it is desirable that identity and experiential knowledge align as closely as possible to produce an authentic representation. Yet the lack of interpreters and hiring practices not inclusive of Deaf consumers often leaves Deaf people no choice for who is available to represent their voice.

Deaf Interpreters. Finally, the role of the interpreter is regularly debated since the model for message accuracy is often in direct conflict with the amount of cultural mediation needed for d/Deaf and hearing parties to understand each other in any given situation. The Deaf Interpreter, a Deaf native sign language user, has developed to resolve cultural misunderstandings and dissimilar language modalities of d/Deaf individuals and hearing sign language interpreters.

Traditional models of interpreting encourage participants in interpreted interactions to focus on the content of language received while acknowledging the presence of the interpreter as little as possible, if at all. Some argue that an interpreter's "invisibility" is impossible and that therefore so is absolute neutrality. As a result, these issues should be included in discussion of the interpreter's role instead of being ignored. Many agree that the role of the interpreter changes to accommodate the parameters of each unique encounter.

Future of Sign Language Interpreters

Technology is a force of change in the field of sign language interpreting. Video technology allows interpreters to provide live simultaneous interpretation services from a remote location and in telephone calls. Interpretation services through a digital interface continue to advance on mobile devices, which have certainly come a long way since the original cumbersome and stationary telecommunications devices designed for the deaf in the mid-20th century. Medical technologies, such as cochlear implants, aim to decrease the incidence of deafness. This, in turn, decreases the need for interpreters. However, Deaf community members continue to fight for the right to use qualified sign language interpreters for language access. As long as there are sign language users, there will be a need for interpreters.

Shannon Moutinho

See also: Alternative and Augmentative Communication; Communication; Language; Speech-Language Pathology

Further Reading

Ball, Carolyn. 2013. *Legacies and Legends: History of Interpreter Education from 1800 to the 21st Century.* Edmonton, AB: Interpreting Consolidated.

Gaiba, Francesca. 1998. *The Origins of Simultaneous Interpretation: The Nuremberg Trial.* Ottawa, ON: University of Ottawa Press.

Humphrey, Janice H., and Bob J. Alcorn. 2007. *So You Want to Be an Interpreter?: An Introduction to Sign Language Interpreting.* Seattle: H & H Publishing.

Lane, Harlen L. 1999. *The Mask of Benevolence: Disabling the Deaf Community.* San Diego: DawnSignPress.

Metzger, Melanie. 1999. "Participant Frameworks: The Role of the Interpreter." In *Sign Language Interpreting: Deconstructing the Myth of Neutrality.* Washington, DC: Gallaudet University Press.

Stokoe, William C. 1960. *Sign Language Structure: An Outline of the Visual Communication Systems of the American Deaf.* Buffalo, NY: Department of Anthropology and Linguistics, University of Buffalo.

Social Capital

"Social capital" is a term used to describe the quality of social relations held by an individual or community. Social capital can be thought of as reflection of *social cohesion.* "Social cohesion" refers to the level of mutual connections, cooperation, and action that occurs among different groups of a society.

Social cohesion and social capital are produced by social relationships, making social capital a group as well as an individual resource. That is, social capital is a feature of the groups to which a person belongs, such as neighborhoods, communities, and institutions, making it a collective characteristic. Groups with high levels of social capital have mutually beneficial levels of interaction and trust, which produce public good that extends beyond the individual person.

What Is Social Capital?

Structural and Cognitive Social Capital. Social capital has been conceptualized in different ways. Some view social capital as having two dimensions that are measured as levels of participation ("structural social capital") and perception ("cognitive social capital"). The *structural* form of social capital involves actions that are taken. At the individual level, such actions might include actual participation in local or voluntary organizations, civic actions, actual support received from neighbors, and contact with family, friends, and neighbors. At the community level, such actions might be measured as per capita group membership and engagement in public affairs. "Cognitive social capital" refers to levels of general trust in others, perceived social support, and sense of community among individuals. From a community perspective, cognitive social capital can be measured as overall trust in the social environment and politicians (Ehsan and De Silva 2015).

Bonding, Bridging, and Linking. Others have conceptualized social capital as existing in three different forms: bonding, bridging, and linking. The *bonding* form of social capital is formed through participation in support groups, local neighborhood associations, advocacy organizations, and other closed networks that share similar ethnic, cultural, or racial identities. When individuals interact across different groups with similar levels of status and power, regardless of group origin or social identity, the *bridging* form of social capital is created. The *linking* form of social capital is developed when individuals or groups who have unequal status and power, as well as different social identities, make connections.

Measuring Social Capital. The different meanings applied to social capital have resulted in a number of measures used to research this concept. Social capital measures include levels of trust in other people as well as "civic trust," which refers to trust in authorities or public institutions. Social capital has also been measured by the "norms of reciprocity" that occur across groups, such as the extent to which neighbors will mutually help one another, a sense of belonging, and "collective efficacy," or the extent to which individuals will act in the interests of a common good. For indicators of social capital, other researchers have looked to participation activities, such as the density, depth, and breadth of contact with family and friends, known as "informal networks"; the density of group memberships (such as religious, sports, hobby, political, and professional groups) and contacts, known as "formal networks"; volunteerism; and voting and political activity. Many of these measures assess individual beliefs or behaviors that are then examined across such groups as neighborhoods, counties, or states.

Important Points to Understand about Social Capital and Disability

Regardless of the conceptualization used, higher levels of social capital have been linked to better education, employment, health, political participation, safety, and well-being outcomes among the general population. Social capital can thus be associated with many of the outcomes desired for persons with disabilities. People with disabilities generally have lower levels of social capital than other people, however (Mithen et al. 2015).

The lower levels of social capital experienced by people with disabilities may be due to several factors. First, certain types of disabilities may limit the ability to form strong social connections. Persons with certain types of mental impairments, such as persons with intellectual or developmental disabilities, have been found to have lower levels of social capital, report higher rates of loneliness, and have increased levels of dependence on family relationships (Condeluci et al. 2008).

Second, discrimination also may result in lower levels of social capital for persons with disabilities. Discrimination that limits participation in educational or vocational activities, for example, subsequently reduces the opportunity to participate in activities that can foster strong social connections.

Lastly, accessibility of the local environment or specific resources may be an issue. To develop high levels of social capital, persons with all types of disabilities, including those with physical and sensory limitations, must be able to participate fully in all aspects of community life.

Summary

As high levels of social capital have been found to be associated with many positive outcomes, including improved health and function, the low levels of social capital that many persons with disabilities experience are cause for concern. Additional research is therefore needed to measure types of social capital and to investigate concrete ways to improve social engagement for Americans with disabilities.

Debra L. Brucker and Amanda Botticello

See also: Community; Poverty; Quality of Life

Further Reading

Condeluci, Al, Melva Gooden Ledbetter, Dori Ortman, Jeff Fromknecht, and Megan DeFries. 2008. "Social Capital: A View from the Field." *Journal of Vocational Rehabilitation* 29, no. 3: 133–139.

Ehsan, Annahita M., and Mary J. De Silva. 2015. "Social Capital and Common Mental Disorder: A Systematic Review." *Journal of Epidemiology and Community Health* 69, no. 10: 1021–1028.

Kawachi, Ichiro, and Lisa F. Berkman. 2000. "Social Cohesion, Social Capital, and Health." In *Social Epidemiology*, edited by Ichiro Kawachi and Lisa F. Berkman, 174–190. New York: Oxford University Press.

Kawachi, Ichiro, Daniel Kim, Adam Coutts, and S. V. Subramanian. 2004. "Commentary: Reconciling the Three Accounts of Social Capital." *International Journal of Epidemiology* 33, no. 4: 682–690.

Mithen, Johanna, Zoe Aitken, Anna Ziersch, and Anne M. Kavanagh. 2015. "Inequalities in Social Capital and Health between People with and without Disabilities." *Social Science & Medicine*, 126: 26–35.

Social Model of Disability

The social (also called the sociopolitical) model of disability originated among disability rights activists in the United Kingdom in the early 1970s. Its primary purpose was to separate the conceptualization of disability from that of impairment—to say that disability was something that was socially created while impairment was merely a biological fact with no cultural values attached to it.

Why Is the Social Model Important?
Under the social model, what became disabling for people was not their inability to walk, see, or hear (for example) but rather the inaccessibility of a physical, social, and cultural environment that remained hostile to their presence in it. As the British Union for the Physically Impaired Against Segregation (UPIAS) explained, disability is "a form of [socially created] disadvantage which is imposed on top of one's impairment, that is, the disadvantage or restriction of activity caused by a contemporary social organization that takes little or no account of people with physical impairments" (quoted in Tremain 2006, 187). Put simply, the social model of disability makes a critical distinction between impairment (body) and disability (society). It roots disabled people's limitations in societal barriers that disable them, not in any individual embodied deficit. Disability studies scholars refer to this system of exclusion as "ableism." They argue that ableism and ableist attitudes are present in all societies that are built by and for nondisabled people (Goodley 2011; 2014).

Historical Overview
Since the 1970s, the social model of disability has come to form the theoretical core of the growing and evolving field of disability studies. Initially, primarily white male researchers who focused on physical and sensory impairments dominated disability studies in the United Kingdom and the United States. Throughout the 1970s and most of the 1980s, sociologists and scholars using sociologically oriented methodologies sought to document and analyze both the causes and the effects of the structural exclusion of disabled people from society in such areas as employment, education, housing, and transportation. Over the remainder of the 20th century and into the 21st century (1985 onward), disability studies scholars went from focusing almost exclusively

on examining the effects of various social forces in the lives of people with physical and sensory impairments to including a much broader range of impairments and a much larger evidence base in their research. Disability studies scholars trained in English and history, as well as other programs, such as American, media, and women's and gender studies built on the foundational literature developed in the field's first decade (1975–1985) by exploring not only the representation of disability and disabled people in culture (e.g., literature, film, art, and popular culture) but also the lived experiences of disabled people throughout history. This new generation of scholars—an increasing number of whom were women; racial or ethnic minorities; lesbian, gay, bisexual, transgender, or queer (LGBTQ) people; and disabled people—were influenced by feminist, queer, and critical race theory. These scholars expanded the range of impairments under their purview to include "mental illness" (often referred to as "madness" by disability studies scholars), intellectual and developmental disabilities, and chronic illnesses (Goodley 2011; 2014). By the first decade of the 21st century, the social model of disability had proved influential in the way international organizations such as the World Health Organization (WHO) defined disability and also helpful in securing rights for people with disabilities through the passing of the Americans with Disabilities Act (ADA) in 1990, the ADA Amendments Act in 2008, and the United Nations Convention on the Rights of Persons with Disabilities (UNCRPD) in 2008. Further, the social model revolutionized the ways in which a growing group of academics, artists, and activists thought about impairment and disability. As Bonnie Smith, professor of women's and gender studies at Rutgers University, noted, "Gone are the days of a simple and dominant physiological or medical definition of disability" (2004, 1).

Impact of the Social Model

By redefining disability as something created in the social world and not through biology (or genes or neurochemistry), the social model of disability enabled scholars (and activists and artists) to move disabled people away from their historical place in society as individuals in need of medical, rehabilitation, welfare, and other services and interventions to that of an oppressed social minority in need of recognition of its civil and human rights. By discarding the notion that disability is negative and rooted in the individual, and by thinking critically about the power of various social arrangements to disable, social model theorists have been able to develop a powerful understanding of what it means to live differently in the world. Part of the success of the social model derives from its ability to expand the definition of disability to include a broad range of impairments, illnesses, and conditions and to show that disability will touch everyone at some point in life. Whether we become disabled or not, all of us at some point in our lives will feel the effects of disability: as we age; as we interact with coworkers, friends, lovers, clients, students, or customers; and as we care for the ones we love. The tremendous diversity among the world's disabled population and the broad range of experiences we all have with disability have been a source of empowerment for disability rights activists and academics alike.

Key Debates About the Social Model

While all disability studies scholars agree on the basic premise of the social model—that disability exists outside of the human body and that it is mediated through the environment and social relations—there are scholars who offer important critiques of some of the social model's finer points. These critiques can be broken down into three general categories, none of which are mutually exclusive (they all overlap). The first seeks to revise our understanding of the social model by critiquing the ways in which it defines impairment as value free. The second values identity politics—as opposed to the more structural approaches of "strict" social model theorists—and urges us to recognize the critical role of class, race, gender, sexuality, and other categories in the formation of disabled people's identities and experiences. A third group of disability studies scholars who focus their work on global disability studies question the usefulness of the social model outside of the five areas that Cushing and Smith (2009) referred to as the Western, English-speaking world: the United States, the United Kingdom, Canada, Australia, and New Zealand. This section will briefly address each one of these critiques of the social model of disability.

Fixed and Value Free vs. Culturally Created. As stated above, the original social model defines impairment as neutral, as a biological reality that exists outside of social relations, politics, and the pathologizing discourses of Western medicine. Initially, disability studies theorists drew an analogy with feminist thinking about sex and gender to describe the difference between impairment and disability: *impairment is to sex as disability is to gender.* Early disability studies theorists held that impairment, like our biological sex, is fixed in our bodies. We have little if any power to control or alter our impairment. It is part of our being, part of who we are; it is real. Disability, on the other hand, is like gender. It is socially created and historically contingent. Because

disability emerges out of the built environment and the social milieu (or environment) within which we live, it changes over time. Disability, like gender, is fluid. We have the power to control what becomes disabling in society by altering the built environment, as well as dominant social relations and cultural perceptions. Disability studies theorists, through their research and writing, seek to promote change in all three areas related to disability: the built environment, social relations, and cultural perceptions.

By the 1990s, feminist and queer theorists from a number of academic backgrounds, including those in disability studies, began challenging the taken-for-granted nature of both biological sex and impairment. They argued that neither is as fixed or as value free as we might assume. Ideas and definitions of both sex and impairment change over time and vary among cultures. For example, a mental illness in one time and place might be a blessing from the gods in another time and place. A missing limb or a lack of sensory perception could evoke stigma and feelings of shame and guilt in one setting and be completely normative in another. One need only look at the shift in language from "mental retardation" to "intellectual and developmental disability" or at the astronomical rise in the diagnosis of autism at the beginning of the 21st century to see the fluidity of impairment categories. A person could be defined as impaired in one historical moment and considered unimpaired in another historical moment. In other cases, people with certain types of impairments might also only experience them sporadically and in varying degrees over the course of their lifetime. Think, for example, of those with multiple sclerosis, lupus, chronic fatigue, or another chronic condition who might have days, weeks, or even months in which they are relatively "symptom-free." Impairment is not as fixed or as static as scholars and activists once presumed. Additionally, disability studies theorists declared that impairment, in most cases, has real disabling effects in the lives of those individuals who live with it. They urged social model theorists and all disability studies scholars to reconcile themselves with the fact that impairment—that is, people's own bodies—can impose real restrictions on their lives, and in some cases those impairments can be deadly. No amount of social activism can alter the lived effects of impairment in some people's lives. Scholars in disability studies refer to these lived realities as the effects of impairment, or *impairment effects*.

Identity Politics. The second critique of the social model has its roots in a particular form of U.S. identity politics (Rembis 2010). Authors writing primarily in the United States argue that a stigmatized and devalued disability identity is one of the powerful legacies of the individualization, medicalization, and pathologization of impairment (Siebers 2008). The result is that disabled people are divided by their impairment. They are divided by medical and rehabilitation professionals, social workers, educators, and a larger society that see them as nothing more than their own individual impairments and treat each one of them as an individual case, patient, or client, different from all the other cases, patients, or clients. The professionals, of course, can find similarities in disabled people's physiology, their neurochemistry, and their symptoms, but disabled people remain isolated and alone, trapped by their own internalization of a depoliticized, pathologized, individualized, and ultimately devalued sense of themselves. That is to say that when people hear the same ableist feedback from the people around them, they begin to believe

it is true about themselves, even sometimes when their experiences tell them otherwise. This phenomenon is known as *internalized ableism*. Only when individuals shed this stigmatized identity can disabled people become free to see the ableist world and their place in it for what it really is; only then can they see the discrimination, segregation, isolation, and outright violence and oppression that they face every day. Disability studies scholars refer to this consciousness-raising process as *claiming* a disability identity or "coming out" as disabled.

According to this form of identity politics, disabled people become empowered when they embrace their disabled identity—when they make it their own and begin to associate, demonstrate, and identify with other disabled people who have done likewise. Once they have experienced this consciousness raising, they are (in most situations) "able" to live life on their own terms. Some of them choose to "let their freak flags fly." Some flaunt their disabled bodies and revel in their sexuality. Others among them choose to "pass," or rather to minimize the extent of their impairment or mute their disabled identities (usually when in the presence of mixed company). Most disabled people, however, choose to live what prominent disability studies theorist Tobin Siebers (2008) calls a *complex embodiment*, which is some mix of all of these extremes. Within this framework, everything disabled people choose to do, every utterance they make, and every cultural artifact they produce gets politicized. The personal lived experience of disability becomes a politicized identity that can be used to enact social and legal change (Siebers 2008).

Critical to this identity-based disability politic, and to its attendant theorizing within disability studies, is the notion of *intersectionality*. Disabled people's complex embodied experience in the world is influenced not only by impairment or the disabling effects of an ableist society but also by the complex interactions and intersections of impairment and disability with the other identities we inhabit, including race, class, gender, sexuality, religion, and other important social and cultural markers. Disability studies scholars interested in identity and identity politics argue that all disability studies research must take into account these important and sometimes conflicting subjectivities (or beliefs) when documenting and analyzing disability history and culture, as well as the daily lives, loves, and experiences of disabled people.

Global Disability Studies. The final major critique of the social model to emerge within disability studies comes from scholars interested in global disability studies. Put simply, disability studies scholars working on non-Western topics and those working outside of the Western, English-speaking world (alternatively referred to as *the global North*) are finding that disability studies theories that are dominant in the West or global North, including the social model, are often ineffective, or in some cases only partially effective, in helping to explain the lived experiences of disabled people in other parts of the world (referred to as *the global South*). Global disability studies theorists make strong arguments for avoiding the uncritical exportation of global North disability studies theories to the global South and, instead, argue for situating analyses of the lived experiences of disabled people in their own local cultural and historical contexts, social relations, and governing structures, as well as larger international political and economic systems. Rather than dismiss global North disability studies, global South scholars encourage collaborative and constructive dialogue between North and

South, which they argue will build stronger disability studies analyses and more powerful disability politics in both parts of the world (Mehrotra 2013).

Summary and Conclusion

Emerging out of the disability rights movement primarily in the United Kingdom and the United States, the social model of disability became the basic tenet of disability studies. A direct critique of the medical model of disability, the social model separated impairment from disability, stating that it was the built environment, social relations, and dominant cultures that disabled people, not necessarily their own bodies. Disability studies scholars have raised important and influential critiques of the social model that have broadened the reach of the field to include a greater number of disability experiences and strengthened the theoretical and methodological foundation upon which arguments were built. As disability studies entered the 21st century, scholars from a number of areas within the field increasingly critiqued the social model's primary focus on white citizens of the Western, English-speaking world, or global North, giving rise to a growing "critical" global disability studies movement. Given the robustness of research and theorization in both the global North and the global South emerging from the social model and its attendant critiques, there is little doubt that the social model of disability, most likely in new and somewhat altered forms, will continue to be influential in a number of academic, social, political, and cultural areas in the future.

Michael Rembis

See also: Americans with Disabilities Act (ADA); Critical Disability Studies; Disability Rights Movement (DRM); Disability Studies;

Disability Studies in Higher Education; Identity; International Classification of Functioning Disability, and Health (ICF)

Further Reading

Cushing, Pamela, and Tyler Smith. 2009. "A Multinational Review of English-Language Disability Studies Degrees and Courses." *Disability Studies Quarterly* 29: 3.

Goodley, Dan. 2011. *Disability Studies: An Interdisciplinary Introduction*. Los Angeles: SAGE.

Goodley, Dan. 2014. *Dis/Ability Studies: Theorising Disablism and Ableism*. New York: Routledge.

Mehrotra, Nilika. 2013. *Disability, Gender and State Policy: Exploring Margins*. Jaipur, India: Rawat Publications.

Rembis, Michael. 2010. "Yes We Can Change: Disability Studies—Enabling Equality." *Journal of Postsecondary Education and Disability Special Issue: Disability Studies* 23, no. 1: 19–27.

Shakespeare, Tom. 2014. *Disability Rights and Wrongs Revisited*. New York: Routledge.

Siebers, Tobin. 2008. *Disability Theory*. Ann Arbor: University of Michigan Press.

Tremain, Shelley. 2006. "On the Government of Disability: Foucault, Power, and the Subject of Impairment" In *The Disability Studies Reader*, 2nd ed., edited by Lennard. J. Davis, 185–196. New York: Routledge.

Note: Portions of this article have been revised and reprinted with permission from: Michael Rembis. (2010) 2015. "Disability Studies." In *International Encyclopedia of Rehabilitation*. Edited by J. H. Stone and M. Blouin. Center for International Rehabilitation Research Information and Exchange. http://cirrie.buffalo.edu/encyclopedia/article.php?id=281&language=en.

Social Security Disability Insurance (SSDI) and Supplemental Security Income (SSI)

The Social Security Administration's (SSA) disability benefits policies are intended to provide income replacement and prevent destitution (or hardship) for those who are born with or acquire disabilities and are unable to work. As the largest disability benefits program in the United States, Social Security disability benefits provide valuable support to many people with disabilities in the form of income replacement, health insurance, vocational rehabilitation, and employment supports.

Social Security Administration Disability Determination

For applicants for Social Security disability, SSA determines both eligibility and entitlement to benefits. "Eligibility" means being qualified and eligible to receive benefits, prior to the determination of whether the person meets the statutory and medical guidelines to be "disabled" for entitlement.

At step one of the disability determination process, SSA determines if the applicant is earning substantial gainful activity (SGA), which is defined as work activity performed for pay or profit at amounts above established levels. For Title II Social Security Disability Insurance (SSDI), a person must have a sufficient work history with earnings having been paid into the program to be eligible and "insured" for benefits. For Title XVI Supplemental Security Income (SSI), a person must demonstrate financial need through limited means and resources to be eligible. A claimant may be entitled for both disability benefits programs. SSDI and SSI have different eligibility guidelines but share an identical disability determination process for entitlement, to be found medically disabled under SSA rules.

Once a person is determined to be eligible, SSA then determines if the person meets the criteria of the SSA definition of disability. SSA's statutory definition of disability is the "inability to engage in substantial gainful activity by reason of any medically determinable physical or mental impairment that can be expected to result in death or that has lasted or can be expected to last for a continuous period of not less than 12 months" (Social Security Administration 2015).

Employment Supports

Employment supports, also known as work incentives, are rules created to allow Social Security beneficiaries to work and continue to receive cash and health care benefits. There exist four categories of employment supports for Social Security disability benefits recipients: SSDI; SSI; SSDI and SSI; and a separate category for "blind." Determining disability and providing employment supports involves determining the value of one's work activity. When a claimant applies for benefits, or when a beneficiary receiving benefits works, SSA makes a substantial gainful activity (SGA) determination that estimates the value of the work that is performed in relation to the actual paid amounts.

Social Security Disability Insurance Employment Supports

The trial work period (TWP) is the primary employment support that allows an individual to test the ability to work for nine months without seeing benefit interruption, regardless of the earned amounts. The month after completion of the TWP plus three grace months, the 36-month extended period of eligibility (EPE) reentitlement period begins. Benefits are suspended for any month where earnings for work are over the SGA level during this period. For the first month that any earnings are over the SGA level after the 36-month EPE, benefits will terminate.

To determine the actual value of a beneficiary's work activity when making a SGA determination involving self-employment income, "unincurred" business expenses, including qualifying business expenses paid or incurred debt, may be deducted from the net earnings. If a beneficiary (or someone receiving benefits) is entitled to Medicare coverage, usually after two years of receiving SSDI, hospital insurance (Part A), supplemental medical insurance (Part B), and prescription drug coverage (Part C) health insurance will continue for at least 93 consecutive months, unless SSA determines medical improvement.

With a goal to help beneficiaries return to employment and minimize barriers to work, work supports continue to evolve and modernize. SSA began testing the Benefit Offset National Demonstration (BOND) in 2010 and is evaluating the gradual reduction of benefits by $1 for each additional $2 earned above the SGA level. This approach to employment support may incentivize returning to work while reducing dependency on entitlement programs, thereby saving the government money and maintaining the safety net of disability benefits.

Supplemental Security Income Employment Supports

In calculating an SSI recipient's benefit payment, SSA may exclude less than one-half of general and earned income. Additionally, for SSI recipient students under the age of 22 attending a school, college, or other training program, SSA may exclude a substantial amount of earned income for the

Student Earned Income Exclusion (SEIE) work support.

In determining continuing eligibility for SSI benefits, SSA excludes certain means, resources, or property under Property Essential to Self-Support (PESS). SSA may exclude some of the equity value of a non-business income-generating property or a nonbusiness property used to make goods or services needed for activities of daily living.

SSI recipients who work and earn above the SGA level may continue to receive benefits under Section 1619(a) if they were eligible for an SSI payment at least a month prior to earning SGA, are still disabled, and meet all of the SSI eligibility rules. Additionally, under Section 1619(b), a person may continue to receive Medicaid benefits if there is need and the earnings are below a certain level, even if SSI cash benefits have been stopped. If a person loses eligibility for SSI benefits because of work and earnings, SSA may reinstate benefits without a new application within 12 months of the stoppage of benefits. Under Section 1619, SSI recipients who are working may continue to receive benefit payments while in a Medicaid or public medical or psychiatric facility for up to two months.

The Plan to Achieve Self-Support (PASS) may allow for deductions in the SGA determination related to expenses for education, vocational training, or business start-up, all for a specified period of time for an individual's reasonable work goal.

Key Concepts in Social Security Disability Insurance

There are employment supports under both SSDI and SSI disability benefits programs. SSA considers the following employment supports that may reduce what is determined to be earned, the value to paid earnings SGA: subsidies, special conditions, unsuccessful work attempts (UWA), and impairment-related work expenses (IRWE). A subsidy is support that is provided by the employer and that results in the employee earning more than the projected value of one's work. Likewise, a special work condition is an employer-provided arrangement and flexibility, such as additional breaks, greater supervision, mentor or job coach assistance, fewer or simpler job duties, all in comparison to other employees performing the same job for the same pay. A person tries to perform substantial work, but an UWA occurs when the work is stopped or reduced within six months or less because of one's impairment or removal of special work conditions required to perform the job. In making the SGA determination, SSA will consider deducting IRWE, impairment-related expenses required to perform the job. Examples of IRWE paid out of pocket include medications, attendant care services, medical devices, and supplies.

The Ticket to Work (TTW) is an underused program that provides reimbursement in the form of a "ticket" for employment networks providing employment, vocational rehabilitation, or other support services related to obtaining or maintaining a job. If a beneficiary is participating in TTW or PASS, a school individualized education program (IEP) or individualized plan for employment (IPE) through a Vocational Rehabilitation Agency prevents the interruption of benefits under the Continued Payment under Vocational Rehabilitation or Similar Program (Section 301) provisions. The benefits may not be terminated until the program is complete, beneficiary participation ends, or SSA determines that the program will not result in "no longer needing benefits" and ultimate disability cessation.

When cash benefits are terminated because of SGA-level work and earnings, expedited reinstatement (EXR) allows for the resumption of temporary cash benefits and Medicare or Medicaid in a provisional period of six months while SSA conducts an expedited medical review. The requirements of EXR include a five-year time limit to file from the date of benefits termination due to SGA work, an inability to perform SGA in the month of EXR filing, and the inability to work at the SGA level due to the original disabling medical condition or one related to it. If the EXR is approved, the beneficiary is authorized an extended work period referred to the initial reinstatement period (IRP) lasting 24 months of payable benefits. During the IRP, any month earning over SGA will not be paid. The 24 months can be consecutive or not, and once the beneficiary has been paid 24 months of benefits, for SSDI, the individual receives a new nine-month trial work period (TWP) and 36-month extended period of eligibility (EPE).

Employment Supports for Persons Who Are Blind

SSDI and SSI benefit recipients who are blind have employment supports with special rules. SSDI beneficiaries who are blind have substantially higher SGA levels than nonblind beneficiaries. SSDI beneficiaries who are blind, age 55 or older, and earning below blind SGA levels may receive benefits indefinitely if work activity uses a lesser level of skill than prior to age 55 or the onset of blindness.

SSI beneficiaries who are blind may deduct a greater variety of work expenses than IRWE, referred to as Blind Work Expenses (BWE). Some examples of BWE include transportation costs, taxes, union dues, service animal expenses, visual and sensory aids, and translation of materials into Braille.

Future of SSDI/SSI

The conceptions of disability and people with disabilities have evolved considerably, and multiple varying definitions of disability have been generated in American social policy. Meanwhile, the SSDI and SSI programs have advanced partly because of legal rulings and medical field progresses in medicine, treatments, and technology. Doubts about Social Security trust fund solvency and clatter about the deservedness of disability benefits (who, when, how, and why) seem to dominate the political discourse today. Legislation has further advanced to provide people with disabilities accommodations in the workplace and protections from discrimination, which may further complicate the disability determination evaluation process. The economy, technology, industries, and workplace dynamics continue to change, bringing further challenges; however, SSA has made consistent efforts in modernizing the programs. While disability is more understood to be "normal," the future is uncertain regarding the extent of generosity of benefits and the strictness of determination rules. Nonetheless, SSDI and SSI remain hallmark programs in the U.S. social welfare system that continue to provide fundamental benefits to people with disabilities.

Richard E. Wharton

See also: Employment, Barriers to; Food; Poverty; Welfare to Work; *Primary Documents*: President Franklin Delano Roosevelt's Statement on the Signing of the Social Security Act (1935); "Social Security Disability: Times for Reform," Comment of Peter Blanck to the Social Security Advisory Board (SSAB) (2013)

Further Reading

Code of Federal Regulations. 2012. "§404.1520, Evaluation of Disability in General." https://www.socialsecurity.gov /OP_Home/cfr20/404/404-1520.htm.

Social Security Administration. "Legislative History." http://www.ssa.gov/history/law .html.

Social Security Administration. "Public Law 98-460-Section 1619." http://www.ssa.gov /OP_Home/ssact/title16b/1619.htm.

Social Security Administration. "The Red Book: A Guide to Work Incentives." http:// ssa.gov/redbook.

U.S. Social Security Administration Benefit Offset National Demonstration. http:// www.bondssa.org/index.php.

Sociology

Sociology is the study of people and the society they live in. Sociology focuses on how people in society interact not only with each other but also with the social structures and institutions that organize that society. The field of disability studies is interdisciplinary, aiming to use approaches from various academic fields to study the social and cultural perspectives that frame the conditions of disabled people. The field has adopted many academic perspectives, including sociological theories, which were critiqued and adapted in order to make them more suitable for the academic advocacy the field seeks to accomplish. It is the task of disability studies to situate disability into traditional sociological theory as a way of encouraging new understandings.

Key Concepts

Collectively, the following foundational theories of sociology have been adopted by disability studies and incorporated to advance the social position of disabled people in society. Each theory marks a particular sociological perspective enlisted in thinking about disability.

Marxism. Marxism is the result of Karl Marx's critique of modern society. In particular, it explores capitalism as an evolving economic system of the modern era. "Surplus population" is a crucial aspect of Marxism because it allows capitalists to profit from the difference between compensation and value of their workers. Surplus population is an unskilled workforce of members who compete against one another for work during periods of limited employment. This population comprises the lowest payed and the most expendable employees in the capitalist system.

A significant amount of the surplus population consists of disabled workers. The low employment rate of people with disabilities is key to an exploration into sociology's relationship to disability because it provides some explanation for why the disabled population is devalued in society, as they are devalued in the capitalist system. Marxism, when put in context with disability, provides some significant explanations for the economic and social condition of the disabled population. While the sociologists who further developed Marxist theory did not specifically align the surplus population with disabled workers, making this link within disability studies provides a historical basis for scholars that illuminates the current condition of disabled people.

Social Constructionism. Social constructionism is a fundamental theory that can be applied to disability to recognize the social aspects of disability. Social constructionism is a concept developed by Peter L. Berger and Thomas Luckmann, who revolutionized the way sociologists and citizens thought about their knowledge of society and their social interactions. Most values and practices are considered socially constructed because institutions (government, education, and the economy) and people consistently adhere to them, reinforcing them as *naturally* occurring. The result of this process is a social belief that these values and practices have always been in place. Irving Zola (1991), a medical sociologist, reflected on his experiences with air travel as a disabled person in the 1950s when he felt he must walk through the airport. However, following the disability rights movement (DRM), Zola felt empowered to use his wheelchair. Zola identified his experience as a social construction because it was the social and historical factors surrounding his experiences, not his actual experiences, that influenced his evolving understanding of the cultural norms around air travel.

Social constructionism has been a crucial theory for disability studies scholars, as the field largely works under the assumption that disability is a socially constructed concept. Yet, it was not until the DRM and disability studies framed disability in social parameters that disability's connection to social construction became widespread in academic research. Using the social constructionism framework allowed scholars and activists to make the radical declaration that people were disabled, not by their bodies, but by the society that oppressed them.

Symbolic Interactionism. The process of socially constructing values and practices occurs through what George Herbert Mead's student, Herbert Blumer, called symbolic interactionism. Blumer's principles of symbolic interactionism state that "people act toward things based on the meaning those things have for them, and these meanings are derived from social interaction and modified through interpretation" (Society for the Study of Symbolic Interaction 2015). It would follow that to have institutions and groups of people reinforcing social values and practices, there has to be a creation of shared meaning. For instance, the blue and white image of a wheelchair for accessible parking is a symbol that has shared meaning because people from diverse groups know that parking spaces with that image painted in the space are reserved for disabled individuals.

Symbolic interactionism is another fundamental sociological theory adopted by disability studies because the shared cultural meaning created about disability is often harmful to disabled people. That shared meaning may express disability as either tragic or inspiring, both of which have been heavily critiqued by the disabled community and scholars. Interactions that influence meaning about disability exist within a structure of normality, a space disability is typically excluded from. Often interactions about disability work to reinforce the belief that disability is not "normal." Understanding how this meaning is created provides a path for scholars' work to remedy the shortcomings of cultural meaning about disability.

Critical Theory. In the broadest terms, critical theory aims to enlighten society to the historical, political, and economic contexts that frame daily life as a path to a less oppressive culture. Critical theorists critique traditional theories for not being dynamic enough to fully realize the depth of knowledge needed for social progress. To remedy this shortcoming, Max Horkheimer, the German sociologist who coined the term "critical theory," determined that in order for a declining society to reach a place of cultural enlightenment, society must use critical theories that are explanatory, practical, and normative. Critical theory determines a social problem, identifies the agents of change, and suggests a solution that is tangible and within the realm of possibility.

Critical theory works to supplement the inadequacies of existing research on and knowledge of disability. In recent years, critical disability studies (CDS) has developed out of a need for a more critical and fluid approach to disability and an effort to move past the binary of disability as either a medical or social issue. Similar to critical theory, CDS strives to be a reflective discipline that is aware of its need to extend theory into practice and to encourage thinking about disability in its complexity. Central to CDS's purpose is the need to align their work with other critical disciplines as a way of broadening the interdisciplinary discourse on disability.

Medicalization. Medicalization represents a shift from understanding certain behaviors as criminal or sinful under religious practice to understanding them to derive from sickness or illness under medical practice. Sociologists began to critique the medical field through the development of medicalization, a process that explains how seemingly unrelated social or behavioral differences become adopted by the medical sphere. Michel Foucault was among the first theorists to highlight the growth of the medical profession in the 18th and 19th centuries and the resulting relationship individuals had with illness. Conrad (2007) divided medicalization critiques into three spheres: the conceptual sphere, where social problems are categorized using medical terms; the influential sphere, in which social movements can adopt medical framing of a social behavior to effect change; and the interactive sphere, where a medical professional shifts a social behavior into the medical realm by diagnosing a patient.

Medicalization is significant to disability studies because the field, like the movement before it, fought against the medicalization of disability in favor of the social model approach to disability. Both the field and the movement could be examples of an effort to demedicalize disability and reframe historical treatment of the disabled population as civil rights injustices. While sociology does critique medicalization, it could be argued that it lacks the social justice element that makes disability studies' use of medicalization meaningful.

Deviance and Stigma. Deviance and stigma are two central sociological concepts that illuminate power dynamics in society. Deviance is a break in obedience to socially acceptable norms. Stigma, then, is the consequence of said deviance that can manifest physically or emotionally. The French sociologist Emile Durkheim originally argued that deviance is essential to a functional society because deviance creates the parameters of conformity. Without deviance, we would not have compliance. Erving Goffman's work on stigma stratifies society into three groups: those without stigma, those with stigma, and those without stigma who can understand the stigmatized condition. These concepts are crucial because society tends to identify disability as a deviation from the norm, which results in disabled individuals being stigmatized. Understanding the stigma of disabled individuals influenced the creation of the field of disability studies.

Key Issues

Identity. Identity is woven into nearly all sociological approaches, perspectives, and theories. While identity is often thought of as being created by individuals or groups, Foucault would disagree. He came to identity from a postmodern perspective (a skepticism toward reality or truth) by which he believed identity *was not* created by individuals and groups for their own purposes but developed by complex social structures and then assigned for the purpose of creating subjects in the machines of modern society. Erving Goffman looked at identity through the lens of symbolic interactionism and framed identity as both a social identity and a personal identity. Goffman claimed that social identity develops out of social interactions, in which each participant interprets social cues of the other participants in the form of appearance, gender, race, disability, etc. This interaction also results in subtler cues in the form of personal attributes, such as integrity, kindness, and compassion. Personal identity, on the other hand, is the understanding that despite the great unifying qualities that effectively work toward erasing identity of individuals, there are still unique traits found in each individual, such as DNA, fingerprints, and handwriting.

Political Economy. Political economy is the relationship between politics and economics that developed out of Marxism. Political economy is useful in understanding why social stratifications exist in capitalist societies, such as the United States. Examining power relations enlightens our understanding of the political economy, because power enables the political economy to effectively assert control over social systems. Using political economy to frame disability reveals that disabled individuals in society are disproportionately unemployed and living in poverty, which further reinforces the power political economy has over disadvantaged populations. Overall, political economy is a major influence in everyday life because it shapes how people are employed and marginalized, how resources are allocated based on class and social structure, and even what goods are available for people to buy.

Conclusion

Sociology is the study of societal structures and the ways people function within those structures. Disability studies has folded the most relevant sociological theories into its scholarship to progress the status of disabled people. While there is much disability studies can critique about sociological approaches to disability, sociology's influence on disability studies cannot be denied. It is the hope of disability studies that the continued interdisciplinary research on disability will inspire prominent academic fields like that of sociology to expand their scholarship on disability as well.

Nicole Sims

See also: Critical Disability Studies; Disability Studies; Identity; Medicalization; Neoliberalism; Stigma

Further Reading

Bohman, James. 2016. "Critical Theory." *The Stanford Encyclopedia of Philosophy.* http://plato.stanford.edu/archives/fall2016/entries/critical-theory/.

Conrad, Peter. 2007. *The Medicalization of Society.* Baltimore: Johns Hopkins University Press.

Macionis, John J. 2012. *Sociology.* New York: Pearson Education.

Society for the Study of Symbolic Interaction. 2015. "Welcome to SSSI!" https://sites.google.com/site/sssinteraction/.

Zola, Irving K. 1991. "Bringing Our Bodies and Ourselves Back In: Reflections on a Past, Present, and Future 'Medical Sociology.'" *Journal of Health and Social Behavior* 32, no. 1: 1–16.

Special Education

Special education is defined as instruction that is altered to meet the unique needs of a child with a disability (Individuals with Disabilities Education Improvement Act §300.39). Special education is federally mandated and an integral aspect of the current educational system that all eligible children with disabilities receive. Key legislation has evolved over the last 40 years to clarify and enhance educational outcomes for students with disabilities.

Purpose of Special Education

The overlying purpose of special education is to allow the child with a disability to access and demonstrate progress in learning the general curriculum—that is, the material all students are to learn. Special education may include instructional adaptations to the content, the use of additional strategies or methods, or changes to how and where information is delivered. Instruction is individualized to accommodate challenges that result from an impairment. This may involve designing adaptations and providing additional services to support the child's educational performance in multiple arenas, including academic, social, emotional, physical, and vocational. Special education may also require teaching skills outside of the school classroom that effectively prepare children and youth for postschool education and employment in addition to life in and access to the community. Some students with disabilities may require related services—that is, services necessary to assist the individual with a disability to benefit from special education. For example, a student who is blind may require related services by a specialist to teach the student how to independently and safely navigate to classes in the school or community settings where specialized instruction occurs. Examples of commonly used related services include transportation, speech-language pathology, occupational therapy, physical therapy, counseling, and school nurse services.

Eligibility. Recent estimates show there are more than 6 million children, youth, and young adults who receive special education and related services in the United States (National Evaluation and Technical Assistance Center 2014). To qualify for special education and related services, a child must be between the ages of 3 and 21. Through the use of multiple assessments, an educational team identifies whether the child meets the requirements for one of 13 disability categories. The disability categories are autism, deaf-blindness, deafness, hearing impairment, intellectual disability, other health impairment, multiple disability, orthopedic impairment, serious emotional disturbance, specific learning disability, speech or language impairment, traumatic brain injury, and visual impairment (including blindness). Finally, for a child to be eligible, the evaluations and observations must demonstrate that the disability adversely affects the child's educational performance.

History and Legislation

The current iteration of special education, as stated in the Individuals with Disabilities Education Improvement Act (IDEIA) 2004, has evolved in several ways since it was first mandated in the Education for All Handicapped Children Act (EHA) of 1975 (PL 94-142). Prior to 1975, the responsibility of educating children with disabilities remained with the states and local school districts (U.S. Department Office of Special Education Programs 2007). Students with intensive needs were often placed in institutions with little focus on teaching academic or social skills. School districts could turn children with disabilities away and refuse to educate them because of cost. For students with disabilities who could attend school, the quality of educational programming varied widely across states and within school districts. Parents were excluded from educational planning for their children. Few teachers were appropriately qualified to teach students with disabilities. Lastly, clear inequities existed with respect to social class and race. For example, African American males were more likely to be labeled as having intellectual disabilities or a serious emotional disturbance.

FAPE and LRE. Resulting from a series of federal legislation and court decisions, as well as pressure from family and professional disability-focused organizations, Congress enacted the 1975 EHA. The EHA provided consistent guidelines to states for the education of all school-aged students with disabilities. The policy ensured that children with disabilities received a *free appropriate public education* (FAPE) that met their unique needs in the *least restrictive environment* (LRE). LRE is considered to be the general education classroom. However, the law clearly established that a continuum of placement options and services should be made available to support the educational needs of each child. The law also mandated that each eligible child with a disability receive an individualized education program (IEP). The IEP was to be developed through a team of educators and the parent of the child with a disability. The EHA also ensured the protection of rights for children with disabilities and their families. Although the major components of the EHA have remained, substantive changes over the past four decades have served to clarify and augment these mandates.

IDEIA (2004) incorporates attention to children with disabilities from birth to three years. Extending FAPE to that group provides a seamless transition from the early intervention system to the school system. Therefore, the federal government has established consistent guidelines to ensure FAPE across the lifespan (birth to 21). Additionally, the LRE mandate has

changed in significant ways. Although it still requires a continuum of placement options and services to meet the individual needs of students with disabilities, there is an increasing trend away from placements in special education–only schools toward educating students with disabilities in their neighborhood schools and alongside same-aged peers without disabilities. Moreover, an increasing number of students with disabilities are being educated for some part of the school day in general education classes. IDEIA (2004) has emphasized that students with disabilities have access to and demonstrate progress in learning the general curriculum.

Key Concepts in Special Education

To ensure meaningful access to general education content, it is critical that children and youth with disabilities be identified early and accurately. Changes in the past several decades have resulted in more effective identification. Discrepancies among students' *intellectual quotient* (IQ) scores in the 1980s and 1990s were primary predictors of a student with a disability receiving special education services. However, researchers began to question the sole use of IQ testing for deciding access to special education services. For example, researchers identified cultural biases in IQ that resulted in disproportionality and inappropriate placement of African American and Hispanic children in certain special education categories. The field now requires multiple assessments in the child's primary language, naturalistic observations of the student, and input from parents and school personnel to accurately identify the disability.

IEP and Transition Planning. Assessments are pivotal to the many improvements related to the IEP planning process. The process now involves a team of personnel to include multiple perspectives and emphasize the importance of parent and student participation. Currently, teams must include a school administrator, general education and special education teachers, related service personnel, and the parent of the student with a disability. The IEP has continued to delineate and increase parental roles and responsibilities. Furthermore, participation for students with disabilities ages 16 and over is now required. That change is consistent with the growing realization of the importance of services to prepare youth with disabilities for life after high school. Transition services became part of the law in 1990, and the IEP now requires transition planning to support adult outcomes in postsecondary education, employment, and, when appropriate, independent living and community participation.

Inclusive Education. The changes made to the law have directly transformed the delivery of special education and related services. Through the 1990s and into the early 2000s, most students with disabilities received education in separate schools or separate classrooms in a school. Even in the same school, students with disabilities spent large portions of the day away from students without disabilities. Students with disabilities are now increasingly included in general education classes; more than 80 percent of students with disabilities spend nearly 60 percent of their school day in general education (U.S. Department of Education 2010). Although educators now emphasize academic achievement for students with disabilities, educational services have expanded to incorporate the development of social-emotional skills, such as developing friendships and networking with peers without disabilities. Inclusion in general education classrooms, therefore, enables students with disabilities to gain access to

the standards-based curriculum and associated resources provided to students without disabilities, receive instruction from qualified general educators, and interact with peers without disabilities. Inclusion in general education classrooms has been identified as a predictor to successful adult outcomes in employment, postsecondary education, and independent living.

Universal Design for Learning. As more students with disabilities attend general education classes, the knowledge and skill sets needed by both general and special educators to promote all students' success changes. Educators are drawing upon new frameworks, such as *Universal Design for Learning* (UDL), and evidence-based practices to enhance access to knowledge for all students. UDL guides educators to attend to the needs of all students in their classrooms. Research continues to emerge that provides teachers with a growing list of research-based practices that can be implemented in integrated settings to support a range of student needs. Most recently, a growing body of culturally relevant practices and strategies to account for variations in student culture and language, skill levels, income disparities, and resource availability in schools has emerged. Furthermore, there is growing awareness that special educators in high schools require knowledge and practices to support youth for postschool success.

Self-Determination and Person-Centered Planning. Collaboration among students, families, and a host of community members has become increasingly pivotal to the individualized delivery of services. Many argue that it must involve cooperation, coordination, and formation of school-home-community coalitions to link services while defraying costs. However, in order for services to reflect the individualized nature of special education, the student's interests and preferences must be a primary focus. Two interrelated practices that are gaining momentum draw on the civil rights of individuals to determine their lives: teaching *self-determination* skills that enable students with disabilities to advocate for themselves and providing services to reflect an individual's hopes and dreams. Another emerging practice is *person-centered planning* (PCP), which involves building a network of family and friends to support the individual to identify and achieve life dreams. PCP is a dynamic planning process that identifies and implements positive ways of supporting the individual in the community over time.

Dilemmas, Debates, and Unresolved Questions

At its core, special education outcomes emerged from the realization that students with disabilities have a right to a free appropriate public education. Over the 40 years of practice and research, many evidence-based practices have evolved. However, enacting them is challenging. One dilemma is balancing educational accountability requirements and testing of students. The law continues to refine guidelines to ensure equitable and consistent access to evaluations, particularly for minority students from culturally and linguistically disenfranchised backgrounds. Additionally, attention to culturally sensitive testing and instruction is now part of the definition of "appropriate" education. Another challenge has emerged from the adoption of the National Common Core Standards by 38 states. Adoption of these standards may benefit students across the United States, as all students are held to the same norms and therefore have access to high-level expectations. Yet the use of those standards also poses significant issues for students with disabilities, as they are entitled to individualized instruction as part of their IEP. Questions arise as to why current federal mandates stretch deeper than ever before into determining the content and instruments on which all students are tested along with the material being tested, the ways it is tested, and the ways data are interpreted. Resolving these issues is interdependent on funding as well. While statutes in the laws are strong and necessary, many requirements are also underfunded or not funded at all. Overlap of services, funding that originates from different revenue streams, and overall rising costs of special education and falling governmental budgets have placed greater demands on individuals with disabilities, their families, service providers, and policy makers.

Lisa S. Cushing and Michelle Parker-Katz

See also: Free Appropriate Public Education; Inclusive Education; Individualized Education Program (IEP); Individuals with Disabilities Education Improvement Act (IDEIA); (In) Exclusion; Section 504 of the Rehabilitation Act; Special Education, Role of the Family in

Further Reading

Individuals with Disabilities Education Improvement Act of 2004. 2004. Pub. L. No. 108-446, §300.39 et seq.

National Evaluation and Technical Assistance Center. 2014. "NDTAC Fact Sheet: Youth with Special Education Needs in Justice Settings." http://www.neglected-delinquent.org/sites/default/files/NDTAC_Special_Ed_FS_508.pdf.

U.S. Department of Education. 2010. "Teacher Shortage Areas Nationwide Listing 1990–91 thru 2010–2011: March 2010." http://www2.ed.gov/about/offices/list/ope/pol/tsa.pdf.

U.S. Department Office of Special Education Programs. 2007. "History: Twenty-Five

Years of Progress in Educating Children with Disabilities through IDEA." http://www2.ed.gov/policy/speced/leg/idea/history.html.

Special Education, Role of the Family in

Families play an important role in the education of their children. When students receive special education services, parents and guardians (hereinafter, use of the term "parent(s)" includes all forms of guardianship) have formal and informal ways of taking part in decisions about their children's school placement and services. However, parents and school personnel may hold different views about what is best for children.

Family Involvement in Special Education

Although most researchers and educators agree that parental involvement in special education is important, the interactions between families and schools are complex. Such interactions are influenced by various factors, including historical narratives about disability and normality; school structures that were originally designed to exclude children with disabilities; problematic special education policies and funding limitations; and uneven power dynamics between families and school professionals. In addition, although special education focuses on the growth of individual students, schools are institutions not only of individual learning but also of socialization and democratization, where children learn to live together in a community. As such, schools must be understood as sites of contestation, where curriculum, teaching, and even the purpose of schooling for children with disabilities are being constantly negotiated.

Parents, whose expertise often is centered in their experiences with their own children, often have different perspectives than educators, whose expertise typically is centered in professional training. Parents may have diverse understandings of disability and the purpose of special education. Further, different parents are in different positions to advocate for their children. Regardless, parents play an important role in special education because they make educational decisions for their children before children are able to do so themselves. Many special education professionals work in a system that is often characterized as using a deficit or *medical model* of disability, which focuses on testing, labeling, sorting, and helping the child to overcome individual impairments or more closely resemble "normal" children. Some parents have reported frustration with this deficit model that focuses on what their children cannot do and how their families are not normal, and prefer instead to embrace a more sociocultural or *social model*, which is concerned with ways that schools and other institutions fail to adequately meet the needs of those with physical or mental impairments (see Lalvani 2015).

Disability studies challenges deficit narratives of disability and questions special education practices that focus on adjusting children to fit within the current education system. Some disability studies scholars, including scholars with disabilities or with children with disabilities as well as critical special educators, have told counternarratives of families living with "dis/ability" that move beyond coping, grief, or interventions to focus on successes and new ways to experience family, community, and interdependence (for example, Ware 2002). Yet, the role of parents in special education has been contested by both educators, who may believe parents lack the expertise to know what is best for their children, and disability studies scholars, some of whom have pointed out that parents also hold deficit notions of their children and, at worst, have neglected or abused their children.

Background and History

Historically, cultural products and research about children contain narratives that unfairly blame mothers for a wide variety of impairments and differences. For example, in the 1970s and 1980s, a number of mothers, labeled "refrigerator mothers" by medical professionals, were thought to have created autism in their children as a result of their cold and neglectful parenting. Contemporary versions of blame include linking behavior problems in children to insufficient parental involvement and school personnel holding preconceived, untested deficit views of families (Harry 2008, 376–77). At the same time, societal conceptions that children who are not viewed as "normal" have less value as citizens can contribute to stigma and isolation for parents of children with disabilities.

Many parents have fought to change the ways in which schools educate children with disabilities. In part because of activism and advocacy of people with disabilities and their parents, the 1975 Education for All Handicapped Children Act guaranteed children a free appropriate public education (FAPE). Prior to the act passing, many parents were expected to educate their children with disabilities outside of the public school system. Later reauthorized and renamed the Individuals with Disabilities in Education Act (IDEA), federal legislation gave parents many formal rights, including the rights to be provided information about their children's education and to be included in decision-making meetings about special education placements and services (Ong-Dean 2009, 1). Unlike families of students without special education labels, parental involvement is written into education policy, which places great responsibility on parents to advocate for their individual children at school.

Dilemmas, Debates, and Unresolved Questions

The Problem with Normal. While public schools (through legislation like the IDEA) guarantee a free appropriate education for each child as well as parental involvement in decision making about children with special education labels, it is well documented that early schools were established with *normative* understandings of children in mind—biased toward white, middle-class, male children developing on the "normal" curve. As such, even as federal policies and local practices change to improve instruction and to make it more inclusive, it is important to note that the structures of most of our schools—including grade-based classrooms, inflexible pacing, and standardized curriculum—were created without considering the needs of students with disabilities. Disability studies scholars have rejected ideas of "normal" versus "abnormal" and advocated for pedagogical and curricular changes that meet the needs of *all* children without segregation or exclusion.

Power Disparities between Parents and Professionals. While parent involvement is written into special education policy as a partnership between families and schools, in practice parents often experience the partnership with special education professionals on unequal terms. Family knowledge gained through experience does not hold the same value as professional knowledge about the child. At the same time, while school professionals are expected to focus on particular aspects of a child's development, parents must think of their children more *holistically*, in terms of their physical and emotional needs, their relationship with their families and communities, and their care throughout the life course. These different ways of viewing the child's needs may create a situation where parents and teachers have competing goals for children.

Research has found that parent involvement is most valued by the school when parents serve as "informants" about their children, providing information that helps teachers work effectively with students, while school professionals retain the power to make decisions about the child's education and placement (Hodge and Runswick-Cole 2008, 638). Many school professionals, including teachers, counselors, psychologists, and therapists, are trained to keep a professional distance from families, and the rules of their engagement are sometimes codified through their professional organizations (Nelson, Summers, and Turnbull 2004, 153–54), which can both create emotional distance from parents and reinforce hierarchies that prevent true partnerships with families.

Different Parents Have Different Positions in Relation to Schools. Schools tend to set the expectations for parent participation, and it is clear that there are still numerous barriers to successful school-family partnerships. Different parents have different opportunities to intervene, and parents with the greatest access to information, resources, and professional knowledge often are best positioned to advocate for their children within school meetings (see Ong-Dean 2009, 3). For immigrant parents or families from a different culture or socioeconomic class from the school

professionals, navigating parental involvement can be frustrating in a setting where white middle-class styles of parental participation are viewed as "natural" or normative. The different ways in which parents of color are perceived within educational systems is especially important in a structure where many children of color with disabilities are both overrepresented and underserved in special education (see Harry 2008).

Labels: Critiques and Values. While many parents and scholars of disability reject the use of labels because they are rooted in deficit notions of disability, some parents, especially those whose children experience nonapparent or "invisible" disabilities, often seek diagnoses or labels because they see them as necessary to get their children the services and accommodations that they need. Some scholars have advocated for more inclusive classrooms that can meet the needs of all students (through, for example, *Universal Design for Learning* programs), which would reduce the need for labeling. However, it is important to note that current funding structures in schools typically tie resources to labels. This is a critical tension that merits further research: how can parents and professionals advocate for children to get the supports they need, while not focusing only on deficits?

Future Directions

Since legislation was instituted in 1975, there have been a number of positive changes to both special education and the rights of parents in regard to their children's education. However, numerous challenges still remain. As evidenced above, there are multiple unresolved issues regarding the role of parents in special education in particular. These issues take place in a context of critiques of the special education system and educational systems more generally. For many parents, as well as critical educators, there is struggle between working within a system not designed for disability and working toward a fundamentally new, inclusive system.

Conclusion

Despite the critiques of special education policies and practices by parents and disability studies scholars, schools remain one of the few institutions serving individuals with disabilities that have guaranteed rights for parents intended to improve educational experiences for students. In any efforts to reform (or recreate) special education, it is clear that people with disabilities and the parents of children with disabilities need to have greater influence on the ways in which schools educate their children. This would require a partnership between schools and families in which desires for schooling and critiques of the system, not just suggestions for how to best fit children into the existing system, are centered.

Gia Super and Kelly Vaughan

See also: Guardianship and Capacity; Inclusive Education; Inclusive Language as Advocacy; (In)Exclusion; Siblings; Special Education

Further Reading

Harry, Beth. 2008. "Collaboration with Culturally and Linguistically Diverse Families: Ideal versus Reality." *Exceptional Children* 74, no. 3: 372–388.

Hodge, Nick, and Katherine Runswick-Cole. 2008. "Problematising Parent-Professional Partnerships in Education." *Disability & Society* 23, no. 6: 637–6347.

Lalvani, Priya. 2015. "Disability, Stigma and Otherness: Perspectives of Parents and Teachers." *International Journal of Disability, Development and Education* 62, no. 4: 379–393.

Nelson, Louise G. Lord, Jean Ann Summers, and Ann P. Turnbull. 2004. "Boundaries in Family and Professional Relationships: Implications for Special Education." *Remedial and Special Education* 25, no. 3: 153–165.

Ong-Dean, Colin. 2009. *Distinguishing Disability: Parents, Privilege, and Special Education.* Chicago: University of Chicago Press.

Ware, Linda P. 2002. "A Moral Conversation on Disability: Risking the Personal in Educational Contexts." *Hypatia* 17, no. 3: 143–172.

Speech-Language Pathology

Speech-language pathology is a health care profession that trains clinicians to advocate, research, evaluate, and provide services in speech, language, social language, cognitive function, and feeding and swallowing, among other areas (Shames and Anderson 2002). This entry will discuss speech-language pathology as well as its intersection with disability and disability studies.

What Is Speech-Language Pathology?

According to the American Speech-Language-Hearing Association (ASHA), which certifies speech-language pathologists and audiologists in the United States, "the overall objective of speech-language pathology services is to optimize individuals' abilities to communicate and swallow, thereby improving quality of life" (American Speech-Language-Hearing Association 2016). To achieve this objective, clinicians, known as speech-language pathologists (SLPs) or speech therapists, are trained to provide services to individuals with various communication-related differences, disorders, and disabilities. Certified, master's-level clinicians work in schools, hospitals, rehabilitation clinics, and many other settings to provide services in speech (e.g., production of sounds, stuttering); language (e.g., grammar, vocabulary); social language (e.g., social skills, idioms); cognitive function (e.g., problem solving); voice (e.g., intonation); and feeding and swallowing, among other areas, across the lifespan.

Because of the variety of settings and services provided by SLPs, these professionals work with individuals with many different disabilities, impairments, and communication differences. While some individuals may have communication disabilities such as disorders of articulation (saying words clearly); receptive language (understanding what is being communicated); and expressive language (conveying thoughts, wants, and needs), others have communication or feeding difficulties as a result of another disability (e.g., cerebral palsy, Down syndrome, stroke, traumatic brain injury), and some experience a combination of both.

People with disabilities and those in disability studies are most likely to interact with SLPs as service providers. Because SLPs work with individuals who are d/Deaf and hard of hearing, people who use augmentative and alternative communication (AAC), and many others who benefit from the skills and services SLPs are trained to provide, SLPs often are present in meetings and on teams in a variety of settings and for a large number of people with disabilities. Additionally, SLPs often participate in advocacy for laws and services that benefit the disability community at large, and these activities may align with those of advocates from the community and within disability studies.

Background

The origins of the field of speech-language pathology might be traced back to ancient Greece and Rome. Early documents indicate that rhetoric, oratory skills, and speech correction were all practiced very early in documented history. For example, Demosthenes, a Greek orator who lived in the 300s BCE, attempted to correct his own speech by speaking with pebbles in his mouth. Interventions in speech correction, as well as efforts to educate and communicate with individuals who were deaf, are recorded from ancient times until the advent of professional organizations.

In the United States, individuals worked toward creating an organization of speech correction teachers in the early 1900s; many of them were most concerned with helping individuals who stutter. During this time, speech-language pathology broke away from medicine and began establishing texts and practices that developed into the field that exists today. Like many allied health professions, speech-language pathology entered the mainstream in the United States after World War II, when veterans returning home required rehabilitation after being wounded in the war (Duchan 2011). This time also signaled a broadening of areas for which speech-language pathologists might provide service. In the mid-1920s, the organization that is now ASHA was founded, though it experienced many name changes before becoming the American Speech-Language-Hearing Association.

Qualifications

Since then, speech-language pathologists in the United States seek certification (called a Certificate of Clinical Competence, or the ASHA Cs) from ASHA to ensure they have completed adequate training and are prepared to work in the field. Clinicians often earn bachelor's degrees in speech-language pathology or communication sciences and disorders, but they cannot be certified by

ASHA to practice in the United States without a master's or doctoral degree, typically in speech-language pathology or speech and hearing sciences.

Recently, changes were made to allow individuals with bachelor-level degrees to apply to be speech-language pathology assistants (SLPAs), which allows them to carry out treatment plans developed by certified SLPs but does not allow them to complete evaluations or design their own treatment plans. The SLPA position was developed to help address the shortage of SLPs, especially in school systems in the United States.

Because SLPs may encounter many different individuals with communication difficulties in their places of employment, ASHA requires that SLPs receive training in all the areas for which they are certified to practice. However, most SLPs will specialize in a specific area, which is often related to their preferred location of practice (American Speech-Language-Hearing Association 2016). For example, a hospital SLP often will have more experience and a higher level of comfort in the areas of feeding and swallowing, as well as cognitive communication differences related to stroke and traumatic brain injury, whereas a school SLP might spend more time on correcting speech errors and developing language and social skills in youth and adolescents.

Wherever SLPs practice, they provide services that are important to the lives of people with disabilities. They are integral in assisting individuals in safely eating by providing feeding and swallowing interventions, in advocating for individuals to receive and gain proficiency in using AAC, and in supporting individuals in developing stronger communication skills. Services such as these may significantly affect the quality of life experienced by an individual with a communication difference or disability.

Dilemmas, Debates, and Unresolved Questions

While the goal of speech-language services is to improve quality of life for individuals, this often is achieved through treatment strategies that subscribe to the medical model of disability, the belief that disability is an individual problem that needs to be modified to achieve normality. Much of the education received by SLPs emphasizes "normal" structures and functions, and treatment goals tend to enforce the need to conform to those structures. Though the medical model is prominent throughout the profession (Boyle et al. 2016), ASHA also encourages SLPs to be advocates for social change and to be aware of cultural and linguistic diversity. As such, SLPs also embrace parts of the social model of disability, the belief that disability is created by structures and systems in society, which create barriers. As a result, the philosophy of SLPs toward disability is varied, and no consistent experiences related to disability models may be apparent.

One area of tension within the field is in interactions between SLPs (and audiologists) and the Deaf community. While SLPs are trained to remediate differences in speech and bolster language skills, they are rarely fluent in American Sign Language (ASL) and may have had little to no experience working or sharing community with those who are culturally Deaf and who may view English as their second language. As a result, SLPs may appear culturally insensitive and might promote practices, such as speech and listening without the use of ASL, that are counter to the preferences of the Deaf community. As with others who are part of disability and ethnic cultures,

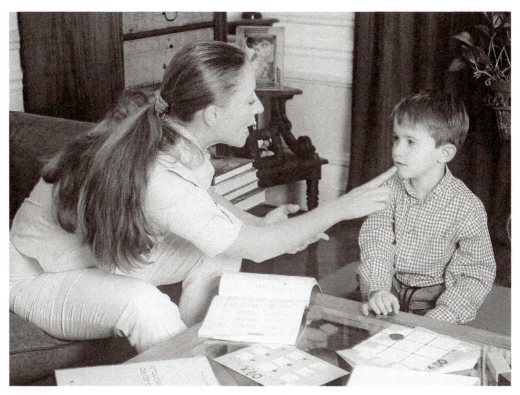

A child works with a speech language pathologist. Some speech language pathology practices remain controversial, especially in work with the deaf community. (BSIP/UIG via Getty Images)

those who identify with Deaf culture benefit from the skill set and services SLPs provide, but typically prefer that clinicians with whom they are working be knowledgeable about and respect their culture and preferences.

Additionally, certain diagnoses and practices are controversial within the field (e.g., apraxia of speech, benefits of oral motor exercises, use of facilitated communication for AAC users). Clinicians of many different generations and levels of experience have varying opinions on these issues and may proceed with evaluation, treatment, and advocacy according to their beliefs or their training in their degree programs. For controversial issues, ASHA may produce position papers, which lay out evidence and serve to guide clinicians. However, while evidence-based practice is encouraged, some controversial topics have varying or contradicting evidence, leaving it up to individuals to decide which practices are best. This ambiguous evidence may be discouraging or frustrating for individuals who are seeking the services of SLPs for diagnoses and practices upon which the field disagrees.

The Future of Speech-Language Pathology and Disability

Speech-language pathology is a well-established allied health field that seeks to improve the quality of life for individuals with communication and feeding needs through the provision of services in a variety of settings. As such, speech-language pathologists should continue to advocate for their clients both locally and nationally, with special attention to the disability community's stance on issues. The field would benefit from increased exposure to and knowledge of disability studies–related concepts, such as the social model of disability and disability culture. In addition to research that is evidence based, increased attention to advocates' perspectives should also be included in research produced by the field.

Cathy Webb

See also: Alternative and Augmentative Communication; Communication; Language

Further Reading

American Speech-Language-Hearing Association. 2016. "Scope of Practice in Speech-Language Pathology." www.asha.org /policy.

Boyle, Michael P., Derek E. Daniels, Charles D. Hughes, and Anthony P. Buhr. 2016. "Considering Disability Culture for Culturally Competent Interactions with Individuals who Stutter." *Contemporary Issues in Communication Science and Disorders* 43: 11.

Duchan, Judith F. 2011. Judy Duchan's History of Speech-Language Pathology. "A History of Speech-Language Pathology: Overview." http://www.acsu.buffalo.edu/~duchan /new_history/overview.html.

Shames, George H., and Noma B. Anderson. 2002. *Human Communication Disorders: An Introduction.* Boston: Allyn and Bacon.

Spirituality

For this entry, the word "spirituality" will refer to the umbrella term that is inclusive of religious beliefs as well as other references to the supernatural. Spirituality is the focus of the section because it includes practices and beliefs associated with religion but is not limited to just these practices and beliefs. Spirituality also includes non-organized thoughts about the supernatural.

Overview

Disability appears as a common theme among religious texts. The Islamic Koran, the Jewish Torah, and the Christian Bible all include references to various disabilities. The Koran refers to disability as both a disadvantage and a deformity. The Torah marks disability as a bodily imperfection and differentiates it from the idealized body. The Christian Bible presents disability as a form of suffering that can be alleviated or healed by God. The Koran, the Torah, and the Bible are all religious texts that guide the beliefs of many spiritual people throughout the world. Most of the world's population adheres to some sort of religious or spiritual belief, and approximately 15 percent of the world's population has a disability (World Health Organization 2011). People with disabilities belong to all of the world's major religions, and many people with disabilities report that spirituality is an important part of their lives. Thus, the spiritual beliefs and views of people with disabilities are important to document. Modern religious congregations are beginning to understand the importance of universal design and inclusion of people with disabilities. Therefore, disability is a relevant topic in religious organizations today, and spirituality is an important topic for the disability community.

History and Models of Disability

Spirituality and disability have had a contentious history. Disability was first defined under moral and religious terms. Because this was the predominant way of thinking for so long, the link between disability and morality has profoundly influenced how disabled people view themselves and how society views persons with disabilities. A framework called the *moral model of disability* incorporates moral values into disability and disabled bodies. The moral model was the reigning way of thinking about disability before the advent of modern medicine, and it still shapes thinking about disability today. The moral model defines disability as a defect caused by sin. It could be caused by one's own sin or the sin of one's ancestors. Disability is then a way that a deity punishes someone for this sin. Historically, the moral model encourages people with disabilities to feel ashamed of their physical conditions because they are a mark of moral lapse.

The *charity model of disability* is the modern evolution of the moral model. There still are moral undertones to this model, but in a seemingly positive way. The charity model views disability as a condition to be pitied and presents people with disabilities as in need of help through the welfare of others. The charity model is consistent with many themes expressed in the various religious texts about disability: that people with disabilities are disadvantaged and that people without disabilities should help people who have disabilities. This model of disability also encourages one to seek purpose and meaning from a disability, especially in a positive way. While this perspective arguably promotes a more compassionate and positive view of disability over a harshly negative one, treating disability as a condition that needs love and care from people without disabilities can promote a disguised stigma toward people with disabilities.

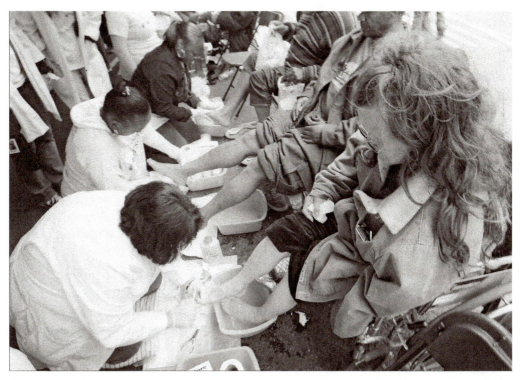

A woman with a disability receives free foot care during the annual Good Friday Easter Event to help the homeless of Skid Row, in Los Angeles, California. Discourse about disability and spirituality is often connected to ideas about charity. (David McNew/Getty Images)

Religious texts often speak directly about disability, often using disability as a metaphor to send a broader message. Some common metaphors in the Bible, Torah, and Koran use disability imagery to refer to spiritual impairment: "deaf ears" or "blind eyes." These metaphors generally associate disability with something negative, indicating the stigma that disability carries.

Disability also serves as "prosthesis" in religious texts. A prosthesis is a device to move along a story's plot and lessons. It is a tool for teaching rather than an independent theme. The use of disability as prosthesis is common in many pieces of literature, not just religious ones (Mitchell 2002). Disability as a narrative prosthesis in religious texts portrays disability as a problem and solves the problem by curing the disability. Absent are the sociopolitical implications of disability; instead, disability is portrayed as one-dimensional.

While a metaphoric interpretation of disability is common, more literal references to disability also appear in religious texts. The Bible and Torah offer several interpretations of how people with disabilities should be viewed and treated within society. In line with the charity model of disability, biblical personalities with disabilities are often seeking help and fulfillment of their goals from nondisabled people and also seeking healing and relief from their disabilities from God. For example, many stories in the Bible involve Jesus healing a person's impairments. Characters with disabilities in the Bible and Torah either are healed miraculously of their disabilities or live suffering from their disability's symptoms. Often, disability is the punishment for sin and is seen as a form of justice when someone does something wrong. Since disability is synonymous with being spiritually impure in Christian, Islamic, and Jewish writings, it often results in a person being morally shunned and unaccepted in the larger society.

Despite the stigma and negativity brought onto disability by religious texts, there are also some positive associations between disability and religion. Most organized religions believe that people with disabilities are worthy of being treated with love and respect. The Bible, Torah, and Koran all illustrate ways in which God wants people to accept people with disabilities openly. The Jewish Talmud specifically illustrates the ways in which disabled people can contribute to society, with and without accommodations. Some scholars argue that because stories about disability in the Bible bring light to issues related to disability and highlight disabled characters, the Bible can help people with disabilities find purpose within their impairments or suffering.

Furthermore, benefits and services for people with disabilities have often been religiously affiliated. Many hospitals and rehabilitation centers aimed at helping people with disabilities began with religious influences. Many services available for people with disabilities today would not have been created if not for the push of religious organizations to help those in need.

Lastly, while many religions preach acceptance of all people, inclusion of people with disabilities into modern religious congregations is still a problem. People with disabilities are often excluded from attending religious services because of inaccessibility of places of spiritual worship. This issue is further exacerbated by the exemption of religious institutions from state and federal disability legislature, including the Americans with Disabilities Act. Accessibility, physical or otherwise, is not a priority for religious places of worship and is rarely discussed among congregations.

Spirituality and the Disability Experience

As mentioned above, there is a clear distinction made between religion and spirituality. Religion, which has been the topic of discussion thus far in this entry, encompasses organized beliefs and practices associated with the supernatural. It includes texts, places of worship, and rituals. Spirituality, on the other hand, refers more broadly to non-organized beliefs about the supernatural that may or may not be associated with a religion. Spiritual identity, then, refers to one's self-given relationship with the divine or with the supernatural. Internalizing one's own relationship with the spiritual is often important for people with and without disabilities.

Analyzing religious texts by themselves often does not give us a good idea of how spirituality is internalized into a sense of a disabled self. Modern interpretations of religious texts and contemporary spiritual practices often differ from the religion's texts and formal preaching. One's spiritual practices do not always coincide with how religious texts say followers of a particular religion should act. A clear example of this from Muslim spirituality is Jinn possession, the idea that Satan can cause one to "go mad." Jinn possession is a popular belief about disability that Muslims hold but that is not found within the Islamic religious book, the Koran. Jinn possession is a conceptualization of disability found in Islamic spirituality that has not been formalized within the religion of Islam.

According to research on disability and spirituality, people's feelings and perceptions about their own disabilities can be influenced by their spiritual beliefs. Although spirituality does not necessarily depend on physical features, physical experiences influence the way people internalize spiritual experiences. Spirituality and spiritual beliefs can encompass both negative and positive feelings about disability. Most stories in religious texts portray disability negatively; however, not all people with disabilities view their disabilities in a negative way. Much of the research on spirituality and disability has shown that people find positive interpretations of the negatively themed texts. In fact, many people with disabilities view their disabilities as a positive aspect of their lives and even choose to identify only with the positive portrayals of disability found in their religious texts.

The literature contains conflicting evidence about whether there is a positive or negative correlation between spirituality and feelings about disability. One mechanism through which spirituality may affect feelings about disability is through coping. "Coping with a disability" refers to dealing with any problems that are related to a disability, reducing stressors caused by these problems, and gaining control over the disability. People can use their spirituality to cope with their disability in both positive and negative ways. In a positive way, spirituality can encourage individuals to engage in more positive health behaviors, provide social support, and help individuals to understand and find meaning in their roles as disabled people. In a negative way, spirituality can promote feelings of anger toward God for causing disability, or people may find it difficult to practice their spirituality because of their disability or feel shame about having a disability because they view disability as a punishment for sin or wrongdoing. Spirituality certainly can influence people's feelings about their disabilities in ways that are both positive and negative. Conversely, there is no evidence that having or acquiring a disability strengthens or weakens religious fervor. People with disabilities practice spirituality in similar ways and at similar rates to people without disabilities.

Modern Theology of Disability

The theology of disability, which is based in Christianity, was developed by Nancy Eiesland (1994). This theology takes the Christian symbols of Christ's crucifixion and the Eucharist and turns them into poignant and respectable evidence that God is indeed disabled, shedding a positive and inclusive light on disability. Some themes are already important in the church and can be further incorporated into a theology of disability. The first of these themes is embodiment. "Embodiment" refers to a person (in this case Christ) who represents an abstract quality (in this case wholeness and connection). Christ must embody disability in a way that promotes wholeness and connection instead of shame and taboo. The second theme is reclaiming religious symbolism. Religious symbols can be reclaimed and used to promote rather than denounce disability. Symbols that are harmful must not just be ignored but rather replaced and reconceived. The symbol of the Eucharist in particular is central to a theology of disability. It is a reminder that Christ's body, which was broken with his crucifixion, is a real connection with wholeness and God. The pinnacle of the Christian religion is in Christ's resurrection with his broken body. Emphasizing embodiment and replacing Christian symbols in a way that embraces disability means that disability is no longer a consequence of individual sin but rather a natural and universal human experience. Disability is then human wholeness.

Eiesland's theology of disability educates followers about the image of God as a disabled being and, therefore, eases the cognitive dissonance (or unease) of Christians with disabilities by using Bible-based curricula. While the theology appears to effectively combine tenets of Christianity and of the social model of disability, it is not well known or well practiced. This theology may prove to be helpful in creating a positive perspective of disability within Christianity.

Kristen Salkas

See also: Historical and Outdated Terminology; Social Model of Disability; Stigma

Further Reading

Eiesland, Nancy L. 1994. *The Disabled God: Toward a Liberatory Theology of Disability*. Nashville: Abingdon.

Mitchell, David. 2002. "Narrative Prosthesis and the Materiality of Metaphor." In *Disability Studies: Enabling the Humanities*, edited by Sharon L. Snyder, Brenda Jo Brueggemann, and Rosemarie Garland-Thomson, 15–30. New York: Modern Language Association.

World Health Organization (WHO). 2011. "World Report on Disability." http://www.who.int/disabilities/world_report/2011/report/en/.

Stigma

Stigma is social construct that involves the recognition of an individual's difference on the basis of some distinguishing characteristic and that results in the devaluation of that individual. This entry will discuss how stigma relates to disability and will explore debates about the concept within the field of disability studies.

What Is Stigma?

Individuals are said to possess a *stigma* when they differ in a significant way from what is considered to be "normal" and socially acceptable. Stigmatized individuals are seen as flawed and even sometimes as being less than human. Stigma can also describe people's outward responses or behavior toward an individual based upon a particular characteristic. Stigma is related to prejudice, or a negative attitude, but whereas prejudice is an internal reaction, stigma is an external process that unfolds in relationships between people in a broad variety of situations. *Visibility* is an important dimension of stigma. When an individual has a visible stigma, people sometimes make attributions or assumptions about that individual based upon the stigmatizing characteristic. For example, if an individual has an obvious disability like blindness, some people may incorrectly assume that the individual is less intelligent than he or she really is, even though blindness and intelligence are not related. Even in the absence of a visible marker, individuals can experience stigma based upon a perceived characteristic or category membership. In this way, people with nonapparent or "invisible" disabilities can often experience stigma too if they reveal their disability.

The degree to which stigmas can be controlled, or managed, affects how they are perceived by others. For example, individuals who are overweight or who are alcoholics may experience more stigma than those with other disabilities because of the assumption that they can regulate their weight or alcohol use, even though this is not always the case.

Historical Overview

The term "stigma" was coined in 1963 by sociologist Erving Goffman. Goffman argued that humans categorize one another as a means of making sense of the world around them. When individuals possess a relatively unique or unusual attribute, they are frequently marked as different and as having a shortcoming. To this end, Goffman defined "stigma" as an attribute that is deeply discrediting. He argued that we often see individuals with stigmas only in terms of the discrediting attribute, that we sometimes view them as "not quite human," and that we "impute many imperfections based upon the original one." Although Goffman referenced several marginalized groups in his writing, he frequently highlighted the experiences of people with disabilities. Goffman was one of the first researchers to discuss the social experiences of people with disabilities, which is why his work is noteworthy in disability studies.

Important Points to Know about Stigma and Disability

Components of Stigma. There are four components to Goffman's theory of stigma. First, Goffman believed that stigmatized individuals tended to *internalize* the negative attitudes toward them that "normals" (his term for nonstigmatized) individuals possess. He suggested that stigmatized individuals frequently experienced shame and self-hatred and that they often worked to avoid contact with "normals." When they did have to interact, they made an effort to seem as typical as possible and worried excessively about how others perceived them. Second, Goffman argued that stigmatized individuals had a responsibility to *integrate* into the larger society as much as possible and that they should attempt to put nonstigmatized individuals at ease and to protect them from a fear of difference. Third, Goffman suggested that in order to combat these problems, stigmatized individuals frequently worked to *conceal* their differences from others as much as possible. Writing that "the greatest rewards are in being considered normal," he argued that individuals should try to "pass" when it is feasible to do so in order to avoid stigmatization (74). Finally, Goffman maintained that even when stigmatized individuals could "pass," they should not go as far as defining themselves as normal (115). Although he argued that "a [stigmatized] individual's 'real' group is his fellow sufferers," he also contended that "to identify with fellow sufferers leads to alienation, separation, and on-inclusivity" (113). He concluded his discussion of stigma by stressing that *stigma management* is a general feature of society, that everyone has experience with stigma to some degree, and that it serves a general purpose of moving society forward.

Disability Critique of Stigma. Even when Goffman's writings had barely been published, criticism of his theory, and particularly the application of his theory to people with disabilities, began mounting. Most notably, in a collection of essays entitled *Stigma: The Experience of Disability*, editor and activist Paul Hunt criticized Goffman's fixation with normality by questioning:

> What kind of goal is this elusive normality? If it does mean simply trying to be like the majority, then it is hardly a good enough ideal at which to aim. Whether they are physically handicapped or not, people need something more than this to work towards if they are to contribute their best to society and grow to maturity. (1966)

Moreover, in his foreword to the collection, Peter Townsend argued that "ordinary people often expect [people with disabilities] to become passive and compliant independents, an isolated category of the pitied who are thrust out of sight at home or in institutions. No wonder they write of the bitterness and frustration involved in playing the role of invalid." Instead, Hunt and other contributors to the volume emphasized the social barriers that people with disabilities encountered, like discrimination in the job market and inaccessible facilities.

As the disability rights movement grew over the next several decades, so did these criticisms. Increased attention to and activism by other marginalized groups (such as women, people of color, and LGBT individuals) also highlighted the ways in which Goffman's thinking was shortsighted and flawed. As Hunt had articulated, "[disabled people] meet fundamentally the same attitude which discriminates against anyone different and shades off into oppression under the right-or rather wrong-conditions" (1966, 12). Activists began to refute Goffman's contention that individuals should passively accept their marginalized status and that it was their responsibility to "manage" their stigma as a means of putting nonstigmatized individuals at ease. Instead, they emphasized the larger social forces that create and sustain disabled people's marginalized status.

Dilemmas, Debates, and Unresolved Questions

Impact on Disability Studies. The expansion of the disability rights movement and the academic field of disability studies have been largely predicated upon dismantling Goffman's theory of stigma and its relevance to people with disabilities. On the one hand, scholars and activists acknowledge that Goffman's discussion of disability in terms of social interaction helped to lay the foundation for the social model of disability. On the other hand, they reject his claims that disability is equated with individual deviance, that disabled people experience shame and self-hatred, and that they always strive toward normality. Instead, disability studies investigates and strives to dismantle the larger social forces that create, sustain, and perpetuate injustice against disabled individuals.

Relevance to Current Scholarship. Within the social sciences, contemporary research on stigma does acknowledge the relevance of both personal values and larger cultural values in the enactments and experiences of stigma. For example, physically disabled individuals who cannot attain our society's high cultural standards of athleticism might instead come to place greater value upon their intellect or their emotional connections with others, taking these as evidence that they are worthwhile individuals. Similarly, nondisabled individuals might be more prone to stigmatizing people with physical disabilities to the extent that they themselves value physical ability. Larger cultural values play a role as well, such that individuals may be more apt to stigmatize and to feel stigmatized according to the strength of the "norm" from which they deviate. In a culture that emphasizes physical fitness and health, overweight individuals may experience more stigma than they would in a culture that does not emphasize these things. Individuals are more likely to stigmatize others if they believe that the differentiating trait is caused by a particular behavior or has the capacity to be controlled in some way. For example, individuals who are considered obese are frequently stigmatized because of the perception that they can control their eating habits but simply choose not to.

Although stigma as a theoretical and academic concept is still frequently employed within psychology and sociology, its relationship to disability studies remains controversial. This is especially true as newer, more nuanced terminology, such as "ableism" and "microaggression," is increasingly used to theorize interactions between disabled and nondisabled individuals. Such concepts acknowledge how these individual interactions are both a product and a reflection of larger social forces that oppress disabled people.

Conclusion and Future Directions

Notably, in 2013 the annual meeting of the Society for Disability Studies convened a plenary session to commemorate the fiftieth anniversary of Goffman's (1963) *Stigma* and to debate its relevance to the field. The presentations built upon several decades of disability studies scholarship but were still fundamentally grounded in Hunt's (1966) and others' original critique. Goffman's, and even more contemporary, discussions of stigma by and large fail to question the concept of "normal" or the idea that everyone should want to achieve it (Garland-Thompson 2013; Schweik 2013; Titchkosky 2013). Perhaps the most astute and all-encompassing criticism was that "Goffman failed to recognize the agency and resistance of disabled people. It is a serious oversight and one that Disability Studies is right to address by focusing on the disability rights movement, disability pride, the adornment of prosthetics, and other topics" (Brune 2013). At the same time, however, several concepts considered fundamental to the field were born out of challenges to Goffman. For example, theoretical discussions of "normality" and the "overcoming narrative" have roots in *Stigma*. In this way, disability studies' very existence as an academic discipline can be attributed to Goffman and the many critiques that his work inspired; thus, *Stigma* will always be relevant.

Kelly Munger

See also: Ableism; Discrimination and Microaggressions; Disability Oppression; Normalization and Discipline; Sociology

Further Reading

Brune, Jeffrey. 2013. "Forum Introduction." *Reflections on the Fiftieth Anniversary of Erving Goffman's Stigma*. Plenary conducted at the Society for Disability Studies.

Garland-Thomson, Rosemarie. 2013. "Roadkill Truths." *Reflections on the Fiftieth Anniversary of Erving Goffman's Stigma*. Plenary conducted at the Society for Disability Studies.

Goffman, Erving. 1963. *Stigma: Notes on Spoiled Identity*. New York: Simon & Schuster.

Hunt, Paul. 1966. *Stigma: The Experience of Disability*. London: Geoffrey Chapman.

Schweik, Susan. 2013. "Stigma management." *Reflections on the Fiftieth Anniversary of Erving Goffman's Stigma*. Plenary conducted at the Society for Disability Studies.

Titchkosky, Tanya. 2013. "Absent Normalcy for Present Stigma: Goffman's provocation." *Reflections on the Fiftieth Anniversary of Erving Goffman's Stigma*. Plenary conducted at the Society for Disability Studies.

Supported Employment

The reauthorization of the Rehabilitation Act in 1992 specified that supported employment was a strategy intended for those individuals with "significant disabilities," whose impairment requires a greater level of support than typically provided through vocational rehabilitation (VR) services. Supported employment is intended for individuals whose needs require long-term, ongoing support to maintain employment. As such, subsequent literature and programs for supported employment often focus on intellectual and developmental disability (IDD) and mental illness.

What Is Supported Employment?

In 2007, during a time when the poverty rate in the United States was at 10 percent in the general population, 25 percent of adults with disabilities living in the community lived in poverty. For individuals with "mental disabilities" (that is, people with mental health conditions, cognitive impairments, or IDD), this rate reached a startling 31 percent (Stats RRTC 2010). Prior to the U.S. economic recession in the first decade of the 21st century, one in four individuals with a disability, and nearly one in three of those with a mental disability, were living in poverty. Unemployment and underemployment are significant factors contributing to a cycle of poverty and disability. The poverty rates reflect a long-term downward trend in disability employment that persisted throughout the recession (Livermore and Honeycutt 2015).

To be gainfully employed, however, people with disabilities need to be able to compete in the labor market. Because employment is recognized as a right, people with disabilities are entitled to protection from discrimination. To this end, antidiscrimination legislation, such as the Americans with Disabilities Act (ADA) and the ADA Amendments Act, make it possible for individuals to pursue *competitive employment* (Blanck 2000; Ozawa and Yeo 2006). Competitive employment involves working in the local labor market wherein an employee is hired, supervised, and paid directly by the business or organization in an integrated setting. In competitive employment, employees receive wages and benefits that are commensurate with their nondisabled coworkers (Wehman, Revell, and Brooke 2003). *Supported employment* is a complementary strategy that can help individuals with disabilities enter into and maintain competitive, gainful

Table 1: Supported Employment Core Values and Quality Indicators

Supported Employment Values	Quality Indicators for Supported Employment Programs
1. Presumption of employment 2. Competitive employment 3. Self-determination and control 4. Commensurate wages and benefits 5. Focus on capacity and capabilities 6. Importance of relationships 7. Power of supports 8. Systems change 9. Importance of community	1. Meaningful competitive employment in integrated work settings 2. Informed choice, control, and satisfaction 3. Level and nature of supports 4. Employment of individuals with significant disabilities 5. Number of hours worked weekly 6. Number of persons from program working regularly 7. Well-coordinated job retention system 8. Employment outcome monitoring and tracking system 9. Integration and community participation 10. Employer satisfaction

Source: Wehman, Paul, W. Grant Revell, and Valerie Brooke. 2003. "Competitive Employment: Has It Become the 'First Choice' Yet?" *Journal of Disability Policy Studies* 14, no. 3: 163–173.

employment (Callahan, Griffin, and Hammis 2011).

Background

Supported employment serves as one of the first integrated employment strategies and provides entry for many individuals with disabilities into competitive employment and community integration. Supported employment aims to limit the impact of one's impairment on productivity in the workplace by providing ongoing support to promote independence and employment stability. Supported employment was first defined in the Developmental Disabilities Act in 1984, and over time it became infused with the philosophy of individualized support strategies and self-determination (Mank et al. 2003; Wehman, Revell, and Brooke 2003). In the wake of the *Olmstead* decision in 1999 and the redefinition of the term "employment outcome" for VR services by the U.S. Department of Education in 2001, there was growing concern that the majority of individuals with disabilities remained employed in segregated work settings. Wehman, Revell, and Brooke (2003) proposed nine values and ten quality indicators to guide supported employment efforts to improve the inclusion of individuals with disabilities in competitive employment:

A 2010–2011 survey of community rehabilitation providers (CRP) found that 14.3 percent of individuals with disabilities being served participated in individual supported employment, and of those individuals, 12.1 percent had IDD (Domin and Butterworth 2013). Researchers also found that group-supported employment, which does not follow the tenets listed in table 1 and which comprises enclaves and mobile work crews, served a smaller but still significant role in employment supports.

Key Concepts

Key strategies used in supported employment include natural supports, job coaching, individual placement and support, and job matching. A brief description of these strategies follows.

Natural Supports. Natural supports comprise the people in one's employment social network who can provide mentoring, friendship, and opportunities to socialize (Office of Disability Employment Policy

2001). While there has been some debate over the definition, natural supports are a form of ongoing support that leverage the relationships formed in everyday life, such as family, friends, and coworkers, but do not eliminate or replace the need for a job coach. (For more information, please see Wehman and Bricout [1999].)

Job Coaching. Job coaching has become an essential support mechanism in providing on-the-job training. A job coach helps employees with work-related tasks, helps provide transportation to and from the job site, and may also help individuals learn and develop personal skills and other skills to maintain employment (O'Day 2009). Job coaches initially remain on-site full-time to teach the individual with disabilities the required job and related skills. Gradually, job coaches lessens their involvement as the supported employee masters job tasks (Nisbet and Hagner 1988). While job coaches remain involved with the supported employee as needed, the goal is for the individual with disabilities to work as independently as possible.

Individual Placement and Support. Individual placement and support (IPS) is an evidence-based best practice for community mental health providers working with individuals with mental illness. IPS-supported employment includes eight core components: (1) eligibility based on client choice; (2) focus on competitive employment; (3) integration of mental health and employment services; (4) attention to client preferences; (5) work incentives planning; (6) rapid job search; (7) systematic job development; and (8) individualized job supports (Luciano et al. 2014).

Job Matching. Job matching emerged to address the problem of underemployment for people with IDD. This process involves individuals with IDD matching their interests and abilities to available jobs in the community rather than choosing from available jobs based on whether or not they have those specific job skills (Kilsby and Beyer 2002). Job matching functions on the premise that interests and abilities are more critical to successful employment outcomes than job skills alone, since individuals who select job opportunities on the basis of interests will likely be more motivated and self-determined. Notably, many people with disabilities entering employment for the first time are often unaware of the options available and may not have the information or experience necessary to gauge their interests and abilities. *Job tasting,* which is a short, unpaid, time-limited work experience that allows people to sample various workplaces and cultures, is one way individuals can determine their job interests and abilities. For example, Project SEARCH, a work-immersion model based at the Cincinnati Children's Hospital that has gained national attention, uses job tasting that leads to job matching (O'Day 2009). Project SEARCH is a full-time program that integrates classroom and training with work experience. The curriculum is customized to an individual's skills and interests and involves a series of work-site internship rotations. Long-term supports, such as job coaching, are also provided to program participants to help them maintain employment afterward.

Debates and Dilemmas

In response to concerns regarding the possible expense of supported employment programs, a series of cost analyses has examined the provision of supported employment compared to sheltered employment. Cimera (2011) found not only that the cumulative costs are significantly lower in supported employment but also that these costs show a downward trend over time. Conversely, the cumulative costs for providing sheltered employment increases over time. While employees in segregated work settings receive services for a longer period of time and work more hours, individuals with disabilities working in supported employment earn higher wages (Cimera 2011). Taken as a whole, the cost analysis of supported employment shows that as an employment strategy it returns a significant net benefit to taxpayers in comparison to segregated employment (Cimera 2012). In other words, not only is supported employment a more cost-effective solution, but it also provides significant social gains.

The model of employment people choose has been found to relate significantly to their reported levels of physical and social integration. The most successful outcomes were reported for those using individual supported employment placements over any form of group support (Jahoda et al. 2008). Further, supported employment can be used as a vehicle for individuals with disabilities not only to maintain the size of their social networks but also to create the opportunity to strengthen and expand their social networks to include others in the community, outside of the disability service system (Eisenman 2007; Forrester-Jones et al. 2004).

Advancements in the Field

Supported employment played a pivotal role in advancing policy such as the Employment First Initiative and the reauthorization of the Workforce Innovation and Opportunity Act (WIOA), which was originally the Workforce Investment Act (WIA) of 1998. The Employment First Initiative, in particular, is a progressive policy shift that requires competitive employment in an integrated setting to be considered first as an option for people with disabilities before any other option (Martinez 2013; Niemiec, Lavin, and Owens 2009). The intent behind this policy is to prevent youth with disabilities from being "tracked" (or automatically placed) into sheltered employment, which pays workers subminimum wage.

Conclusion

In 2014, Wehman, Chan, Ditchman, and Kang conducted a study to examine the effect of supported employment interventions on the employment outcomes of transition-age youth with IDD served by the public vocational rehabilitation system using a case-control study design. The results indicated that the effect of supported employment was especially strong for youth who were Social Security beneficiaries, special education students, and individuals with intellectual disabilities or autism who were high school graduates. These findings suggest that supported employment is an effective service for enhancing the vocational rehabilitation outcomes of young adults and provides valuable information for policy makers, health care providers, rehabilitation counselors, and educators.

Kate Caldwell

See also: Customized Employment; Employment, Barriers to; Employment First; Vocational Rehabilitation; Workers' Cooperatives; Youth with Disabilities, Employment of

Further Reading

Blanck, Peter. 2000. *Employment, Disability, and the Americans with Disabilities Act: Issues in Law, Public Policy, and Research, Psychosocial Issues.* Evanston, IL: Northwestern University Press.

Callahan, Michael, Cary Griffin, and Dave Hammis. 2011. "Twenty Years of Employment for Persons with Significant Disabilities: A Retrospective." *Journal of*

Vocational Rehabilitation 35, no. 3: 163–172.

Cimera, Robert Evert. 2011. "Supported versus Sheltered Employment: Cumulative Costs, Hours Worked, and Wages Earned." *Journal of Vocational Rehabilitation* 35, no. 2: 85–92.

Cimera, Robert Evert. 2012. "The Economics of Supported Employment: What New Data Tell Us." *Journal of Vocational Rehabilitation* 37, no. 2: 109–117.

Domin, Daria, and John Butterworth. 2013. "The Role of Community Rehabilitation Providers in Employment for Persons with Intellectual and Developmental Disabilities: Results of the 2011 National Survey." *Intellectual and Developmental Disabilities* 51, no. 4: 215–225.

Eisenman, Laura T. 2007. "Social Networks and Careers of Young Adults with Intellectual Disabilities." *Intellectual and Developmental Disabilities* 45, no. 3: 199–208.

Forrester-Jones, Rachel, Samantha Jones, Sophie Heason, and Michele Di'Terlizzi. 2004. "Supported Employment: A Route to Social Networks." *Journal of Applied Research in Intellectual Disabilities* 17, no. 3: 199–208.

Jahoda, Andrew, Jeremy Kemp, Sheila Riddell, and Pauline Banks. 2008. "Feelings about Work: A Review of the Socio-Emotional Impact of Supported Employment on People with Intellectual Disabilities." *Journal of Applied Research in Intellectual Disabilities* 21, no. 1: 1–18.

Kilsby, Mark S., and Stephen Beyer. 2002. "Enhancing Self-Determination in Job Matching in Supported Employment for People with Learning Disabilities: An Intervention Study." *Journal of Vocational Rehabilitation* 17, no. 2: 125–135.

Livermore, Gina A., and Todd C. Honeycutt. 2015. "Employment and Economic Well-Being of People with and without Disabilities Before and After the Great Recession." *Journal of Disability Policy Studies* 26, no. 2: 70–79.

Luciano, Alison, Robert E. Drake, Gary R. Bond, Deborah R. Becker, Elizabeth Carpenter-Song, Sarah Lord, Peggy Swarbrick, and Sarah J. Swanson. 2014. "Evidence-Based Supported Employment for People with Severe Mental Illness: Past, Current, and Future Research." *Journal of Vocational Rehabilitation* 40, no. 1: 1–13.

Mank, David, Andrea Cioffi, Paul Yovanoff, and Steven J. Taylor. 2003. "Supported Employment Outcomes across a Decade: Is There Evidence of Improvement in the Quality of Implementation?" *Mental Retardation* 41, no. 3: 188–197.

Martinez, Kathleen. 2013. "Integrated Employment, Employment First, and US Federal Policy." *Journal of Vocational Rehabilitation* 38, no. 3: 165–168.

Niemiec, Bob, Don Lavin, and Laura A. Owens. 2009. "Establishing a National Employment First Agenda." *Journal of Vocational Rehabilitation* 31, no. 3: 139–144.

Nisbet, Jan, and David Hagner. 1988. "Natural Supports in the Workplace: A Reexamination of Supported Employment." *Journal of the Association for Persons with Severe Handicaps* 13, no. 4: 260–267.

O'Day, Bonnie. 2009. "Project SEARCH: Opening Doors to Employment for Young People with Disabilities." *Disability Policy Research Brief: Center for Studying Disability Policy.* https://www.mathematica-mpr.com/our-publications-and-findings/publications/project-search-opening-doors-to-employment-for-young-people-with-disabilities.

Office of Disability Employment Policy. 2001. "Small Business and Self Employment for People with Disabilities: A World In Which People with Disabilities Have Unlimited Employment Opportunities." https://www.dol.gov/odep/about/strategic_plan_contents.htm.

Ozawa, Martha N., and Yeong Hun Yeo. 2006. "Work Status and Work Performance of

People with Disabilities." *Journal of Disability Policy Studies* 17, no. 3: 180–190.

Stats RRTC. 2010. "Annual Disability Statistics Compendium." http://disabilitycompendium.org/.

Wehman, Paul, and John Bricout. 1999. "Supported Employment and Natural Supports: A Critique and Analysis." http://www.worksupport.com/documents/article15.pdf.

Wehman, Paul, W. Grant Revell, and Valerie Brooke. 2003. "Competitive Employment: Has It Become the 'First Choice' Yet?" *Journal of Disability Policy Studies* 14, no. 3: 163–173.

Supportive Housing

What Is Supportive Housing?

Supportive housing is a living situation that explicitly connects affordable housing for people with disabilities with services that support independent living. Instead of viewing housing and services as separate issues, supportive housing interconnects these two necessities, ensuring that supportive services are accessible within the living situation. The main goal of supportive housing is to increase the number of housing options that support people with disabilities living independently in the community.

People served by supportive housing include those with developmental disabilities, mental illness, and physical disabilities because these groups benefit from having stable community-based housing with wraparound services. People with developmental disabilities gain self-sufficiency from targeted case management services. For those with mental illness, stable housing and case management can be the key to recovery. Having an accessible unit can help someone with a physical disability become more independent.

Supportive housing is a broad category used to describe multiple types of housing and can include many kinds of services. It may also be called special-needs housing, supported housing, permanent supportive housing, or affordable housing for persons with disabilities. In addition, depending on how services are linked into the housing, familiar supportive housing models include group homes for people with mental illness or developmental disabilities, residential treatment programs for those with mental illness, and community-integrated living arrangements (CILA) for people with developmental disabilities.

There are many issues to consider when creating supportive housing. Housing issues include price (is it affordable?); location (is it safe? near transit?); ownership (is it a rental? owned by the individual, his or her parents or guardians?); and funding program (are there special rules based on how it is funded?). Housing affordability is especially important since lower-income households, especially those with disabilities, often cannot afford to pay the full value of what housing is worth on the market. Service issues include the service provider (family member, volunteer, direct support worker?); intensity (what level of supports are needed?); frequency (how often are supports provided?); and funding source (family, government, etc.?) Services offered vary according to a person's changing needs, can be provided formally by an agency or informally by family and friends, and can be provided at work or in the home.

Supportive housing provides people with disabilities with opportunities for safe, accessible housing and integrated services to support living as independently as possible. This living situation also allows for adaptability as individuals' needs for support change over time. Supportive housing can be structured in many different ways but ultimately provides a combination of affordable housing with wraparound supportive services tailored to an individual's needs.

How Did It Develop?

Supportive housing emerged in response to multiple factors: increasing numbers of people with disabilities, deinstitutionalization and the efforts of the independent living movement, changing public attitudes toward services for people with disabilities, and federal court cases (e.g., *Olmstead v. L. C.*).

Public health and medical improvements have contributed to longer lifespans for the entire population and specifically people with disabilities. Children with disabilities reaching adulthood in the 1980s were the first generation of people with disabilities who were likely to outlive their parents or primary caregivers. People with disabilities and their family members have advocated for appropriate community-based housing options with a focus on access to services in community-based housing situations that promote independence and involve a small number (six or fewer) of individuals living together. During the 1980s, the disability industry went through a period of deinstitutionalization, in which people with disabilities moved out of institutions and into less intensive settings. The *Olmstead* decision required state governments to provide meaningful options for community living for people with disabilities.

How Available Is It (How Is Access Distributed)?

Supportive housing is unevenly available throughout the United States. Data on supportive housing is difficult to determine because of varying definitions and minimal tracking. There is currently no overarching

federal policy for how much supportive housing is needed or where it should be located. Consequently, local groups have taken the lead on creating supportive housing to meet the needs of people with disabilities.

Supportive housing is an innovative solution to the housing needs of individuals, and therefore there is not just one model. Additionally, supportive housing is generally owned and operated by private agencies rather than local government agencies. As a result, there is no central listing for supportive housing resources, making it difficult to locate available options when seeking them. The Corporation for Supportive Housing is a national organization that advocates for increased access to supportive housing opportunities and is a resource for families looking for options.

Supportive housing can be offered in multiple types of dwellings (e.g., apartments, townhomes, and houses) and can be located almost anywhere in most communities. While some municipalities have zoning restrictions for group homes, most supportive housing is physically no different from traditional housing and is not zoned any differently, so it can be located anywhere there are residential units.

What Policies Support Supportive Housing?

Supportive housing is not the standard form of housing available to individuals with disabilities in the United States. Special permissions are often needed to use federal or state programs to fund supportive housing for an individual or small group. Typically, government housing agencies and human service agencies are administratively and financially separate, making it difficult to implement supportive housing.

Some states have applied for special waivers to their state Medicaid programs to pay for supportive housing services. The Affordable Care Act also contains provisions for supportive housing within certain rules. HUD's Permanent Supportive Housing program funds the costs of development and services for people who are both homeless and disabled. At the state level, there are affordable housing financing programs that often have preferences or incentives for creating supportive housing units. State human service departments have various programs that permit or encourage services to be offered in community-based settings.

How Is Supportive Housing Evaluated?

Supportive housing is evaluated by its ability to provide someone with an affordable home that allows them to access needed supportive services. Housing and services each have important options to consider regarding the who, what, when, where, and how of supportive housing. Housing can be separated into types based on size, location, occupancy, ownership, and financing. Services can be categorized by frequency, intensity, provider, and source. Table 1 illustrates the major supportive housing options: housing type, housing ownership, housing funder, service funder, service

level, and service provider, with housing considerations in the left three columns and service decisions in the three right columns. Within each column, the rows begin with the least intense and least public option and move progressively toward more services and public support.

What Are the Benefits to Supportive Housing?

The primary benefit of supportive housing is increased quality of life for residents. Being community based with adaptable services means that someone with a disability can decide how to live and receive assistance as needed. Supportive housing residents are able to work and play in their community and be near family members and friends as they choose.

There are also significant financial benefits to supportive housing, which costs significantly less than hospitalization or institutionalization. Living in a nursing home or institution can cost upward of $100,000 each year. Supportive housing costs a fraction of that to operate because of operating efficiencies and reduced intensity.

Finally, supportive housing is a benefit to families and communities because it is

Table 1: Supportive Housing Options Matrix

Housing type	Housing ownership	Housing funder	Service funder	Service level	Service provider
House	Single family	Individual	Individual	Call-in	Family
Apartment	Condo	Family	Family	Weekly	Roommate
Group home	Joint ownership	Donors	Donors	Part-time daily	Neighbor
Shared apartment	Rental	Agency	Agency	Full-time daily	Volunteers
Room	Organization	Bank	State	24-hour daily	Nonprofit
Dormitory	Government	Government	Federal	2 FTE	Government

a long-term solution. Parents who are the primary caregivers of adult children with disabilities can know that their family members will be cared for after they are unable to provide the care. People with disabilities on their own can access a support network. With supportive housing, those individuals with low incomes can still receive high-quality care and housing.

Obstacles to Supportive Housing

Supportive housing aligns with the desires of individuals who want to live in the community, leads to increased quality of life, and is more cost-effective. However, there are still barriers to developing and widely implementing these options. Supportive housing requires coordinating across agencies for funding, which is difficult. Additionally, entrenched interests, including the nursing home and home health agency lobbies, are well funded and often able to oppose changing policy to support this innovation. Lastly, it can be difficult to find champions within existing policy structures to implement supportive housing, which is a more tailored model rather than a one-size-fits-all model.

Richard Koenig

See also: Community Living and Community Integration; Group Homes; Independent Living

Further Reading

Braddock, David, Richard Hemp, Emily S. Tanis, Jiang Wu, and Laura Haffer. 2017. *The State of the States in Intellectual and Developmental Disabilities: 2017.* Washington, DC: American Association on Intellectual and Developmental Disabilities.

Corporation for Supportive Housing. 2013. "CSH Dimensions of Quality Supportive Housing, Second Edition." http://www.csh.org/wp-content/uploads/2013/07/CSH_Dimensions_of_Quality_Supportive_Housing_guidebook.pdf.

Corporation for Supportive Housing. 2017. "Toolkit for Developing and Operating Supportive Housing." http://www.csh.org/qualitytoolkit_TOC.

Koenig, Richard. 2015. "Supportive Housing for Persons with Disabilities: A Framework for Evaluating Alternative Models." *Housing Studies* 30, no. 3: 351–367.

Olmstead v. L. C. 1999. 527 U.S. 581.

Ridgeway, Priscilla, and Anthony Zipple. 1990. "The Paradigm Shift in Residential Services: From Linear Continuum to Supportive Housing Approaches." *Psychosocial Rehabilitation Journal* 13, no. 4: 11–32.

Tabol, Charity, Charles Drebing, and Robert Rosenheck. 2010. "Studies of 'Supported' and 'Supportive' Housing: A Comprehensive Review of Model Descriptions and Measurement." *Evaluation and Program Planning* 33, no. 4: 446–456.

T

Theater

Theater and performance exist as places for storytelling. Disability has had its place in this system, but it has often been a mistaken representation. The acts of performance and storytelling were some of the first ways society shared and educated and are still major ways of reaching mass audiences. From the time of the ancient Greeks, plays have included characters with disabilities, but these characters have been outcasts and undesirables. Most characters with a disability are written to focus on their hardships and rouse feelings of pity or disgust in the audience. Here, the focus is on this inner sense of turmoil, not normality and inclusion. Disability in theater often presents "disabledness" in the form of a person, rather than presenting a person who also has a disability.

Background

Tobin Siebers, the author of *Disability Theory*, points out that an able-bodied performer portraying a disabled character is a type of drag. This disability drag is often seen as acceptable in theater. Often, such performances are considered particularly award-worthy, as evidence of an actor's skill. For example, Alex Sharp won a Tony for his role as Christopher Boone in *The Curious Incident of the Dog in the Night-Time* in 2015, playing an autistic character when he himself is not autistic. That same year, Bradley Cooper, who played the title role in *The Elephant Man*, was also nominated for a Tony. The disconnect between reality and acting ability shows how inefficient the portrayals are. Both the performance and the audience attempt to substitute a palpable fantasy for the reality that the actor actually lives. Casting disabled actors helps align these performances with reality, but this is rarely done.

Disability at the Theater

Before the Americans with Disabilities Act (ADA) of 1990, it was difficult for disabled audience members to know if it was even possible to patronize a theater. Despite the work of the ADA, many places continue to be inaccessible. Accessible stages, backstages, and audience seating need to be part of how society thinks about inclusion of disabled people in all areas of theater.

It is rare to find disabled designers, technicians, and managers in the theater industry. There are few of these professionals working and making a living in the field. Prejudice and discrimination play a major factor in the employment of people with disabilities in the theater industry as well as in the lack of access behind the scenes. One organization having this conversation is the U.S. Institute for Theatre Technology. This organization has included disability in its diversity initiative and in its Gateway Mentorship Program. This program is bridging the connection between education and employment for the underrepresented people behind the scenes.

Inclusive Disability Theater

Currently, it is not common practice to include disability in a theater's inclusion and diversity initiative. However, one company that does include disability in its diversity initiative is the Oregon Shakespeare Festival. This company, based out of Ashland, Oregon, not only casts actors with disabilities but also includes technicians with disabilities in their staff. Working backstage with a wheelchair user technician helped open their minds to the possibility of disabilities onstage as well.

Smaller community theater organizations that have been developed just for disability inclusion include the following: *Tell'in Tales Theatre*, in Chicago, founded by Tekki Lomnicki in 1994; *AXIS Dance*, in Oakland, California, founded by Thais Mazur in 1987; *The DisAbility Project*, in St. Louis, cofounded by Joan Lipkin and Fran Cohen in 1996; and *Phamaly Theatre Company*, in Denver, founded in 1989 by five disabled actors who wanted to perform. Day programs for adults with intellectual disabilities around the country have also developed acting programs to develop social skills and life skills.

Case Study: Phamaly Theatre Company. In the Phamaly Theatre Company, all of the performers have disabilities. In its production

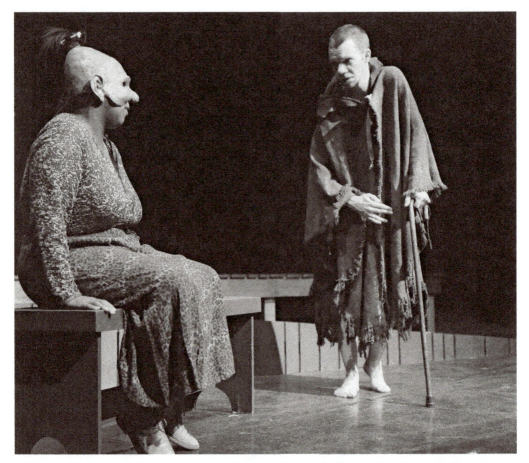

A dress rehearsal of Phamaly Theatre Company's production of *The Elephant Man*, at the Aurora Fox Arts Center in Aurora, Colorado. Although plays that include characters with disabilites are common, disabled actors are rarely cast for such parts. (Cyrus McCrimmon/The Denver Post via Getty Images)

of *Man of La Mancha*, Regan Linton was cast as the character of Dulcinea. They used her physical situation to add new depth to the character by ripping the actress out of her wheelchair during the scene in which Dulcinea is raped. This made the audience unquestionably aware of how vulnerable she was with her inability to escape the situation because of her paralyzed legs. She then dragged herself back on stage to sing "Aldonza." From this perspective, the lines "to a creature who'll never do better than crawl" are more invested with meaning than as originally written—exhibiting how Phamaly has found ways to imbue originality into plays that may be thought to have been done in every way possible.

Designing for Disability

All designers bring their individual perspective to a production, and a designer with a disability is not any different. In the case of a designer with a disability, working with a performer with a disability means that aspects of understanding can be easily navigated. Most able-bodied designer reactions are to correct or hide a body's imperfections. Such design removes much of the uniqueness that the disability of the performer brings to a piece.

When designing for the disabled actor, awareness of the technicalities of a disability is critical. For instance, a person with a spinal cord injury may have difficulty regulating his or her body temperature. This may mean that the actor is unable to wear hats or wigs because of potential overheating. When sign language is the primary method of communication, easy hand visibility in front of the costume necessitates wise color and pattern choices. Wheelchairs can go up ramps, but the set designer needs to be aware of what that movement looks like and the energy it takes. People with

visual impairments are often talented at moving easily through space, but knowing how they do this can help a scenic designer. There are only a handful of designers with a disability who are currently working professionally and who understand these nuances. Very few were disabled before going into their profession.

Conclusion

Witnessing a performer with a missing a limb or in a wheelchair is only distracting for a short period of time, until the viewer becomes familiarized—this is where normalizing disability starts. Having disabled artists in a performance setting puts the subject on the table to begin discussion and to promote conversation. Without room for disabled artists to show their skills in the roles afforded them, society's understanding of disability will not progress. Disabled theater professionals have not expected the industry to change for them; they only ask for accommodations so they may access their craft. Theater, performance, and entertainment are powerful educational tools that can make the goal of social inclusion a reality.

Mallory Kay Nelson

See also: Contemporary Art; Disability and Performance in Everyday Life; Fine Arts; Poetry

Further Reading

Considine, Allison. 2015. "Theatre Artists with Disabilities Are Ready, Willing, and, Yes, Able." *American Theatre*, October 20. http://www.americantheatre.org/2015/10/20/theatre-artists-with-disabilities-are-ready-willing-and-yes-able/.

Davies, Telory. 2009. *Performing Disability: Staging the Actual*. Saarbrücken, Germany: VDM, Verlag Dr. Müller.

Dziemianowicz, Joe. 2015. "*Spring Awakening*'s Stroker Bway's First Wheelchair Actor." *New York Daily News*, September 15. http://www.nydailynews.com/entertainment/theater-arts/ali-stroker-broadway-history-spring-awakening-article-1.2361740.

Fraser, Mat. 2017. "Mat Fraser: All Theatres Should Cast at Least One Disabled Actor a Year." Opinion. *The Stage*, May 10. https://www.thestage.co.uk/opinion/2017/mat-fraser-all-theatres-should-cast-at-least-one-disabled-actor-a-year/.

Genzlinger, Neil. 2017. "A Wheelchair on Broadway Isn't Exploitation. It's Progress." *New York Times*, March 24. https://www.nytimes.com/2017/03/24/theater/a-wheelchair-on-broadway-isnt-exploitation-its-progress.html.

Kuppers, Petra. 2003. *Disability and Contemporary Performance: Bodies on the Edge.* London: Routledge.

Linton, Regan. 2009. Personal interview. November 20.

Sandahl, Carrie, and Philip Auslander. 2005. *Bodies in Commotion: Disability and Performance.* Ann Arbor: University of Michigan Press.

Siebers, Tobin. 2008. *Disability Theory.* Ann Arbor: University of Michigan Press.

Therapeutic Recreation

Therapeutic recreation is a professional field that seeks to develop recreation and leisure skills for people with disabilities throughout their lifetime. They serve as community builders for people with disabilities, including individuals who have an illness or disabling condition who are seeking psychological and physical health recovery and well-being. This entry will examine therapeutic recreation for people with disabilities.

What Is Therapeutic Recreation?

Therapeutic recreation strives to create opportunities for people with disabilities to engage in their communities with equal access and enjoyment while learning new skills and pursuing lifetime leisure interests. Individuals with disabilities encounter many social barriers that require adaptation and change for equal access to exist. One can also encounter physical barriers, such as inadequate transportation, assessable doors and walkways, and adaptive equipment, that can make it difficult for someone with a disability to have equal access. These are referred to as structural barriers.

Background and History

Emergence of Therapeutic Recreation. The use of recreation for therapeutic purposes has been present throughout history. In the United States, following World War I and World War II, soldiers began showing signs of what doctors would come to know as post-traumatic stress disorder (PTSD) from their traumatic experiences in war. The Red Cross helped create games and exercises to engage patience for healing purposes, in addition to their correctional facilities and psychiatric institutions. This became a significant emerging point for the field of therapeutic recreation through the late 1930s and 1940s.

Medicalization and Recreational Therapy. During this time period, the way recreation therapy had been taught began to shift to the medical and psychological way of training for the field. This created two paths of understanding about where recreation therapists practice, the medical model versus the social model of disability. The first, very much influenced by the medical model of disability, is in hospital settings. This model looks at individuals with disabilities and their limitations first. The *medical model* seeks adaptations to help individuals interact with society as society deems appropriate. This model is counter-positioned to the *social model* of disability, which argues that disability is not something within one individual and instead places responsibility on society for creating disabling barriers—social and environmental disadvantages from structures and rules that limit access.

Therapeutic Recreation in the Community. In the 1960s, a movement started to make recreation more organized with member organizations. When the National Parks and Recreation Association (NRPA) formed in 1965, there was finally a voice for the importance of recreation in the lives of all people. By 1967, the NRPA approved the National Therapeutic Recreation Society, which created a public space for people bringing recreation programs to individuals with disabilities in their communities. Throughout the 1970s and 1980s, the field established a national credentialing body, called National Council for Therapeutic Recreation Accreditation, and a body for continued research development and best practices to reinforce the important impact of therapeutic recreation services provided in clinical settings.

At the same time, some states sought to seek more equality in recreation participation for people with disabilities. In 1968, Eunice Kennedy Shriver helped to create the Special Olympics and hosted the first Special Olympics Games at Soldier Field in Chicago, Illinois. Illinois would continue the effort to enhance opportunities for people with disabilities in their communities by creation of the first Special Recreation Association (SRA) in 1970. Through cooperation with neighboring communities,

recreation programming for individuals with disabilities addresses important barriers in recreation participation by facilitating better trained professional staff, access to buildings with appropriate program adaptations, and an identifiable resource that caters to the needs of individuals.

Important Points to Understand about Therapeutic Recreation

Impact of Legislation. During the late 1960s and early 1970s, national legislative movements were taking form to address social justice. Their goals were to reinforce the social movement for equity and address inequity in various public institutions. Some key pieces of legislation that affect therapeutic recreation included the following:

- PL 93-112 Rehab Act (1973)
- PL 94-142 Education for All Handicapped Children Act (1975)
- PL-100-146 Developmental Disabilities Bill of Rights Act Amendment (1987)
- PL 100-407 Technology Related Assistance for Individuals with Disabilities Act (1988)
- PL 101-336 Americans with Disabilities Act (1990)
- Title I Employment
- Title II Government Services
- IIA (change rules, policies and practices; remove architectural, transportation, and communication barriers; provision of auxiliary aids and services)
- IIB: Public Transit
- Title III Public Accommodations
- Title IV Telecommunications (relay services, translation)

Each law and section of law attempted to confront disparities and inequities in the lives of people with disabilities in the

United States. These laws helped strengthen the Illinois legislature's design of law to provide "Recreation for the Handicapped" and continue to define the inclusiveness of those services to be fitted to each community in identifying their needs and priorities. Funding from this legislation is only available if there is a cooperative agreement between neighboring communities. The funds can only be used to the benefit of the provision of recreation and leisure opportunities for members of the community.

Shift toward Inclusive Practices. Through the 1980s, special recreation associations partnered closely with Special Olympics and with community vocational providers who largely served individuals with intellectual disabilities in community-based programs. A significant shift toward inclusive practices became an important point of emphasis with the 1990 Americans with Disabilities Act (ADA). However, inclusive practices, promotion, and reimbursement vary widely in different communities, which leads to fewer opportunities for recreation in poorer communities.

Social Ecological Model. Lewin's (1951) social ecological model (SES) is relevant in examining the disparity of opportunities created by the success or lack of success in the inclusion movement during this period. The model highlights challenges such as fiscal resources, resistance to change in policy, and institutional bureaucracy as barriers to access. In the recreation world, these are all applicable barriers to community inclusion in programs afforded to nondisabled peers. Therapeutic recreation professionals can play a large role in design of community access and integration. They can also advise businesses and community-based recreation agencies about barriers that inhibit program accessibility for people with disabilities.

ADA Accessibility Guidelines. Providers continued to be challenged to eliminate barriers through public mandate. Chapter 10 of the 2010 Americans with Disabilities Act Accessibility Guidelines (ADAAG) noted nine recreation areas: amusement rides, boating facilities, exercise equipment, fishing piers, golf and mini-golf facilities, play areas, swimming pools, spas, and shooting facilities. New policies were required as well—in particular, a service animal policy and a policy for other power-driven mobility devices (OPDMD). New policies may create the need to attempt to raise additional revenue through increased user fees, increased tax levy for programs funded through public resources, and grants and partnerships.

Dilemmas, Debates, and Unresolved Questions

Professional Profiles. The field of therapeutic recreation is trending toward overwhelmingly white and female instructor positions, as well as students. This trend creates a particularly narrow lens in academic preparation to translate to more diverse populations with their own cultural views and needs. Another risk in the lack of diversity is in service itself. The SRA's mission is to serve people with all disabilities in their member communities. However, if staff cannot use or understand sign language and do not have ready access to interpreter services, people who are in the Deaf community may dismiss providers as resources.

This barrier exists through cultural difference and can create other barriers like language or even cultural representation in the field. This is a problem parks and recreation professionals have yet to solve and at times do not fully acknowledge.

Community Building Role. The future role of therapeutic recreation providers is evolving and includes an appreciation of a multicultural community identity. Partnerships with other family unit building agencies like Lekotek are important to the process of overcoming the resource issues that poorer communities face. Lekotek is a toy-lending library that offers play sessions to its member families, so that they learn to play as a family unit with their family member with a disability. Membership fees to these programs may still be a barrier. Therefore, providing scholarships or larger play groups at discounts may ensure that children with disabilities acquire skills and have toys to engage in play with family and friends.

Many different partnerships need to be maintained in order to ensure access to recreation from a provider. A therapeutic recreation program can only be seen as a resource if it is believed to be an asset to a community. Communities such as the Deaf, veterans with disabilities, aging populations with disabilities, adult athletes with physical disabilities, and many more may not believe an agency that publicizes Special Olympics in its program will have resources for them as well.

Another important component connected with community resource building involves institutional partnerships with schools. Providing leisure education in classrooms and working with educational partners helps to develop understanding of leisure and the relationship among leisure, lifestyle, and society. The development of recognition of personal interest is important to social growth, as is the ability to share those interests and engage in them with peers and mentors.

A foundational community partner that is perhaps underused is the Forest Preserve and Department of Natural Resources system, particularly in urban communities.

There has to be a philosophical dedication to ensuring that nature-based programs are represented in the leisure education programs. Finally, therapeutic recreation should seek to guide in the development of culturally welcoming programs that overcome disparities.

Conclusion and Future Direction
Therapeutic recreation professionals play a vital role in the development and inclusion of people with disabilities in their communities. They can design around and review barriers and risks to recreation participation, and they can also work with the people with disabilities they serve and disability studies ethicists to ensure diverse programs that meet the needs of people with disabilities. Policies, procedures, and program design must continue to evolve in order to serve the diversifying needs of all people in communities.

Michael McNicholas

See also: Community Living and Community Integration; Social Model of Disability; Therapist, Role in Activities of Daily Living (ADLs)

Further Reading

Bullock, Charles C., and Michael J. Mahon. 2017. *Introduction to Recreation Services for People with Disabilities: A Person-Centered Approach.* 4th ed. Urbana, IL: Sagamore-Venture Publishing.

James, Ann. 1998. In *Perspectives in Recreational Therapy: Issues of a Dynamic Profession,* edited by Frank Brasile, Thomas Skalko, and Joan Burlingame. Enumclaw, WA: Idyll Arbor.

Mansfield, Jeffrey A., compiler. 2017. "Recreational Therapy History by Categories." Therapeutic Recreation Directory. http://www.recreationtherapy.com/history/rthistory4.htm.

Reiner, Larry. 1997. "History of SRAs." Illinois Parks and Recreation. http://www.lib.niu.edu/1997/ip970945.html.

Therapist, Role in Activities of Daily Living (ADLs)

Therapists often play a big part in maintaining the health and functioning of people with various disabilities. Therapists can often help individuals to restore or maintain their ability to participate in a wide range of activities of daily living (ADLs). ADLs are the basic activities involved in caring for oneself. ADLs typically include bathing, toileting, dressing, eating, mobility, hygiene and grooming, taking care of personal devices (such as hearing aids, glasses), and sexual activity.

What Are Activities of Daily Living?

Assistance with ADLs can include helping an individual with all of the skills involved in carrying out a specific activity. ADLs are the personal care skills of bathing or showering, toileting and related hygiene, getting dressed, eating, functional mobility, caring for personal devices, personal grooming and hygiene, and sexual activity (American Occupational Therapy Association [AOTA] 2014, S19). ADLs include functional mobility, or the ability to get from one place or position to another (such as transferring into the bathtub), wheelchair mobility, and movement in bed (AOTA 2014 S19). Care of personal devices involves the use, cleaning, and maintenance of personal devices, such as prosthetics, and adaptive equipment (AOTA 2014 S19). Another ADL includes sexual activity, or activities used to achieve sexual satisfaction (AOTA 2014 S19).

Age and ADLs. People of all ages may need assistance learning and performing ADLs. Children with sensory processing or sensory integration difficulties may have challenges performing the motor aspects of ADLs, and oversensitivity to sensory stimuli may cause children to avoid participating in ADLs (Koenig and Rudney 2010). Children with mild impairments, including developmental coordination disorder, sensory integrative dysfunction, learning disabilities, and disabilities affecting attention (e.g., ADHD), also may have symptoms that interfere with their ability to carry out ADLs (Gantschnig et al. 2013). Individuals with disabilities who have challenges with fine or gross motor skills, cognitive impairments (such as memory), visual impairments, or hearing impairments may have difficulty learning and carrying out ADLs independently. Finally, as they age, older adults are the most likely to need help with ADLs.

Assessing Activities of Daily Living

When people are unable to carry out ADLs independently, they may need instruction to learn to perform the activities, help from others or assistive devices, or changes to their environment. *Occupational therapists* most often evaluate a person's ability to perform ADLs and plan interventions to address challenges in the health care setting. Assessment methods can include observation of the person performing an activity or completion of a rating scale or checklist of skills. Both formal and informal methods can be used to evaluate an individual's ability to perform ADLs. Commonly used formal assessments include the Functional Independence Measure (FIM), the Hawaii Early Learning Profile, the Pediatric Evaluation of Disability, and the Vineland Adaptive Behavior Scales (Asher 2013).

Promoting the Development of Activities of Daily Living

In schools, ADLs may be included as part of a functional life-skills curriculum designed for students with disabilities. Educational personnel, such as special education teachers, may be involved in assessing and teaching ADLs in the school setting. Teachers and school support staff may assist students in carrying out ADLs (such as eating or toileting) during the school day. Task analysis, prompting, and video modeling are strategies that can be used to teach individuals to perform ADLs more independently. Assistive technology and environmental modifications can be used to maximize an individual's participation in ADLs.

Task Analysis. Task analysis is the process of breaking a complex skill into smaller steps. Some ADLs, for example brushing teeth, consist of several steps that must be carried out in sequence to complete the activity. The individual steps can be taught using prompting strategies.

Prompting Strategies. A *prompt* is an extra cue given to encourage a person to perform an action. An individual can be prompted to perform a step by physical touch or guidance, verbal cues, gestures, or modeling. Steps may be taught by beginning with the first step (known as "forward chaining") or last step (known as "backward chaining") and teaching additional steps as those are mastered or by working on all of the steps at once (known as "total task instruction"). There are different prompting techniques that can be used to teach ADLs. These methods can be used to teach activities with several steps or one step. Prompts can be delivered starting with more intensive types of prompts and fading to less intensive prompts as the person masters the steps (known as "most-to-least prompting"). Alternatively, prompts can be given starting with less intensive prompts and increasing assistance until the person performs the step correctly (known as "least-to-most prompting"). The amount of time

between an instruction or natural cue and a prompt can also be varied when teaching with prompts. In *simultaneous prompting*, the prompt is given immediately, which should result in errorless learning, as the learner is not given a chance to make a mistake. Another option is using *time delay*, which involves waiting for the individual to respond before providing a prompt. With all prompting strategies, the goal is to eventually fade the prompts so that the ADL is performed independently.

Video Modeling. Videos can be used as a tool for teaching ADLs to individuals with severe disabilities. Video modeling involves a person watching a video of an activity being performed and then copying what was shown in the video. A form of video modeling is *video self-modeling*, in which the person watches a video of him- or herself doing the activity. *Video prompting* is another way to teach with videos. In video prompting, the video is shown in smaller clips in which each represents one step of the activity. Examples of ADLs that can be taught using videos include hygiene and grooming activities like brushing teeth, dressing skills like zipping a zipper, and personal device care, such as cleaning glasses (Bellini and Akullian 2007).

Assistive Technology. Assistive technology (AT) can be used to help individuals perform ADLs with greater independence, particularly for those who have difficulty performing the physical skills required for ADLs. AT is an adaptive device (or service) that helps people increase their participation or independence in their daily life. AT can range from low tech to high tech. Examples of AT used for ADLs include eating utensils with thicker grips that make them easier to grasp, electric toothbrushes that reduce the need to manually move the toothbrush, and shower chairs that allow a person to sit while bathing. Use of AT can increase a person's independence in performing ADLs and reduce reliance on others for help with these tasks.

Environmental Modifications. Environmental modifications can be put in place so that people with disabilities can perform ADLs with greater independence. Environmental modifications are physical changes to a person's home, workplace, or school that are needed to ensure safety and help one function more independently. Changes can be made to a bathroom or kitchen so that an individual can carry out ADLs like bathing, toileting, performing personal hygiene, and eating with greater independence. Examples include a raised toilet, kitchen lighting that allows a person to see better and eat more independently, and grab bars in a bathroom. Other physical changes can be made to buildings, such as widening doorways to allow a wheelchair to pass through or installing ramps so that individuals can access environments where they perform ADLs.

Other Skills for Living Independently

While ADLs encompass basic personal care skills, there are additional activities involved in being able to live independently and take care of oneself without help. First and foremost, it is vital that therapists assist with the instrumental activities that are of personal import to the individual. Instrumental activities of daily living (IADLs) are "activities that support daily life within the home and community and that often require more complex interactions than those used in ADLs" (AOTA 2014, S43). IADLs includes activities such as taking care of others (such as children, parents, and pets); communicating; driving and getting around the community; managing finances; managing

health conditions (such as exercising or taking medication); performing household chores; shopping; preparing meals; engaging in spiritual activities; and remaining safe (AOTA 2014). IADLs are often activities that can be carried out by another person (such as dining out instead of cooking, or hiring a housekeeper). Some people with disabilities may require or desire support only for certain ADL or IADL needs. Other individuals may need support for a combination of both ADL and IADL tasks.

Conclusion

Therapists can often play an important role in assisting with ADLs and IADLs to help a person with a disability live independently. The ability to perform ADLs may be linked to positive results for students with disabilities after they complete their education. Self-care and acquisition of independent living skills are predictors of postschool success in the areas of employment, education, and independent living (Test et al. 2009). Thus, providing direct support to meet the ADL and IADL needs of individuals with disabilities is essential for optimal postschool outcomes.

Lauren Mucha

See also: Activities of Daily Living (ADLs); Independent Living; Occupational Therapy; Wellness and Health Promotion

Further Reading

American Occupational Therapy Association. 2014. "Occupational Therapy Practice Framework: Domain and Process." *American Journal of Occupational Therapy* 68: S1–S48.

Asher, Ina Elfant. 2007. *Occupational Therapy Assessment Tools: An Annotated Index.* Bethesda, MD: American Occupational Therapy Association.

Bellini, Scott, and Jennifer Akullian. 2007. "A Meta-Analysis of Video Modeling and Video Self-Modeling Interventions for Children and Adolescents with Autism Spectrum Disorders." *Exceptional Children* 73, no. 3: 264–287.

Buning, Mary Ellen, Joy Hammel, Jennifer Angelo, Mark Schmeler, Stephanie Doster, Kristi Voelkerding, Eileen R. Garza. 2004. "Assistive Technology within Occupational Therapy Practice (2004)." *The American Journal of Occupational Therapy: Official Publication of the American Occupational Therapy Association* 58, no. 6: 678–680.

Gantschnig, Brigitte E., Julie Page, Ingeborg Nilsson, and Anne G. Fisher. 2013. "Detecting Differences in Activities of Daily Living between Children with and without Mild Disabilities." *American Journal of Occupational Therapy* 67, no. 3: 319–327.

Koenig, Kristie Patten, and Sarah G. Rudney. 2010. "Performance Challenges for Children and Adolescents with Difficulty Processing and Integrating Sensory Information: A Systematic Review." *American Journal of Occupational Therapy* 64, no. 3: 430–442.

Test, David W., Valerie L. Mazzotti, April L. Mustian, Catherine H. Fowler, Larry Kortering, and Paula Kohler. 2009. "Evidence-Based Secondary Transition Predictors for Improving Postschool Outcomes for Students with Disabilities." *Career Development for Exceptional Individuals* 32, no. 3: 160–181.

Transition from High School

Preparing youth for life after high school has become increasingly driven by accountability procedures and mandates. States, school districts, and individual schools are now under the microscope to produce not only graduates but also citizens who are career and college ready with a rigorous set of academic knowledge and skills.

What Is Transition?

For youth with disabilities, current legal policies have put heavy emphasis on statewide accountability measures, including procedures for tracking data on transition planning, goals, services, and postschool outcomes. Under the Individuals with Disabilities Education Improvement Act (IDEA) of 2004, transition services are defined as follows:

A coordinated set of activities for a child with a disability that: (a) Is designed to be within a results-oriented process, that is focused on improving the academic and functional achievement of the child with a disability to facilitate the child's movement from school to post-school activities, including post-secondary education, vocational education, integrated employment (including supported employment); continuing and adult education, adult services, independent living, or community participation; (b) is based on the individual child's needs, taking into account the child's strengths, preferences, and interests; and (c) includes instruction, related services, community experiences, the development of employment and other post-school adult living objectives, and, if appropriate, acquisition of daily living skills and functional vocational evaluation. (118 Stat. 2658)

Given this federal definition, at the age of 16 (younger depending on state law), individualized education programs (IEPs) for students with disabilities are written with a focus on services, supports, and post-school outcomes in three distinct areas: (1) postsecondary education and training; (2) employment when deemed appropriate by the IEP team; and (3) independent living. States are mandated to report annually on certain quality indicators in secondary transition to monitor compliance with IDEA 2004. State performance plans require data on postschool outcomes (Indicator 14) and the documentation of how those outcomes are reached (Indicator 13). Indicator 13, or the quality of documentation of the transition process, is measured by the "percent of youth age 16 and above with an IEP that includes coordinated, measurable, annual IEP goals and transition services that will reasonably enable the child to meet the post-secondary goals" (20 U.S.C. 1416(a)(3)(B)). To evaluate the maintenance of post-school outcomes, data are required for Indicator 14, or the "percent of youth who had IEPs, are no longer in secondary school and who have been competitively employed, enrolled in some type of postsecondary school, or both, within one year of leaving high school" (20 U.S.C. 1416(a)(3)(B)).

Background and History

Employment-Centered Education. Today, students with disabilities are supported and monitored in their pathway from school to young adulthood. In the past, however, students with disabilities were often segregated from general education or did not participate in education at all. In 1975, the Education for All Handicapped Children Act was passed to give a "free appropriate public education" (FAPE) to all students with disabilities, regardless of the severity of the disability. In 1983, the U.S. Department of Education's National Commission on Excellence in Education published the report *A Nation at Risk: The Imperative for Educational Reform.* This report asserted that youth did not have the skills to enter the labor market and that a high school education should prepare youth for a career and citizenship. In the wake of transition now being looked at as a federal initiative, Madeleine Will, the assistant secretary of the U.S. Office of Special Education and Rehabilitative Services at the time, defined transition as follows:

An outcome oriented process encompassing a broad array of services and experiences that lead to employment. Transition is a period that includes high school, the point of graduation, additional postsecondary education or adult services, and the initial years of employment. Transition is a bridge between the security and structure offered by the school and the risks of life. (Will 1984, 1)

In this employment-centered definition, Will identified three different levels of services that an individual with a disability might need in order to move from high school and obtain the desired employment outcome. These levels of services include the following: no special services, time-limited services, and ongoing services.

Shift to Community Living. In 1985, Andrew Halpern expanded Will's definition to include that successfully living in one's community was the primary goal of transition. Halpern's (1985) model defined successful adjustment to a community setting as having three main components: residential environment, employment, and social and interpersonal networks. This model was based on the premise that all three areas contributed to a successful transition and that deficiencies in one area threatened the success in another area. Halpern maintained the three levels of services established by Will (1985), noting that general services, limited special services, or ongoing special services were needed for youth with disabilities to smoothly transition from high school to successful adjustment in their communities.

Emergence of Transition Services and Supports. In 1990, the Education for All Handicapped Children Act was amended and renamed the Individuals with Disabilities Education Act (IDEA), giving students with disabilities the opportunity to be equal to students without disabilities by improving support services and resources. The 1990 and 1997 reauthorization of IDEA included improvements that mandated transition services for students with disabilities. In conjunction with this legislation, the leading professional organization for research and practice in special education, the Council for Exceptional Children, established a subdivision entitled Division on Career Development and Transition (DCDT) and published a position paper that defined transition as follows:

> Transition refers to a change in status from behaving primarily as a student to assuming emergent adult roles in the community. These roles include employment, participating in post-secondary education, maintaining a home, becoming appropriately involved in the community, and experiencing satisfactory personal and social relationships. The process of enhancing transition involves the participation and coordination of school programs, adult agency services, and natural supports within the community. The foundations for transition should be laid during the elementary and middle school

years, guided by the broad concept of career development. Transition planning should begin no later than age 14, and students should be encouraged, to the full extent of their capabilities, to assume a maximum amount of responsibility for such planning. (Halpern 1994, 117)

Taking into account an even broader scope of what transition entails and what supports are necessary to achieve these benchmarks in adult life, DCDT's definition paved the way for the current comprehensive definition put forth by the most recent reauthorization of IDEA in 2004.

Important Points to Know about Transitions from High School

Data on Transition from High School. The National Longitudinal Transition Study-2 (NLTS2) (Wagner et al. 2005) has provided the largest bank of data that illustrates a broad understanding of the experiences of high school students with disabilities as they progress through early adulthood. The NLTS2 collected information over a 10-year period from a nationally representative sample of high school students with disabilities who were receiving special education services under IDEA in the 2000–2001 school year. The report indicates that only 43 percent of youth with disabilities were employed during the period immediately after high school, compared to 63 percent of their peers without disabilities. In addition, certain populations of youth with disabilities are at an even greater risk of experiencing poor employment outcomes, such as African Americans and females. The type and severity of the disability is also related to employment outcomes. Employment rates range from 9 percent for those with significant disabilities to 75 percent for those with learning disabilities. Compared to their peers without disabilities, young adults with disabilities are less likely to receive a high school diploma (62 percent vs. 88 percent), three times as likely to drop out of school (31 percent vs. 11 percent), and only one-fifth as likely to enroll in postsecondary education (Wagner et al. 2005).

Benefits of Transition Services. However, despite the large gap in outcomes between students with and without disabilities, providing individualized transition services to students with disabilities allows them to be supported in their pathway to a fulfilling adulthood. For example, individuals with disabilities who graduate from postsecondary education or training programs are more likely to be employed, earn a higher wage, use a checking account, have a driver's license or permit, and engage in social activities (Newman et al. 2011). Therefore, the process of developing and implementing responsive school-to-work transition services, supports, and policies for young adults with disabilities is imperative to successful outcomes in adult life.

Taxonomy for Transition. Conceptualizing the structure of transition in the context of schools, Kohler (1996) proposed a taxonomy for transition programming based on effective transition practices that includes five areas: (1) student-focused planning, such as students participating in the development of the IEP; (2) student development, such as learning employment skills; (3) family involvement, such as training families about their legal rights; (4) program structure, such as resources provided for transition service delivery in the classroom and other environments; and (5) interagency collaboration, such as referral to an adult service provider agency. This taxonomy is typically utilized to organize best practices because it is widely used as the foundational framework for delivery of comprehensive transition services in schools.

Organizational Model. Another prominent organizational model of best practices addresses transition within standards-based education and school reform (Morningstar and Clark 2003). This model aligns secondary education and special education, bridging the practices that should be used not only in special education but inclusively in secondary education settings for students with and without disabilities. Morningstar and Clark (2003) proposed this model of practices in the context of training general secondary and special educators with the same knowledge and skills in transition for all students moving from high school to adult life. Their model is structured with tiered supports. The practices include components that *all* students should be provided (few supports), *some* students should be provided (moderate supports), and only a *few* students should be provided (most intensive supports). The organizational model has five broad domain areas: (1) curriculum focused on postsecondary outcomes; (2) collaboration within school and community; (3) family involvement; (4) instruction that promotes independence and engagement; and (5) assessment for student-focused planning. A tiered example in the domain of curriculum focused on postsecondary outcomes would be as follows: (a) *all* students should receive curriculum that is connected to careers and postsecondary educational goals; (b) *some* students will need more moderate supports such as supplemental transition or academic or behavioral curricula; and, c) *few* students will need the most intensive supports, such as specific curricula individualized to their needs (Morningstar and Clark 2003).

Dilemmas, Debates, and Unresolved Questions

Technical Assistance for Transition Services and Support. In addition to effective program organizational models, there has been a national effort to streamline the dissemination of transition research, practices, and resources in an accessible format. The National Secondary Transition Technical Assistance Center (NSTTAC) was a dissemination center funded by the U.S. Department of Education's Office of Special Education Programs (OSEP). NSTTAC is now housed at the National Technical Assistance Center on Transition (NTACT) and is regarded as the national leader in technical assistance in secondary transition. NSTTAC disseminates evidence-based practices and policies to support students with disabilities as they transition from secondary education to college, other postsecondary education and training options, and employment.

Evaluating Transition Practices. In an effort to improve service provision and compliance, NSTTAC performed a systematic review of the literature in secondary transition to determine the evidence base for instructional practices. NSTTAC identified evidence-based practices in secondary transition using quality indicator checklists developed to rank studies with experimental and single-subject research designs and literature reviews (Test et al. 2009). Depending on the number of high- or acceptable-quality studies (as indicated by using a quality indicator checklist), strategies were rated to have strong, moderate, or potential levels of evidence. These practices have been categorized using Kohler's (1996) Taxonomy for Transition Programming. Evidence-based practices were found in the taxonomy areas of student-focused

planning (such as *The Self-Directed IEP* by Martin, Marshall, Maxson, and Jerman [1996]); student development (such as teaching academic skills focused on postsecondary education goals using technology); family involvement (such as using training modules to promote parent involvement in transition); and program structure (such as including paid internship opportunities in high school).

Lack of Evidence-Based Practices. To date, no evidence-based practices have been identified in the area of interagency collaboration. A large portion of the research supporting many of the evidence-based practices identified by NSTTAC has samples of students with moderate to severe disabilities. While the evidence-based practices identified are considered to be effective interventions, more research is needed with students with mild disabilities to further establish the body of literature (Test et al. 2009). Additionally, very few studies specifically examined the impact of these interventions on students from culturally linguistically diverse (CLD) backgrounds. All evidence-based practices in transition should be used with the principles of individualization and cultural competence when working with CLD youth with disabilities.

Conclusion

A significant variable in postschool outcomes for students with disabilities is quality trained special educators prepared with specific knowledge and skills in secondary transition to facilitate services and supports for students' successful movement from high school to adult life (Benitez, Morningstar, and Frey 2009). Research has shown that after receiving coursework or professional development in transition, teachers feel more effective and are more likely to implement transition practices (Benitez, Morningstar, and Frey 2009). This research supports the idea that the more knowledge, resources, and pedagogical skills teachers are privy to, the more they will use the information and implement skills with students and their families. Given the increasing emphasis on state accountability of transition services, and a growing body of research on models of service delivery and best practices, significant focus should be on preparing teachers to implement high-quality transition supports. Not only should rigorous research continue to bolster evidence of promising transition practices, but comprehensive teacher preparation in transition will enhance quality services and linkages that create the foundational bridge to successful student outcomes.

Joanna Keel

See also: Americans with Disabilities Act (ADA); Every Student Succeeds Act (ESSA); Individuals with Disabilities Education Improvement Act (IDEIA); Natural Supports; Schoolwide Systems of Supports

Further Reading

Benitez, Debra T., Mary E. Morningstar, and Bruce B. Frey. 2009. "A Multistate Survey of Special Education Teachers' Perceptions of Their Transition Competencies." *Career Development for Exceptional Individuals* 32, no. 1: 6–16.

Halpern, Andrew. 1985. "Transition: A Look at the Foundations." *Exceptional Children* 51, no. 6: 479–486.

Halpern, Andrew S. 1994. "The Transition of Youth with Disabilities to Adult Life: A Position Statement of Division on Career Development and Transition." *Career Development for Exceptional Individuals* 17, no. 2: 115–124.

Kohler, Paula D. 1996. "A Taxonomy for Transition Programming: Linking Research and Practice." Champaign: Transition Research Institute, University of Illinois. http://www.ed.uiuc.edu/sped/tri/institute.html.

Martin, James E., Laura H. Marshall, Laurie Maxson, and Patty L. Jerman. 1996. *The Self-Directed IEP*. Longmont, CO: Sopris West.

Morningstar, Mary E., and Gary M. Clark. 2003. "The Status of Personnel Preparation for Transition Education and Services: What Is the Critical Content? How Can It Be Offered?" *Career Development for Exceptional Individuals* 26, no. 2: 227–237.

National Commission on Excellence in Education. 1983. "A Nation at Risk: The Imperative for Educational Reform." http://www2.ed.gov/pubs/NatAtRisk/index.html.

National Secondary Transition Technical Assistance Center, University of North Carolina–Charlotte. 2012. National Secondary Transition Technical Assistance Center. http://www.nsttac.org/.

National Technical Assistance Center on Transition. 2015. http://www.transitionta.org/.

Newman, Lynn, Mary Wagner, Anne-Marie Knokey, Camille Marder, Katherine Nagle, Debra Shaver and Meredith Schwarting. 2011. "The Post-High School Outcomes of Young Adults with Disabilities up to 8 Years after High School: A Report from the National Longitudinal Transition Study-2 (NLTS2)." National Center for Special Education Research. http://www.nlts2.org/reports/2011_09_02/index.html.

Test, David W., Valerie. L. Mazzotti, April L. Mustian, Catherine H. Fowler, Larry Korterig, and Paula Kohler. 2009. "Evidence-Based Secondary Transition Predictors for Improving Post School Outcomes for Students with Disabilities." *Career Development for Exceptional Individuals* 32, no. 3: 160–181.

Wagner, Mary, Lynn Newman, Renée Cameto, Nicolle Garza, and Phyllis Levine.

2005. *After High School: A First Look at the Post School Experiences of Youth with Disabilities: A Report from the National Longitudinal Transition Study-2.* Menlo Park, CA: SRI International.

Will, Madeline. (1984). *OSERS Programming for the Transition of Youth with Disabilities: Bridges from School to Working Life.* Washington, DC: U.S. Department of Education. Office of Special Education and Rehabilitative Services.

Transitional Experiences of Students with Disabilities

In this entry, the transitional experience of students with disabilities is discussed. Transitional experiences are the experiences of students with disabilities as they graduate from high school and enter educational, employment, or independent living environments. I will explain the transition experience, components of transition preparation, racial differences in transition experiences, and the examination of the transitional experience in the disability studies in education field.

What Is Transitional Experience of Students with Disabilities?

Transitional experience can be defined as the process of students with disabilities leaving K–12 education and going into adulthood. During this process, students also experience a change in disability policy structures that provide support. When students with disabilities are in K–12 education, students receive educational support and services provided through the Individuals with Disabilities in Education Act (IDEA) of 1990, reauthorized in 1997 and 2004. Under this government mandate, they are provided with evaluations to determine eligibility for services; individualized

education programs (IEP) created by a team of individuals (principals, counselors, school psychologists, special education teachers, general education teachers, parents, and the student); and specialized services to meet their educational needs.

After students with disabilities graduate from high school, their rights fall under the Americans with Disabilities Act (ADA) of 1990, amended in 2008, in which students must initiate acquisition of supports and structures to help them access their job, school, daily living, or participation in the community. They also are responsible for creating communication loops of support providers to ensure everyone is informed. If students desire and give written consent, they can provide their parents with access to their education or employment information. Whereas in K–12 education, the parents were the biggest stakeholders and a team convened to ensure students' needs were met, after graduation, this responsibility shifts to the students. The differences in disability policies in high school and after graduation (IDEA and ADA) can be seen in table 1.

Having a successful transition experience can help students with disabilities live meaningful lives. Ideally, students will be able to live and experience life according to their personal dreams and visions rather than the dictates of others' views of their abilities. This topic is vital to disability studies to bring about understanding of the conditions that support and challenge the ability of people with disabilities to live their lives prior to and after the transition to adulthood.

Background and History

According to the original Individuals with Disabilities Education Act (IDEA) of 1990, amended in 1997 and reauthorized in 2004, transition planning is supposed to begin well before a student's graduation or the age

Table 1: Differences between Disability Policies in K–12 Education and after Graduation

IDEA (K–12)	ADA (After High School)
• Focus on success. • School's responsibility to provide evaluation and determination for special education eligibility. • Individualized Education Plan (IEP) with specific goals, accommodations and/or modifications, and other services to meet student's need educational needs. • Services are provided until student graduates or turns 21 years of age. • Provided with a team of school professionals and parent or caregiver to create support and structures at school. • Parent or caregiver has access to student records.	• Focus on ensuring access. • Individual's responsibility to disclose disability and provide evaluation paperwork. • Individuals must be able to talk about how their disability affects their ability to perform tasks. • Focus on providing equal access to individual. • Individuals are provided accommodations based on evaluation to complete desired task (employment, education, independent living). • Written Consent for Parent participation or access to records is required.

of 21. By the time a student is 14, schools are required to begin developing in IEPs transition goals that reflect what the student wants to do after graduation. The transition plan is required to go into effect at age 16 and be reviewed on a yearly basis. All decisions regarding the transition process are supposed to be based on the strengths, preferences, and skills of the student.

Students are supposed to be involved in these meetings with hope that they will develop self-determination skills needed for after graduation. These skills include being able to talk about their disability, understanding its impact on their participation in academic or social activities, and advocating for accommodations to help them go to school, work, live independently, or participate in the community. These transition goals are related to going to college, getting a job, or living outside the homes of parents or caregivers.

Important Points to Know about the Transition Experiences

The race of a student with a disability may have implications that affect transition experience and outcome. Research has shown that African Americans and Hispanic students with disabilities are more likely to be unemployed after high school than white students with disabilities. According to the National Longitudinal Transition Study-2, which in 2009 surveyed previous students with disabilities who attended school in the 2000–2001 school year, Hispanic students with disabilities made the lowest hourly wage, while African Americans had the lowest benefit packages (Newman et al. 2011, 15–151). At the time, 63 percent of white students with disabilities were living independently after graduating high school, compared to 52 percent of Hispanic students with disabilities and 47 percent of African American students with disabilities. White (94 percent) and Hispanic (98 percent) students with disabilities were more likely to be enrolled in postsecondary school than African American (77 percent) students with disabilities.

The transition experience of African American students with disabilities has been affected by a number of factors that often predict success. African American students with disabilities make up the largest proportion of students in special education when considering the general population and are found to participate less and have less parental involvement in transition IEP meetings than white and Hispanic students (Cameto, Lavine, and Wagner 2004, 5–6). Transition program participation was found to be a key predictor of success of students with disabilities in college or work after graduation (Test et al. 2009, 178–80).

Because of their lack of involvement in the transition process, students with disabilities are found to initially have inadequate self-determination skills needed to successfully participate in postsecondary activities (Banks 2014, 37–38). However, after experiencing some form of failure in their postsecondary progress, they are able to understand and effectively use these skills in their education or employment. African Americans are more likely to inform their employer of the need for accommodations than white or Hispanic students with disabilities but are less likely to receive accommodations at work.

Dilemmas, Debates, and Unresolved Questions

One issue with the transitional experiences of students with disabilities is that there is not a set process or system of providing postsecondary accommodation services for students with disabilities. Higher education institutions, employers, independent living homes, and community agencies are not obligated to adhere to strict guidelines in the same manner that K–12 educators do. Also, students go from having services and plans created for them by multiple adult stakeholders to immediately having to be responsible for finding stakeholders, forming lines of collaboration and communication, and attempting to obtain accommodations for

activities they participate in. The transition is sudden for students who may have had special education services provided for them since kindergarten.

Another dilemma is often the unavailability of information during the transition process. While representatives from work, school, or the community are involved in setting up the transition process and plan for students with disabilities, students may not know what specific organizations or institutions offer. For example, some employers or universities may have programs for specific disability categories. Students may be unaware that these programs exist and may spend additional time after graduation moving from job to job or residence to residence until they are able to find a suitable job or home.

Conclusions

The transition experience of students with disabilities varies across races and is affected by the IEP transition process. While the intention of the IEP transition process was to promote postsecondary success in independent living, college, work, or community participation, not all students are prepared for life after high school. The transition experience of students with disabilities is an important factor that influences their livelihoods. Students with disabilities want to be able to make decisions that result in positive outcomes for their lives. This process begins during the transition experience, in which students can begin to acquire skills and techniques that will allow them to provide and advocate for themselves without depending on others. Students with disabilities want to live healthy and productive lives, and the path to this outcome begins with an effective transition experience.

Warren Whitaker

See also: Employment, Barriers to; Every Student Succeeds Act (ESSA); Individuals with Disabilities Education Improvement Act (IDEIA); Self-Determination in Education; Transition from High School

Further Reading

Banks, Joy. 2014. "Barriers and Supports to Postsecondary Transition: Case Studies of African American Students with Disabilities." *Remedial and Special Education* 35, no. 1: 28–39.

Cameto, R., P. Levine, and M. Wagner. 2004. "Transition Planning for Students with Disabilities: A Special Topic Report of Findings from the National Longitudinal Transition Study-2 (NLTS2)." National Center for Special Education Research.

Newman, Lynn, Mary Wagner, Anne-Marie Knokey, Camille Marder, Katherine Nagle, Debra Shaver, and Xin Wei. 2011. "The Post-High School Outcomes of Young Adults with Disabilities up to 8 Years after High School: A Report from the National Longitudinal Transition Study-2 (NLTS2). NCSER 2011-3005." National Center for Special Education Research.

Test, David W., Valerie L. Mazzotti, April L. Mustian, Catherine H. Fowler, Larry Kortering, and Paula Kohler. 2009. "Evidence-Based Secondary Transition Predictors for Improving Postschool Outcomes for Students with Disabilities." *Career Development for Exceptional Individuals* 32, no. 3: 160–181.

U.S. Department of Education. 2007. "IDEA Regulations Secondary Transitions." https://www2.ed.gov/about/offices/list/ocr/transitionguide.html.

U

United Nations Convention on the Rights of Persons with Disabilities

The United Nations Convention on the Rights of Persons with Disabilities identifies the human rights of persons with disabilities and the obligations of states to respect, protect, and fulfill those human rights. For many years, disability organizations and nongovernmental organizations have fought for a formal recognition of the human rights of persons with disabilities in international law. Finally, in the late 1990s, the global disability rights movement took part in the drafting of an international disability rights agreement. On December 5, 2006, the United Nations General Assembly unanimously adopted the Convention on the Rights of Persons with Disabilities (CRPD).

What Is the CRPD?

The CRPD is a convention, which is an international and legally binding agreement among nation-states. The CRPD establishes the human rights of persons with disabilities and the corresponding obligations on "member states" (those nation-states that have chosen to adopt the CRPD) to promote, protect, and fulfill these human rights. The CRPD also sets out the national and international institutions necessary for implementing and monitoring the Convention (United Nations Human Rights Office of the High Commissioner 2014, module 2, 23). The CRPD does not create new rights, but it applies existing human rights to the specific situation of persons with disabilities.

Human Rights Approach to Disability. The CRPD is the first convention that details the concrete steps that member states must take to prohibit discrimination and achieve real equality for persons with disabilities (Lord et al. 2012, part 1, 17). For many years, traditional approaches to disability have been based on treatment and cure, drawing upon the medical model of disability, as well as on charity approaches. The CRPD illustrates a paradigm shift, as it moves away from these disability models. Instead, the CRPD builds upon the social model of disability and introduces a new international disability rights paradigm. The overall aim of this human rights model of disability is to make societies more inclusive. The human rights model therefore provides guidance on interventions that are necessary for persons with disabilities to exercise their human rights and enjoy their true equality (Harpur 2012, 4).

Historical Overview

Persons with disabilities were victims of gross human rights violations during World War II. Still, there was no mentioning of persons with disabilities in the United Nations Charter when the United Nations was established in 1945. That was also the case when the Universal Declaration of Human Rights was adopted by the United Nations General Assembly in 1948.

Human rights are rights that a person has simply because he or she is a human being. On that basis, persons with disabilities have always been protected by general international human rights—because of the fact that they are humans. In essence, the human rights approach to disability considers people with disabilities as holders of rights and not as objects of charity or treatment. It clarifies that individuals are more often disabled by the physical and attitudinal barriers societies erect to exclude and stigmatize them than by their own physical or mental conditions (Kanter 2015, 846). Thus, it is vital to have a specific convention on the rights of persons with disabilities, and the CRPD indicates that governments should be involved in the protection of disability rights (United Nations Human Rights Office of the High Commissioner 2014, module 2, 22–23). By October 2017, 174 countries had ratified the convention. The United States is one of only a few members of the United Nations that have not ratified the CRPD.

Key Concepts

Coverage. The purpose of the CRPD is set out in article 1, which makes it clear that persons with disabilities have the same human rights as all other persons. There is no specific definition of disability or disabled persons in the CRPD to describe the covered group of persons, such as with the Americans with Disabilities Act. However, article 1 of the CRPD broadly explains and describes disability as a complex and evolving concept:

> Persons with disabilities include those who have long-term physical, mental, intellectual or sensory impairments which in interaction with various barriers may hinder their full and effective participation in society on an equal basis with others.

The CRPD sees disability as a result of interactions between persons with impairments and external barriers hindering their participation in society. This illustrates that the CRPD builds upon the social model of disability. Therefore, the notion of disability is not a rigid notion, as it depends on surrounding environments and, in any case, might change from one society to the next (United Nations Human Rights Office of the High Commissioner 2014, module 2, 24).

Equality. The CRPD is fundamentally a nondiscrimination convention, stating that people with disabilities have the same human rights as everybody else and are entitled to treatment on an equal basis with all other persons. However, the convention does not say that everybody should be treated the same. Rather, the CRPD is about treating people in such a way that the outcome for each person is equal. Such a *substantive equality* would sometimes demand different treatment for those people who may or may not be equally situated. The goal of substantive equality requires societies to rethink their structures, norms, and attitudes to achieve greater equality for all (Kanter 2015, 844).

Human Rights Articulated

The CRPD contains 50 articles, and the *Optional Protocol* includes 18 articles. Each article is important and relates closely to the others, as all human rights are indivisible, interdependent, and interrelated (Lord et al. 2012, part 1, 17). The general principles and obligations in the first 9 articles of the CRPD are particularly cross-cutting and have a broad impact on all the other articles. Articles 1–9 deal with issues like dignity and autonomy, equality and nondiscrimination, participation and inclusion, women and children with disabilities, awareness raising and accessibility. Articles 10–30 address the individual rights of the CRPD, such as the following:

Article 10, right to life

Article 11, situations of risk and humanitarian emergencies

Article 12, equal recognition before the law

Article 13, access to justice

Article 14, liberty and security of the person

Article 15, freedom from torture or cruel, inhuman, or degrading treatment or punishment

Article 16, freedom from exploitation, violence, and abuse

Article 17, protecting the integrity of the person

Article 18, liberty of movement and nationality

Article 19, living independently and being included in the community

Article 20, personal mobility

Article 21, freedom of expression and opinion, and access to information

Article 22, respect for privacy

Article 23, respect for home and the family

Article 24, education

Article 25, health

Article 26, habilitation and rehabilitation

Article 27, work and employment

Article 28, adequate standard of living and social protection

Article 29, participation in political and public life

Article 30, participation in cultural life, recreation, leisure, and sport

In most cases, these rights correspond to rights found in other human rights conventions. Their importance in the CRPD is that they explain the individual human right in the specific context of disability.

Member State Obligations

The member states have the responsibility to respect, protect, and fulfill the human rights of the CRPD (Lord et al. 2012, part 1, 9).

Respect. The obligation to *respect* means that states must not violate the human rights of the convention and must also eliminate laws, policies, and practices that are contrary to the CRPD. To mention an example, states must not discriminate against persons with disabilities when it comes to the allocation of public social services.

Protect. The obligation to *protect* means that states must protect persons with disabilities against violations of rights by nonstate actors like individuals, businesses, medical professionals, and private organizations. To mention an example, states must protect persons with disabilities against discrimination in the private labor market and must enact laws prohibiting such discrimination by private employers.

Fulfill. The obligation to *fulfill* means that states must take positive action to ensure that persons with disabilities can exercise their human rights in real life. To mention an example, states must allocate the necessary resources and reasonable accommodation to children with disabilities for them to enjoy their right to inclusive education.

Implementation of the CRPD

Committee on the Rights of Persons with Disabilities. The CRPD features strict requirements of how the implementation of the human rights of persons with disabilities should be monitored at both the international and national level. At the international level, according to CRPD article 34, the *Committee on the Rights of Persons with Disabilities* has been tasked with reviewing the implementation of CRPD. The committee is a body of 18 international and independent experts. It reviews periodic country reports on the member states' implementation of the convention. It also reviews shadow reports from disability rights and disabled people's organizations supplementing or rebutting the official periodic country reports. Given that background information, the committee holds a hearing and finally issues *concluding observations* to the country in question. Concluding observations are conclusions, concerns, and recommendations regarding the rights of persons with disabilities in that particular country.

The committee furthermore issues *general comments* on particular issues. General comments are interpretations by the committee on individual articles of the convention—one example being General Comment No. 3 on women and girls with disabilities and CRPD article 6. Finally, with regard to countries having ratified the Optional Protocol, the committee may hear individual complaints of human rights violations and may undertake inquiries regarding gross human rights violations in specific countries.

Monitoring at the National Level. The CRPD is unique in that it also deals with monitoring and implementation at the national level. According to CRPD article 33, states must set up coordination mechanisms within governments and national focal points. States must also set up independent monitoring mechanisms, which will usually be independent national human rights institutions or ombudsman's offices. Finally, the convention underlines that civil society, in particular persons with disabilities and their representative organizations,

shall be involved and participate fully in the monitoring process.

Dilemmas, Debates, and Unresolved Questions

Does the CRPD Have the Potential for Creating Change? The CRPD establishes a number of general obligations, prompting national legal reform as well as comprehensive actions like educating and raising awareness of disability rights. The convention also requires the establishment of effective national monitoring mechanisms, which must include national *disabled people's organizations* (Lord and Stein 2008, 456). Thus, with the help of human rights norms as primary drivers, the CRPD creates a potential for change, culture building, and social transformation in individual member states (474, 479).

In reality, there are, however, a lot of obstacles to genuine implementation and enforcement of the CRPD. Key obstacles to change and improvements of the human rights situation of persons with disabilities at the national level can briefly be described as follows (Mittler 2016, 41):

- lack of political will and commitment by national governments to develop a time-tabled roadmap for CRPD implementation
- constraints on national disabled people's organizations
- lack of awareness and research
- lack of data for monitoring and evaluation

International Monitoring. At the international level, when it comes to monitoring, there is no international "police authority" enforcing the convention. If governments do not take criticism and recommendations from the international CRPD Committee seriously, there is not much more for civil society and the international community to do than naming and shaming the country in question.

Advocacy and Empowerment. Despite these challenges, it is important to underline that the CRPD provides a powerful advocacy tool for disabled people's organizations and other disability and human rights organizations—either individually or in coalitions. By legal commitment, most states and governments all over the world have promised to respect, protect, and fulfill the human rights of persons with disabilities. The CRPD provides a mechanism to keep these governments accountable and to maintain an empowering focus on disability rights.

CRPD in the United States. The United States has a poor record of ratifying international human rights conventions. Although numerous other countries have ratified the CRPD, the United States has still not done so. President Barack Obama signed the CRPD in 2009 and worked for its ratification. However, in 2012 ratification was denied by U.S. Senate vote. The opposition in the U.S. Senate had to do with a number of issues, including the following:

- opposition to international human rights conventions in general
- concern regarding the CRPD's intrusion into U.S. sovereignty
- concern that the CRPD would undermine the parental right to homeschool children (Kanter 2015, 868).

Conclusion: The Future of CRPD

With the CRPD, member states have accepted the social model of disability and acknowledged that people with disabilities are entitled to human rights like everyone else. The CRPD clarifies how those rights should be realized and requires a voice

for disability rights organizations when it comes to implementation of the convention. Researchers, organizations, and individuals all over the world can use the CRPD to advocate for change. In the United States, the major current challenge is to support the ratification of the CRPD.

Pia Justesen

See also: Americans with Disabilities Act (ADA); Disability Rights Movement (DRM), History and Development of; Globalization; U.S. International Relations; *Primary Documents*: Statement of Senator Robert J. Dole on the Convention on the Rights of Persons with Disabilities before the Senate Foreign Relations Committee (2013)

Further Reading

Harpur, Paul. 2012. "Embracing the New Disability Rights Paradigm: The Importance of the Convention on the Rights of Persons with Disabilities." *Disability & Society* 27 (1): 1–14.

Kanter, Arlene S. 2015. "The Americans with Disabilities Act at 25 Years: Lessons to Learn from the Convention on the Rights of People with Disabilities." *Drake Law Review* 63: 819–883.

Lord, Janet E., Katherine N. Guernsey, Joelle M. Balfe, Valerie L. Karr, Allison S. deFranco, and Nancy Flowers. 2012. *Human Rights. Yes! Action and Advocacy on the Rights of Persons with Disabilities.* Minneapolis: University of Minnesota Human Rights Center.

Lord, Janet, and Michael Ashley Stein. 2008. "The Domestic Incorporation of Human Rights Law and the United Nations Convention on the Rights of Persons with Disabilities." *Washington Law Review* 83: 449–479.

Mittler, Peter. 2016. "The UN Convention on the Rights of Persons with Disabilities: Implementing a Paradigm Shift." In *Disability and Human Rights: Global*

Perspectives, edited by Edurne Iriarte, Roy McConkey, and Robbie Gilligan, 33–48. London: Palgrave.

United Nations Human Rights Office of the High Commissioner. 2014. "The Convention on the Rights of Persons with Disabilities: Training Guide." *Professional Training Series* no. 19.

United Nations. "United Nations Division for Social Policy and Development Policy, Convention on the Rights of Persons with Disabilities Homepage." https://www.un.org/development/desa/disabilities/convention-on-the-rights-of-persons-with-disabilities.html.

Universal Design

"Universal design" (UD) is defined by the Center for Universal Design as "the design of products and environments to be usable by all people, to the greatest extent possible, without the need for adaptation or specialized design." Wide application of UD holds promise for making a more welcoming and accessible world for everyone.

UD has a rich history in making buildings and the surrounding environment more accessible. An example of UD is curb cuts that make sidewalks accessible to individuals using wheelchairs, but also to those pushing baby strollers and delivery carts. Retrofitting inaccessible sidewalks with curb cuts is expensive, but when included in the original sidewalk design process, they add little cost to the construction project. The savings when UD is incorporated in the beginning of a project has also been found to be the case in the application of UD to a wide variety of commercial products, technology, services, and environments. Thus, UD holds promise for making a more welcoming and accessible world for everyone.

Access, Accommodation, and Universal Design

How we think about accommodations is deeply rooted in our culture and institutional practices. An accommodation occurs when an adjustment or modification is made to a product or environment so that it is accessible to an individual with a disability. A focus on accommodations is grounded in a "medical model" or "deficit model" of disability, in which a professional identifies an individual's functional limitations or "deficits" and prescribes a cure, rehabilitation, or adjustments that allow the person to access an established environment or use an existing product. For example, in college, a student with a disability may be required to provide documentation of the disability to a specified office at the institution before requesting accommodations. A staff member within the office determines what accommodations are reasonable and shares this information with appropriate faculty teaching courses in which the student is enrolled. Examples of accommodations in educational settings include materials in alternative formats (such as Braille or accessible electronic documents), extra time on exams, sign language interpreters, and movement of classes to wheelchair-accessible locations. Thus, the institution views the student's "deficit" (the disability) as the access "problem" and offers an accommodation as a "solution" to that person's problem.

An alternative perspective is to see ability on a continuum, where each human being is more or less skilled in seeing, hearing, walking, using the hands, reading, processing information, paying attention, etc. This approach supports the view of disability as a diversity issue, like those defined by gender, race and ethnicity, sexual orientation, etc. Disability is thus considered one aspect of a spectrum of human variations. Some have even argued for terminology that reflects this view—for example, referring to characteristics of people who have neurological conditions such as those on the autism spectrum as "neurodiversity." Focusing on difference rather than deficit aligns with the social model of disability, which considers variations in ability to be a normal part of the human experience and encourages society to remove access barriers caused by the inaccessible design of products and environments. UD is consistent with the social model of disability.

Key Concepts in Universal Design

UD has emerged as a paradigm to address diversity and equity in the design of a broad range of applications, including facilities, software, on-site and online instruction, and services. It has been most widely applied in the "built environment"—that is, physical structures such as curb cuts, ramps into buildings, and other structural features that make spaces accessible to people with a wide range of mobility skills. The proactive practice of UD encourages consideration of the great diversity of characteristics that users possess, such as ability, language, race, ethnicity, culture, gender, sexual orientation, and age. UD challenges individuals and institutions to make their products and environments welcoming to, accessible to, and usable by everyone. For example, a woman could be black, five and one-half feet tall, forty years old, a poor reader, and deaf. All of these characteristics, including her deafness, should be considered when developing a product or environment she, as well as individuals with many other characteristics, might use. Infusing UD into all aspects of human life can be an important step toward destigmatizing disability,

ensuring equity, and making all members of a community feel welcome.

The "universal" in UD represents an ideal with respect to the audience for a specific product or environment. However, no application will be fully usable by every human being; in many cases that is not even desirable. For example, designing an electric drill that can be easily operated by a young child is not desirable. UD does, however, require that designers address access and use issues related to diverse characteristics of members within the broadly defined population for whom the application is intended. These considerations include race; ethnicity; culture; native language; socioeconomic status; gender; age; learning style; dexterity; and ability to hear, see, move, read, and pay attention. With this view, the traditional view of a person "having a disability" or "not having a disability" is too simplistic to be useful; the goal is to simply design a product or environment so that it is usable by a broad audience.

UD is a proactive process rather than a reactive one. Universally designed products and environments have built-in features that anticipate the needs and preferences of a diverse group of users. When products and environments are developed, they should be designed to reduce or eliminate characteristics that make them inaccessible to some individuals or segregate certain groups of people. Different names for similar proactive approaches to design include "barrier-free design," "accessible design," "inclusive design," and "usable design," in addition to UD. Proactive design, however, predates the use of any of these terms. The common thread in all these approaches is that a diverse group of potential users can fully benefit from a product or environment in an inclusive setting.

Application of UD

With UD, the user is not expected to adjust to the limitations of an inflexible product or environment; rather, the application is expected to adjust to the needs and preferences of the vast majority of its potential users. UD seeks to make it possible for everyone to participate in an inclusive setting without being singled out. For example, providing steps into a building makes it inaccessible to some people, while adding a separate ramp for wheelchair users is a step toward accessibility. However, providing a wide sloping ramp for all individuals to use promotes inclusion. In this last example, a person using a wheelchair and someone who does not can enter the building together. Similarly, suppose the director of admissions for a kindergarten program anticipates that a parent who is blind may at some time need to register a child. The director can then instruct their technical staff to employ Web site design features to ensure that the online registration system is designed to be accessible to a parent who is blind and using screen reader technology to access the text on the screen.

A typical service counter in a place of business is not accessible to everyone, including those of short stature, those who use wheelchairs, and those who cannot stand for extended periods of time. Applying UD principles results in multiple heights for a service counter—the standard height designed for individuals within the average range of height and who use the counter while standing up and a shorter height for those who are shorter than average, use a wheelchair for mobility, or prefer to interact with service staff from a seated position.

An example of a product that includes UD features is the modern mobile telephone, which includes speech output, allows users to adjust the size of characters on the screen, and can interface with assistive technology such as Braille embossers used by individuals who are blind. Another example of UD in the design of technology can be found in Web site design. A universally designed Web site will include alternative text (alt text) for images that can be read by screen readers for people who are blind. Documents included on the Web site can also be formatted in such a way that screen readers and voice synthesizers used by individuals who are blind, and by those who have learning disabilities that make it difficult for them to read text, can read aloud the text presented on the screen. When instructors apply UD to an on-site or online course, they consider the great diversity of potential students (such as anyone who meets the entrance requirements of the course) and ensure that learning activities are relevant to students from different cultures, whose primary language is not the one in which the course is taught, who have different reading abilities, or who have different levels of sensory abilities.

A key feature of UD is that making a product or an environment accessible to people with disabilities often benefits others. Automatic door openers benefit individuals using walkers and wheelchairs but also benefit people carrying groceries and holding babies, as well as elderly citizens. When television displays in airports and restaurants are captioned, programming is accessible not only to people who are deaf but also to others who cannot hear the audio in noisy areas. The captions also benefit people in a quiet environment, such as near someone who is sleeping, as well as those who wish to know the spelling of terms spoken in the video presentation. Thus, UD does not replace other design considerations but, in concert with those considerations, makes a design, a course, a building, a recreational facility, and technology better.

Summary and Conclusion
Designing any product or environment involves the consideration of many factors, including issues related to aesthetics, engineering, environmental impact, safety, and cost. Rather than focus on the average user, UD encourages designers to consider a broad range of user characteristics, including disability. Rather than an individual adjusting to an inaccessible world, UD requires that facilities, commercial products, technology, instruction, services, and resources be designed to be welcoming to and usable by a diverse audience that includes people with disabilities. UD is an attitude, goal, and process that values diversity, equity, and inclusion; promotes best practices and high standards; is proactive; can be implemented incrementally; benefits everyone; and minimizes the need for accommodations.

Sheryl Burgstahler

See also: Classroom Accommodations; Community Living and Community Integration; Social Model of Disability

Further Reading
Burgstahler, Sheryl. 2015. *Universal Design in Higher Education: From Principles to Practice.* Boston: Harvard Education Press.

Center for Applied Special Technology (CAST). 2017. www.cast.org.

Center for Universal Design. 2008. https://www.ncsu.edu/ncsu/design/cud/.

Center for Universal Design in Education. 2017. www.uw.edu/doit/programs/center-universal-design-education/overview.

Rose, David, and Anne Meyer. 2012. *Teaching Every Student in the Digital Age:* *Universal Design for Learning.* Alexandria, VA: Association for Supervision and Curriculum Development.

Urban Education

Disability in urban education exists among the complexities of race, culture, language, socioeconomic status, and disability within the educational context. While many in the field of education segregate disability within *special education*, disability remains pervasively integrated into the current understanding and experience of schooling in the urban context.

What Is Disability and Urban Education?
Neighborhoods are segregated across racial and socioeconomic boundaries. Thus, the individuals who attend urban schools are typically of lower socioeconomic status and belong to a minority race or culture (Blanchett, Klinger, and Harry 2016). This school segregation creates inequality in educational delivery. Education and educational outcomes are often very different in urban schools than in suburban or rural schools (Blanchett, Klinger, and Harry 2016). Disability in urban education exists among the intersections of race, culture, disability, and socioeconomic status in our current educational system.

While attention is being placed on the role of race and ethnicity in our current educational system, the narrative of disability is often silenced or, at best, isolated. To obtain a holistic understanding of schooling in an urban context, one must understand how race, disability, socioeconomic status, and culture interact. Students with disabilities in urban contexts are living and learning at the intersections of these identities. The interplays between disability, race, economic status, and culture have explicit and implicit effects on an individual's everyday educational experiences.

Background and History

To understand the complexities of disability and urban education, it is important to identify some of the key historic events in the United States that have affected how students are educated in urban contexts. These events expose the entanglement of race and disability in U.S. history.

Race and Disability. Slavery was often justified under the guise of "blackness" being a "defect" of the human condition (Annamma et al. 2016). "Blackness" existed synonymously with disability. These ideas were also seen in the pseudo-sciences of phrenology and physiognomy, which attempted to correlate facial structure, brain size, and other physical features with personality traits and mental abilities (Annamma et al. 2016). While these ideas lost popularity in the late twentieth century, some argue that remnants of their impact are still present. The assumption that all students of color are "at risk" for school failure on the basis of their skin tone is a way in which modern-day society still equates physicality with ability (Annamma et al. 2016). Additionally, educational researchers have suggested that the utilization of "evidence based" testing, which many contest is culturally biased, has led to unfair identification and placement of certain minority groups into special education (Annamma et al. 2016).

Separate and Unequal. The interplay between disability, race, culture, and schooling is also evident throughout federal judiciary hearings. The historic 1954 *Brown v. Board of Education* Supreme Court decision stated that the segregation of children in specific schools on the basis of the color of their skin was unconstitutional. This court decision dismantled the dominant ideology that separate was equal. While this court decision had obvious implications for the structures of public schooling at the time, disability advocates used the ruling to dismantle similar segregation of students with disabilities into separate schools and classrooms. Years later, the 1970 *Diana v. State of California* case ruled that students had the right to be tested for special education placement in their native language to prevent the overrepresentation of language minorities in special education. Similarly, in the 1972 case *Larry P. v. Riles*, the Supreme Court ruled that the use of cognitive tests caused discrimination against African Americans, resulting in their overrepresentation in special education. As a result, the American Association of Mental Deficiency (AAMD) lowered the required IQ standard score for a classification of intellectual disability from 85 to 70 (Annamma 2016; Blanchett, Klinger, and Harry 2016). The Supreme Court continues to make determinations in cases that are representative of the complexities of the intersections of race, culture, disability, and schooling in the United States.

Education Policy

Several key laws and policies also guide the education of students with disabilities in the United States. The first federal law related to mandatory education for all students with disabilities was entitled the Education for All Handicapped Children (1975). The bill was renamed the Individuals with Disabilities Education Act (IDEA) in 1990. One of the tenets of this law protects children from testing and identification bias by ensuring that discrimination does not occur during testing procedures. Additionally, parent participation in the assessment and placement process was included to protect the rights of students with disabilities and their parents. Mandates regarding discipline of students with disabilities were added to protect students with disabilities from being removed from their current setting for extended periods of time without certain processes and protections. These features of the law have particularly important implications for students with disabilities living in the urban setting.

Important Points to Understand about Urban Education and Disability

Contextual Factors. Students with disabilities in urban settings are shaped by the contexts in which they live. Their lives outside of the school building can significantly affect their performance in the classroom. Research has suggested that living in chronic lifelong poverty can have detrimental effects on the brain development and cognition of children (Blanchett, Klinger, and Harry 2009). Additionally, women who live in poverty are less likely to have access to adequate prenatal care and nutrition. Greater risks of exposure to alcohol, drugs, or tobacco during pregnancy can also negatively affect cognitive development. Children born into poverty are more likely to be born at a lower birth weight and face a greater risk of exposure to lead (Blanchett, Klinger, and Harry 2009). All of these contextual factors can prevent children from developing typically and affect their ability to perform in the academic settings.

Cultural Factors. Along with contextual factors, children also possess cultural identity. Different cultures hold varying belief systems regarding disability. Urban schools are typically composed of families from diverse cultural backgrounds, and these families may hold ideas about disability that

are not dominant in white mainstream culture. The Individuals with Disabilities Education Act is derived from American principles of individualism, equity, and choice. Cultures that hold opposing values may not benefit from IDEA in ways that predominantly white middle- and upper-class citizens do (Blanchett, Klinger, and Harry 2009). If service providers, teachers, and other school personnel fail to acknowledge and understand these different perspectives, services can be delivered in culturally inappropriate and, thus, ineffective ways.

Structural Factors. Coupled with the context and identity of the child, the current structure of American schooling affects students with disabilities in urban schools. Teachers and schools are facing increasing accountability for the academic performance of their students. At the end of the 20th century, federal legislation began holding school districts accountable for the academic growth of their students with disabilities. At the same time, the systemic failure of schools in urban areas made them susceptible to state intervention if adequate yearly progress was not made. In turn, states increasingly began to determine teacher pay and retention by students' scores on standardized state tests. For many, this increased accountability was a sign of progress for students with disabilities. For the first time in this nation's history, the learning of students with disabilities mattered. Others argue, however, that this accountability has had negative ramifications for students with disabilities in urban settings. For teachers to remain employed and schools to stay open, they must have students who perform well on standardized tests. Students with disabilities are historically and traditionally low performers on state assessments. Therefore, a disincentive was created for inclusion of students with disabilities in schools and general education classrooms (Annamma et al. 2016).

Dilemmas, Debates, and Unresolved Questions

Achievement Gap. In our current educational system, there are a number of concerning trends involving students with disabilities in urban schools. One notable issue is the *achievement gap*. The achievement gap is the trend in education in which certain groups of students academically outperform other groups of students. Generally, white students living in rural or suburban areas outperform their minority peers living in urban areas. Researchers have found that teachers in urban schools are less likely to employ best academic practices or have advanced degrees than teachers in other settings. This disparity in educational outcomes and educational practices also extends to student with disabilities from minority cultures. Hence, some suggest that individuals with disabilities from minority cultures and races experience a different quality of education than their disabled white peers (Blanchett, Klinger, and Harry 2009).

Postschool Outcomes. Students with disabilities in urban contexts also face less favorable postschool outcomes. While more students with learning disabilities are entering into college than ever before, the vast majority of these students are from affluent households with incomes of $100,000 or greater (Annamma et al. 2016). Students with disabilities in urban contexts have lower rates of graduation and higher percentages of unemployment (Blanchett, Klinger, and Harry 2009). Some critics argue that these statistics point to a system that is not preparing all students for success after completion of traditional schooling.

School-to-Prison Pipeline. Another current issue in education is the *school-to-prison pipeline*. The school-to-prison pipeline refers to a current trend in educational data that suggests that students who experience discipline and academic failure in school are being funneled into the juvenile justice system (Mallett 2014). The data suggests that students of color are disciplined more harshly in the school environment (Annamma et al. 2016). African Americans who have an "emotional disturbance" classification are more likely to be removed from school through suspensions, expulsions, and arrests than their white peers with similar labels (Annamma et al. 2016). Thus, students who are black and disabled are disproportionately represented in the number of students who are part of this pattern (Mallett 2014).

Overrepresentation of Minorities. Finally, minority youth are overrepresented in special education categories (Blanchett, Klinger, and Harry 2009). Black students are overrepresented in nine of thirteen disability classifications (Ferri and Conner 2005). This overrepresentation is more clearly observed in subjective disability categories, such as specific learning disabilities (SLD) or emotional disturbance (ED), rather than sensory disabilities, like blindness or physical impairment. Subjective disability categories are determined by team consensus, in contrast with an observable biological problem or medical diagnosis (Annamma et al. 2016). The introduction of *response to intervention* (RTI) as the new determination of an educational diagnosis of SLD was, in part, a response to the overidentification of minority students (Artiles, Bal, and King Thorius 2010). However, critics of RTI still argue that the system fails to consider the unique cultural, linguistic, and social structures that individuals living in urban areas may face (Artiles, Bal, and King Thorius 2010). Once entered into special education, students of color with disabilities are more likely to be placed in segregated special education settings. Their disabled white peers, however, are more likely to spend time in the general education classroom (Annamma et al. 2016; Blanchett, Klinger, and Harry 2009).

The Future Directions in Urban Education

Both the past and the present of disability in urban education suggest that fundamental differences in education exist for students with disabilities who do not belong to white majority culture. While much research has been produced over the past few decades identifying the deficits and gaps in education, the problem still persists. As reforms are made toward creating a more egalitarian educational system in the United States, it will be necessary to critically examine the role of disability in our current educational system. It is necessary for policymakers, advocates, researchers, and educators to identify ways in which to address the dilemmas that affect students with disabilities in urban settings. Effective and efficient education reform for urban schools will occur when a holistic approach to understanding students with disabilities is adopted.

Julie Vryhof

See also: Classroom Accommodations; Individuals with Disabilities Education Improvement Act (IDEIA); (In)Exclusion; Intersectionality of Race, Gender, and Disability; Learning Disabilities; Schoolwide Systems of Supports

Further Reading

Annamma, Subini Ancy, David Conner, and Beth Ferri. 2016. *DisCrit: Disability Studies and Critical Race Theory in Education.* New York: Teacher College, Columbia University.

Artiles, Alfredo J., Aydin Bal, and Kathleen A. King Thorius. 2010. "Back to the Future: A Critique of Response to Intervention's Social Justice Views." *Theory into Practice* 49, no. 4: 250–257.

Blanchett, Wanda J., Janette K. Klinger, and Beth Harry. 2009. "The Intersection of Race, Culture, Language, and Disability: Implications for Urban Education." *Urban Education* 44, no. 4: 389–409.

Ferri, Beth A., and David J. Connor. 2005. "Tools of Exclusion: Race, Disability, and (Re)segregated Education." *Teachers College Record* 107, no. 3: 453–474.

Mallett, Christopher A. 2014. "The 'Learning Disabilities to Juvenile Detention' Pipeline: A Case Study." *Children & Schools* 36, no. 3: 147–154.

U.S. International Relations

Disability has always been a part of U.S. international relations, but it is often ignored by analysts and policy makers. Increasingly, policy makers have acknowledged disability's part in international relations and its changing significance. At various times and in different circumstances, disability in international relations has been framed as tragedy, charity, social progress, rights, liberation, oppression, or a combination of these themes.

The Role of Disability in U.S. International Relations

Analysts of U.S. foreign policy disagree over how much importance attaches to group (such as disabled people), national (such as the United States), and universal human interests. At each of these levels of interest, disability is an increasingly important part of programs, yet analysts and policy makers question the nature and value of a disability focus.

Victims and Agents of Change. Disabled people are often victims of international relations, with death and economic hardship being frequent results of both direct violence (such as war) and structural violence (such as barriers to medical care). Primarily in the early 20th century, but often today as well, charitable organizations emphasized the hardships of disability. Increasingly, disabled people's participation has played a role in change, especially with the evolution of the disability rights movement. The disability rights movement challenged analysts and policy makers who assumed that tragedy of disability was inevitable damage from war and development. Some organizations and policy makers now recognize important international disability-related dimensions of education, recreation, and transfer of technology. Analysts may once have perceived killings of Tanzania's albino population, discrimination against Chinese people with AIDS, or the U.S. prison and police abuse of disabled people as purely internal matters rather than as global issues.

State and Nonstate Policy Makers. The disability dimensions of international relations are evident in governmental policy, but especially in transnational activity. A 20th- and 21st-century global movement of nonstate actors has called attention to disability issues: from the International Society for Crippled Children (later Rehabilitation International) to Amnesty International and Human Rights Watch to Disabled Peoples' International. Their work through the United Nations started a shift from a passive, deficit view of disability to one reflecting such new concepts as *universal design*. In addition, local and subnational disabled people's organizations (DPOs) acquired global significance with attention from disability activists, the World Bank, and other international institutions.

The U.S. State Department prepares country reports on human rights conditions that now include a section on disability rights (U.S. International Council on Disabilities 2017). During the Obama administration, the State Department created a "special advisor for international disability rights" within the Bureau of Democracy, Human Rights, and Labor (DRL). It is unclear whether and to what extent this position will continue under the current administration. However, several United Nations bodies, including the World Health Organization, the World Bank, and the Office of the United Nations High Commissioner for Human Rights, have instituted major disability-related programs.

Background and History

Perspectives on international relations led to analysts and policy makers ignoring or emphasizing disability within many overlapping issues, including war and peace, rehabilitation and development, and human rights. The emphasis sometimes detrimentally affected, and at other times benefitted, disabled people.

War and Peace. Policy has unevenly addressed tensions following war, rehabilitation, education, and travel. Toward the end of the 20th century, disability-related war and peace concerns became global, as evidenced by the Landmine Survivors Network and the Convention on the Prohibition of the Use, Stockpiling, Production and Transfer of Anti-Personnel Mines and on Their Destruction (Mine Ban Treaty) (Rutherford 2011). Analysts and policy makers' increasing reference to human security and peace building adds a dimension of civilian disability, which activists articulated.

Rehabilitation and Development. Humanitarian or charity approaches to disability inspired such events as the 1922 founding of the International Society for Crippled Children, now known as Rehabilitation International (Groce 1992). The United Nations Sustainable Development Goals for 2015–2030 incorporates disability in five items, including education and employment. Development strategies such as tourism and export promotion may have both positive and negative effects on disabled people.

Rights. Many analysts, policy makers, activists, and media now conceptualize disability issues in terms of rights. The independent living movement (ILM) has grown from a grassroots movement in Berkeley, California, to hundreds of centers for independent living, many of them outside the United States. In 1983, ILM pioneers Ed Roberts, Judy Heumann, and Joan Leon cofounded the World Institute on Disability. Many leaders who shaped the Americans with Disabilities Act (1990) were influenced by international experiences and principles (in Pelka 2012). Examples include Justin Dart Jr.'s work on Japan and Vietnam and John Lancaster's post-Vietnam War activism with Paralyzed Veterans of America.

Key Concepts in International Relations and Disability

Very important parts of the international relations-disability nexus include the importance of nongovernmental actors and intersections with other social groups. Both factors have varied over time but are likely to be especially important in the 21st century.

NGOs, DPOs, PVOs, and International Relations. International relations are changing, and the rise of global disability politics is part of that change. Disabled Peoples'

International (as a collective of national disabled people's organizations, or DPOs) and Amnesty International (as a leading human rights nongovernmental organization, or NGO, with disability rights activities) aspire to transform a hierarchical global order. Their structures are based on national chapters or affiliates, which results in there being much stronger organizations in some regions than others. Many other countries have private voluntary organizations (PVOs) that carry out disability-related programs funded by the U.S. Agency for International Development. These programs will change some aspects of international relations while reinforcing others.

Intersections. Some analysts and policy makers have come to appreciate disability's intersection with gender, race and ethnicity, sexuality, class, age, urbanization, and other factors as key in international relations. Coalitions between disabled people and other groups can bridge or exacerbate tensions. For example, in postconflict peace building and in international development, participation or exclusion of disabled women often determines effectiveness.

Dilemmas, Debates, and Unresolved Questions

In the United States and elsewhere, organizations and policy makers sometimes associate their activities with specific diagnoses, such as learning disability, intellectual disability, AIDS, hearing or vision loss, spinal cord injury, or post-traumatic stress disorder. At other times, they may adopt a *cross-disability* approach, emphasizing the prominence of multiple disabilities and common issues of discrimination. Organizations frequently form cross-disability coalitions to devote themselves to named purposes (such as disabled people's participation in development strategies or disability rights promotion at the United Nations) while continuing to pursue specific interests.

Additionally, "independent living" as a social movement began in the United States, and disability rights activists worldwide have praised disability rights policy such as the Americans with Disabilities Act. On the other hand, the United States has not ratified the United Nations Convention on the Rights of Persons with Disabilities (CRPD), the Mine Ban Treaty (Rutherford 2011), or the Inter-American Convention on the Elimination of all Forms of Discrimination against Persons with Disabilities.

The aforementioned State Department country reports on human rights reflect U.S. leadership in the field but also reflect its great unevenness in disability rights promotion. Additionally, war, tourism, and economic globalization generally will have varying effects on the world's disabled people. International policy can contribute to widespread discrimination and suffering; it also can foster change, participation, and well-being. All of these tendencies will be present in the global future, but some factors will become increasingly important and others less so.

Future Directions and Conclusion

Disability will be a factor in future international relations, but it is uncertain what that role will be. The significance of disability can be greatest in approaches envisioning a changed global system with increasing importance for some transnational actors, particularly NGOs and DPOs. Some disabled people will benefit from international relations and policy, while others will continue to be excluded. States, institutions, movements, and competing values will continue to involve power, social justice, participation, and wealth. Disability in international relations will be subject to both global backlash and global progress. Because of major changes in global society, disabled people will be active shapers, not just passive observers, of that future.

Art Blaser

See also: Americans with Disabilities Act (ADA); Globalization; Neoliberalism; Poverty; United Nations Convention on the Rights of Persons with Disabilities

Further Reading

Groce, Nora. 1992. *The U.S. Role in International Disability Activities: A History and a Look towards the Future.* New York: Rehabilitation International.

National Council on Disability. 2003. "Foreign Policy and Disability: Legislative Strategies and Civil Rights Protections to Ensure Inclusion of People with Disabilities." https://ncd.gov/rawmedia_repository /38402a3d_fead_4182_84cb_7558dd07e190 .pdf.

Pelka, Fred. 2012. *What We Have Done: An Oral History of the Disability Rights Movement.* Amherst: University of Massachusetts Press.

Rutherford, Ken. 2011. *Disarming States: The International Movement to Ban Landmines.* Santa Barbara, CA: Praeger.

U.S. International Council on Disabilities. 2017. "Consolidated Disability Findings from the 2016 United States Department of State Reports on Human Rights and Practices." http://usicd.org/doc/Complete%20 2016%20Human%20Rights%20Reports %20Disability%20Citations%20.pdf.

V

Veterans

The problem of disability for veterans can be linked to a wide range of social issues and interrelated problems that are not always addressed by disability policy studies. Veteran unemployment, which is nearly twice the national average, and homelessness, which is nearly one-third of homeless persons in the United States, exemplify how problems that coincide with disability often elude the focus of disability studies. The Veterans Affairs Administration (VA) is the primary federal-level agency responsible for administering comprehensive care to eligible military veterans. Yet, the VA has become infamous for its bureaucracy, which often makes it difficult for military servicemembers to obtain care and file medical disability claims. This development is especially troubling, considering that approximately one out of every three veterans returning from the wars in Iraq and Afghanistan have posttraumatic stress disorder (PTSD) and that veteran suicides remain at an all-time high.

Background

Recent studies have made veteran policy issues a central line of focus, where they call attention to different problems, including those that involve institutions like the VA (Wool 2015). Scholars, it should be noted, have pointed out a troubling development that focuses on disabled veterans themselves, who are designated to be the problem, rather than on the policies themselves (Gerber 2012). Complicating matters

is the fact that there is no single literature or subdisciplinary area of research dedicated to the study of disability and veterans. This development reflects a general trend across the social and medical sciences, where military studies and problems that affect military-affiliated social groups are not characteristically core areas of focus.

Important Points to Understand about Veterans with Disabilities

Twenty-first-century wars, in spite of their increased use of smart weapons and surgical strikes, have only increased the physical demands placed on soldiers and their bodies. Veteran support services have been taxed beyond the limits of their intended effectiveness, though studies of these developments remain limited and tend to be restricted to a small group of research specialists focused on institutional problem solving.

Interdisciplinarity and Diverse Perspectives. The interdisciplinary nature of the topic in this instance means that scholars and experts, writing from diverse perspectives that include history, science, and cultural studies, have pursued more critical approaches to understanding veterans and disability. This work, although not policy centered, offers important contributions to understanding problems associated with disability. David Serlin (2002; 2004) and Heather Perry (2002) trace the history of the development of prosthetics in their work, which documents the history of war, wounding, and disability and its impact on veterans. Noteworthy here is how both

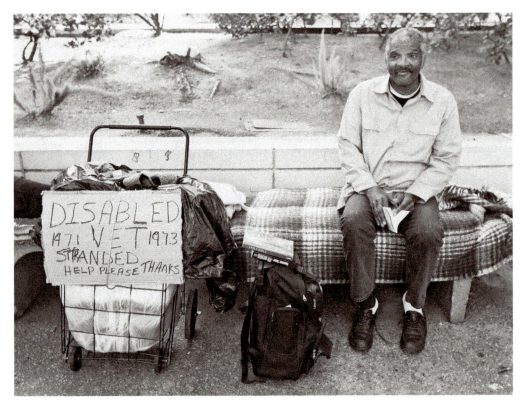

A disabled and homeless Vietnam veteran in downtown Los Angeles, California. Veterans face a number of social challenges that are often overlooked in disability policy. (Ted Soqui/Corbis via Getty Images)

authors highlight the role played by gender, social class, and other social identity dynamics insofar as it helped shape the postwar lives of veteran amputees.

Sandra Trappen (2013a; 2013b) challenges the *medical model* of disability when she looks at how combat casualties are bound within a political economy that operates intrinsic to war and medical progress. Trappen's analysis highlights that combat injuries and the radical undoing of bodies in connection with war are not mere "accidents." Rather, as it is argued, they have become infrastructural to medical social organization and progress. She invites readers to rediscover the critical tradition, where social theory might be called upon to explain the transformation of bodies, which

is becoming accelerated because of developments wrought by war and global capitalism. Trappen's critique asks us to engage with what some might consider a radical idea: to think about the different ways wounded soldiers serve as medical test subjects. John Kinder (2015) is similarly critical of the medical model of disability. His work looks at what he calls "the veteran problem" within a historical context, where it addresses the social construction of veteran identity since the time of the U.S. Civil War. The collective work of this group of authors bridges disciplinary boundaries to contribute a historical critical vocabulary to the study of veterans and disability, as they situate disability within a dynamic historical sociocultural context.

Dilemmas, Debates, and Unresolved Questions

Although it seems somewhat contradictory, taking into consideration the overwhelming public passion for "supporting the troops," disabled veterans are known to struggle upon their return home when they attempt to access medical care and rehabilitation. This development, as Trappen and Kinder point out, is not exceptional, but it is part of a historic pattern where wounded veterans are shown to embody problematic social identities upon their return from war.

Contradictions in Depiction. Variously violent, addicted, homeless, and maladjusted, such depictions are at odds with the more seemly renderings of soldiers "overcoming" their physical limitations imposed as a result of injury. As scholars note, the social contradictions produced as a result of U.S. foreign policy have in this sense become fully embodied. "Wounded warrior" social identities, as they have come to be known, are potentially problematic. Such depictions are often employed to manipulate the sentiments of people through the use of patriotic symbols, imagery, and discourses. In this case, Trappen argues that the privileging of American exceptionalism through rehabilitation narratives celebrates military service without calling into question the military interventionist foreign policies that produce wounded soldiers. One way (perhaps the best way) to address the problems associated with combat injury and disabled veterans, she argues, is to simply stop making them (Trappen 2013b).

Contradictions in Advocates and Allies. Disabled veterans are supported by a large network of disability rights advocates, who work to advance health care, support services, research and education, and veterans' benefits and rights. The most well known among them, the private nonprofit "Wounded Warrior Project" (WWP), has come under criticism, as its activism and expense allocation stirred debate about the proper role of government supporting veterans upon return from war. The WWP controversy centers on the fact that the organization, arguably one of the more high-profile veterans' advocacy groups, is privately funded by donations. This stands in contrast with traditional sources of support for wounded veterans, which historically have been the responsibility of the Veterans Administration, an organization that is publicly funded through tax dollars. This brings up a question asked by Kinder (2015): "What are the nation's obligations to those who fight in its name?" More to the point, why is the government subcontracting and privatizing veteran support services while simultaneously underfunding institutional obligations and support mandates for the VA?

Gender Inequality. Issues of gender inequality in connection with injury and disability have also surfaced as a problem. Research indicates that women veterans are disadvantaged compared to their male counterparts, in terms of the rate and types of injury suffered. For example, gender-based differences in PTSD services were documented by one study, which conducted a longitudinal study of disability recipients over a 10-year time period. The study found that women veterans, when compared with male veterans, were less likely to gain and more likely to lose their service connection for PTSD disability claims over the 10-year period (Sayer et al. 2014). Military sexual trauma (MST) emerged as a serious problem as a result of the wars in Iraq and Afghanistan. In what is termed "in-service" sexual trauma, a new front was opened in the battle for disability benefits, which has proved daunting for many women veterans.

MST can trigger long-term mental health conditions like PTSD as well as other major depressive and anxiety disorders, all of which potentially make the transition back to civilian life for veterans more challenging. The VA provides screening for MST diagnosis; however, efforts to obtain follow-up care and claims filing for disability benefits face obstacles. Bureaucratic inefficiencies, claim delays, and inaccurate adjudications have in many instances prevented access to care, thereby adding to the trauma already experienced by injured soldiers. Studies have, furthermore, shown how veterans who report sexual trauma and seek compensation are more likely than others to face discrimination, loss of security clearances, and career repercussions.

Lawsuits brought by the Service Women's Action Network, American Civil Liberties Union (ACLU) Women's Rights Project, and the ACLU of Connecticut, with support from the Veterans Legal Services Clinic at Yale Law School, who served as lead counsel, argued successfully that women claimants were not being addressed by the Veterans Administration. In what is perhaps the most significant development resulting from the lawsuits, the VA was forced to turn over never-before-released data on mental health disability benefit claims filed by veterans who claimed they suffered from rape, sexual assault, and sexual harassment in connection with their military service. The data further revealed other disparities in terms of treatment outcomes and access. The VA granted disability claims for post-traumatic stress disorder (PTSD) caused by in-service sexual trauma at significantly lower rates than it has granted claims for PTSD arising from other causes. Moreover, the data confirmed there was significant variation among VA regional offices in the treatment of MST-related mental health claims; here again, unequal treatment based on gender was discovered and documented by the ACLU/Yale study (ACLU 2017).

Conclusion

The United States is presently without rival in terms of the ability to finance and wage war. Sadly, as research demonstrates, the men and women who serve and fight the wars are too often treated as disposable assets; their minds and bodies are regarded as mere collateral damage. Aside from supporting veterans and thanking them for their service, there is not much evidence to suggest that public support translates into effective policy for disabled veterans. In light of this, researchers and policy advocates must continue their efforts to advocate for veterans' policy issues and lobby for institutional change.

Sandra Trappen

See also: Individualism and Independence; U.S. International Relations; Vocational Rehabilitation

Further Reading

American Civil Liberties Union. 2013. "ACLU Report." https://www.aclu.org/sites/default/files/assets/lib13-mst-report-11062013.pdf.

Gerber, David A., ed. 2012. *Disabled Veterans in History.* Ann Arbor: University of Michigan Press.

Kinder, John M. 2015. *Paying with Their Bodies: American War and the Problem of Disability.* Chicago and London: University of Chicago Press.

Perry, Heather R. 2002. "Re-Arming the Disabled Veteran: Artificially Rebuilding State and Society in World War One Germany." In *Artificial Parts, Practical Lives: Modern History of Prosthetics,* edited by Katherine Ott, David Sterlin, and Stephen Mihm, 75–101. New York and London: New York University Press.

Sayer, Nina A., Emily M. Hagel, Siamak Noorbaloochi, Michele R. Spoont, Robert A. Rosenheck, Joan M. Griffin, Paul A. Arbisi, and Maureen Murdoch. 2014. "Gender Differences in VA Disability Status for PTSD Over Time." *Psychiatric Services* 65, no. 5: 663–669.

Serlin, David. 2002. "Engineering Masculinity: Veterans and Prosthetics after World War Two." In *Artificial Parts, Practical Lives: Modern Histories of Prosthetics*, edited by Katherine Ott, David Sterlin, and Stephen Mihm, 45–74. New York and London: New York University Press.

Serlin, David. 2004. *Replaceable You: Engineering the Body in Postwar America*. Chicago: University of Chicago Press.

Trappen, Sandra. 2013a. "Mayberry R.F.D. Will Not Be Presented Tonight." *Social Text Periscope*. https://socialtextjournal.org/periscope_article/mayberry-r-f-d-will-not-be-presented-tonight/.

Trappen, Sandra. 2013b. "War and Disability." *The Feminist Wire*. http://www.thefeminist wire.com/2013/11/war-and-disability/

Wool, Zoe H. 2015. *After War: The Weight of Life at Walter Reed*. Durham, NC: Duke University Press.

Vocational Evaluation

The vocational evaluation process is an organized and individualized approach for accurately predicting the consumers' vocational functioning potential, developing meaningful vocational objectives, and ultimately finding successful employment for consumers. This process involves an individualized assessment that takes multiple factors into consideration. The ultimate goal of vocational evaluation is to meet the specific needs of each individual .

Background and History

Historically, people with disabilities are underrepresented in the workforce. Census data suggests that the employment rate for people with disabilities is only 18 percent, compared to 69 percent for nondisabled workers (Bureau of Labor Statistics U.S. Department of Labor 2013). Since the development and implementation of the Americans with Disabilities Act (ADA), the alarmingly high employment gap for people with disabilities has not meaningfully changed. There are several possible reasons for the large disparity in employment rates between people with disabilities and those without disabilities. Research suggests a combination of multiple barriers can make it extremely difficult for people with disabilities to find or maintain successful employment. Often, people with disabilities face more than one barrier at a time. Common barriers faced by individuals with disabilities include attitudinal, communication, physical, social, and transportation barriers (Centers for Disease Control and Prevention [CDC] 2016).

VR Process. To address some of these issues, the U.S. federal government developed the Vocational Rehabilitation (VR) program to assist persons with disabilities in becoming gainfully employed. Upon opening a case, the VR "customer" is assigned a counselor at no cost to the customer. These counselors offer a variety of services to ensure that customers can secure employment that is consistent with their unique strengths, resources, priorities, concerns, abilities, interests, and informed choices. These services traditionally include conducting *vocational evaluations*, assisting with applications for higher education, and referring customers for training, assistive technology evaluations, job placement services, and other supportive programs. Every customer who opens a case with VR has a certain amount of case funds allocated to them that can be used to cover training costs, transportation costs, and other costs relating to their successful vocational rehabilitation. In general, a successful vocational outcome is achieved once the VR customer is hired for a 90-day consecutive period for at least 30 hours a week at minimum wage or greater. An outcome like this is recognized as a successful closure (or "status 26"), which is credited to the VR counselor.

What Is Vocational Evaluation?

A comprehensive vocational evaluation is the cornerstone of most successful VR closures. A person's goals are documented in the client's *individualized plan for employment* (IPE). Depending on the goals documented in the IPE, the client could be referred to such services as higher education, vocational training, or self-employment services. It is critical that VR customers receive a *comprehensive* vocational evaluation if they are to develop an effective IPE goal. However, the level of comprehensiveness should be relative to the individual customer. Some customers may not need any level of formal evaluation service beyond collecting relevant information in a portfolio; others may require much more intensive, continuous evaluation services (Sitlington and Clark 2007).

Types of Vocational Evaluations

The initial interview is the first vocational evaluation where the customer has a face-to-face meeting with the VR counselor for the purpose of building rapport and gathering information. The customer provides the counselor with information pertinent to goal planning and the IPE. The counselor and customer discuss the customer's long-term vocational goals and discuss possible vocational evaluations or referrals to other services on the basis of individual needs.

Behavioral Observations. Behavioral observations include descriptions of behaviors observed by the VR counselor during the evaluation process. Behavioral observations are important when making decisions about customers who may be unable to maintain successful employment or when assessing a customer's interpersonal skills. Best practices suggest that the counselor use clinical language and describe accurate and unbiased observations. In cases where the customer is referred to a training program or is receiving *on-the-job evaluation* (OJE) services, a vocational instructor or supervisor can provide feedback to the counselor about the customer's behavior as well. Continuous feedback between counselors, training programs, and employers can yield long-term benefits for all parties involved, as parties will be able to understand each other's needs better.

Psychometric Testing. Psychometric testing is a standardized instrument for evaluation that assesses a variety of vocational interests, cognitive abilities, academic achievement levels, etc. The customer completes a paper questionnaire or test, which is then evaluated by a VR counselor. Best practices for psychometric testing include that each test is reliable, standardized, and culturally/gender unbiased and that it assesses current levels of knowledge. It is important for vocational training programs to offer industry-specific evaluative metrics and vocational interest assessments to provide to VR customers as well. In practice, vocational instructors and job coaches spend more hands-on time with VR customers than the counselor does. Hence, there should be open lines of communication between the VR agency and the vocational training program to ensure that as much meaningful information is documented and communicated as possible. It is critical that mental health is not overlooked throughout the vocational evaluation process. Many state VR agencies have a developed referral network of psychologists and other mental health service providers who can provide counseling or administer additional psychological tests for VR customers as needed.

Work Sample. Work sample is a diagnostic evaluation that assesses the vocational aptitude, strengths, limitations, and other personal characteristics necessary for success in the workplace. A VR counselor, vocational instructor, or job coach observes the customer completing workplace activities and determines critical information for the individual's vocational prognostics. Vocational instructors and job coaches who observe the customer report the customer's performance and progress to the VR counselor at predetermined times. Examples of work samples include *cluster trait* (multiple tasks), *simulation*, and *single trait* (one task) samples, which assess different skills depending on the client job interest and ability. Best practices for work samples include that the work sample selected must be considered in direct relationship to the client's vocational goals, should be standardized whenever possible, and must be valid, meaning that the work sample should be directly related to a specific job.

Assistive Technology. An assistive technology device is defined by the Individuals with Disabilities Education ACT (IDEA) as "any item, piece of equipment, or product system, whether acquired commercially off the shelf, modified, or customized, that is used to increase, maintain, or improve functional capabilities of a person with a disability" (Authority 20 U.S.C. 1401(1)). For individuals with certain physical or sensory disabilities, technology may be required to make a work environment accessible. Examples include screen magnifiers for people with visual impairments; computer joysticks or head mice for people who experience frequent body spasms or have difficulty with fine motor control; and communication devices for people who have difficulty speaking or articulating. In many cases, these technologies are highly advanced, and they could be expensive or require an expert to install and provide instruction or training. Because of this combination of factors, nearly all assistive technology devices, setup costs, and other associated expenses are covered in full by VR. For a customer to receive the appropriate assistive technology, the VR counselor makes a referral for an assistive technology assessment. These assessments are typically conducted by an outside agency or specialist.

Job Analysis. Job analysis is the understanding of what a worker does when performing a specific job, as obtained by breaking the job down into specific tasks. It is slightly different from the other vocational evaluations listed above, as it is primarily conducted by a vocational instructor or a job coach rather than a VR counselor. The vocational instructor should have the knowledge and ability to analyze different jobs to determine the physical requirements and vocational preparation required for an individual to perform each job. Job analysis is essential to providing accurate recommendations to clients and completing successful vocational evaluations.

Barriers to Standardized Practice

It is important to note that the manner in which vocational assessments and evaluations are conducted varies. First, there is a degree of subjectivity inherent to the process of selecting which assessment and evaluation instruments to administer and how to interpret the results. To account for this, many vocational assessments and evaluations are conducted by a multidisciplinary team (Perry, n.d.). Differences in vocational assessment and evaluation practices may also vary based on location. In the United States, VR is a federal program, but each state has its own VR agency with its own respective policies and procedures. As a result, each agency faces unique financial and resource constraints, political climates, social climates, and other considerations. Globally, changes in the economic landscape, advances in technology, and evolving employer needs make identifying appropriate vocational goals a moving target.

Goals in Vocational Rehabilitation

As mentioned earlier, working 30 hours a week at minimum wage or greater generally constitutes a successful closure. However, for many individuals—especially those with severe physical disabilities—such a workload could be too physically taxing to be a realistic IPE goal. In these cases, a comprehensive evaluation can be used to not only identify a work environment that minimizes barriers and aligns with their interests and abilities but also ensure that the VR counselor can receive proper recognition for services provided. Given the large caseloads that many counselors manage, it is critical that there is a meaningful relationship between effort and reward, to ensure that all VR customers receive the same level of service, regardless of their disability.

Future Directions

Many people with disabilities pursue self-employment at some point during their lives. In fact, people with disabilities are nearly twice as likely to be self-employed as the general population (Bureau of Labor Statistics 2013; Parker Harris, Caldwell,

and Renko 2014). The Office of Disability Employment Policy (ODEP) points out that people with disabilities often consider self-employment because they get to be independent, set their own pace and schedule, reduce transportation problems with a home-based business, and receive continued support from Social Security Disability Insurance (SSDI) or Supplemental Security Income (SSI), along with health care, provided that their assets and income are within the program requirements (ODEP 2005). Given these benefits, there are tangible financial and social incentives to pursue self-employment. However, there is a general lack of standardized metrics and procedures used to evaluate self-employment skills in a vocational evaluation setting. Given the individualized nature of self-employment and the wide variety of business structures and possibilities, it is inherently challenging to develop one-size-fits-all evaluation measures and progress measures. As such, it is important that the prospective entrepreneur has a business mentor and a strong support system (Parker Harris, Caldwell, and Renko 2013). These individuals should be involved in the continuous vocational evaluation process and should communicate with the entrepreneur's VR counselor to ensure that appropriate supports and resources are being provided to ensure the continued success of the business enterprise.

Sarah M. Osier and Aaron A. Maass

See also: Employment, Barriers to; Employment First; Vocational Rehabilitation

Further Reading

Bureau of Labor Statistics. U.S. Department of Labor. 2013. "Persons with a Disability: Barriers to Employment, Types of Assistance, and Other Labor-Related Issues—May 2012." http://www.bls.gov/news.release/pdf/dissup.pdf.

Centers for Disease Control and Prevention. 2016. "Common Barriers to Participation Experienced by People with Disabilities." http://www.cdc.gov/ncbddd/disabilityand health/disability-barriers.html.

Parker Harris, Sarah, Kate Caldwell, and Maija Renko. 2013. "Accessing Social Entrepreneurship: Perspectives of People with Disabilities and Key Stakeholders." *Vocational Rehabilitation* 38, no. 1: 35–48.

Parker Harris, Sarah, Kate Caldwell, and Maija Renko. 2014. "Entrepreneurship by Any Other Name: Self-Sufficiency versus Innovation." *Journal of Social Work in Disability & Rehabilitation* 13, no. 4: 1–33.

Perry, D. "The Basics of Vocational Assessment: A Tool for Finding the Right Match between People with Disabilities and Occupations." *International Labour Organization.* http://www.ilo.org/public /english//region/asro/bangkok/ability /download/voc_assessment.pdf.

Sitlington, Patricia L., and Gary M. Clark. 2007. "The Transition Assessment Process and IDEIA 2004." *Assessment for Effective Intervention* 32, no. 3: 133–142.

Vocational Rehabilitation

The purpose of vocational rehabilitation (VR) is to help individuals with a disability (congenital or acquired) find gainful employment. Consumers are assigned a VR counselor. The counselor assists consumers in determining what type of work they want to pursue, if they would like to further their education so that they can find a more advanced or skilled job, or if they would like to start their own business.

Background and History

Vocational rehabilitation can be traced back to post–World War I, with the Soldiers Rehabilitation Act of 1918. Many veterans in the war were coming home from Europe injured with physical or mental disabilities. Congress examined other state-offered programs for injured individuals to return to work. Later, they expanded the Soldiers Rehabilitation Act to include nonveterans who had been injured on the job. However, at that point, not all disabilities were covered by the federal legislation. The Barden-LaFollette Act of 1943 included individuals with mental illness and intellectual disabilities in addition to allowing states to choose to create a separate agency for the blind. In 1954, the National Institute on Disability and Rehabilitation Research (NIDRR) was created. The 1970s were considered the "golden age of rehabilitation." The Vocational Rehabilitation Act of 1973 established the VR program in all states, introducing counselors to work with people with severe disabilities in an individualized context to help them pursue employment or educational goals. Since 1973, several additions to vocational rehabilitation legislation have been added, streamlining the application process to serve a larger number of individuals.

What Is Vocational Rehabilitation?

Individualized Plan for Employment. When clients are assigned a VR counselor, they develop an *individualized plan for employment* (IPE). The IPE can be modified as needed to meet the needs of the consumer. If the consumer would like to find gainful employment quickly, the counselor will work with him or her on interviewing and job seeking skills. The counselor and the state agency typically have connections with employers willing to hire persons with disabilities. They may also utilize a *job developer.* The job developer's goal is to network with potential employers for consumers and refer them for interviews. Some state agencies may have a full-time job developer while others rely on the counselor's vocational expertise.

Return to School. In cases where consumers want to return to school, consumers must have a specific end goal they would like to achieve. Finding that goal can be difficult, as many people change careers multiple times in their lives. It is up to the VR counselor and VR management to determine if paying for school is an effective component of the IPE. It is unlikely that the state would agree to send a consumer to medical school, as that is a very expensive and lengthy process. However, if the consumer had already been enrolled in medical school, it would provide a much better financial incentive. The counselor and supervisor would likely agree upon having the state pay for a consumer's trade school or vocational school. This approach represents a highly successful mode of VR. If consumers can become plumbers or electricians in two years, they would likely be more financially stable than at minimum wage jobs, although a minimum wage job may be easier to obtain. Figuring out the potential future financial stability is part of the negotiating process that takes place during the development of the IPE.

Self-Employment. VR also offers counseling and financial incentives for consumers who want to start their own business. Consumers may be eligible for state grants after they develop a thorough, promising business plan. VR counselors do not generally come from a business background and do not have the knowledge to advise the consumer on how to develop a business. Consumers may seek out their own business mentor, or VR counselors may be able to provide someone with business experience.

Important Points to Understand about Vocational Rehabilitation

Vocational Rehabilitation Requirements. To be eligible for VR services, individuals must have a physical or mental impairment that hinders their ability to find or retain gainful employment. The individual could have been injured on the job or may have a chronic disability (such as multiple sclerosis, HIV/AIDS, or schizophrenia) that is causing them difficulties in completing their current tasks at their job. They may also be disqualified from working for their current employer because of the inability to complete the minimum amount of work necessary. If the employer cannot provide *reasonable accommodations* for the employee with a disability to continue working, the employee can turn to the state VR agency for assistance. It is first recommended that if the employee incurs a disability on the job, the employer provides an accommodation, thus eliminating the need for VR to become involved. However, if this accommodation is not possible or is too costly for the employer, VR services begin.

Vocational Rehabilitation Offices. Individuals with disabilities can seek VR services at their local Department of Rehabilitation Services (DRS/DORS) office. Depending on where individuals live, they will be assigned to their nearest office. All offices are required by law to adhere to the Americans with Disabilities Act's (ADA) *public accessibility standards.* Many offices have bilingual staff and culturally competent counselors. Some offices may have specific counselors trained in sign language to work with deaf individuals. If the office does not, the state may pay for a contractor to provide translation services as needed. Blind and visually impaired individuals may seek services at the Bureau of Blind Services, which is part of the Department of Rehabilitation Services in many states and which specializes in serving individuals with visual impairments.

Services Provided. The primary goal of VR services is to help individuals with disabilities find gainful employment. Several other services are often provided as well. The individual may be paired up with a *job coach* in addition to a counselor. The job coach can help the client with specific job-related questions and concerns, such as asking for reasonable accommodations in the workplace. They may also visit work sites to determine that the accommodations are acceptable for the employee. VR offers multiple services, including independent living skills, assistive technology, career training, on-the-job training, career counseling, and home modifications.

The services available through VR programs vary widely depending on the state. They can include assessment to determine the strengths and challenges of the individual; vocational interests, counseling, and guidance; referral to services from other agencies; vocational and other types of postsecondary education and training (including self-determination and self-advocacy training); interpreter and reader services; rehabilitation technology services and other job accommodations; placement in suitable employment; employer education on disability issues, such as the ADA and job accommodations; services to family members; and other goods or services necessary to achieve rehabilitation objectives identified in the IPE.

Independent Living Skills. Independent living skills are often used in cases of individuals moving into new housing recently after being released from a nursing home or hospital. The focus on these skills is especially common when working with individuals with intellectual and developmental disabilities. The vocational rehabilitation team may help the client secure housing or assist them in being more independent through activities of daily living, such as eating, grooming, and cleaning. In some states, another agency has been designed to support individuals with independent living.

Assistive Technology and Home Modifications. Assistive technology is utilized when an individual with a disability needs help purchasing a wheelchair, walker, cane, hearing aid, or any other adaptive device or technology. The counselor works with the client in submitting a request to Medicaid or Medicare to fund the necessary equipment and works with a third-party supplier to ensure that the equipment is delivered timely and accurately. Home modifications are based on the requirements of the Americans with Disabilities Act. The VR agency could pay a contractor to provide different types of reasonable accommodations to promote independent living. Examples include an accessible ramp for someone who uses a wheelchair, a more durable railing on the stairs, or an electronic seat that allows for multiple-floor access.

Conclusion

Vocational Rehabilitation is an investment. The original justification of VR was that money spent on rehabilitating persons with disabilities will allow them to become taxpayers in the workforce. Through paying taxes, they will support VR and other government services. Ideally, the U.S. economy would see a net positive gain, and VR would pay for itself.

David Goldberg

See also: Customized Employment; Employment, Barriers to; Employment First; Supported Employment; Vocational Evaluation

Further Reading

Riggar, T. F., and Dennis R. Maki. 2004. *Handbook of Rehabilitation Counseling.* New York: Springer Publishing Company.

U.S. Congress. 1973. "Rehabilitation Act of 1973 Public Law, 112." http://paradigm-healthcare.com/wp-content/uploads/2013/03/REHABILITATION-ACT-OF-1973.pdf.

Voting Rights

Voting gives Americans a say in their government and in the laws that affect their daily lives. For people with disabilities, voting is an important way to make sure elected leaders protect disability civil rights. However, persons with disabilities might have trouble voting because of discrimination, inaccessible polling places, or state voting laws.

Voting Rights for Disabled People

The right to vote is a key citizenship right for Americans. Voting gives Americans a way to participate in their democracy by choosing their leaders and weighing in on policies that affect them. Voting is a human rights issue for people with disabilities. People with disabilities may especially want to vote to elect politicians who support disability rights. Voting can help disabled people get fellow people with disabilities and allies into positions of power. Voting is an essential way to advance the disability rights movement and to get a say in important discussions that affect disabled people's lives.

When they try to vote, people with disabilities may face unfair laws, negative public attitudes, accessibility issues, and financial challenges. Each of these issues makes it more difficult for people with disabilities to exercise their right to vote. Despite the barriers facing people with disabilities as they try to cast their ballots, voting is one of the most important things people with disabilities can do to improve policies that affect them.

Background and History

The U.S. Constitution, the Voting Rights Act, the Help America Vote Act (HAVA), the Americans with Disabilities Act (ADA), and several other federal laws protect the right of people with disabilities to vote. There are only a few ways a person can legally lose the right to vote. In most states, people with disabilities can only lose their right to vote if a court decides they are not capable of voting. Any time that a person loses the right to vote, it is a decision made by lawyers or government officials in a court. Guardians, health care providers, nursing home staff, and polling place workers do not have the right to deny someone the chance to vote (Bazelon Center for Mental Health Law [BCMHL] 2016). If someone with a disability shows up to vote and the polling place workers doubt his or her right to vote, the person with a disability still has the protected legal right to cast a ballot. In states with laws preventing some people with disabilities from voting, polling place workers can challenge the vote before or after the fact, but they are not allowed to prevent the person with disability from voting on election day (BCMHL 2016).

Important Points to Understand About Voting Rights and Disability

In some states, people with mental illness or intellectual disabilities can be denied their right to vote. Many states have laws allowing a court to take away that right. Some states have laws that prevent people who are under guardianship from voting. Several other states have outdated and unclear laws preventing people who are "insane" or mentally incompetent from voting. Some states have no laws against people with disabilities voting. Even in these states, sometimes people with disabilities are prevented from voting by caregivers, health care providers, or polling place workers.

Barriers to voting are very common for people with disabilities. Many people with disabilities across the country report difficulties with accessibility both when entering their polling place and once inside their polling place (National Council on Disability 2015).

Caregiver and Health Provider Interference. Sometimes, the person caring for a person with a disability might decide that the person with a disability is not capable of voting. This issue has been reported across the country. A family member, caregiver, or health provider might prevent the person with a disability from registering to vote, getting information about the election, getting an absentee ballot, or traveling to a polling place. In many nursing homes or mental institutions, health providers have stopped election workers trying to enter the facility. In these cases, the institution staff often claim that the people with disabilities in the facility are "not competent" or "too demented" to vote (BCMHL 2016). This behavior is illegal and reflects negative attitudes about disability in our society. Some people still hold on to the belief that people with disabilities need help and charity rather than civil rights. In some nursing homes, staff might be motivated to keep their disabled residents from feeling empowered and independent, because nursing homes and institutions profit from keeping people with disabilities dependent on their services. In some institutions, voting might be seen as a threat. Nevertheless, voting is a civil right, and caregivers or health providers do not have the right to take it away.

Accessibility at Polling Places. Access is another common issue for people with disabilities who wish to vote. Despite federal laws mandating that polling places be accessible, a large percentage of people with disabilities have difficulty accessing their polling place. A person's assigned polling place might be an apartment building, a business, or another private location that is not wheelchair accessible. In these cases, people with disabilities have the right to "curbside voting," in which a polling place worker brings a ballot outside the building to allow the person to vote (Equip for Equality 2014). Curbside voting might be a good solution for some people, but it can also make it more difficult to keep ballots secret. Many people with disabilities report that they have not been able to vote privately and independently in recent elections (National Council on Disability 2015).

If people with disabilities are able to enter the polling place, access issues may continue. The voting booths are most often designed for people who are standing rather than sitting in a wheelchair. In addition, some disabled voters might need assistance reading or marking their ballot. Disabled voters have a legal right to receive help filling out their ballot (BCMHL 2016; Equip for Equality 2014). However, some polling places have denied disabled voters this right. In fact, health providers, caregivers, and election officials have a legal duty to help people with disabilities with voting if requested. In the past, some polling place workers have prevented people with disabilities from bringing personal assistants, friends, or other helpers with them to assist with reading and marking (BCMHL 2016). This action is illegal and might occur because polling place workers do not understand the law or because they believe that "independence" is required to be "competent" to vote. Many disabled voters report facing physical barriers or attitudinal barriers inside their polling places (National Council on Disability 2015).

Absentee Voting. Absentee voting is another option that is available to persons

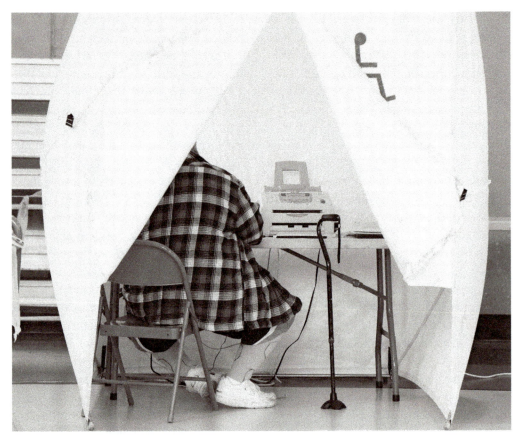

An accessible voting booth in use during the 2014 general election in Manchester, New Hampshire. Inaccessible polling places prevent people with disabilities from exercising their voting rights. (Darren McCollester/Getty Images)

with disabilities. Absentee voting is an ideal option for many people with disabilities, as it allows them to complete the ballot at home with any assistance, accommodations, or extra time they might need. However, disability rights groups are still advocating for polling place accessibility to ensure equal access for all.

Voter ID Laws. Some states require photo identification to vote. Getting a photo ID can be expensive and difficult, especially for people with disabilities. Voter ID laws may decrease the number of disabled people who are eligible to vote (BCMHL 2016). These laws are even more of a barrier for

disabled people who are classified as low income or are immigrants.

Dilemmas, Debates, and Unresolved Questions

Many of the ways that society prevents people with disabilities from voting come from traditional ideas about *citizenship*. Early citizenship theories claimed that only individuals who were rational, independent, and contributing to society (usually though traditional work and family expectations) deserved the rights of citizenship. These ideas about citizenship were used in the past to prevent women from voting, and they are used today to prevent disabled persons from voting (Carey 2009). Only giving voting rights to certain people with disabilities (for example, people with physical disabilities but not with intellectual disabilities) can create divisions in the disability community.

To avoid the problems with these old ideas of citizenship, modern thinkers in disability studies are thinking about citizenship and rights in terms of *universal human rights.* Instead of citizens "earning" rights through their ability to follow society's rules and expectations, all humans deserve rights simply because they are human. A universal human rights approach can help argue for rights for all people with disabilities. The 2012 United Nations Convention on the Rights of Persons with Disabilities (CRPD) is an important document that describes ways that countries should protect the human rights of persons with disabilities. In article 29, the CRPD clearly says that voting rights are human rights for people with disabilities. The CRPD declares that people with disabilities have a right to accessible polling stations, private voting, and assistance with voting as needed.

The right to vote can be considered both a citizenship and a human rights issue. Some people argue that citizenship should only be a right for people with a certain intellectual or ability level. Disability advocacy groups will continue to argue that voting and other parts of citizenship should be rights for all humans. The debates over who has rights to citizenship will continue in the future.

The Future of Voting Rights

Disability rights organizations will continue to advocate to end discriminatory state laws, including "competence" laws and voter ID laws. Disability rights groups will also advocate for the United States to ratify the CRPD, which would encourage the United States to increase voting rights protections for people with disabilities. To help people with disabilities overcome the current access barriers, organizations can assist with voter registration and absentee voting. Trainings and information about voting rights can be shared with people with disabilities, health care providers, family members, and election officials. Reducing voting barriers for people with disabilities is an important advocacy goal, as voting rights are key to participation in American democracy.

Elizabeth Adare Harrison

See also: Americans with Disabilities Act (ADA); Citizenship; Community Living and Community Integration; Guardianship and Capacity; Independent Living, "Nothing about Us without Us"

Further Reading

Bazelon Center for Mental Health Law. 2016. "A Guide to the Voting Rights of People with Mental Disabilities." http://www.bazelon.org/portals/0/voting/voting%20rights%20guide%202016.pdf.

Carey, Allison. 2009. *On the Margins of Citizenship: Intellectual Disability and Civil Rights in Twentieth-Century America.* Philadelphia: Temple University Press.

Equip for Equality. 2014. "Exercising Your Right to Vote." http://www.equipforequality.org/wp-content/uploads/2014/03/12_Voting_Rights_Overview_03.pdf.

National Council on Disability. 2015. "Experiences of Voters with Disabilities during the 2012 Election Cycle." http://www.ncd.gov/publications/2013/10242013.

United Nations. 2008. "Convention on the Rights of Persons with Disabilities." http://www.un.org/disabilities/convention/conventionfull.shtml.

W

Welfare to Work

Most people, including people with disabilities, would prefer to work rather than receive government benefits or various welfare services. However, people with disabilities face a number of barriers when moving from welfare to work. In other countries, notably the United Kingdom and Australia, there are specific policies known as "Welfare to Work" for people with disabilities. In the United States, there is not one policy that encompasses the idea of "welfare to work." Rather, welfare to work is a concept that is located at the intersections of and interplay between many specific pieces of policy and the rules that govern them.

The End of "Welfare as We Know It"

Bill Clinton ran for president on the promise to "end welfare as we know it," and in 1996, he signed the Personal Responsibility and Work Opportunity Reconciliation Act (PRWORA). The central piece of this legislation transformed Aid to Families with Dependent Children into Temporary Aid for Needy Families (TANF) benefits. This shift was characterized by time limits during which an individual could receive benefits from the government and work requirements that a person had to fulfill to maintain eligibility. PRWORA is generally regarded as a success, at least in moving people off welfare and into work. However, inequality has continued to grow, primarily because most of the jobs that TANF beneficiaries obtained paid a low wage and most people affected by the legislation have not been able to end the cycle of poverty.

PRWORA reasserted the importance of paid employment within American ideology and encouraged beneficiaries to take whatever employment they could. Many states implemented various employment service and training programs to help people receiving benefits find employment or gain the skills they need to secure a job. Critics of the law argue that it is racist and misogynist, because the people primarily affected by the reforms were people of color and women. Further, the law favored two-parent households over single mothers or fathers. Many scholars have noted that PRWORA works to separate the "deserving poor" (such as widows or older people) from the "undeserving poor," with the aforementioned groups labeled as "undeserving poor." There was a strong push to end welfare dependency, where people stayed on welfare benefits rather than obtaining a job because if they worked they would lose eligibility for other benefits, such as food stamps or child care assistance. Thus, with the shift to TANF, PRWORA ended the idea that welfare benefits were an entitlement or a right within U.S. policy and replaced it with the notion of responsibility. People had to fulfill responsibilities to enjoy their rights (in this case, people had the responsibility to be employed or fulfill work-related obligations to receive welfare benefits).

People with Disabilities and Barriers to Employment: Welfare *or* Work

Most people with disabilities were not affected by PRWORA (unless a person with a disability claimed TANF rather than benefits through the Social Security Administration on the basis of that disability); rather, people with disabilities were regarded as part of the "deserving poor." The potential of people with disabilities to contribute to the labor market has not been a priority within U.S. policy; while "welfare to work" affected most people without disabilities receiving benefits, a person with a disability receiving Social Security Administration (SSA) benefits was not subject to the same time limits or work requirements. People with disabilities faced many barriers if they wanted to leave welfare benefits and enter the labor market. The primary barriers were policy related, although people with disabilities also face barriers related to inaccessible public places and transportation; low levels of training and education; and the attitudes of the public, especially employers.

In particular, the interplay between Social Security Administration benefits and Medicaid or Medicare prevented many people with disabilities from even trying to find employment. Again, the centrality of work in U.S. policy is clearly evident. Before people with disabilities become eligible for Supplemental Security Income (SSI) or Social Security Disability Insurance (SSDI) through the SSA, they have to prove straight medical eligibility that includes the "inability to engage in any substantial gainful activity by reason of any medically determinable physical or mental impairment which can be expected to result in death or which has lasted or can be expected to last for a continuous period of not less than 12 months." Furthermore, eligibility for Medicaid is linked with eligibility for SSI, while Medicare is linked with SSDI. Therefore, to be eligible for either income benefits or health care benefits, people with disabilities first have to show that they are unable to work. Although the SSA programs do allow recipients to work up to a certain amount

before losing their benefits, eligibility for SSA programs and the link with health care create an "all or nothing" situation.

People with disabilities were hesitant to attempt to enter the workplace for two primary reasons. First, entering the workplace meant losing the SSA benefits and the Medicaid or Medicare that came along with them. The jobs that people with disabilities received would have to have health care benefits along with them (which much entry-level, low-paid work does not include). Second, there was no guarantee that people who left SSA benefits would regain eligibility. Often, the eligibility process took well over one year. Eligibility, especially the medical criterion of being unable to work, may have been harder to establish if a person had left benefits to attempt to work recently. For these reasons, most people with disabilities were concerned with choosing welfare *or* work; the piecemeal amalgamation of policies in the United States and the interplay between them prohibited most people with disabilities from even thinking about how to move from welfare to work.

Ticket to Work and Voluntary Welfare to Work

In 1999, the United States adopted the Ticket to Work and Work Incentives Improvement Act (TTW), which provided welfare-to-work services to people with disabilities on a voluntary basis. The number of people and amount of money spent on SSA disability programs had been expanding exponentially, and this act was an effort to take a more active approach to labor market policy for people with disabilities by facilitating the move from welfare to work for those individuals who wanted it. Wittenburg and Loprest (2004) asked, "How do you provide return-to-work services to a population of participants who must show a permanent inability to work at the time of application to qualify for benefits?"

TTW addresses barriers to employment for people with disabilities receiving SSA benefits on two fronts. First, the "ticket to work" part of the act's title refers to a training program developed to provide skills and other employment resources to people with disabilities. Eligible beneficiaries received a ticket that they could redeem for these employment services at providers known as employment networks (ENs) across the country. The law has been expanded so that vocational rehabilitation centers can also serve as ENs. This program is voluntary, people with disabilities do not have to use their ticket if they do not want to (as opposed to the work requirements placed on TANF beneficiaries under PRWORA). However, TTW is also a voluntary program for ENs; they are not required to work with a person trying to redeem a ticket. Many people with disabilities have reported difficulty finding an EN to work with them or accept their ticket, which is not surprising because ENs are only paid for their services when they achieve an employment outcome with an individual. This payment scheme leads to "creaming," where providers only work with people who are close to the labor market and are likely to reach one of the employment milestones that the EN will be paid for.

The other part of TTW's title, "Work Incentives Improvement," refers to the incentives that the act created for people with disabilities to try to move into the labor market. Many of these focus on removing policy barriers. For instance, TTW introduced expedited reinstatement processes to return individuals to benefit eligibility if they try to work and find that they cannot. SSI beneficiaries also receive a nine-month trial work period, during which they remain eligible for and receive benefits without losing any of their income. The act also extended eligibility for medical services when a beneficiary leaves SSA; Medicare beneficiaries retain their eligibility for Medicare for 93 months, while Medicaid beneficiaries are allowed to buy into a state plan at a reduced cost to maintain their health insurance. (The Affordable Care Act also helps in this regard, as people with disabilities are now less likely to be in a position where they cannot afford health insurance even if they do not get it through their place of employment.)

Conclusion: Impact of Welfare to Work on the Employment of People with Disabilities

Welfare to work for people with disabilities in the United States is still voluntary. This is consistent with a rights-based approach, and people with disabilities can choose whether to transition into the labor market. However, it still reflects the status of people with disabilities as part of the "deserving poor" and reveals that society still does not expect them to contribute to the labor market. TTW had a very meager goal: to double the proportion of people receiving disability benefits who move into the labor market (prior to TTW, only about 0.5 percent of beneficiaries transitioned into the labor market). While TTW met that goal, not everyone can access TTW benefits equally, especially because ENs vary across the country and because they have the option to work with a person or not.

TTW has not had a substantial impact on the employment of people with disabilities, which still lags far behind that of people without disabilities. More work on facilitating transitions from welfare to work for people with disabilities is necessary in the United States.

Randall Owen

See also: Employment, Barriers to; Employment First; Neoliberalism; Poverty; Vocational Rehabilitation

Further Reading

Owen, R., R. Gould, and S. Parker Harris. 2015. "Disability and Employment in the United States: The Intersection of Healthcare Reform and Welfare to Work Policy." In *Disabled People, Work and Welfare: Is Employment Really the Answer?,* edited by C. Grover and L. Piggot, 127–44. Bristol, UK: Policy Press at the University of Bristol.

Parker Harris, S., R. Owen, R. Jones, and K. Caldwell. 2013. "Does Workfare Policy in the United States Promote the Rights of People with Disabilities?" *Journal of Vocational Rehabilitation* 39, no. 1: 61–73.

Thornton, C., R. Weathers, and D. Wittenberg. 2007. "Ticket to Success? Early Findings from the Ticket to Work Evaluation." *Journal of Vocational Rehabilitation* 27, no. 2: 69–71.

Wittenburg, D., and P. Loprest. 2004. "Ability or Inability to Work: Challenges in Moving towards a More Work-Focused Disability Definition for Social Security Administration (SSA) Disability Programs." Briefing paper prepared for the Ticket to Work and Work Incentives Advisory Panel. www.ssa.gov/work/panel/panel_docu ments/pdf_versions/Disability%20Defini tion%20Draft2.pdf.

Wellness and Health Promotion

Wellness and health promotion represent the processes by which individuals control and improve their health. The focus is on individual behavior as well as the interaction between the individual and the environment.

Historically, people with disabilities were not considered "healthy," simply because they had disabilities. While many conditions associated with the disability label are health related, it is also true that many people with disabilities can be healthy and, like all persons, can play an important role in optimizing their health. Health promotion is especially important for people with disabilities because of an increased risk of having chronic health conditions, such as diabetes, heart disease, and obesity, when compared to people without disabilities (Dixon-Ibarra and Horner-Johnson 2014).

Engaging in health behaviors is one avenue where people with disabilities can promote their own health. The most common types of health behaviors include physical activity, healthy eating, smoking cessation, and visiting a health care provider.

Many individual, social, environmental, and policy factors play a role in promoting or limiting an individual's ability to perform health behaviors and can involve individual characteristics or decisions, social or environmental context, and community-level policies. Individual factors include attitudes and beliefs toward a behavior. Examples of social and environmental factors could be the effect on health promotion behaviors by a person's interpersonal relationships, or barriers presented by the physical structure of facilities. Finally, policies toward persons with disabilities within a facility or a community can affect health.

Physical Activity

Physical activity is any bodily movement that works muscles and requires more energy than resting. There are three types of physical activity: (1) exercise; (2) leisure activity; and (3) general daily activity.

Exercise is any physical activity that is both planned and structured with the purpose of improving one's health. There are four types of exercise: aerobic, strength, balance, and flexibility. The Centers for Disease Control and Prevention (CDC) recommends that adults get at least 150 minutes per week of aerobic activity, such as brisk walking or rolling, playing basketball, or dancing. They also recommend at least two days of strength activity that works all the major muscle groups (legs, hips, abdomen, chest, shoulders, and arms). These recommendations are the same for people with and without disabilities (U.S. Department of Health and Human Services 2008).

Despite the many health benefits that result from being physically active (improved mental health; reduced risk of falls; and lowered risk of heart disease, some cancers, type 2 diabetes, and obesity), people with disabilities are less likely to engage in the recommended amount of physical activity when compared to people without disabilities (Carroll et al. 2014). While many of the reasons for not engaging in adequate physical activity are common for all people regardless of disability status, some factors are unique to people with disabilities.

Attitudes and beliefs toward physical activity play a significant role in whether or not anyone is physically active. For example, if people dislike physical activity or believe that physical activity is "hard work," they are less likely to be active and participate in physical activity programs. One factor that is unique to people with disabilities is the belief that their disability prevents them from being active. Family, friends, and health care professionals play an important role as well. Having friends and family who are supportive, encouraging, and available to exercise with is associated with increased chances of being physically active. Health care professionals have been found generally to be less likely to recommend physical activity to people with disabilities, associating the disability with poor health (Carroll et al. 2014). When a health care professional does recommend activity, the person with disability is far more likely to be physically active. Fitness centers offer a unique opportunity for people with disabilities to be active. However, most fitness centers do not meet the accessibility guidelines as stipulated in Title III of the Americans with Disabilities Act (Arbour-Nicitopoulos & Ginis 2011). Examples of accessibility include exercise equipment with seats that move out of the way for someone in a wheelchair, and a swimming pool with a lift to assist people getting in and out of the pool. Staff may assume people with disabilities do not have the capability to be active and may not offer support or assistance. In the management of access barriers, community policies have a direct impact on physical activity. For example, sidewalks must be level and free from cracks, and traffic lights in the community should allow sufficient time for crossing the street.

Healthy Eating

Healthy eating is an essential type of health behavior. The Dietary Guidelines for Americans has three overarching goals: (1) balancing calories with physical activity to manage weight; (2) increasing the consumption of seafood, fruits, vegetables, whole grains, and low-fat or nonfat dairy; and (3) decreasing the use of salt, bad fats (trans fat or saturated fat), sugar, and refined grains. Like most Americans, people with disabilities are not following Dietary Guidelines for Americans, and they are significantly less likely to follow these dietary guidelines than people without disabilities (Hall, Colantonio, and Yoshida 2003).

Subtle barriers can prevent an individual with a disability from having access to healthy food and drink options. For example, accessibility barriers can prevent participation in cooking classes, and grocery stores in urban environments are generally not accessible because they lack suitable entrances for wheelchair users (e.g., ramps or automatic doors). In the store, healthy foods, such as fresh fruits and vegetables, may be out of physical reach for a person in a wheelchair. Grocery store layouts change at the request of the suppliers, and items can be relocated to another part of the store without notice. While this may be a minor issue for most, it is problematic for those with a visual impairment who must navigate unfamiliar routes to healthy food options within the store. Thus, accessibility is also important to the development of positive eating habits for people with disabilities (Mojtahedi et al. 2008).

For those persons with intellectual disabilities, it has been necessary to develop specialized programs to teach and promote healthy eating habits. Such programs work extensively with families, friends, and other professionals who work with the individuals. Often only minor accommodations are necessary, such as providing more time to eat or sharing potluck dinners with more nutritional options. A key goal of many programs is simply to increase awareness of the nutritional options and decisions made by people with intellectual disabilities.

Health Care Access

The provisions of the Americans with Disabilities Act (ADA) should facilitate accessible health care for people with disabilities. Being able to access health care is a key component of health promotion and wellness. However, many health care facilities and services remain inaccessible because of physical barriers and the lack of familiarity by health care professionals in adapting care practices on behalf of people with various disabilities (Mudrick et al. 2012).

With regards to physical barriers, the layout and equipment in health care facilities often present barriers. For example, women with disabilities have lower rates of mammogram and clinical exams, which could be attributed to inaccessibility of examination tables and diagnostic equipment. Additionally, hallways to examination rooms may not be wide enough for wheelchairs in some cases (Peterson-Besse et al. 2014).

Familiarity with disability and knowledge about accommodations by health care providers can play an integral role in the quality of health care. In the past, physicians, nurses, and other health providers rarely encountered people with disabilities in their routine practices. For this reason, programs were developed to improve the skills and comfort level of health professionals in providing care to people with disabilities. There are many examples of the integration of disability topics into medical school training. However, widespread adoption has yet to be realized.

Summary and Conclusion

It is important that health promotion initiatives work toward developing strong partnerships between people with disabilities and health providers to ensure not only that people with disabilities receive the highest quality health care but also that they are empowered to take control of their health. The quality of health care is dependent on how well people with disabilities are able to access care, how well their health providers are trained to provide care to people with disabilities, and how well health promotion programs are able to educate people with disabilities about the importance of accessing health care so that they are able to control and maintain good health.

Many factors affect the ability of people with disabilities to take control of their health care and health promoting behaviors. When someone wants to take part in health promoting behaviors and programs, it is important that social, environmental, and policy factors are taken into account. Health promotion is complex, and it requires individuals to interact with social and physical environments. This interaction can promote or hinder the quantity and quality of health promotion for people regardless of whether or not they have a disability.

Vijay Vasudevan and Natasha A. Spassiani

See also: Food; Health and Fitness, Access to; Health Care, Barriers to for Minorities; Health Determinants; Preventive Health Care

Further Reading

Arbour-Nicitopoulos, Kelly P., and Kathleen A. Martin Ginis. 2011. "Universal Accessibility of 'Accessible' Fitness and Recreational Facilities for Persons with Mobility Disabilities." *Adapted Physical Activity Quarterly* 28, no. 1: 1–15.

Carroll, Dianna D., Elizabeth A. Courtney-Long, Alissa C. Stevens, Michelle L. Sloan, Carolyn Lullo, Susanna N. Visser, Michael H. Fox, et al. 2014. "Vital Signs: Disability and Physical Activity—United States, 2009–2012." *Morbidity and Mortality Weekly Report* 63, no. 18: 407–413.

Dixon-Ibarra, Alicia, and Willi Horner-Johnson. 2014. "Disability Status as an Antecedent to Chronic Conditions: National Health Interview Survey, 2006–2012." *Preventing Chronic Disease* 11: E15.

Hall, Lynda, Angela Colantonio, and Karen Yoshida. 2003. "Barriers to Nutrition as a Health Promotion Practice for Women with Disabilities" *International Journal of Rehabilitation Research* 26, no. 3: 245–247.

Mojtahedi, Mina C., Patty Boblick, James H. Rimmer, Jennifer L. Rowland, Robin A. Jones, and Carol L. Braunschweig. 2008. "Environmental Barriers to and Availability of Healthy Foods for People with Mobility Disabilities Living in Urban and Suburban Neighborhoods." *Archives of Physical Medicine and Rehabilitation* 89, no. 11: 2174–2179.

Mudrick, Nancy R., Mary Lou Breslin, Mengke Liang, and Silvia Yee. 2012. "Physical Accessibility in Primary Health Care Settings: Results from California On-Site Reviews." *Disability and Health Journal* 5, no. 3: 159–167.

Peterson-Besse, Jana J., Emily S. Walsh, Willi Horner-Johnson, Tawara D. Goode, and Barbara Wheeler. 2014. "Barriers to Health Care among People with Disabilities Who Are Members of Underserved Racial/Ethnic Groups: A Scoping Review of the Literature." *Medical Care* 52: S51–S63.

U.S. Department of Health and Human Services. 2008. "Physical Activity Guidelines for Americans." http://www.health.gov /paguidelines/guidelines/default.aspx.

Workers' Cooperatives

Workers' cooperatives are an organizational system made up of individuals coming together to accomplish an overall, common goal or set of goals, as any other organization does. Cooperative organizations are peculiar in terms of ownership; they are owned and self-managed by its workers. Cooperative models are of growing interest for the employment of people with disabilities. The flexibility of the arrangement and the unique structures make it an attractive employment option. Furthermore, workers may bypass discrimination that is often encountered in the competitive labor market.

History of Workers' Cooperatives

The historical roots of workers' cooperatives can be traced back to a number of self-managed organizations in the early 19th century in Europe. Workers' cooperatives emerged from the unprecedented rapid social changes generated by the Industrial Revolution taking place all across Europe. The new market economy made changes at all levels of social-cultural life; the way basic goods were produced and traded was reshaping people's status and roles in society. Many workers were unhappy with capitalist practices that favored competition and the maximization of profit over worker input or happiness. The rapidly growing market economy led many people to seek alternative models for ownership and production.

Workers' cooperatives aim to organize production in anticapitalistic ways, by sharing the ownership and the profits among the workers themselves. Workers' cooperatives place a high value on job security and favor such ideas as workers' democratic control over production and common ownership of the means of production. Growing skepticism about workers' roles in the capitalist system was the basis for the development of the labor movement, the socialist workers' movements, and the development of *cooperative economic activities* across the world. Collaborative efforts among workers to find alternative organizational structures and defend their labor wages and working conditions began to multiply across Europe.

Cooperatives and the Economy

Workers' cooperatives started as one of those new alternatives to a purely competitive employment market and also claimed to be a healthier organizational model capable of competing in a capitalist economy. The model benefits workers simultaneously by recognizing individual ownership and by distributing shares of equity.

A workers' cooperative puts the emphasis on exerting control over the organizational processes in a number of ways. For example, democratically elected employee representatives usually form part of the executive committee or managing board that makes the final decisions about production, marketing, financing, and all other relevant aspects of the organization. The consequences of such organizational controls are what differentiate a for-profit enterprise from a cooperative enterprise. A cooperative enterprise allows every worker/owner to participate in the decision-making process by sharing ideas with the representatives on the board. A cooperative's guiding principles focus on the organization's sustainability, the quality of the product, workers' safety, and the profitability of the cooperative as a way to guarantee fair wages to the worker/owners and support expansion or quality upgrades in the production. An example of this work can be seen in the way workers' cooperatives select their managers and administration: they are all democratically elected by every worker/owner.

Another peculiarity of workers' cooperatives is that managers are considered and treated as any other worker of the firm, and these companies usually employ far fewer managers than traditional organizations because the workers are personally invested in maximizing productivity for the betterment of the cooperative and so require minimal supervision. Moreover, in traditional forms of workers' cooperatives, the workers themselves hold all the firm's shares, with no outside owners, and each member has one voting share.

There are multiple types of cooperatives, such as traditional industrial organizations;

consumer cooperatives (for all types of goods and services); food cooperatives (which function like supermarkets that offer discounts to its members); and agricultural cooperatives (sharing resources and labor that will add value to food production), which are very common in developing countries. In all cases, a cooperative becomes a viable alternative for individuals who have little financial, political, or intellectual capital to overcome employment barriers. Most of the examples in the literature describe people involved in cooperatives as individuals facing systemic barriers or social disadvantages—like individuals with disabilities—and explain how the cooperative model offers an opportunity to overcome such disadvantages (International Labour Organization 2012; Schultze 2002; Altus et al. 2001). Regardless of the nature of the collaborative endeavor, a cooperative just requires the use of individuals' social capital and skills to organize their work as a means of employment and economic development.

Workers' Cooperatives in the United States

In the United States, formal workers' cooperative experiences started in the year 1842, when the Supreme Court established that labor unions had a right to exist. Unions immediately grew throughout the East into the U.S. territory. Literature describes workers' cooperative experiences in the United States flourishing rapidly after the Supreme Court decision, particularly in the food industry. By 1867, there were close to 200 cheese businesses, creameries, farms, and textile co-op factories in North America (Schultze 2002; Cord 2000). These labor experiences have been replicated and improved across time, but just a few of them have been carefully studied. Today, work

done by the International Labour Organization (ILO), recognizes the cooperative form of enterprise as a means for sustainable employment, which can lead to improved livelihood and social inclusion. As of 1991, there were more than 150 workers' cooperatives producing goods and services in the United States.

Literature on the subject provides numerous examples of cooperative businesses started by people with disabilities. Sperry, Brusin, and Seekins (2002) provide a wide range of examples that have been crafted into disability-oriented cooperative businesses, such as medical billing, woodworking, lawn care and snow removal, word processing and secretarial firms, graphic design, used-clothing stores, home inspection, glass installation, auto body repair, dog biscuit manufacturing, bicycle shops, commercial fishing, welding, and tree farming. These examples are evidence of how people with disabilities may create their own enterprise through cooperatives to achieve self-employment. The success of the cooperative model in meeting the needs of people with disabilities lies in the values and principles that guide the cooperative movement: nondiscrimination, equality, equity, and solidarity. In addition, the model's emphasis on the training and education of members shows the strong concerns for the overall development and improvement of the community of worker/owners.

Conclusions

To conclude, people with disabilities have historically experienced discrimination in the labor market, and the workers' cooperative approach offers an alternative for them to overcome employment barriers and to improve their life conditions. A number of collaborative initiatives have demonstrated that workers' cooperatives have the potential to improve people's lives and change society. By participating in a cooperative enterprise, people with disabilities can take control of their lives, become productive workers in an organization, contribute to the improvement of their community, and regain self-esteem by becoming worker/owners of their company (Sperry, Brusin, and Seekins 2001). Workers with disabilities engaged in cooperative enterprises have the chance to gain access to the labor market through collaboration with others in similar situations.

Luciano Berardi

See also: Apprenticeships; Customized Employment; Employment, Barriers to; Vocational Rehabilitation

Further Reading

Altus, D., L. Egrstrom, G. van Dijk, P. Bos, and D. Muhm. 2001. "Consumer Co-ops: A Resource Guide for Consumers with Disabilities." *Utopian Studies* 12, no. 2: 246–250.

Cord, X. E. 2000. "Textiles and Cooperative Commerce in Colonial America: The Example of William McCormick." *Uncoverings* 21: 27–55.

International Labour Organization. 2012. "A Cooperative Future for People with Disabilities." Issue brief. http://www.ilo.org/skills/pubs/WCMS_194822/lang--en/index.htm.

Melnyk, G. 1985. *The Search for Community: From Utopia to Co-operative Society.* Montreal: Black Rose Books.

Nadeau, E. G., and David J. Thompson. 1996. *Cooperation Works!: How People Are Using Cooperative Action to Rebuild Communities and Revitalize the Economy.* Rochester, MN: Lone Oak Press.

Schultze, G. E. 2002. "Work-Ownership & Catholic Social Thought. Special Feature: Mondragon Cooperatives." *Social Policy* 32, no. 2: 12–16.

Shaffer, J. 1999. *Historical Dictionary of the Cooperative Movement.* Lanham, MD: Scarecrow Press.

Sperry, C., J. Brusin, and T. Seekins. 2001. "Rural Economic Development: Work Cooperatives and Employment of People with Disabilities: Part One." *Scholar Work at University of Montana, Employment* 3. http://scholarworks.umt.edu/ruralinst_employment/3.

Y

Youth with Disabilities, Employment of

When students graduate from secondary school, outside agencies such as vocational rehabilitation (VR) or other community agencies can provide case management support to young adults with disabilities. *Transition* in VR refers to the process of preparing high school students with disabilities for adult living and employment. Transition services have positive impacts, but more transition services and supports are needed for youth with disabilities to benefit fully.

Background

Occupational, rehabilitation, and health practitioners have long recognized that unemployment has adverse effects on health, such as depression and anxiety, alcohol abuse, and poor physical well-being. Despite efforts to increase adulthood outcomes, students with disabilities are not reaching their employment and postsecondary education goals at the same rate as youth without disabilities. There is a stark difference in employment rates of youth with and without disabilities. As of August 2014, the employment rate for youth 16 to 19 years was 17 percent for youth with disabilities and 30 percent for youth without disabilities, and for those 20 to 24 years, it was 32 percent for youth with disabilities and 65 percent for youth without disabilities (U.S. Department of Labor 2015).

Postsecondary Education. Further, the U.S. Department of Education reported in 2007 that students without disabilities were enrolling in postsecondary education at twice the rate of students with disabilities. In addition to lower rates of enrollment in postsecondary education, there is also a discrepancy between the kinds of programs youth with and without disabilities pursue. Research has shown that youth without disabilities often enroll in bachelor programs whereas students with disabilities attend either training/certificate or associate's degree programs, which put them at employment and financial disadvantages after graduation. Therefore, legislation has been developed to ensure that students with disabilities receive appropriate and adequate preparation for their transition to adulthood.

The Introduction of Transition Planning. VR originated in special education settings in the early 1980s, when there was a growing concern about employment prospects for youth with disabilities. The Rehabilitation Act of 1973 and the Education for All Handicapped Children Act of 1975 were in place, but they did not provide enough stimulus for schools and state VR agencies to adequately prepare youth to transition from school to work or post–high school educational opportunities. A combination of unique physical and emotional changes during youth, the reality of zero-to-minimal work experience, and the level of education rendered transition-age youth with disabilities in crucial need of individualized plans for moving from school to work. Advocacy efforts for including transition planning in the educational plan for all high school students with disabilities eventually led to the establishment of mandated transition services in the Individuals with Disabilities Education Act of 1990 (IDEA). IDEA further required that transition planning begin at age 14. The rationale was that students, in conjunction with their transition-plan adviser or counselor, should articulate a plan at the earliest appropriate age and refine it during high school to reflect updated knowledge of the labor market as well as changes in personal interests. The transition plan is a physical document within the *individualized education program* (IEP), which details the supports and services needed by each student along with how and who will deliver each. The transition plan is a document developed with the school system, student, his or her family, and outside agencies that focus on preparing and training students with skills necessary to transition to adulthood (employment, education, independent living) (IDEA 2004). The transition plan is required to be measurable, specific, step-by-step, and must include services and supports the students can access. Four main linear steps should be followed to create effective transition plans for students with disabilities: (1) conducting transition assessments; (2) identifying present levels of performance; (3) setting postsecondary outcomes and goals; and (4) planning transition services delivery. In addition, transition planning services should include linking youth with disabilities and their families to other services offered in the community, including VR, to help the youth reach their full potential after graduating from high school.

Factors Influencing Employment among Youth with Disabilities

There are several individual, family, and larger system-level factors that either support or inhibit youth with disabilities attempting to achieve their potential after graduating from high school. For example, research has shown that boys are more likely to find jobs and that girls are more likely to pursue postsecondary education programs attending two- or four-year colleges (Balcazar, Oberoi, and Keel 2013). Type and severity of disability also plays a role. For example, one year after graduating from high school, students with intellectual disabilities have lower rates of employment and college or training program attendance compared to students with physical disabilities. For most students with disabilities, the importance of family involvement in their in-school and post–high school success cannot be overstated.

Interacting Service Systems. In addition, youth with disabilities and their families have to navigate multiple levels of systems, such as the school system and outside agencies like VR. This process can serve as both a barrier and a facilitator to the post–high school student's goals. The amount of resources at the schools that these youth attend and the quality and support from their teachers play important roles in the development of students with disabilities, particularly when they transition to adulthood. However, teachers have expressed a need for more emphasis on delivering transition content in their teacher preparation programs, requesting instruction in employment services, postsecondary education, assessment, and ways to build effective partnerships with outside agencies. Youth with disabilities and their families also interact with VR. Accounts of practices implemented by successful school districts have found that one contributing factor was a positive and symbiotic relationship with VR. Involving outside agencies in students' transition planning is required by the IDEA of 2004.

Some strategies these districts implement are professional development between the school system and VR counselors, regular interagency gatherings, and face-to-face engagement among students and their families, the school system, and VR counselors. Based on the success of these districts and the utilization of VR services for students with disabilities, it is clear that interagency collaboration between these two systems can contribute to successful student outcomes when implemented properly.

Recommendations for Improving Employment Outcomes

Transition planning is a time-consuming process that is essential for students with disabilities because it makes them aware of and provides them with the supports and services necessary to reach their adulthood goals. Youth with disabilities who completed work preparation programs as part of their transition plans have been shown to be more likely to secure employment after graduation, and when they do so, they tend to earn higher salaries than those who do not finish such programs. However, there are still a few challenges to ensuring effective transition services to all students with services, such as lack of funding, ineffective transition planning, poor access to services by outside agencies, and confusion about how to apply for postsecondary educational supports.

Systemic Programming and Partnerships. The implementation of promising programs to serve students with disabilities in transition service delivery, such as paid internships, require a strong partnership between high schools, state agencies, employers, and the students and their families (Balcazar, Oberoi, and Keel 2013). Such systemic programming requires a high investment of effort and open communication. However, it ensures a real-life employment experience for the students and increased awareness and understanding from the employers who get to see the youth working in their business. There are other benefits of such partnerships: students and families gain knowledge and understanding of how to access available services; employers develop awareness of accommodation needs and the skills the youth with disabilities can bring to the job; school systems create real work experiences for students; and students engage in postschool connections with outside agencies like VR (Balcazar, Oberoi, and Keel 2013). However, given the complex nature of the transition process and the number of parties that need to be involved, it is important to communicate continually. Best practices for achieving post–high school goals for youth with disabilities recommend open communication in the collaboration process between these parties—rehabilitation service providers, students and families, and secondary educators.

Other Strategies. Besides strong interagency partnership between VR services and school systems, some other recommendations for successful adulthood outcomes (employment, education, and independent living) for youth with disabilities are an active and early participation of VR in the IEP plan development and the transition process; an increased understanding among transition planners of policies and procedures within schools, particularly those relevant to students with disabilities; increased awareness among school staff of available transition services through state VR agencies; the creation of seamless procedures for transferring students from transition VR services to adult services; and cultural competency development to better serve minority and diverse youth with disabilities.

Conclusion

Youth with disabilities have much lower employment and postsecondary education achievements than youth without disabilities, and they require more supports and services to adequately transition to adulthood. Several individual factors, such as gender, age, disability type and severity, and family involvement, impact successful transition after high school graduation. Systemic contributors, such as employment and postsecondary education programs and services received, the school system, and the state VR system, can also affect transitions. Research has shown that when the school system and the VR agencies collaborate closely to ensure services and supports to students with disabilities, students have better transition outcomes, particularly in employment. Therefore, improvements to interagency partnerships are recommended.

Ashmeet Kaur Oberoi

See also: Employment, Barrier to; Individualized Education Program (IEP); Online Social and Professional Networks and Work; Transition from High School; Vocational Rehabilitation

Further Reading

Balcazar, Fabricio E., Ashmeet Oberoi, and Joanna M. Keel. 2013. "Predictors of Employment and College Attendance Outcomes for Youth in Transition: Implications for Policy and Practice." *Journal of Applied Rehabilitation Counseling* 44: 38–45.

Newman, Lynn, Mary Wagner, Renee Cameto, and Ann-Marie Knokey. 2009. "The Post-High School Outcomes of Youths with Disabilities up to 4 Years after High School: A Report from the National Longitudinal Study-2." Menlo Park, CA: SRI International. https://files.eric.ed.gov/full text/ED505448.pdf.

U.S. Department of Education Office of Special Education and Rehabilitation Services. 2014. "36th Annual Report to Congress on the Implementation of the Individuals with Disabilities Education Act, 2014." Washington, DC: U.S. Department of Education. http://www2.ed.gov/about/reports/annual /osep/2014/parts-b-c/36th-idea-arc.pdf.

U.S. Department of Labor, Office of Disability Employment Policy. 2015. "Youth Employment Rate." http://www.dol.gov /odep/categories/youth/youthemployment .htm.

Leaders and Key Figures in Disability

Muhammad Ali (1942–2016)

Muhammad Ali was a professional boxer. Ali's record was impressive, with 56 wins, only 5 losses, and 37 knockouts. He was also an Olympic gold medalist. He was named Sportsman of the Century by *Sports Illustrated* and Sports Personality of the Century by BBC (Ali 2017). In 1990, he was inducted into the International Boxing Hall of Fame. In addition to being one of the greatest boxers of the 20th century, Ali was an activist within the civil rights, religious freedom, and antiwar movements. He is often referred to as a leader in black and African American communities but is less often thought of in relation to his disability experiences.

Born Cassius Clay, Ali changed his name to Muhammad Ali after converting to the Nation of Islam. Journalists and sport announcers often ignored his name change at the time, even though he referred to the name Cassius Clay as his "slave name." One of his friends and mentors was civil rights leader Malcolm X, who encouraged Ali to use his position to influence politics and fight for civil rights. According to Randy Roberts and Johnny Smith, "Under Malcolm's tutelage, (Ali) embraced the world stage, emerging as an international symbol of black pride and black independence" (2016, xviii).

In 1967, Ali incited outrage when he refused to serve in the U.S. Armed Forces and spoke out against the Vietnam War. Ali was one of the first public figures to protest the war (AFP 2016). Ali stated, "My conscience won't let me go shoot my brother, or some darker people, or some poor hungry people in the mud for big powerful America. . . . And shoot them for what? They never called me nigger, they never lynched me, they didn't put no dogs on me, they didn't rob me of my nationality, rape and kill my mother and father. . . . Shoot them for what? How can I shoot them poor people? Just take me to jail" (Calamur 2016). Ali's opposition to the Vietnam War led to arrest, and he was stripped of his boxing titles. However, Ali was able to avoid jail time and was permitted to return to boxing in the 1970s. Although Ali lost his first fight after returning to boxing, he worked hard and won the heavyweight champion title in 1974. President Barack Obama described Ali as "the man who believes real success comes when we rise after we fall."

As a child, Ali struggled with reading and was diagnosed with dyslexia. Ali recalled, "As a high school student, many of my teachers labeled me dumb. I could barely read my textbooks" (Slipper 2014). Ali refused to let his teacher's opinions of him define him, but his experiences in

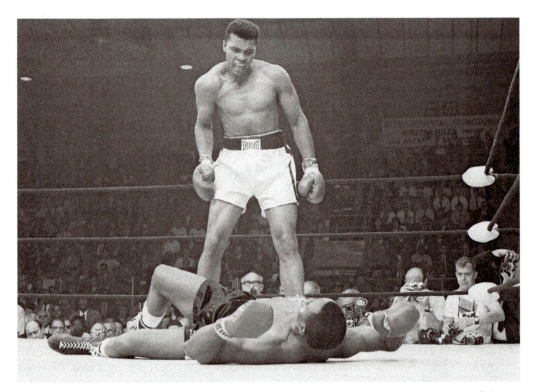

Heavyweight champion Muhammad Ali stands over Sonny Liston during their title fight in Lewiston, Maine, on May 25, 1965. Ali's advocacy and experience with dyslexia and Parkinson's disease are often overlooked when speaking about his legacy. (Bettmann/Getty Images)

school influenced him to support literacy programs later in life. In 2006, Ali and his wife, Lonnie Ali, partnered with Scholastic Books to create "Go the Distance," a curriculum designed to motivate and inspire young black readers.

In 1984, Ali announced that he had been diagnosed with Parkinson's disease. Thereafter, he worked to raise awareness about Parkinson's disease and expand research efforts. Ali remained an activist to the end of his life. He supported Palestine and the Black Lives Matter movement, and he continued to advocate for religious freedom and civil rights. Ali passed away on June 3, 2016.

Further Reading

Ali, Muhammad. 2017. "The Greatest of All Time." https://muhammadali.com/.

Calamur, Krishnadev. 2016. "Muhammad Ali and Vietnam." *The Atlantic*, June 4. https://www.theatlantic.com/news/archive/2016/06/muhammad-ali-vietnam/485717.

Roberts, Randy, and Johnny Smith. 2016. *Blood Brothers: The Fatal Friendship between Muhammad Ali and Malcolm X.* Philadelphia: Basic Books.

Slipper, Dan. 2014. "The Dyslexia Factor." BBC. http://www.bbc.co.uk/ouch/features/high_achieving_dyslexics.shtml.

Nura Aly

Nura Aly is a disabled musician and disability advocate. Aly was born with spina bifida and uses a wheelchair. She was exposed to advocacy at an early age because her mother, Mary Mrugalski, had to fight for

Aly to receive adequate school services, particularly during budget cuts. Mrugalski frequently had to drive Aly to school because the accessible school bus was late. When the only elevator at Aly's school broke down and the school decided she could just be excused from those classes, Mrugalski carried Aly up the stairs to ensure she did not fall behind. Eventually, Mrugalski was able to rally the school to hire a teacher to assist Aly (Vansickle 2002). Her mother's dedication to ensuring she received an education paved the way for Aly to become involved in disability advocacy.

Aly began playing violin when she was eight years old, and she has performed at Victory Gardens Theater and Access Living in Chicago, Illinois. She received a bachelor of arts in music from DePaul University and K–12 music teacher certification from Northeastern Illinois University.

Aly volunteers with JJ's List, which is a communications and marketing social enterprise that seeks to guide businesses in better meeting the needs of employees and customers with disabilities (JJ's List 2017). Aly leads disability awareness training and blogs about her experiences as a disabled woman. Aly is passionate about using disability awareness training to educate nondisabled people about disability. She explains, "People see me rolling down the street and sometimes they'll see me struggle with a curb cut or something in the sidewalk, and they'll see me struggling and come and push me. . . . But a lot of the time, they push me without asking. And if you push me without asking and I don't know you're coming, it actually is dangerous for me, I could fall. So, for me, it's really important that if you want help, it's okay to go ahead and ask" (Sanders 2015). By teaching more people about disability, Aly hopes to create more accessible and inclusive communities for people with disabilities.

Further Reading

JJ's List. 2017. "About jjslist.com." http://www.jjslist.com/pages/about/4.php.

Sanders, Hosea. 2015. "Group Spreads Awareness of Disability Interaction." http://abc7chicago.com/society/group-spreads-awareness-of-disability-interaction/840756/.

Vansickle, Abbie. 2002. "Struggling to Get in the Door." http://dailynorthwestern.com/2002/05/22/archive-manual/struggling-to-get-in-the-door/.

Patty Berne

Patty Berne is a disabled, queer, and Japanese-Haitian activist, writer, and filmmaker. Berne is the cofounder and director of Sins Invalid, a performance project that centers artists with disabilities, particularly those who are further marginalized by race, gender, and sexuality. Sins Invalid's performance work focuses on disability, beauty, and sexuality (Sins Invalid, n.d.).

In 2008, Berne wrote about the history and work of Sins Invalid in the anthology *Telling Stories to Change the Word*. In 2013, Berne produced the documentary film *Sins Invalid: An Unashamed Claim to Beauty*. The film exposed the work of Sins Invalid to a much wider audience and received international critical acclaim from the Kansai Queer Film Festival in Japan and the Inside Out Film Festival in Canada.

Berne's art and activism centers disability justice. She explains: "I think Disability Justice as a framework understands disability within a social justice context, understanding that we all live in multiple power relations. So, within white supremacy, within patriarchy, within capitalism, within heteronormativity, within enforced interbinaries . . . Structural oppressions interact with each other" (Disability Visibility Project 2015).

In 2009, the National Gay and Lesbian Task Force honored Berne with the Empress | Jose Sarria Award for Uncommon Leadership in the field of LGBTQI and disability rights.

Further Reading

Disability Visibility Project. 2015. "DVP Interview: Patty Berne and Alice Wong." https://disabilityvisibilityproject.com /2015/12/14/dvp-interview-patty-berne -and-alice-wong/.

Sins Invalid. n.d. "Mission." http://www.sinsin valid.org/mission.html.

Marca Bristo

Marca Bristo is a cofounder and the current president and chief executive officer (CEO) of Access Living, Chicago's center for independent living. In 1977, at age 23, Bristo became a quadriplegic in a diving accident and was treated at the Rehabilitation Institute of Chicago. Just two years later, Bristo played a key role in establishing Access Living and leading the newly formed

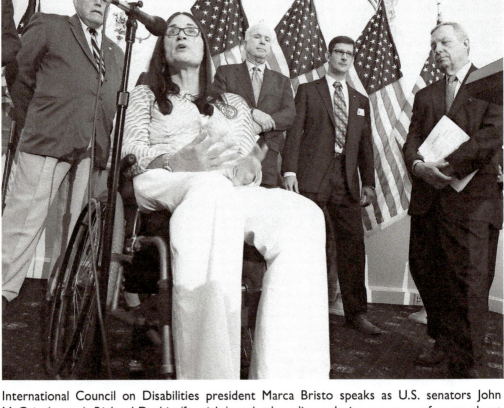

International Council on Disabilities president Marca Bristo speaks as U.S. senators John McCain (center), Richard Durbin (far right), and others listen during a news conference about the United Nations Convention on the Rights of Persons with Disabilities in Washington, D.C., on July 12, 2012. Bristo has helped to craft national and international reforms to protect the rights of people with disabilities. (Alex Wong/Getty Images)

independent living center. In her early years at Access Living, Bristo and other disability activists lobbied the Chicago Transit Authority (CTA) to ensure all buses were wheelchair accessible and fought to improve the accessibility of Chicago Public Schools (McKeough 2008).

Since her early activism in the late 1970s, Bristo has been an influential disability rights activist. She has been involved in implementing local, state, national, and international disability rights legislation and policies. As a member of the U.S. Task Force on the Rights and Empowerment of Americans with Disabilities, Bristo was instrumental in writing and passing the Americans with Disabilities Act of 1990. As a result, Bristo was bestowed with the Americans with Disabilities Act Award and the Distinguished Service Award of the President of the United States.

In 1994, Bristo was appointed as chair of the National Council on Disability, which is the entity that advises the president and Congress on disability policy. Bristo was the first disabled person to serve on the National Council on Disability in this capacity.

Later, Bristo took part in negotiation sessions for the United Nations Convention on the Rights of Persons with Disabilities (CRPD), which the United Nations adopted in 2006. Bristo currently serves as president of the U.S. International Council on Disabilities, which is a collection of U.S. disability rights organizations that seeks to support disability rights around the world. Bristo is leading a campaign that advocates for the United States to ratify the CRPD (Access Living 2014).

On the importance of disability advocacy, Bristo stated: "The things we've been advocating for are not just for a marginal group of people; they're for the society as a whole. Disability affects all of us. It's time that we normalize and accept it rather than perceive it to be at the margins of our society" (McKeough 2008). Bristo noted that her disability has played a role in her accomplishments and success, explaining, "That's part of the disability experience: taking risks and having a tenacious sense of can-do-it-ness" (McKeough 2008).

Further Reading

Access Living. 2014. "Marca Bristo, President & CEO: BIO." https://www.accessliving.org/138JK95.

McKeough, Kevin. 2008. "Spirit Triumphant." *Chicago Magazine*, January. http://www.chicagomag.com/Chicago-Magazine/January-2008/The-Transformers/Marca-Bristo/.

Lydia X. Z. Brown

Lydia X. Z. Brown is a genderqueer, transracially/transnationally adopted East Asian autistic activist, organizer, writer, speaker, and educator. Brown focuses on radical disability justice, with a particular emphasis on violence against multiply marginalized disabled people, including policing, abuse, institutionalization, and incarceration (Brown, n.d.).

Recalling how they became involved in activism, Brown stated:

A number of different scenes and events that . . . led to my work . . . included numerous cases of abuse of Autistic people, learning about the deaths of some Autistic people, learning about the existence of institutions like the Judge Rotenberg Center . . . learning about organizations like Autism Speaks . . . that claim to represent Autistic people in the complete absence of any Autistic leadership whatsoever. And the accumulation of all of these themes, all of

these . . . consistently recurring incidents of violence against people like
me—simply for having neurologies
like mine—led me to the conviction
that . . . I must [do] something to benefit
my community. (Brown, n.d.)

Brown served as an intern, project assistant, and policy analyst for the Autistic Self
Advocacy Network from 2013 to 2015. She
has also served as a legal intern for the Disability Law Center of Massachusetts and
as a Holley Law Fellow for the National
LGBTQ Task Force.

Brown is currently a public interest law
scholar at Northeastern University School
of Law. She is also the copresident of TASH
New England, a disability organization that
promotes social justice and human rights for
people with significant disabilities. Additionally, she is chair of the Massachusetts
Developmental Disabilities Council and
a board member of the Autism Women's
Network. In 2017, Brown received the Zola
Emerging Scholar Award from the Society
for Disability Studies.

Brown writes regularly about autism,
disability, and intersectional social justice
issues on their blog *Autistic Hoya*. Additionally, Brown was the lead editor of *All
the Weight of Our Dreams*, the first ever
anthology of writings and artwork by autistic people of color.

Further Reading

Brown, Lydia X. Z. n.d. "About." https://
autistichoya.net/bio/.

Lawrence Carter-Long

Lawrence Carter-Long is a disability activist and media critic. Carter-Long is currently
a public affairs specialist for the National

Council on Disability. Prior to working
with the National Council on Disability, he
served as the director of advocacy and the
executive director for the Disabilities Network of New York City.

Carter-Long is a well known and highly
sought expert on disability and media and
has been featured in the *New York Times*,
BBC, NBC's *The Today Show*, National
Public Radio, and CNN.

From 2006 to 2010, Carter-Long founded
and curated the disTHIS! Film Series,
which aimed to show disability "through
a whole new lens" and promoted films by
emerging filmmakers and performers that
broke stereotypes of disability (disTHIS!
Film Series 2010). "The disTHIS! Film
Series screened movies which evoked pride
instead of pity, character over charity and
direction rather than diagnosis. disTHIS!
screenings were funny, sexy and even a
little startling; always provocative, never
quite what you'd expect" (disTHIS! Film
Series 2010).

Carter-Long also produced and co-hosted
the New York City radio show *The Largest
Minority* and later curated and cohosted *The
Projected Image: A History of Disability in
Film* on the Turner Classic Movies network
(Harlan-Simmons, n.d.).

In 2016, Carter-Long coauthored a
groundbreaking report about media coverage of police-related killings of people
with disabilities. *The Ruderman White
Paper on Media Coverage of Law Enforcement Use of Force and Disability*, published by the Ruderman Family Foundation,
revealed that while up to half of people
killed by the police have disabilities, the
media largely ignores disability as a factor
(Ellis 2016).

Carter-Long has received a number
of awards recognizing his work, including from New York City mayor Michael

Bloomberg and from the American Association of People with Disabilities (Harlan-Simmons, n.d.)

Although critical of disability representation in mainstream media, Lawrence believes American culture is at a possible turning point. He explains:

We're at a very interesting time in our history and in our culture regarding the depictions of people with disabilities in the media. You don't have the teachers or the preachers or the social workers sort of pushing the agenda, but more and more there are opportunities—whether it's via the Internet, YouTube, Facebook—for people to blog, to put their own stories out there. And so I think what's happening now is we're seeing a change in the types of stories that are being told. . . . We're seeing more complexity in those stories, more depth in those stories, more authenticity in those stories, and as a result, we've become less lazy and they've become more interesting, because the nuances are all there in ways that we really haven't seen before. (Harlan-Simmons, n.d.)

Further Reading

disTHIS! Film Series. 2017. "disTHIS! Film Series." https://www.facebook.com/pg/disthis/about/?ref=page_internal.

Ellis, Justin. 2016. "Media Missing the Story: Half of All Recent High Profile Police-Related Killings Are People with Disabilities." http://www.rudermanfoundation.org/blog/in-the-media/media-missing-the-story-half-of-all-recent-high-profile-police-related-killings-are-people-with-disabilities.

Harlan-Simmons, Jane. n.d. "Lawrence Carter-Long on the Media, Arts, and Disability."

http://www.artsworkindiana.org/index.php?pageId=174&newsId=258.

Hyler, Steven E., Glen O. Gabbard, and I. Schneider. 1991. "Homicidal Maniacs and Narcissistic Parasites: Stigmatization of Mentally Ill Persons in the Movies." *Hospital and Community Psychiatry* 42, no. 10: 1044–48.

Judi Chamberlin (d. 20I0)

Judi Chamberlin was an activist and educator in the psychiatric survivors movement, which later evolved into the mad pride movement. In the 1960s, Chamberlin experienced a miscarriage and became severely depressed. Her doctors advised she seek treatment in a psychiatric hospital, and so she voluntarily admitted herself. However, after several voluntary admissions, Chamberlin was diagnosed with schizophrenia and subsequently involuntarily admitted (Shapiro 2010). Trapped in the psychiatric institution for five months, Chamberlin experienced numerous forms of abuse. She and other patients were secluded as a form of punishment for resistance, medicated against their will, and forbidden to leave the premises of the institution.

After being released, Chamberlin authored the book *On Our Own: Patient-Controlled Alternatives to the Mental Health System*, which advocated for humane and person-centered mental health treatment. She later collaborated with the National Council on Disability to coauthor the human rights report *From Privileges to Rights: People Labeled with Psychiatric Disabilities Speak for Themselves*. Chamberlin served as the cochair of the World Network of Users and Survivors of Psychiatry, and in this role, she advised the United Nations on disability from 2001 to 2014.

When asked what the most critical issue for people with psychiatric disabilities was, Chamberlin responded:

The issue of mental illness and violence. It's so linked in people's minds and it distorts what most people with psychiatric disabilities are like. Because while the research shows over and over again that people with psychiatric diagnoses are not more violent than anybody else, that's not what people believe, and it's hammered in all the time with crime shows—that this is what people with psychiatric disabilities are like—they're unpredictably violent in a way that justifies all this forced treatment. (Goldberg 2009)

Chamberlin is credited with promoting the reclaiming of the word "mad." According to Shapiro (2010), her work "changed [mad] from a word that was a pejorative word . . . [to a word] that was saying to the world at large: We are worthy individuals, and our minds our worthy, and they're to be respected."

Chamberlin passed away in 2010 at the age of 65, but her legacy lives on through the Mad Pride movement.

Further Reading

Goldberg, Carey. 2009. "A Talk with Judi Chamberlin." http://archive.boston.com/bostonglobe/ideas/articles/2009/03/22/a_talk_with_judi_chamberlain/.

Shapiro, Joseph. 2010. "Advocate for People with Mental Illnesses Dies." http://www.npr.org/templates/story/story.php?storyId=122706192.

Eli Clare

Eli Clare is a writer, speaker, activist, teacher, and poet who focuses on the intersections of gender, race, sexuality, and disability. Clare has written extensively about his experiences as a white, disabled, and genderqueer person. His work embraces intersectionality and discusses disability, queer and trans identities, the politics of the body, and social justice.

Clare has written two books of creative nonfiction. The first, *Exile and Pride: Disability, Queerness, and Liberation*, was first published in 1999 and was a finalist for the ForeWord's Book of the Year Award in 2009. The second, *Brilliant Imperfection: Grappling with Cure*, was published in 2017. Clare has also written a collection of poetry, *The Marrow's Telling: Words in Motion*, which was a Lambda Literary Award finalist in 2008. Clare travels around the United States providing multimedia talks, trainings, workshops, classroom presentations, lectures, keynotes, readings, and retreats to university and community groups.

Clare advocates for the power of storytelling as a way of countering shame and social oppression. He stated: "A politics that resists shame can emerge from . . . storytelling. So much of what we know in various communities about resistance has come through story. It is through listening to and collecting stories that we begin to notice oppression patterns and systems and develop strategies of rebellion and resistance" (Fritsch 2009).

In addition to his scholarly pursuits, Clare is heavily involved in activism. In the late 1980s, he walked almost 4,000 miles across the United States over eight and a half months for global nuclear disarmament. He credits the experience with teaching him about intersectional politics and direct action. He explained; "We ended up talking to people we would never have had access to otherwise. It was an important set of lessons to learn about how to bring people together to have challenging conversations" (Fritsch 2009).

Clare has also coordinated a rape prevention program, assisted in organizing the inaugural Queerness and Disability Conference, and led workshops that seek to challenge white supremacy in disabled communities and the disability rights movement.

Further Reading

Fritsch, Kelly. 2009. "Resisting Easy Answers: An Interview with Eli Clare." *Upping the Anti* no. 9. http://uppingtheanti.org/journal/article/09-resisting-easy-answers/.

Rebecca Cokley

Rebecca Cokley is a disability rights activist who has influenced the direction of modern disability-related policies and practices. Her activism is closely informed by her disability experience and identity. Cokley was born with achondroplasia, the most common form of dwarfism, which has also affected the past three generations of her family. After graduating from the University of California Santa Cruz with a BA in political science in 2001, Cokley started her career with the Institute for Educational Leadership, where she developed resources for youth with disabilities. In 2009, Cokley was appointed to the Obama administration and served in a variety of roles in the Office of Special Education and Rehabilitative Services, the Presidential Personnel Office, and the Administration for Community Living. She continued her service to the executive office as the executive director of the National Council on Disability from 2013 until 2017.

Cokley was inducted into the Susan M. Daniels Disability Mentoring Hall of Fame in 2015, on the 25th anniversary of the Americans with Disabilities Act, to honor her contributions to the field of disability rights. Currently, Cokley serves as a senior fellow for the Center for American Progress, where she continues to focus on disability-related policy. Cokley has also shared her expertise through numerous opinion articles in the *Washington Post*, CNN, and Talk Poverty. These pieces address a wide range of topics that affect disability: family building, genetic editing, and the problematic, colloquial use of terms related to mental illness to discredit others. In her CNN opinion piece addressing her personal and familial experiences, Cokley said:

> I am who I am because I have dwarfism. Dwarfs share a rich culture, as do most disability groups. We have traditions, common language and histories rich in charismatic ancestors. I can honestly say that I may not have been able to work in the White House doing diversity recruitment for President Barack Obama had I not been born a little person. It allowed me to understand discrimination, isolation and society's lowered expectations. (Cokley 2017)

Further Reading

Cokley, Rebecca. 2017. "Please Don't Edit Me Out." *Washington Post*, August 10. https://www.washingtonpost.com/opinions/if-we-start-editing-genes-people-like-me-might-not-exist/2017/08/10/e9adf206-7d27-11e7-a669-b400c5c7e1cc_story.html?noredirect=on&utm_term=.37279dd5075d.

Diane Coleman

Diane Coleman, JD, is the president, CEO, and founder of Not Dead Yet. Coleman is a person with neuromuscular disabilities, and she has been a wheelchair user since childhood. Coleman established Not Dead Yet in 1996, to ensure that disability perspectives were represented in debates about assisted suicide and euthanasia and to oppose the legalization of these practices.

Not Dead Yet contends that assisted suicide and euthanasia are "deadly forms of discrimination against old, ill, and disabled people" (Not Dead Yet 2017a). Not Dead Yet argues that assisted suicide is discriminatory because our culture devalues life with a disability. Consequently, disabled people are encouraged by physicians, health insurance companies, family members, and society at large to engage in assisted suicide, whereas nondisabled people who express a desire to die typically receive suicide prevention and support. Coleman and other members of Not Dead Yet advocate for society to support disabled people's lives rather than their deaths.

Coleman is a highly regarded speaker and writer on assisted suicide and euthanasia. She has authored numerous op-eds and articles for local, regional, and national outlets, including the *Chicago Tribune* and the *Wall Street Journal* (Not Dead Yet 2017b). She also has been featured as a guest on national television news broadcasts for ABC, CBS, CNN, MSNBC, and NPR (Not Dead Yet 2017b).

Coleman has testified four times before subcommittees of the U.S. House of Representatives and Senate (Not Dead Yet 2017b). Additionally, she has coauthored amicus briefs, which are legal documents that advise courts of additional perspectives or arguments. These briefs were written on behalf of Not Dead Yet and other national disability rights organizations and were filed in numerous state courts and in the U.S. Supreme Court.

Prior to founding Not Dead Yet in 1996, Coleman was the director of advocacy at the Center for Disability Rights in Rochester, New York, for 3 years and was the executive director of Progress Center for Independent Living in Forest Park, Illinois, for 12 years (Not Dead Yet 2017b). Coleman has also served as an adjunct faculty member at the University of Illinois at Chicago and taught graduate courses in disability ethics.

Further Reading

Not Dead Yet. 2017a. "Who We Are." http://notdeadyet.org/about.

Not Dead Yet. 2017b. "Not Dead Yet-Staff." http://notdeadyet.org/about/staff.

Kitty Cone (1944–2015)

Kitty Cone was a civil rights and disability rights activist who focused on policy and law reform to support long-term change. Cone was diagnosed with muscular dystrophy (MS) around the age of 15, after previously being misdiagnosed with cerebral palsy and polio. She reported experiencing extensive discrimination at boarding schools in her youth and at a university as a young adult. In addition to these experiences, Cone noted that exposure to racial segregation in her youth while living in Georgia further fueled her political activism. Cone went on to organize massive protests regarding racial segregation, women's rights, and the Vietnam War. Her extensive résumé of political organizing skills impressed Ed Roberts, and Cone was offered a position with the Center for Independent Living shortly after moving to California in 1974 (Cone 1996–1998).

Cone may be best known for her organization and participation in the San Francisco 504 sit-in in 1977. In 1973, Section 504 of the Rehabilitation Act was signed into law, providing people with disabilities federal civil rights protection for the first time. The Department of Health and Education Welfare (HEW) was tasked with producing regulations, defining both disability and discrimination, for this law to be effective. The HEW produced a draft of proposed regulations in 1977 when the Carter presidency began. Delayed publication and leaked information concerning a review of these regulations revealed that changes that weakened the mandate had been installed. As a result, the American Coalition of Citizens with Disabilities (ACCD) called for sit-ins in eight HEW headquarters. Cone was a key leader, organizer, and participant in the 28-day sit-in that took place in the San Francisco HEW building. She forged coalitions and garnered community support, allowing demonstrators to sustain their efforts long past any of the sit-ins at other HEW headquarters. The persistence of Cone and her fellow demonstrators eventually paid off when the HEW secretary, Joseph Califano, signed the original, unchanged regulations for implementation. Cone reflected on this experience in the documentary *The Power of 504*: "The signing of the regulations signified the public birth of the disability rights movement. It ushered in an era of disability activism, empowerment, and legislative victories based on the legal concepts of nondiscrimination and integration embodied in Section 504." (Disability Rights Education and Defense Fund 2015).

See also *Primary Documents*: Kitty Cone's "Short History of the 504 Sit In" for the Twentieth Anniversary of the Sit In (1997)

Further Reading

Disability Rights Education and Defense Fund. 2015. "Celebrating Kitty Cone: 1944–2015." https://dredf.org/2015/03/25 /celebrating-kitty-cone-1944-2015/.

Vladimir Cuk

Vladimir Cuk is a disability advocate and scholar. He currently serves as the executive director for the International Disability Alliance (IDA). The IDA comprises more than 1,100 organizations of people with disabilities and their allies across eight global and six regional networks (International Disability Alliance, n.d.). These organizations work together to "promote the rights of persons with disabilities across the United Nations' efforts to advance human rights and sustainable development" (International Disability Alliance, n.d.). The foundation of the IDA's efforts is the United Nations Convention on the Rights of Persons with Disabilities (CRPD), which is a human rights treaty that aims to provide and protect the rights of persons with disabilities throughout the world. Cuk is also involved in the implementation of the United Nations' 2030 Agenda on Sustainable Development, which is a framework that seeks to end extreme poverty, promote peace, protect the human rights of all people, and care for the planet (United Nations Population Fund 2015).

Cuk has a long history of advocacy for the rights of people with disabilities. Prior to serving with the IDA, Cuk was the director of the Association of Students with Disabilities of Serbia, which focused on youth with disabilities in Serbia and four other countries in southeastern Europe. In this role, he promoted the rights of youth with disabilities, focusing specifically on providing access to education and eliminating architectural barriers.

Cuk received a master's of science in disability and human development from the University of Illinois at Chicago. He speaks at international meetings and forums to include the perspectives of people with disabilities in human rights discussions at the local, national, and international levels.

Further Reading

International Disability Alliance. n.d. "Who We Are." http://www.internationaldisability alliance.org/about.

United Nations Population Fund. 2015. "Transforming Our World: The 2030 Agenda for Sustainable Development. http://www .unfpa.org/resources/transforming -our-world-2030-agenda-sustainable -development.

Justin Dart Jr. (1930–2002)

Justin Whitlock Dart Jr. is widely regarded as an icon within the disability rights movement and is often remembered as the "father" of the Americans with Disabilities Act (ADA). Dart came from a wealthy background, as his father was the president of Dart Industries and his grandfather founded Walgreens. Dart himself was a successful entrepreneur, having established several businesses in Mexico and Japan in

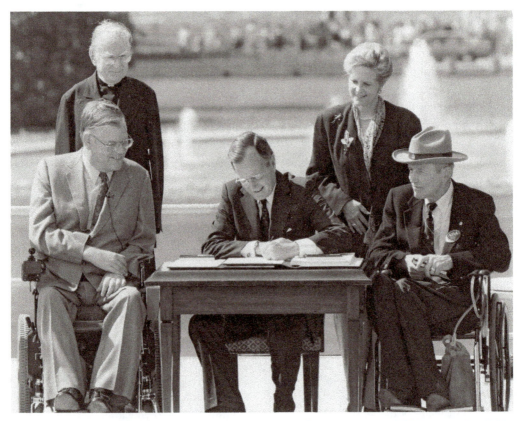

President George H. W. Bush signs the Americans with Disabilities Act of 1990, on July 26, 1990, in Washington, D.C. Standing (left to right) are Reverend Harold Wilkie and Sandra Parrino of the National Council on Disability, and seated (left to right) are Evan Kemp, chairman of the Equal Employment and Opportunity Commission, President Bush, and Justin Dart Jr., chairman of the President's Committee on the Employment of People with Disabilities. Dart is often referred to as the "father" of the ADA for his advocacy in creating the civil rights legislation. (Fotosearch/Getty Images)

the 1950s and 1960s. During these ventures, he advocated for the rights of women and people with disabilities. Dart eventually left the business world in 1967, devoting the entirety of his time to human rights causes.

Dart's political interests were informed by his disability identity. After contracting polio at the age of 18, Dart experienced paralysis in his lower body and became a wheelchair user. Dart worked for various state and federal disability commissions and was appointed the vice chair of the National Council on Disability in 1981 by President Ronald Reagan. During his tenure as vice chair, Dart and his wife undertook a "Road to Freedom" expedition. Dart traveled to every state and interviewed individuals with disabilities to better understand what they wanted from the U.S. government. The feedback provided by these citizens was used to draft a national policy that called for the protection of civil rights of people with disabilities. This policy draft was the foundation for the landmark Americans with Disabilities Act of 1990 (ADA).

Dart worked at the federal level in a number of capacities, leading the Rehabilitation Services Administration and chairing the Congressional Task Force on the Rights and Empowerment of Americans with Disabilities. While working with the government, Dart was known to vocalize criticism of agencies and their approaches to policy development. After the ADA was signed in 1990, Dart supported the development of organizations devoted to disability rights. Notably, he founded Justice for All in 1993 and was among multiple founders of the American Association of People with Disabilities in 1995. Dart was awarded the Presidential Medal of Freedom from President Bill Clinton in 1998 for his extensive contributions to the disability community and the United States. Up until his passing,

Dart worked on a political manifesto on empowerment. Some of his last written words included the following: "I call for solidarity among all who love justice, all who love life, to create a revolution that will empower every single human being to govern his or her life, to govern the society and to be fully productive of life quality for self and for all" (Fay and Pelka 2002).

Further Reading

Fay, Fred, and Fred Pelka. 2002. "Disability Rights Hero Completes His Mission; Justin Dart Obituary." *Ability Magazine.* https://abilitymagazine.com/JustinDart _remembered.html.

Peter Dinklage

Peter Dinklage is an American actor best known for his role as Tyrion Lannister in *Game of Thrones*. In the beginning of his career, Dinklage found himself frustrated with the limited roles available to someone with dwarfism, as the roles were typically limited to elf or leprechaun (Kois 2012). He was able to finally break into acting after playing a lead in the independent film *The Station Agent*, which won the Audience Award at Sundance (Kois 2012).

Dinklage won two Emmy Awards for Outstanding Supporting Actor in a Drama Series and a Golden Globe Award for Best Supporting Actor for his role in *Game of Thrones*. He appreciates the role, not only because of its success, but also because the character he plays turns stereotypes of little people "on its head. No beard, no pointy shoes, a romantic, real human being" (Kois 2012).

Dinklage has used his platform to be an outspoken disability activist, particularly critical of treatment of people of short stature. He explains that little people "are still the butt of jokes. It's one of the last bastions of acceptable prejudice. Not just by people who've had too much to drink in England and want to throw a person. But by media, everything" (Kois 2012).

Further Reading

Kois, Dan. 2012. "Peter Dinklage Was Smart to Say No." http://www.nytimes.com /2012/04/01/magazine/peter-dinklage -was-smart-to-say-no.html.

Carlos Drazen (d. 2011)

Carlos Drazen was a disability studies scholar and activist. As a black disabled woman, Drazen advocated for the field of disability studies to explore the intersections between race and disability.

During her childhood, Drazen lived in an institution for children with disabilities in Chicago, Illinois. When the institution closed, the building was acquired by University of Illinois at Chicago (UIC), and it became the Department of Disability and Human Development. As an adult, Drazen became a student in the Department of Disability and Human Development, and she studied and researched in the same building in which she was once institutionalized. Drazen earned a master's of science in disability and human development, and she was working on her doctorate in disability studies when she suddenly passed away in 2011.

Drazen was a dedicated scholar and activist. "Her special passion was grappling with issues of race and disability, mixed identities, injustices of all forms, and always asking the very big questions" (Department of Disability and Human Development 2017). She served two terms on the board of Access Living, Chicago's independent living center (Access Living 2011). As a board member,

Drazen provided direction and feedback on many of Access Living's programs and initiatives, particularly those involving disabled communities of color (Access Living 2011). Drazen also published a chapter, "Both Sides of the Two-Sided Coin: Rehabilitation of Disabled African American Soldiers," in the seminal disability studies text *Blackness and Disability.*

Drazen's memory, vision, and passion are recognized and honored through the Carlos Drazen Memorial Scholarship. This scholarship is awarded to a graduate student in the Department of Disability and Human Development at UIC who studies the intersections of race and disability (Department of Disability and Human Development 2017).

Further Reading

Access Living. 2011. "In Memory of Board Member Carlos Drazen." https://www .accessliving.org/118ga49.

Department of Disability and Human Development. 2017. "Drazen Scholarship Application Open." https://ahs.uic.edu/inside-ahs /news/drazen-scholarship-application -open/.

Tammy Duckworth (1968–)

Dr. Tammy Duckworth is a U.S. senator who represents Illinois. She was born in Thailand to a Thai and Chinese mother and an American father. Her family eventually moved to Hawaii, where she graduated from high school and earned her bachelor's degree in political science from the University of Hawaii.

In 1990, while working toward a master's degree in international affairs from George Washington University, Duckworth joined the Army Reserve Officers' Training Corps. In 1992, she was recognized as

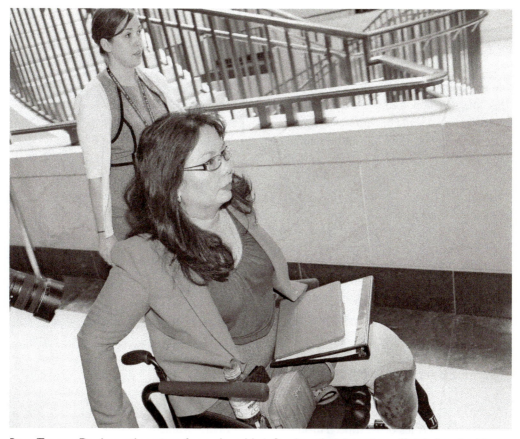

Rep. Tammy Duckworth arrives for a closed briefing by administration officials for the House Armed Services Committee and the Intelligence Committee on Syria on September 9, 2013, in the Capitol Building in Washington, D.C. (Mandel Ngan/AFP/Getty Images)

a commissioned officer, and she decided to pursue a job as a helicopter pilot, as it was one of the only combat positions open to women. Duckworth later transferred to the Army National Guard. In 2004, while working toward a doctorate in political science at Northern Illinois University, Duckworth was deployed to Iraq. When a helicopter she was copiloting was struck by a rocket-propelled grenade, Duckworth lost both her legs and became a double amputee. As a result of the incident, she received a Purple Heart and was promoted to major (Duckworth, n.d.).

In 2006, Duckworth was the Democratic nominee in Illinois for the U.S. House of Representatives but lost to her Republican opponent. She was then appointed director of the Illinois Department of Veteran Affairs. During her tenure as director, she created programs for veterans with brain injury and post-traumatic stress disorder (PTSD). In 2009, President Barack Obama nominated Duckworth to be an assistant secretary at the U.S. Department of Veteran Affairs (Duckworth, n.d.). In 2012, Duckworth ran again for U.S. House of Representatives and won, becoming the first disabled woman and first person born in Thailand to be elected to Congress. As a representative, Duckworth served on the Committee for Armed Services and the Committee on Oversight and Government Reform.

In 2015, Duckworth retired from the army as a lieutenant colonel and finished her doctorate in human services. She then began campaigning for U.S. Senate. Her contentious race with incumbent Mark Kirk became a national controversy when Kirk made remarks about her ethnic background. Duckworth won the race and became the second Asian American woman senator in U.S. history.

Further Reading

Blahovec, Sarah. 2017. "Someone Should Help Disabled People Run for Office." *NOS Magazine*. http://nosmag.org/someone-should-help-disabled-people-run-for-office/.

Duckworth, Tammy. n.d. "Meet Tammy." http://tammyduckworth.com/meet-tammy/.

Roger Ebert (1942–2013)

Roger Ebert is widely considered one of the greatest film critics of all time. Throughout his career, he worked as a journalist, television host, screenwriter, and author. In 2002 and 2003, Ebert underwent treatment for cancer in his thyroid and salivary glands. In 2006, his cancer returned in his jaw. After having part of his jaw removed, Ebert began using a computerized voice system to communicate.

After becoming disabled, Ebert continued to work as a film critic. Access Living, the independent living center in Chicago, noted, "By continuing the work he loved after acquiring a disability, Ebert sent a message to the world that disability is a natural part of life that will impact everyone in some way at some point in his or her life. Just as important, Ebert sent the message that disability doesn't change who we areand doesn't stop us from pursuing what we love" (Access Living 2013).

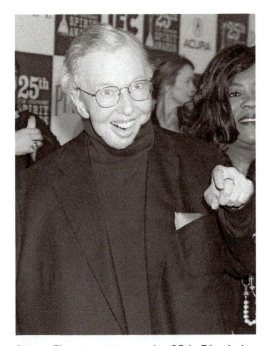

Roger Ebert arriving at the 25th Film Independent Spirit Awards, in Los Angeles, California, on March 5, 2010. (Carrienelsonl/Dreamstime.com)

Ebert worked to make it known that disability is a part of humanity. He once stated, "I consider empathy to be the cornerstone of our existence as human beings. It allows us to place ourselves in the place of another person, and care about what it means to live in their shoes. Too many people look at a disabled person and think that whatever they see defines that person. That doesn't even begin to tell us who that person is, and what they are capable of" (Access Living 2013).

Due to his contributions and influence, Ebert was named the most powerful pundit in America by *Forbes* magazine in 2007. He also is the only film critic in history to receive a star on the Hollywood Walk of Fame. Ebert continued to use his platform to speak out on disability issues and promote the work of fellow disability rights advocates until his death in 2013.

Further Reading

Access Living. 2013. "Access Living Mourns Loss of Roger Ebert." https://www .accessliving.org/118ga316.

Mike Ervin

Mike Ervin is a Chicago-based writer and disability activist, well known for his *Smart Ass Cripple* blog and books, as well as his leadership in organizing protests against the Jerry Lewis telethons. Ervin has muscular dystrophy (MD), and at the age of six years, he and his sister served as poster children for the Jerry Lewis telethon. This annual event (1966–2010) raised money for the Muscular Dystrophy Association (MDA) by showcasing children with MD (referred to as "Jerry's kids") in a tragic light and eliciting viewer sympathy. As an adult, Ervin started the organization Jerry's Orphans to oppose the telethons and their presentation of people with MD as pitiable. He organized picket protests of the event starting in 1991 and continued them for over a decade. These efforts are detailed in the documentary *The Kids Are All Right*, in which Ervin explains, "Doing something is always better than doing nothing. If you get one person to listen that's accomplishing something." The Jerry Lewis telethon was eventually rebranded and later discontinued altogether.

In addition to founding Jerry's Orphans, Ervin founded the Chicago chapter of ADAPT and served on the board of directors for Access Living and the Council for Disability Rights. Ervin has written multiple plays and short stories and has had more than 1,000 articles and essays published with a variety of news outlets. He is a regular contributor to The Progressive, a news forum dedicated to championing progressive politics. For his personal blog, *Smart Ass Cripple*, and his associated books, *Smart Ass Cripple's Little Red Book* (2011) and *Smart Ass Cripple's Little Yellow Book* (2012), Ervin relied on a sarcastic brand of humor to capture the attention of readers and drive home points related to political, civil, and disability rights.

Further Reading

Smart Ass Cripple. n.d. http://smartasscripple .blogspot.com/.

Fred Fay (1944–2011)

Dr. Frederick Fay was a respected disability rights advocate and key organizer of disability communities throughout his lifetime. Fay sustained a spinal cord injury at the age of 16 and subsequently began using a wheelchair. Twenty years later, a cyst developed on Fay's brain stem, and he traded his wheelchair for a motorized bed that allowed him to remain flat on his back. Fay discussed ideas about disability community and identity in a 1998 *Boston Globe* edition, where he explained, "Disability is an equal opportunity . . . anyone can qualify at any moment" (Disability Action Center 2011).

Shortly after he became a wheelchair user, Fay cofounded a counseling and information center for people with disabilities called Opening Doors. This development was the first of many in Fay's lifetime. In 1963, Fay codeveloped the Washington Architectural Barriers Project with a mission of making the Washington, D.C., public transport systems accessible for all people. His activism greatly influenced the passing of the Architectural Barriers Act of 1968. Fay's political impact was extensive. He promoted the passing of Section 503/504 of the Rehabilitation Act of 1973, the Individuals with Disabilities Education Act in 1975, and the Americans with Disabilities Act in 1990.

Fay cofounded the Boston Center for Independent Living in 1974 and acted as the director of research and training at Tufts University's Department of Rehabilitation Medicine. Among all his accomplishments, Fay was heralded for being an effective communicator who could bring people of diverse communities together. This strength is best illustrated by his development of the Massachusetts Coalition of Citizens with Disabilities and the larger American Coalition of Citizens with Disabilities. Fay was also a strong proponent of the movement toward improved assistive technology. His efforts and achievements were publicly recognized when he was awarded the Henry B. Betts Award in 1998.

Further Reading

Disability Action Center. 2011. "Fred Fay." https://actionctr.org/resources/profiles-in -courage/fred-fay/.

Lex Frieden

Lex Frieden is a disability rights activist and professor who was instrumental in conceiving and drafting the Americans with Disabilities Act of 1990 (ADA). The ADA is largely considered the most important antidiscrimination law for people with disabilities in the United States.

In the 1970s, a few years after acquiring a spinal cord injury, Frieden became involved in the independent living movement, working closely with other disability activists considered severely disabled. In the 1980s, Frieden served as executive director of the National Council on the Handicapped (now the National Council on Disability), an independent federal agency that provides policy recommendations to Congress and the president. As executive director, Frieden oversaw the drafting of the ADA (Frieden, n.d.).

From 2002 to 2006, Frieden returned to the National Council on Disability once President George W. Bush appointed him as the agency's chair. He later went on to serve on the United Nations Panel of Experts on Standard Rules for Disability and became president of Rehabilitation International (Frieden, n.d.).

Frieden is currently a professor of biomedical informatics and professor of physical medicine and rehabilitation at the University of Texas Health Science Center at Houston, as well as an adjunct professor of physical medicine and rehabilitation at Baylor College of Medicine (Frieden, n.d.). He is also the director of the Independent Living Research Utilization Program (ILRU), which is a research, training, and technical assistance program for people with disabilities and seniors (Frieden, n.d.).

Frieden has been widely recognized for his work improving the status of persons with disabilities around the world. He has been honored with two Presidential Citations for his involvement in disability rights, and he received the Henry B. Betts Award in 1998 for "efforts that significantly improve the quality of life for people with disabilities" (Frieden, n.d.).

Further Reading

Frieden, Lex. n.d. "Lex Frieden." http:// lexfrieden.com/_lfrieden/lex1.html.

Haben Girma

Haben Girma is a civil rights lawyer, a disability activist, and the first Deafblind woman to graduate from Harvard Law School. Girma became a civil rights lawyer to help expand access to digital information, including books, for people with disabilities. Girma recognizes her experiences as the daughter of refugees, a black woman, and a person with disabilities as assets in her pathway to success.

Girma was inspired to litigate civil rights law after an experience in college. Although nondisabled people often take the everyday choice of what to eat for granted, Girma was denied the opportunity to do so because her college provided her with a plate of food rather than allowing her to choose what she would like to eat. Initially, although she was not happy about possibly missing out on foods like chocolate cake, Girma hesitated to take action about the issue. Demanding menu choice felt trivial to her, especially in relation to her mother's experiences as a refugee from Eritrea. She explained, "I'd grown up hearing stories about the war in Eritrea, limited resources, people struggling to survive. It was hard for me to make a fuss about access to cafeteria menus. At the same time, I realized after months of not getting access that if I didn't do anything, other students with disabilities would face a similar barrier" (Shapiro 2015). Girma explained to the cafeteria managers that under the Americans with Disabilities Act, a reasonable accommodation was required to ensure she had access to the same choices as nondisabled students. The managers complied, and Girma experienced firsthand the importance of enforcing the ADA and other civil rights laws.

After Girma graduated from Harvard Law School, she began practicing as a disability rights attorney. In a recent case, she represented the National Federation of the Blind in a lawsuit that sought to require the digital library Scribd to ensure that its software and services were accessible. The court ruled in favor of the National Federation of the Blind, and Scribd agreed to make all documents and books accessible. After the victory, Girma stated, "Working on this groundbreaking case to help blind readers gain access to books was one of the most rewarding moments in my legal career" (Girma, n.d.).

Girma has been named a Champion of Change by President Barack Obama, a BBC Women of Africa Hero, and a Forbes 30 under 30 Leader. She was also selected to introduce President Obama at the ceremony marking the 25th anniversary of the Americans with Disabilities Act. Girma continues to work advocating for the rights of people with disabilities.

Further Reading

Girma, Haben. n.d. "Frequently Asked Questions." https://habengirma.com/faq/.

Shapiro, Joseph. 2015. "She Owes Her Activism to a Brave Mom, the ADA and Chocolate Cake." http://www.npr.org/sections/goatsandsoda/2015/07/31/428075935/she-owes-her-activism-to-a-brave-mom-the-ada-and-chocolate-cake.

Temple Grandin (1947–)

Temple Grandin is an autistic educator, scientist, and author. Named one of the 100 most influential people in the world by *Time* magazine in 2010, Grandin has written and lectured extensively about her experiences as an autistic person. Grandin is recognized as one of the first well-known people to publicly disclose she was autistic (Silberman 2015). Additionally, Grandin has published several books about how she views the world as an autistic person and what she experiences with autism. Her efforts to educate others about autism have served to address some of the stigma, prejudice, and discrimination autistic people face.

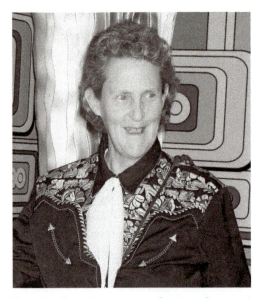

Temple Grandin is a professor of animal science and an expert on animal welfare in large-scale farming operations. She is also a spokeswoman for autism and a best-selling author. (Carrienelsonl/Dreamstime.com)

Grandin emphasizes the importance of neurodiversity, stating, "The world is going to need . . . different kinds of minds to work together" (Grandin 2010).

Grandin, who has a doctorate in animal science, initially rose to prominence in the scientific and animal farming community because of her contributions to the improvement of livestock farms and slaughterhouses. Grandin has described the ways autism affects how she experiences the world. Rather than process information verbally, she processes it visually. This way of thinking allowed her to better understand the experiences of farm animals and provide recommendations to make farms and slaughterhouses more humane. She also designed livestock-handling equipment and created an animal welfare and productivity scoring system to assess animal well-being (Grandin, n.d.). Her equipment and rating scale have been adopted by many large corporations.

As an autistic person, Grandin has served as a subject of curiosity and fascination for many people. She has been the focus of several television programs and movies, including an Emmy Award–winning semi-biographical HBO film. However, Grandin is a contentious figure within the autistic community. Some autistic people have criticized Grandin for overgeneralizing the experiences of autistic people, not accurately portraying autism, and supporting applied behavioral analysis, a controversial form of therapy widely accepted in the scientific community.

Further Reading

Grandin, Temple. 2010. "The World Needs All Kinds of Minds." Filmed February. TED video. https://www.ted.com/talks/temple _grandin_the_world_needs_all_kinds _of_minds.

Grandin, Temple. n.d. "Biography: Temple Grandin, Ph.D." http://www.grandin.com /temple.html.

Silberman, Steve. 2015. *NeuroTribes: The Legacy of Autism and the Future of Neurodiversity.* New York: Avery Publishing.

Laura Hershey (1962–2010)

Laura Hershey was a widely published poet, accomplished consultant, and persistent activist known for her commentary on women's and disability rights. Born with a form of muscular dystrophy (MD), Laura grew up using a wheelchair. She achieved a bachelor's degree in history from Colorado College and went on to earn a master's degree in creative writing from Antioch University in Los Angeles, California. A significant portion of Hershey's written work involved themes concerning the preservation of dignity.

"You Get Proud by Practicing" is one of Hershey's most famous works; throughout seven stanzas, this poem encourages people to be proud of themselves, despite social standards and norms. In it, Hershey writes, "You do not need / To be able to walk, or see, or hear, / Or use big, complicated words, / Or do any of those things that you just can't do / To be proud." In addition to poetry, Hershey published the book *Survival Strategies for Going Abroad: A Guide for People with Disabilities*, as well as numerous news columns. In one such column, "From Poster Child to Protester," Hershey details her experiences being used as a poster child for the Jerry Lewis Telethon and later protesting the annual event. The Jerry Lewis Telethon (1966–2010), later called the Love Network (2011) and the MDA Show of Strength (2012–2014), was an annual event that raised money for the Muscular Dystrophy Association (MDA). Disability rights activists, such as Hershey, criticized the event for painting the experience of MD as tragic and presenting people with MD as indebted to the charitable acts of strangers (Hershey 1997). Hershey was cited for trespassing in a 2001 protest of the event.

Hershey engaged in a wide range of activism. She was associated with organizations such as ADAPT and Not Dead Yet, and she advocated for the improvement of community-based services and increased visibility of LGBTQ persons with disabilities, among other topics. In 1998, Hershey was awarded the President's Award from the Committee on Employment of People with Disabilities.

See also *Primary Documents*: Laura Hershey's Poem *"You Get Proud by Practicing"*

Further Reading

Hershey, Laura. 1997. "From Poster Child to Protester." *Spectacle*, Spring/Summer. https://www.independentliving.org/docs4/hershey93.html.

Judy Heumann

Judith "Judy" Heumann is an internationally recognized American disability rights activist. Heumann was raised in New York City by two Jewish immigrant parents. When she was 18 months old, she contracted polio, and she has used a wheelchair for much of her life. Heumann was initially exposed to advocacy after her local public school prohibited her from attending, claiming her wheelchair created a fire hazard. Heumann's mother contested the school's decision, and Heumann was finally able to start attending a segregated school for people with disabilities in fourth grade. Although Heumann is critical of segregated camps and schools for children with disabilities, she also recognizes that these experiences allowed her to create community with other disabled children and encouraged her to begin thinking about organizing and activism (Disabled in Action, n.d.).

After completing her K–12 education, Heumann attended Long Island University, where she majored in speech and minored in education. Heumann aspired to become a teacher but faced disability discrimination in the educational system yet again when the New York State Teaching Board would not grant her a teaching license, claiming that she "failed" the medical examination because of her disability. Heumann successfully sued the board and became the first wheelchair user to teach in New York City public schools (Disabled in Action, n.d.).

In 1970, Heumann cofounded the activist group Disabled in Action. She stated:

We were really interested in looking at creating something that had the influence of younger people more, that was more cross disability and that really dealt more with the issues that we had been discussing since we were kids. . . . One of the important parts of the Independent Living Movement [is] we see ourselves as being a part of society. . . . It is the ability to come together as disabled people and be supportive of each other and really articulate what the problems are and what the solutions to those problems are and then work on removing the barriers. So it is a rights movement. (Disabled in Action n.d.)

After a few years, Heumann left teaching to fully commit to disability rights activism and disability policy. From 1975 to 1982, she served as the deputy director for the Independent Living Center in Berkeley, California, the first independent living center for people with disabilities in the world. During that time, she played an instrumental role in the sit-ins at the U.S. Department of Health, Education, and Welfare (HEW) offices in San Francisco and around the nation. The protests eventually led to the signing of the regulations of Section 504 of the Rehabilitation Act, which was the first antidiscrimination legislation for people with disabilities. In 1983, Heumann cofounded the World Institute on Disabilities, and she served as the codirector until 1993. From 1993 to 2001, she worked as the assistant secretary to Office of Special Education and Rehabilitation Services for the United States. From 2002 to 2006, she was the first ever adviser on disability and developments to the World Bank. In 2010, under the Obama administration, Heumann was appointed as special adviser for international disability rights for the U.S. State Department. She served in this role until 2017.

Heumann assisted in drafting the Education for All Handicapped Children Act (now the Individuals with Disabilities Education Act) and contributed to writing the regulations that would eventually become the Americans with Disabilities Act. Heumann has won numerous awards and accolades for her national and international disability rights activism and contributions to policy.

See also *Primary Documents*: Remarks of Judith E. Heumann, Assistant Secretary, U.S. Department of Education, at the White House upon the Signing of the Individuals with Disabilities Education Act (IDEA) (1997)

Further Reading

Disabled in Action. n.d. "A Discussion with Judy Heumann on Independent Living." http://www.disabledinaction.org/heumann.html.

Stevie and Annie Hopkins

Stevie and Annie Hopkins are siblings with disabilities who founded 3E Love, which is "a social entrepreneurial experiment to change the perception of disability" (3E Love, n.d.). 3E represents the company's mission, which is to educate, embrace, and empower. The company designs and prints T-shirts, stickers, bracelets, and other merchandise with 3E Love's trademarked International Symbol of Acceptance, also referred to as the Wheelchair Heart. The logo depicts a traditional wheelchair symbol but replaces the typical wheel with a heart.

Annie Hopkins initially designed the logo in 2004 for a residence hall T-shirt while she and Stevie were undergraduate students at the University of Illinois. Later, Annie had the symbol tattooed on her shoulder.

After many disabled activists praised the tattoo, Annie and Stevie realized it represented a powerful symbol, and they decided to form 3E Love in 2007. According to 3E Love, "The symbol is an attitude and a lifestyle. It's accepting one's abilities and rallying around that diversity and turning it into strength. It's loving and living life to the fullest no matter who you are and what you look like, no matter what you can or cannot do" (2011).

Sadly, just two years after the venture began, Annie passed away suddenly in 2009 at age 24. Stevie was determined to continue Annie's legacy and celebrate her passion for advocacy and disability studies. In order to encourage disability scholars, he established the Annie Hopkins Scholarship at the University of Illinois at Chicago and at the University of Illinois Urbana-Champaign. Also, he continued to build the 3E company and spread Annie's symbol of acceptance and diversity. Since then, 3E Love has sold merchandise with the International Symbol of Acceptance to tens of thousands of people from all around the world.

As another tribute to his sister, Stevie designated January 20 as the International Day of Acceptance in 2010. "Acceptance is created from an Empowered movement that Educates others to Embrace diversity and Love Life by seeing beyond abilities" (3E Love, n.d.). Eight years later, the movement continues and has since been cosponsored by a significant number of disability activists, advocates, and organizations. As 3E Love continues to grow, their long-term vision is to be an inclusive disability social media and marketing company.

Further Reading

3E Love. 2011. "Meaning of Symbol." http://www.3elove.com/pages/meaning-of-symbol.

3E Love. n.d. "International Day of Acceptance." http://threeellc.com/idoa/.

Roland Johnson (d. 1994)

Roland Johnson was a black disabled man who advocated for the rights of people with intellectual and developmental disabilities (IDD). In 1958, when Johnson was 12 years old, his parents placed him in Pennsylvania's Pennhurst State School and Hospital for the Mentally Retarded because they were struggling to care for him. During that time, many people believed that disabled people could not live at home and were better served living in a hospital or institution full-time. Pennhurst was an institution now infamous for its neglect and abuse of the thousands of people with disabilities who lived there.

Johnson spent 13 long years at Pennhurst, enduring physical, verbal, and sexual abuse. He said, "Pennhurst didn't meant (sic) nothing to me. Pennhurst was me with sorrows and grief. I didn't like it at all" (Johnson 1994, 11). Johnson also experienced a complete loss of control over his life at Pennhurst. He recalled, "When I was in Pennhurst . . . I had people who controlled my life. I had people control me and tell me what to do, tell when to get up, tell me when to go to bed, tell me what not to do" (Johnson 1994, 21). Because of these experiences, after he was released from Pennhurst, Johnson became a devoted advocate for deinstitutionalization, the movement to move people out of institutions and into community settings. In addition to sharing his traumatic experiences at Pennhurst, Johnson emphasized that people with disabilities had a right to control their own medical treatment and lives.

Johnson was also a prominent leader in the self-advocacy movement, the rights and empowerment campaign for and by people with IDD. He cofounded and served as the president of Speaking for Ourselves, a self-advocacy organization that is now known as Self Advocates Becoming Empowered (SABE). He observed, "I have a lot of people tell us that sometimes people just don't listen. . . . So we have to waken people up and make people understand that we are in control of our own life" (Johnson 1994, 21). Johnson passed away in 1994, but his legacy of self-advocacy lives on.

Further Reading

Johnson, Roland. 1994. "Lost in a Desert World." http://www.disabilitymuseum.org/dhm/lib/detail.html?id=1681&&page=21.

I. King Jordan

Dr. Irving King Jordan is a Deaf educator and advocate who made history when he was selected as Gallaudet University's first Deaf president after the Deaf President Now! protest. Jordan was born hearing to hearing parents but lost his hearing at the age of 21 after an automobile accident (Gallaudet University, n.d.).

In 1970, Jordan earned a bachelor of arts in psychology from Gallaudet. He then transitioned to University of Tennessee, where he earned a master of arts in psychology in 1971 and a doctorate in psychology in 1973. Jordan returned to Gallaudet as a faculty member in the Department of Psychology. In 1983, he became chair of the department, and in 1986, he was appointed dean of the College of Arts and Sciences (Gallaudet University, n.d.).

In 1988, Jordan applied to be president of Gallaudet University. Although he was qualified, a hearing candidate, Elisabeth Zinser, was selected instead. The students of Gallaudet contested the decision and engaged in a large-scale protest known as Deaf President Now! The protest lasted six days, at which point Elizabeth Zinser resigned and Jordan was selected as the new president. Afterward, Jordan advocated for the rights of Deaf people and people with disabilities around the world. He has been internationally recognized for his scholarship and has received 11 honorary degrees (Gallaudet University, n.d.).

In 1990, President George H. W. Bush appointed Jordan as vice chair of the President's Committee on Employment of People with Disabilities. In 1993, President Bill Clinton reappointed him. In 2006, Jordan retired from his position of president. In 2010, President Barack Obama appointed Jordan to serve on the Commission of Presidential Scholars, which selects outstanding citizens to honor for their achievements in academics, the arts, education, and public service.

Further Reading

Gallaudet University. n.d. "Dr. I. King Jordan Jr." https://www.gallaudet.edu/history/presidents/jordan-iking.html.

Bob Kafka

Bob Kafka is a disability rights activist who has an extensive history of using direct action and nonviolent civil disobedience to address both local and national disability-related issues. Kafka grew up in a politically progressive family but was drafted for the Vietnam War in 1966. After serving in Vietnam, Kafka returned to the United States and earned a bachelor of arts in economics from the University of Houston in 1971. Two years later, Kafka sustained a neck injury in a car accident and began using a wheelchair for mobility. When pursuing a master's degree in education, Kafka became involved with disability service organizations, eventually holding leadership positions in the Texas Coalition of Citizens with Disabilities and the Southwest Wheelchair Athletic Association.

After engaging in a 1984 national ADAPT protest regarding public transit accessibility, Kafka and his wife, Stephanie Thomas, founded the Texas branch of ADAPT. Kafka continues to be a national organizer for ADAPT but has offered his organizational and experiential expertise to various disability rights groups throughout the years. Kafka served as the director of the Handicapped Student Services at University of Houston (1974–1980), as the executive director of the Texas Paralyzed Veterans Association (TPVA) (1978), and later as president of TPVA (1987–1991). Kafka supported Houston's Coalition for Barrier Free Living and the Coalition of Texans with Disabilities (1981–1987), and he was elected to the American Coalition of Citizens with Disabilities in the mid-1980s.

Further Reading

"Bob Kafka." 2009. October 24. http://www .thegeneanddaveshow.com/bob-kafka/.

Helen Keller (1880–1968)

Helen Keller was an author, an educator, and a prominent figure in disability history. At 19 months of age, Keller was affected by an illness and became both blind and deaf. At age 6, Keller was connected with teacher Anne Sullivan, who worked with Keller for the rest of her own life. Keller developed a variety of communication skills, first learning to connect felt objects with associated words that she spelled by finger tapping on her palm. She attended the Perkins Institution to learn Braille and learned to speak with the support of Sarah Fuller at the Horace Mann School. Keller also learned to read lips and sign language by touching the speaker with her hands. Keller eventually attended and graduated from Radcliffe College in 1900, becoming the first blind and deaf person to earn a bachelor's degree.

Keller was a political and disability rights activist as well as a prolific writer. Some of her most famous works include *The Story of My Life* (1903), *Optimism* (1903), *The World I Live In* (1908), *My Religion* (1927), *Helen Keller's Journal* (1938), and *The Open Door* (1957). In the work *Optimism*, Keller highlights her belief in possibilities for persons with disabilities, writing, "Optimism is the faith that leads to achievement; nothing can be done without hope" (American Foundation for the Blind 2018). Keller was also a notable public speaker, presenting in various countries. Over 475 of Keller's speeches and essays can be found in the Helen Keller Archives of the American Foundation for the Blind. In addition, Keller cofounded the American Civil Liberties Union, promoted the organization of commissions for blind people in more than 30 states, and raised extensive funds for the American Foundation for the Blind. She was awarded the Presidential Medal of Freedom in 1964 and was elected to the National Women's Hall of Fame in 1965.

See also *Primary Documents*: Letter from Alexander Graham Bell to Annie M. Sullivan (1903)

Further Reading

American Foundation for the Blind. 2018. "Helen Keller Biography." http://www.afb

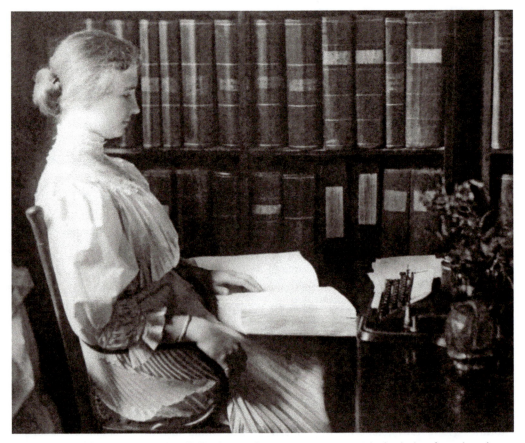

Blind and deaf from birth, Helen Keller learned to communicate with the help of teacher Anne Sullivan. Keller become a respected writer and social activist. (Library of Congress)

.org/info/about-us/helen-keller/biography -and-chronology/biography/1235.

Riva Lehrer

Riva Lehrer is a disabled artist, writer, and curator. Born with spina bifida, Lehrer recalls being told in art school, "Bodies like yours are not acceptable subject matter for art" (Lehrer 2015). Lehrer has strongly resisted this idea by creating work that centers people who are stigmatized because of their disability, gender identity, or sexuality. At the forefront of disability arts and culture, Lehrer is best known for her paintings of disabled people.

One of her most successful bodies of work, Circle Stories, is a collection of portraits of disabled scholars, activists, and artists with physical disabilities. The title of the Circle Stories series refers to the process, symbolism, and intent. Lehrer created the portraits through a cooperative process with her subjects, with the intent of producing a representation of their relationship to their bodies and their lives. She extensively interviews her participants and discusses their lives, work, and understanding of disability. She explains, "Through this collaborative process, we seek imagery that is a truthful representation of their experience" (Lehrer, n.d.). Lehrer also draws on the symbol of the circle as a representation of a wheelchair, which is the universal symbol for disability. She notes, "A wheel . . . transforms the ordinary object of the chair into the mark of physical and social difference" (Lehrer, n.d.). Lastly, Lehrer's art is political and resists dominant ideas about disability and the body. She states, "My work aims to chart the existence of a community of disabled innovators who provide support and context for the work of redefinition of disability in the 21st century" (Lehrer, n.d.).

Lehrer's work has been featured in the Smithsonian, United Nations, and National Museum of Women in the Arts, among others. Lehrer has also received a number of awards and fellowships recognizing her work. In addition to creating visual art, she has written many pieces on disability culture, sex and disability, and gender identity. She has also been featured in a number of different documentaries about art and identity, such as *The Paper Mirror*, *Variations*, and *Code of the Freaks*. She is currently a faculty member at the School of the Art Institute of Chicago and an instructor at Northwestern University.

Further Reading

Lehrer, Riva. 2015. "Valuable Bodies." TEDxGrandRapids. June 30. https://www.youtube.com/watch?v=cjAzDqDRyK4.

Lehrer, Riva. n.d. "Circle Stories." http://www.rivalehrerart.com/circle-stories.

Victoria Ann Lewis

Victoria Ann Lewis is a disabled writer, director, actress, and educator. Her experiences as a disabled woman in the performing arts have strongly influenced her scholarship and activism.

Lewis became disabled after contracting polio as a child. She eventually learned to walk again, with the support of a leg brace. Rather than shelter their disabled daughter, her parents encouraged her to achieve. Her father, who was a singer and a clown, inspired Lewis's interest in performing arts. When Lewis decided she wanted to be an actress, her parents enrolled her in drama school (Churnin 1993).

As an adult, Lewis pursued professional acting. She was cast in numerous supporting roles in television programs, including the popular series *Knots Landing*. She was also cast in supporting and starring roles in various successful plays, such as *Light Sensitive* at San Diego's Old Globe Theatre.

In addition to acting, Lewis served as Artist in Residence at the Mark Taper Forum Theatre in Los Angeles, California. For 12 years, she partnered with diverse communities, such as blue-collar workers, black and Latina teen mothers, and people with disabilities, to create documentary plays (University of Redlands 2017). During this time, she produced a documentary titled "Who Parks in Those Spaces?" The documentary featured disabled people and highlighted their experiences, emotions, humor, ambition, and sensibility (Oppenheim 1985). For her work on the documentary, Lewis received a 1985 Los Angeles Area Emmy nomination for Best Public Affairs Special by an Independent Station (International Movie Database 2017).

Lewis went on to complete a doctorate in theater from the University of California, Los Angeles in 2000 and is currently a professor of theater at the University of Redlands. Much of Lewis's scholarship focuses on the inclusion of disabled people in the performing arts. She coedited an anthology of plays by disabled artists, titled *Beyond Victims and Villains: Contemporary Plays by Disabled Playwrights*. In addition, she has published and presented extensively about disability and access in the performing arts and about the need for more diverse types of characters with disabilities that go beyond stereotypes. She also advocates for accessible performing arts education and training and for nontraditional casting practices that include disabled performers.

Further Reading

Churnin, Nancy. 1993. "Theater: Seeing The 'Light': Victoria Ann-Lewis Wins Acclaim in a Breakthrough Old Globe Role That She Landed Because of—and in Spite of—Her Disability." *Los Angeles Times*, February 21. http://articles.latimes.com/1993-02-21 /entertainment/ca-943_1_victoria-lewis.

International Movie Database. 2017. "Victoria Ann Lewis." http://www.imdb.com/name /nm0507859/.

Oppenheim, Irene. 1985. "Disabled Actors Reach Out on TV." *New York Times*, December 1. http://www.nytimes.com/1985/12/01 /arts/disabled-actors-reach-out-on-tv .html?mcubz=2.

University of Redlands. 2017. "Victoria Lewis." http://www.redlands.edu/study /schools-and-centers/college-of-arts-and -sciences/undergraduate-studies/theatre -arts/meet-our-faculty/victoria-lewis2/.

Paul Longmore (d. 2010)

Paul Longmore was an author, historian, professor, and disability rights activist. When he was 7 years old, Longmore acquired polio and subsequently lost use of his hands and used a ventilator to breathe at night and during part of the day.

Longmore wrote by holding a pen in his mouth and punching a keyboard with it. He used this method to write his first history book, *The Invention of George Washington*. Shortly after the book was published in 1988, Longmore received national attention when he burned a copy of it in front of the Federal Building in Los Angeles, California, to protest Social Security policies that created disincentives for disabled people to work. Such policies limited the amount of income disabled people could earn and still receive medical equipment, personal care assistance, and other necessities for independent living. Longmore was in jeopardy of losing services because of his earnings from book royalties, and his protest highlighted the ways legislation forces disabled people to choose between employment/independence and survival. Later, the Longmore Amendment was added to Social Security policy in order to allow disabled people to earn royalties and still receive Social Security benefits.

Longmore was a key figure in establishing disability studies as a field of study. In the early 1990s, he became a professor at San Francisco State University, where he wrote about the history of disability and the disability rights movement. He was a leading contributor to many areas of inquiry in disability studies, including stereotypes in film and television, assisted suicide, and the social model of disability.

Longmore highlighted the ways in which disabled people have revolutionized how society views and treats disabled people. He stated, "Previously, disability was defined as a set of limitations in the abilities of people with disabilities to function in society because of some pathology in us. The disability rights movement redefined disability as a problem mainly out there in society—not . . . in our bodies and minds but in society" (Shapiro 2010). Hence, Longmore argued, society needed to change to support the independence and rights of disabled people.

Longmore passed away in 2010, shortly after the 20th anniversary of the Americans with Disabilities Act. After his passing, San Francisco State University renamed their Institute on Disability, which Longmore cofounded, the Paul K. Longmore Institute on Disability in order to celebrate his significant contributions to the field of disability studies.

Further Reading

Shapiro, Joseph. 2010. "Paul Longmore, Historian and Advocate for the Disabled, Dies." http://www.npr.org/sections/health-shots/2010/08/11/129127432/paul-longmore-historian-and-advocate-for-disabled-dies.

Kathy Martinez

Kathleen "Kathy" Martinez is a blind lesbian Latina and Native American disability rights activist. She began her career advocating for women and immigrant farm workers (Newsham 2014). She then shifted to disability rights, particularly focusing on the employment gap, which she views as a major barrier to equality for people with disabilities. She explained, "If we don't have money to spend, if we're not employed, we'll still be marginalized. So employment, really, [has] been my life's work" (Newsham 2014).

Martinez lectures and publishes on issues related to disability employment and has been featured in *Diversity Inc.*, *Boston Globe*, and the *Washington Post*. Martinez discusses many aspects of employment for disabled people but is particularly concerned with addressing prejudice and discrimination. She observed, "The biggest barriers [to employment] are not architectural, but attitudinal. There are a lot of misconceptions out there . . . There are people who don't think those of us with disabilities can work." Martinez also uses her own personal experience to discuss the importance of instilling youth with disabilities with the belief that they can—and will—work.

In 2002, Martinez was appointed by President George W. Bush to the National Council on Disability, an independent federal agency that advises Congress and the president on disability policy issues. Then, from 2005 to 2009, she was the executive director at the World Institute on Disability, where she managed a number of initiatives, including Proyecto Visión, a national technical assistance center that aimed to increase employment opportunities for Latinxs with disabilities in the United States.

In 2009, Martinez was nominated by President Barack Obama to serve as the assistant secretary of labor for the Office of Disability Employment Policy. In this role, she worked with federal contractors to ensure more people with disabilities were hired, retained, and promoted.

In 2015, Martinez transitioned to Wells Fargo as a senior vice president, leading the company's Disability Market Segment and Strategy. As a strategist, Martinez works to improve and expand Well Fargo's ability to serve people with disabilities and their families.

Further Reading

Bureau of Labor Statistics. 2017. "Persons with a Disability: Labor Force Characteristics Summary." https://www.bls.gov/news.release/disabl.nr0.htm.

Newsham, Jack. 2014. "Seven Things You Should Know about Kathy Martinez." https://www.bostonglobe.com/business/2014/06/28/seven-things-you-should-know-about-kathy-martinez-assistant-secretary-labor/5NPG8CCyMi6Z1RbjqaDEPO/story.html.

Marlee Matlin

Marlee Matlin is a Deaf American actress. Matlin reached critical acclaim for her performance in *Children of a Lesser God*, for which she won a Golden Globe Award and

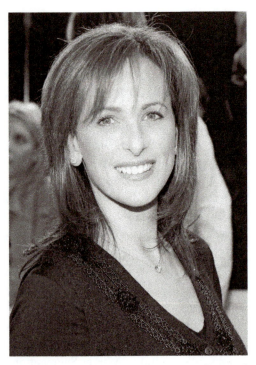

Marlee Matlin is an award-winning film and television actress and an activist for the Deaf involved with a number of charitable organizations. (Starstock/Dreamstime.com)

an Academy Award. She went on to participate in many groundbreaking roles in such works as *The West Wing* and *The L Word*, performing in both American Sign Language and spoken language. She has since been nominated for more than 20 awards and has won 6 major awards.

During the 2007 and 2016 Super Bowls, Matlin interpreted "The Star-Spangled Banner" in American Sign Language. Other notable work includes participation in the Deaf revival of the musical *Spring Awakening*, *Dancing with the Stars*, and *Celebrity Apprentice*, where she raised $1 million for charity in one episode alone. Her participation in *Celebrity Apprentice* sparked controversy years later when it was revealed during the 2016 presidential campaign that President Donald J. Trump allegedly made fun of

Matlin and often referred to her as "retarded" during her stint on *Celebrity Apprentice*. In response, Matlin published a statement explaining: "The term [retarded] is abhorrent and should never been used. The fact that we are talking about this during a very important moment in American history has upset me deeply. I am Deaf. There are millions of Deaf and hard of hearing people like me, in the United States and around the world who face discrimination and misunderstanding on like this on a daily basis. It is unacceptable" (Resnick and Suebsaeng 2016).

Matlin has been an outspoken disability rights activist and has advocated for the inclusion of more Deaf and disabled people in television and film. She has also recently teamed up with the American Civil Liberties Union (ACLU) to help Deaf people know their rights when it comes to law enforcement (ACLU, n.d.).

Further Reading

American Civil Liberties Union. n.d. "Marlee Matlin on Deaf and Police Interaction." https://www.aclu.org/video/marlee-matlin-deaf-and-police-interaction.

Davis, Lennard. 2009. "Let Actors with Disabilities Play Characters with Disabilities." *Huffington Post*. http://www.huffingtonpost.com/lennard-davis/let-actors-with-disabilit_b_380266.html.

Resnick, Gideon, and Asawin Suebsaeng. 2016. "Donald Trump Called Deaf Apprentice Marlee Matlin 'Retarded,' Three Staffers Say." http://www.thedailybeast.com/articles/2016/10/13/donald-trump-called-deaf-apprentice-marlee-matlin-retarded.html.

Tatyana McFadden

Tatyana McFadden is one of the most accomplished Paralympic athletes of all time. McFadden was born with spina bifida and spent the first six years of her life in a Russian orphanage. During that time, she was not provided with a wheelchair and was forced to move around using only her arms. She was then adopted by Deborah McFadden, the commissioner of disabilities for the U.S. Department of Health, and her partner (McFadden, n.d.).

McFadden had a difficult transition to the United States, and her health consequently declined. Her mothers enrolled her in sports, hoping it would assist her in building strength and confidence. After trying a wide range of accessible sports, McFadden fell in love with wheelchair racing. Because of her passion for the sport, she excelled at wheelchair racing. At age 15, she became the youngest Paralympian representing the United States at the 2004 Paralympics in Athens, Greece.

Tatyana has the unique ability to perform well at short-distance races, such as the 100 meters, as well as long-distance races, such as the 5,000 meters or the marathon. This skill has led McFadden to dominate the sport of wheelchair racing. At age 27, she has participated in the 2004 Paralympics in Athens, Greece; the 2008 Paralympics in Beijing, China; the 2012 Paralympics in London, England; and the 2016 Paralympics in Rio, Brazil. She has earned 17 medals, 7 of which are gold. She has also won 15 World Championship medals and 16 marathons around the

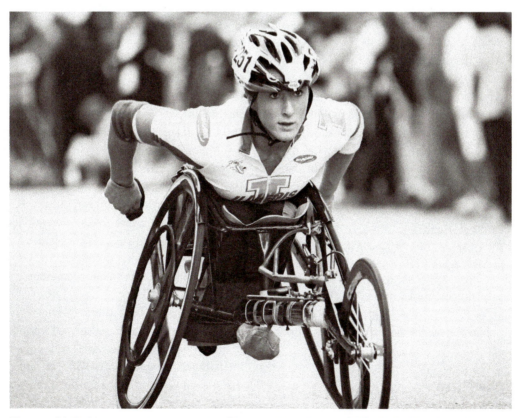

Tatyana McFadden participating in the Chicago Marathon in 2010. McFadden is an internationally acclaimed athlete and advocate for the rights of people with disabilities. (Cafebeanz Company/Dreamstime.com)

world. In 2014, she also participated in the Winter Paralympics in Sochi, Russia. She won a silver medal in cross-county skiing and was ecstatic to win in her home country.

Reflecting on the role athletics has played in her life, McFadden said, "Sports has been my life; ever since I was six, it's just been my passion. . . . I worked very hard to become the best. I usually don't let anything stand in my way. . . . Sports did save me, and made the strong and determined person I am today" (BP America 2012).

In addition to excelling in sports, McFadden advocates for access and rights for people with disabilities. In high school, she and her mother Deborah sued her school district to win the right to practice on the track with her nondisabled classmates. The lawsuit led to the Maryland Fitness and Athletics Equity for Students with Disabilities Act, which required schools to provide students with disabilities with equal opportunity to compete in athletics (McFadden, n.d.). After this victory, McFadden advocated for similar legislation on the national level, which was passed in 2013 (McFadden, n.d.). McFadden is also a lifetime member of the Girls Scouts and is on the Board of Directors of Spina Bifida of Illinois.

Further Reading

BP America. 2012. "A Day in the Life: Tatyana McFadden." Filmed July 2012. YouTube video, 3:09. Posted July. https://www.youtube.com/watch?v=Fy3df8X726Y.

McFadden, Tatyana. n.d. "About Tatyana." http://tatyanamcfadden.com/about-tatyana/.

Mia Mingus

Mia Mingus is an activist, writer, and educator who focuses on disability justice and transformative justice. Her scholarship and activism is closely linked to her identity as a queer, physically disabled Korean woman, a transracial and transnational adoptee from the Caribbean.

Mingus highlights disability justice as an inclusive and radical movement that works toward the liberation of all people. She encourages everyone, regardless of their specific causes, to center disability in their work. According to Mingus, "Understanding disability and ableism is the work of every revolutionary, activist and organizer—of every human being. Disability is one of the most organic and human experiences of the planet. We are all aging, we are all living in polluted and toxic conditions and the level of violence currently in the world should be enough for all of us to care more about disability and ableism" (Mingus 2017).

Mingus is a survivor of child sexual abuse and has worked toward ending child sexual abuse for disabled and nondisabled children for over a decade. She founded the Living Bridges Project, which collects stories about everyday people's responses to child sexual abuse with the goal of offering inspiration, support, and resources. Mingus is also a cofounder and core member of the Bay Area Transformative Justice Collective (BATJC), which is a group in the Bay Area of California that seeks to create and sustain transformative justice responses to child sexual abuse that do not lead to more violence but rather promote accountability, healing, and resiliency.

Mingus has a blog titled *Leaving Evidence*, and her writing has also been featured in numerous magazines and anthologies, including *Criptiques*; *The Wind Is Spirit: A Bio/Anthology of Audre Lorde*; and *Dear Sister: Letters from Survivors of Sexual Violence*.

Mingus has received numerous awards and accolades for her activist work. In 2008, she was honored with the Creating Change Award by the National Gay and Lesbian Task Force; in 2013, she was recognized by the White House as a Champion for Change; and in 2016, she was named a Just Beginnings Collaborative Fellow.

Further Reading

Mingus, Mia. 2017. "Access Intimacy, Interdependence, and Disability Justice." https://leavingevidence.wordpress.com/2017/04/12/access-intimacy-interdependence-and-disability-justice/.

Leroy Moore Jr.

Leroy Moore Jr. is a black disabled artist, activist, and educator. Moore was born with cerebral palsy. Although he was raised in an activist family, he noted, "At an early age I realized that both of my communities, Black and disabled, did not recognize each other and because of this fact I continued to search for some kind of balance with my two identities" (Moore 2008).

After studying black and African American disabled musicians and learning from what he has referred to as the black disabled movement, Moore founded Krip-Hop Nation. "Krip-Hop Nation's Mission is to educate the music, media industries and general public about the talents, history, rights and marketability of Hip-Hop artists and other musicians with disabilities" (Krip-Hop Nation 2017). Krip-Hop Nation creates numerous products, including mixtapes featuring disabled musicians from around the world, resource pamphlets, books, performances, presentations, radio shows, magazine articles, and blog posts (Krip-Hop Nation 2017). Additionally, Krip-Hop seeks to support hip-hop artists and other musicians with disabilities by connecting them with agents and assisting them with breaking into mainstream media outlets.

In addition to establishing Krip-Hop Nation, Moore is a cofounder of Sins Invalid, which is "a performance project that incubates and celebrates artists with disabilities, centralizing artists of color and queer and gender-variant artists" (Sins Invalid, n.d.). The goals of Sins Invalid include forwarding the disability justice movement, providing politically engaged spaces, promoting the work of multiply marginalized people with disabilities, and developing coalitional relationships with different communities.

In addition to his work with Krip-Hop Nation and Sins Invalid, Moore engages in activism related to police brutality against and wrongful incarceration of disabled people and people of color. He also is an internationally known lecturer on issues of race and disability, and he writes a regular column in *Poor Magazine*, a grassroots publication led by poor people and indigenous people.

Further Reading

Banton, Martin, and Gurnam Sinh. 2004. "'Race,' Disability and Oppression." In *Disabling Barriers, Enabling Environments*, 111–117. Thousand Oaks, CA: Sage.

Krip-Hop Nation. 2017. "Who Is the Krip-Hop Nation?" http://kriphopnation.com/.

Moore, Leroy Franklin, Jr. 2008. "Krip-Hop Project's Leroy F Moore on Being Black and Disabled." http://www.amoeba.com/blog/2008/07/jamoeblog/krip-hop-project-s-leroy-f-moore-on-being-black-disabled.html.

Sins Invalid. n.d. "Sins Invalid: An Unashamed Claim to Beauty in the Face of Invisibility." http://www.sinsinvalid.org/.

Swain, John. 2004. *Disabling Barriers, Enabling Environments*. Thousand Oaks, CA: Sage.

Lillibeth Navarro

Lillibeth Navarro is the founder and executive director of Communities Actively Living Independent and Free (CALIF), the independent living center in Los Angeles, California. As a disabled Filipina woman, Navarro has engaged in disability activism and advocacy in the Philippines and United States. Navarro is a polio and cancer survivor who considers herself a person with a severe disability (CALIF 2011).

Navarro is recognized as a pioneer of the disability rights movement in Southern California. Her work has focused on community living, independence, services and supports, and access to public transportation and public space. According to Navarro, "When a particular minority group is always asked to justify their existence, their right to health care, to transportation, their right to housing, their right to a personal care attendant, there is no word for it but discrimination" (Navarro 2006). A committed activist, Navarro has been arrested more than 30 times in the struggle for disability rights.

Navarro led the fight for accessible public transportation in Southern California and was a central figure in the disability rights organization Americans Disabled for Attendant Programs Today (ADAPT). ADAPT engaged in numerous protests and demonstrations to advocate for public transportation for disabled people.

Later, Navarro advocated for the Americans with Disabilities Act of 1990 (ADA). Once the civil rights law passed, Navarro used the ADA to ensure disabled people received the right to accessible public transportation and public spaces. She led a class action lawsuit against a California bus company, arguing that the company's inaccessible buses were a violation of the ADA. Although the case was initially dismissed, an appeal eventually led to a settlement from the bus company. In 2015, Navarro was also part of a class action lawsuit against the city of Los Angeles because of their significant number of broken sidewalks, which were difficult if not impossible to use with mobility devices such as wheelchairs. The city of Los Angeles settled and agreed to spend billions of dollars to bring the city's sidewalks into compliance with the ADA.

Navarro also has engaged in advocacy with Not Dead Yet, the grassroots disability rights organization opposed to assisted suicide and euthanasia. Assisted suicide and euthanasia are controversial issues within the disability community, and Navarro believes that support for assisted suicide is often based on the desire to cut costs and the ableist belief that life with a disability is not worth living.

Further Reading

Communities Actively Living Independent and Free (CALIF). 2011. "Administration." http://califilc.webs.com/administration.htm.

Navarro, Lillibeth. 2006. "From All Sides." https://calif-ilc.blogspot.com/.

Ari Ne'eman

Ari Ne'eman is the cofounder of the Autistic Self Advocacy Network (ASAN), an advocacy group for and by autistic people. ASAN's aim is to ensure autistic people have the same rights as nondisabled people. ASAN has focused on key issues such as equal employment opportunities, community living, inclusion, and the end of discrimination. Ari served as president of ASAN from 2006 to 2016.

Currently, Ne'eman serves as the CEO of MySupport.com, which is an online platform that aims to empower disabled people and elders to self-direct their own personal support services. He is also a board member of the American Association of People with Disabilities and the World Institute on Disability.

In 2009, President Barack Obama appointed Ne'eman to the National Council on Disability, which is a federal agency that advises Congress and the president on issues related to disability policy. Some controversy ensued as a result of the nomination. Ne'eman is against the movement to "cure" autism, as he believes autism is not a disease but rather a neurological difference and a part of neurodiversity. Consequently, some people disapproved of Obama's selection of Ne'eman, claiming that he is high functioning and thus cannot understand the difficulties the parents of autistic children with more severe impairments face. Ne'eman rejected these claims, calling on society to become more accepting of autistic people and support them in living more independently. He stated:

In America we've spent over a billion dollars on autism research. What have we got for that? We've not seen anything that's appreciably impacted the quality of life of autistic people, regardless of their place on the spectrum. . . . The average person . . . [thinks]: am I going to be able to find a job, to communicate, to live independently, either on my own or with support? Those are the real priorities. (Hannaford 2013)

Despite the criticism, he was confirmed to the National Council on Disability in 2010 and served until 2015. During his tenure, he chaired the council's Committee on Entitlements Policy.

In addition, Ne'eman previously served as a member of the Department of Labor's

Advisory Committee on Increasing Competitive Integrated Employment of People with Disabilities, a member of the Interagency Autism Coordinating Committee, vice chair of the New Jersey Adults with Autism Task Force, and adviser to the DSM-5 Neurodevelopmental Disorders Workgroup convened by the American Psychiatric Association.

Further Reading

Hannaford, Alex. 2013. "Andrew Wakefield: Autism, Inc." *The Guardian*, April 6. https://www.theguardian.com/society/2013/apr/06/what-happened-man-mmr-panic.

Tia Nelis

Tia Nelis is a leader in the U.S. self-advocacy movement for individuals with developmental and intellectual disabilities. She currently is the director of policy and advocacy for TASH, a national organization that advocates for human rights and inclusion for people with significant disabilities and support needs. She is a leader in the field, and she previously held a number of roles, including self-advocacy specialist at the Rehabilitation Research and Training Center on Developmental Disabilities and Health within the Institute on Disability and Human Development at the University of Illinois at Chicago. She also is one of the past chairs of the National Organization of Self Advocates Becoming Empowered (SABE). She describes her role as a self-advocate as helping the world "to get rid of the labels that hurt people." People with disabilities, she says, are people first—not just "patients and clients, but friends and neighbors."

Nelis was personally invited to the White House to celebrate the 25th anniversary of the Americans with Disabilities Act

(ADA). In his speech honoring the ADA anniversary, President Barack Obama specifically noted her accomplishments in self-advocacy, alongside fellow leader Ricardo Thornton. Obama remarked, "I want to thank some of the activists who are here—folks like Ricardo Thornton and Tia Nelis. In 1999, the Supreme Court ruled that institutionalizing people with disabilities—isolating them, keeping them apart from the rest of the community—is not just wrong, it is illegal. Ricardo and Tia have pushed to make sure that ruling is enforced."

Nelis was also spotlighted as one of the leaders of the disability rights movement by tech giant Google. Google published a story and video about her pivotal role in the self-advocacy movement for people with intellectual and developmental disabilities. Google also had Nelis's image painted up a set of stairs in Washington, D.C., to mark the advances made by people with disabilities since the passage of the ADA. The painting of the stairs was a nod to the historic Capitol Hill crawl, where disability activists crawled up the steps of the Capitol in order to get the ADA passed.

Further Reading

Council on Quality and Leadership. n.d. "Tia Nelis." https://www.c-q-l.org/files /2018Documents/2018-CQL-Board-of -Directors.pdf.

TASH. n.d. http://tash.org/.

Susan Nussbaum

Susan Nussbaum is a disabled playwright, novelist, and disability rights activist. Nussbaum acquired a disability in her 20s, after being struck by a car on her way to acting class in Chicago, Illinois. At the time, Chicago was extremely inaccessible.

Although a family friend provided her with employment, she had to use a urinal in a broom closet because the women's restroom was upstairs. There was no accessible public transportation, so she was required to use an ambulance to get to and from work every day. She recalled, "Through the rage and shame I carried with me like a straining dog on a leash, I dimly saw that what I was experiencing in the streets, at my job, my seemingly futile search for accessible housing, in every corner of my new life, was unjust" (Nussbaum 2013a). However, despite this feeling of injustice, Nussbaum continued to think of disability as an individual, medical problem.

Then, she learned of Access Living, Chicago's independent living center. She applied for a job and was hired, which allowed her to form community with other disabled people. Through their collective activism, Nussbaum began to understand disability as a systemic issue rather than an individual one. She said, "I understood at last, and set aside my anger and shame. It wasn't personal. It was political" (Nussbaum 2013a).

Nussbaum founded one of the first groups for girls with disabilities, the Empowered Fe Fes. The Empowered Fe Fes teaches young girls with disabilities about disability rights, women's rights, and the ways in which the issues of women and disabled people intersect (Access Living 2017). It also provides peer support and assists girls with disabilities in forming community. Because of her work with disabled girls, Nussbaum was recognized as one of 50 Visionaries Who are Changing Your World by *Utne Reader* in 2008.

Nussbaum is also a celebrated playwright and novelist. Her work centers on authentic, diverse disabled characters and focuses on the disability experience. Her first novel,

Good Kings Bad Kings, tells the story of teenagers with disabilities living in an institution in the Chicago area. The novel explores such issues as disability identity, disability community, disability rights, and the segregation and abuse that occur in institutions. *Good Kings Bad Kings* was awarded the prestigious PEN/Bellwether Prize for Socially Engaged Fiction (Nussbaum 2013b).

Further Reading

Access Living. 2017. "The Empowered Fe Fes: Group for Young Women." https://www.accessliving.org/index.php?tray=content&tid=top845&cid=180.

Nussbaum, Susan. 2013a. "My Disability Was Nothing Personal." https://www.psychologytoday.com/blog/one-true-thing/201309/susan-nussbaum-my-disability-was-nothing-personal.

Nussbaum, Susan. 2013b. "Susan Nussbaum." http://www.susannussbaum.com/.

Corbett O'Toole

Corbett O'Toole is an activist, writer, and educator who focuses on feminist, queer, and disability issues. O'Toole has been disabled since she acquired polio as a one-year-old. She now identifies as having multiple disabilities, quipping, "I love the disability community so much I've added a few more disabilities along the way" (Nichols 2013).

As a young adult, O'Toole joined a disabled women's consciousness-raising group in Berkeley. She recalled:

It was the first time I had the experience of going from being isolated about my disability and thinking everything that had happened to me was my responsibility and/or my fault, to realizing that what had happened to me was actually part of a systemic model of what was happening to all of us. . . . I got very angry. I got . . . in touch with all of the years that I had not been able to talk about or deal with all of the oppression around my disability. (O'Toole and Sherer Jacobson 1998)

O'Toole channeled her newfound awareness of disability oppression and indignation into activism. She began working at the Berkeley Center for Independent Living, which was a hub for the disability rights movement.

In 1977, she participated in a protest calling for regulations for Section 504 of the Rehabilitation Act. Although the Rehabilitation Act was signed in 1973, it could not be implemented without the regulations. O'Toole explained, "In 1973, one sentence was added to a rehabilitation bill, in Section 504. That one sentence gave disabled people in the United States their first civil rights law, but the law could not be enforced until the federal government wrote down what that one sentence did and did not cover" (2015, 54). Approximately 150 disabled people and allies occupied the Department of Health, Education, and Welfare building in San Francisco, California. The sit-in lasted 28 days, making it the longest occupation of a federal building in U.S. history. The protest ended after the regulations were signed, which was a significant victory for the disability rights movement.

O'Toole later focused her disability activism on the intersections between disability, gender, and sexuality. In 1980, she formed the National Disabled Women's Education Equity Project, which conducted research and held conferences about disability and gender. In response to homophobia and the cultural invisibility of disabled lesbians within the disability community and in broader society, O'Toole also began writing about queer disability identity and advocating for disabled lesbian women's health (O'Toole and Sherer Jacobson 1998). After adopting a daughter from Japan, O'Toole also began raising awareness about disabled parenthood.

O'Toole has been a leader in organizing multiple groundbreaking symposiums and conferences, including the Disabled Women's Symposium, the International Conference on Parents with Disabilities and their Families, Funding All Women: Including Women and Girls with Disabilities, and the world's first International Queer Disability Conference.

In 2015, O'Toole published her memoir, *Fading Scars: My Queer Disability History*, which was nominated for a Lambda Literary Award in the category of LGBT Nonfiction.

Further Reading

Nichols, Meriah. 2013. "Cool Cat: Corbett O'Toole." http://www.meriahnichols.com/cool-cat-corbett-otoole/.

O'Toole, Corbett. 2015. *Fading Scars: My Queer Disability History*. Fort Worth, TX: Autonomous Press.

O'Toole, Corbett, and Denise Sherer Jacobson. 1998. "Advocate for Disabled Women's Rights and Health Issues: Corbett O'Toole." http://content.cdlib.org/view?docId=kt4779n6sq&brand=calisphere&doc.view=entire_text.

Michael Phelps

Michael Phelps is widely recognized as one of the greatest swimmers and Olympic athletes of all time. As a child, Phelps was diagnosed with attention deficit hyperactivity disorder (ADHD). He initially became involved in swimming as an outlet for his excess energy due to his ADHD.

When Phelps was 15 years old, he qualified for the 2000 Olympics in Sydney, Australia, becoming the youngest male swimmer to qualify in 68 years. Although he did not win a medal in his first Olympics, he went on to compete in the Olympics five more times. As of the 2016 Olympics in Rio de Janeiro, Brazil, Phelps had won a total of 28 medals, making him the most decorated Olympian of all time. Additionally, he holds a large number of world records in swimming.

Phelps has elected not to take medication for his ADHD and rather to use swimming and behavioral modifications to manage his disability. He made a controversial statement regarding his decision not to take medication, claiming, "Your mind is the strongest medicine you can have. . . . You can overcome anything if you think you can and you want to" (Wedge 2012). Several

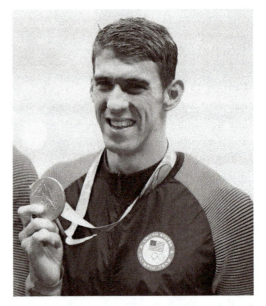

U.S. Olympic champion swimmer Michael Phelps celebrates victory after the 4 x 100-meter medley relay at the 2016 Summer Olympics in Rio de Janeiro, Brazil. Phelps has been outspoken about his experience with ADHD. (Zhukovsky/Dreamstime.com)

disability rights activists, psychologists, and psychiatrists have challenged this position and noted that ADHD is a neurological disability and thus an integral part of who someone is rather than a condition that can be overcome. On the other hand, such overcoming narratives are often critiqued as problematic within disability communities, as such narratives pathologize those who do choose to take medication. At the same time, Phelps serves as a role model to children and adults with ADHD, many of whom are stigmatized and told they cannot achieve their dreams because of their disability.

Further Reading

Wedge, Marilyn. 2012. "From ADHD Kid to Olympic Gold Medalist: How an Olympian Beat ADHD and Then Beat the World's Best Swimmers." *Psychology Today.* https://www.psychologytoday.com/blog/suffer-the-children/201209/adhd-kid-olympic-gold-medalist.

Leah Lakshmi Piepzna-Samarasinha

Leah Lakshmi Piepzna-Samarasinha identifies as a queer, disabled, nonbinary femme writer, artist, and activist of Burgher/Tamil Sri Lankan and Irish/Roma descent. Her writing and art highlight the experiences of queer and transgender people of color, as well as themes of abuse and violence. Piepzna-Samarasinha has authored the memoir *Dirty River: A Queer Femme of Color Dreaming Her Way Home* (2015), as well as collections of her poetry in *Bodymap* (2015); *Love Cake* (2011, Lambda Literary Award 2012); and *Consensual Genocide* (2006). She has had countless other works published in a range of poetry anthologies, and she coedited *The Revolution Starts At Home: Confronting Intimate Violence within Activist Communities* (2011).

Additionally, Piepzna-Samarasinha works as a freelance journalist, and she has performed spoken word for the last two decades. In the latter arena, Piepzna-Samarasinha organized Browngirlworld, a series for queer people of color. She also is a leading artist with Sins Invalid, a performance collective devoted to disability justice. On her Web site, Piepzna-Samarasinha described a 2016 show put forth by Sins Invalid entitled *Birthing, Dying, Becoming Crip Wisdom* as being about "being too old to die young, about not being a supercrip or a better-off-dead-pathetic victim, but about being all of our complicated, real, evolving disabled lives" (Piepzna-Samarasinha 2018).

Further Reading

Piepzna-Samarasinha, Leah Lakshmi. 2018. "Leah Lakshmi Piepzna-Samarasinha." https://www.brownstargirl.org/.

Victor Pineda

Victor Santiago Pineda is a disability rights activist, educator, and scholar who focuses on accessibility and policy. Pineda was born in Venezuela. When he was two years old, he began experiencing progressive weakening of his skeletal muscles. As a result, he was denied access to schools, and his mother was forced to homeschool him. As a child, Pineda immigrated to the United States. He was able to attend school, although he faced prejudice and discrimination from his peers. When Pineda was in middle school, the Americans with Disabilities Act of 1990 (ADA) was passed. He credits the ADA with providing him with opportunities he otherwise would have been denied as a disabled person.

After graduating from high school in 1997, Pineda participated in the California Youth Leadership Forum for Students with Disabilities and discovered he was passionate about education and advocacy for disabled people. Pineda attended the University of California, Berkeley, where he received bachelor's degrees in political economy and business administration, as well as a master's degree in city and regional planning. Pineda then went on to receive a doctorate in urban planning and social policy development from the University of California, Los Angeles.

Because of his background in urban planning, Pineda's activism and scholarship have focused on inclusion, with a particular emphasis on the ways built environments can either disable or enable people. In an interview with the Disability Visibility Project, Pineda explained, "What's really disabling to me are the ways in which the cities that we build have a conception of what is the standard body, what is the standard levels of function" (Wong 2014). When asked to imagine how to design an ideal city that is welcoming to all types of people, he suggested:

I think it's based on three key principles. One is . . . equal access and equal opportunity. . . . Two . . . engaged, thriving communities that interact, because I think that's where I think you're really able to have social consciousness. . . . And the third, which I think is the most important, which is really an opportunity for constantly revisiting your history so that you have a real sense of where you come from. (Wong 2014)

Pineda engaged in a wide range of political work. He helped negotiate the United Nations Convention on the Rights of Persons with Disabilities (CRPD). He has presented his scholarship to the U.S. Senate, Department of Justice, and Treasury. He also has spoken to the United Nations and World Bank, and to international governments, such as those of Cuba, Qatar, and Thailand, about increasing accessibility and inclusion for disabled people. In 2015, President Barack Obama named Pineda to the U.S. Architectural and Transportation Barriers Compliance Access Board, which is a federal agency that provides leadership regarding accessible design and compliance to the ADA.

Pineda is currently the president of World Enabled, an international nonprofit that promotes the rights of people with disabilities, and is a senior research fellow at the Haas Institute at the University of California, Berkeley.

Further Reading

Wong, Alice. 2014. "DVP Interview: Victor Pineda and Alice Wong." https://disability visibilityproject.com/2015/04/26/dvp -interview-victor-pineda-and-alice-wong/.

Christopher Reeve (1952–2004)

Christopher Reeve was an American actor well known for his portrayal of Superman in the 1978 movie titled after his character. Reeve also acted in numerous acclaimed films, such as *The Bostonians* (1984), *Street Smart* (1987), *The Remains of the Day* (1993), and *Rear Window* (1998). Reeve acquired a disability in 1995 after an equestrian accident resulted in his cervical spinal injury; thereafter, he used a wheelchair and portable respirator. Reeve's acquired disability garnered national attention and commentary due to his existing celebrity status.

Reeve continued to work in the entertainment industry but devoted much of his time

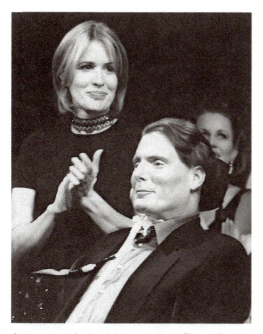

Actress and disability activist Dana Reeve and her husband, actor Christopher Reeve, appear at a fundraiser for the Actor's Fund and the Christopher Reeve Foundation in New York City, on June 12, 2000. Christopher Reeve was one of the most famous and most controversial figures in disability during the 1990s. (Laurence Agron/Dreamstime.com)

to rehabilitation and the support of spinal cord injury research. Specifically, Reeve called for more progressive and urgent stem cell research that could lead to cures for spinal cord injuries. Reeve's advocacy focused on the possibility of a cure, asserting that "every scientist should remove the word 'impossible' from his lexicon" (Groopman 2003). In 1999, Reeve partnered with the American Paralysis Association to establish the Christopher and Dana Reeve Foundation, which continues to work toward the mission of funding innovative research on spinal cord injury. In 2002, under Reeve's foundation, the Paralysis Resource Center was developed to help people living with paralysis acquire support and advice.

Reeve's legacy remains controversial in disability communities. Reeve's stance on "curing" disability attracted criticism from many members of the disability community. Critics argue that people with disabilities are most importantly in need of, not curing, but rather improved community and technological supports. Many disability activists believe that Reeve perpetuated a tragic perspective of disability and consequently endangered struggles for people with disabilities to be recognized and respected as first-class citizens (Brown 1996).

Further Reading

Brown, Steven E. 1996. "Super Duper? The (Unfortunate) Ascendancy of Christopher Reeve." Independent Living Institute. https://www.independentliving.org/docs3/brown96c.html.

Groopman, Jerome. 2003. "The Reeve Effect." *The New Yorker,* November 10.

Ed Roberts (1939–1995)

Edward (Ed) Roberts was a disability rights activist and is widely referred to as the founder of the independent living movement. After contracting polio at age 14, Roberts experienced paralysis from the neck down and began using a wheelchair for mobility and an iron lung respirator to breathe. Roberts soon became accustomed to adversity and to challenging it. For instance, he and his mother had to petition his high school in order for him to be awarded his earned diploma.

Roberts was later accepted to the University of California (UC), Berkeley in 1962; however, Berkeley attempted to rescind their offer of admittance when they became aware of Roberts's disability and support needs. Some of Roberts's mentors at a local college took his story to the media, which pressured UC Berkeley into providing the maximum amount of aid possible to support Roberts's attendance. Roberts moved into Cowell, the university hospital, which housed more students with disabilities in following years.

Roberts was a pioneer for independence and accessibility at Berkeley, founding the Physically Disabled Students Program. Roberts influenced the organization's development because of his peers' desire to live independently in apartments. the organization was led by students with disabilities, and it provided a variety of services, such as wheelchair repairs, peer counseling, and attendant recommendations. It was this program that inspired, and served as a foundation for, the Centers for Independent Living (CIL), which served the larger community. Roberts worked as the executive director of the CIL and was instrumental in developing and providing attendant and interpreter referrals, accessible housing options, and training on mobility, benefits education, and advocacy efforts.

Roberts was appointed the director of the California Department of Rehabilitation in 1975, and he fought for enforcement of Section 504 of the Rehabilitation Act during this tenure. He was awarded a MacArthur grant, and he cofounded the World Institute on Disability (WID). After his passing in 1995, the Ed Roberts Campus was designed in Berkeley, California. This campus is a universally designed space that houses numerous disability organizations.

Further Reading

Levine, Daniel S. 2017. "Ed Roberts, Activist: 5 Facts You Need to Know." Heavy. https://heavy.com/news/2017/01/ed-roberts-activist-google-doodle-quotes-bio graphy-history/.

Franklin Delano Roosevelt (1882–1945)

Franklin Delano Roosevelt served as the 32nd president of the United States from 1933 until his death in 1945. Roosevelt was elected to a record four terms as president, leading the United States through the majority of the Great Depression as well as World War II. A member of the Democratic Party, Roosevelt helped define many modern liberal beliefs. For example, he implemented a series of federally funded work programs in response to the economic crisis of the Great Depression. Many people from racial, ethnic, and religious minority backgrounds were strong supporters of Roosevelt's social politics. Roosevelt established

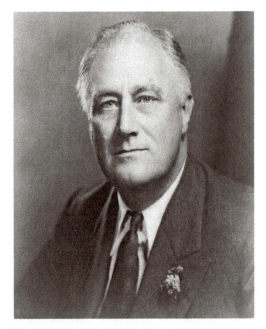

Franklin D. Roosevelt, the nation's longest serving president, was first elected in 1932 and remained in office until his death in 1945. Roosevelt contracted polio at the age of 39 but was seldom seen publicly or photographed using a wheelchair or other mobility aids. (Library of Congress)

the United States' first social insurance program, through the Social Security Act, which provided federal aid for older adults, people who were unemployed, youth, and people with disabilities. Social justice was considered a priority; in 1932, Roosevelt claimed, "In these days of difficulty, we Americans everywhere must and shall choose the path of social justice . . . the path of faith, the path of hope, and the path of love toward our fellow man" (National Park Service 2018).

Roosevelt was affected by polio in 1921 and experienced paralysis from the waist down. To date, he is the only known person with a disability to serve as the president of the United States. However, Roosevelt did not use his wheelchair in public or at public events. When providing speeches, Roosevelt supported himself by gripping the lectern with his hands. It has been reported that members of the Secret Service regularly interfered with members of the press who tried to capture pictures of the president while he was using his wheelchair. The presentation, or concealment, of his disability and the significance of his choices have been chronicled and debated by historians. Prior to his presidency, Roosevelt established a rehabilitation center for people affected by polio in Georgia, at a space he personally frequented. In 1938, he founded the National Foundation for Infantile Paralysis, which is now referred to as the March of Dimes. The foundation continued to fund patient care, research, and support for vaccine development.

See also *Primary Documents*: President Franklin Delano Roosevelt's Statement on the Signing of the Social Security Act (1935); Franklin Delano Roosevelt's Announcement on Founding of the National Foundation for Infantile Paralysis (1937)

Further Reading

National Park Service. 2018. Franklin Delano Roosevelt Memorial. https://www.nps.gov /frde/learn/photosmultimedia/quotations .htm.

Amber Smock

Amber Smock is a disability rights activist and advocate. Smock is currently the director of advocacy and external affairs for Access Living, the center for independent living in Chicago, Illinois. Smock leads Access Living's disability advocacy efforts, which include one-on-one advocacy for individuals, community organizing, public relations, and policy analysis (Smock 2016). Access Living's advocacy strategy focuses on numerous disability issues, such as housing, health care, education, employment, and transportation, and also includes multiply marginalized people with disabilities, such as women, Latinxs, and youth. Smock is also a lobbyist, and works with state officials to advocate for increased budgeting for services and supports and independent living for people with disabilities.

Reflecting on her work at Access Living, Smock stated:

Disability status has always been relevant to human rights work, but it has not always been a recognized or visible component of this work. I have been especially fortunate to work at Access Living . . . and gain a front line role in the disability movement. . . . As a person with hearing loss, engaged in the Deaf world, I can affirm that I have been personally transformed by the advocacy work I do, and I Wish to carry that forward to others. (Access Living 2016)

Smock is proud of her identity as a Deaf woman. As a child, she wore hearing aids and read lips. Then, in her 20s, she learned American Sign Language (ASL), which allows her to be in community with other Deaf people and to use access tools such as ASL interpreters and video relay. She presently serves as the chair of the Illinois Deaf and Hard of Hearing Commission.

Prior to going to Access Living, Smock cofounded and led an activist group for women with disabilities, Feminist Response in Disability Activism (FRIDA). She also worked for the disability rights organization ADAPT, serving as a trainer for the National ADAPT Youth Summit and the chair of the National ADAPT Media Committee.

Smock has received numerous accolades for her work, including the American Association of People with Disabilities Paul G. Hearne Leadership Award and the Chicago Foundation for Women's Founder's Award (Smock 2016). She was also voted the Best Deaf Activist in Illinois by Deaf Illinois (Smock 2016).

Further Reading

Access Living. 2016. "Amber Smock Appointed to Cook County Commission on Human Rights." https://www.accessliving .org/1410ga509.

Smock, Amber. 2016. "About Amber Smock." https://ambersmock2016.blogspot.com/p /about-amber-smock.html.

Vilissa Thompson

Vilissa Thompson is a disability rights activist, writer, and consultant. She is the founder and CEO of Ramp Your Voice!, an organization that promotes self-advocacy and empowerment among people with disabilities, particularly black disabled women.

After becoming a licensed social worker, Thompson started blogging and quickly realized that few blogs discussed disability and that even fewer considered the intersections between race, gender, and disability. This discovery motivated her to create Ramp Your Voice! She recalls, "I created Ramp Your Voice in 2013 to bridge a gap I saw—the lack of voices from disabled people of color, particularly Black disabled women" (Melancon 2017). Thompson uses Ramp Your Voice! to discuss disability issues through an intersectional and personal lens. She has covered such topics as racism, dating, education, and politics.

In 2016, Thompson created the #DisabilityTooWhite hashtag to address the lack of diversity and white supremacy within the disability community. The hashtag quickly went viral and prompted numerous disabled people of color to voice their experiences. Thompson also wrote the Black Disabled Women Syllabus, a compilation of books, essays, articles, speeches, and music that seeks to center the voices of black disabled women and educate others on the experiences of black disabled women. Thompson explained:

When I go out in the world, they see a Black woman in a wheelchair and make assumptions about my humanness and abilities without knowing my name. Being multiply and visibly marginalized has shaped me in ways that I did not realize until I became an advocate. The erasure and invisibility of Black disabled people, and Black disabled women specifically, led me to this work (Melancon 2017).

Thompson has been featured in *Huffington Post*, *New York Times*, *Buzzfeed*, *Bitch Media*, *Upworthy*, *Black Girl Nerds*, and the *Atlantic*.

Further Reading

Melancon, Trimiko. 2017. "Ramp Your Voice: An Interview with Vilissa Thompson." http://www.aaihs.org/ramp-your-voice-an -interview-with-vilissa-thompson/.

Maria Town

Maria Town is a disability rights advocate who focuses on disability policy and community engagement. After working in the White House under the Obama administration, she became the director of the Mayor's Office for People with Disabilities in the city of Houston.

Town first became connected to disability studies and disability activism at Emory University, where she developed relationships with such leading scholars as Benjamin Reiss and Rosemarie Garland-Thomson. After graduating, Town worked in the Provost's Office at Emory, where she promoted diversity initiatives and worked on community building.

Town then joined the U.S. Department of Labor's Office of Disability Employment Policy. As a policy adviser on the Youth Policy Team, Town promoted leadership and career development for adolescents and young adults with disabilities.

After almost five years as a policy adviser, Town became an associate director for the Office of Public Engagement in the White House during the Obama administration. Town explained, "Our job is to make sure that real people can connect with the White House and have their voices heard and [to make sure] that the president is aware of what the people are saying" (Perry 2017). Town worked to inform the administration of disability issues and engage the disability community in policy.

Town emphasizes the importance of disability community in her work and activism. She said, "Growing up with a disability, you're often encouraged to try to be as 'normal' as possible and to 'pass' [as nondisabled]. But when I was finally able to connect with other people with disabilities and see how cool the community was . . . I realized that there's a power in that, and I wanted to make sure that other people could feel that power and experience it too" ("Amy Poehler's Smart Girls" 2016).

Town also has a blog called *CP Shoes*, in which she discusses her experiences as a woman with cerebral palsy. The blog explores disability, fashion, and design, and Town shares her nearly lifelong quest to find fashionable, durable, and affordable shoes that work for a person with cerebral palsy.

Further Reading

"Amy Poehler's Smart Girls Facebook Page." 2016. Facebook.com. Last modified December 3, 2016. https://www.facebook .com/amypoehlersmartgirls/videos /10155429156694338/.

Perry, David M. 2017. "The Future of Disability Rights in the White House." *Pacific Standard*, January 26. https://psmag.com /news/the-future-of-disability-rights-in -the-white-house.

Harriet Tubman (1822–1913)

Harriet Tubman is one of the most well-known abolitionists and civil rights activists, although she is less frequently recognized as a person with a disability. Tubman is most famous for helping to rescue slaves through the Underground Railroad, but she also made substantial contributions to support the care of older adults and people with disabilities after the Civil War.

Tubman was born into slavery on a plantation in Maryland. Tubman was enslaved by Edward Brodess. Brodess hired her out

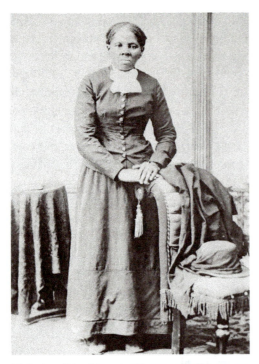

Hailed as "the Moses of her people" because of her courageous rescue of hundreds of slaves on the Underground Railroad, Harriet Tubman was a living symbol of the resistance of African Americans to slavery in the United States. Her experience with epilepsy is an often overlooked aspect of her identity. (Library of Congress)

to other landowners, who treated her cruelly and often brutally whipped her. As a teenager, she protected another slave from harm and was struck with a weight that fractured her skull and nearly killed her. Tubman was forced to return to work just two days after the injury, despite the fact that her head was still bleeding and she had received no medical care. The head trauma resulted in Tubman developing narcolepsy, epilepsy, hallucinations, and migraines (Caring Voice Coalition 2013).

Initially, Tubman struggled with manual labor, and she was consequently returned to Brodess. She eventually began to recover and regained some of her strength. Then, in 1849, Brodess died and left his family deep in debt.

Fearing she would be sold to settle the debt, Tubman escaped to freedom in Philadelphia, traveling approximately 90 miles by foot.

Tubman was able to return to free her family. Later, she made more trips to Maryland to guide other enslaved people, leading approximately 70 people to freedom. During the Civil War, she also served as a scout and spy for the Union army.

Tubman also established the Harriet Tubman Home for the Aged in Auburn, New York (Caring Voices Coalition 2013). Perhaps because of her own injury, Tubman recognized the need for African American elders with disabilities to receive care and compassion. When Tubman reached old age and began experiencing frailty, she received care in the home she had founded. She passed away in 1913.

Tubman has been posthumously honored for her humanitarian and abolitionist work through a number of national monuments and historic site designations. Her immense contributions were most recently recognized when the Obama administration announced she would be added to the $20 bill, which would enter circulation in 2020. As of 2018, however, it was unclear whether the Trump administration would carry through with those plans. Tubman would be the first woman of color to appear on U.S. paper currency.

Further Reading

Caring Voice Coalition. 2013. "Night Vision." http://www.caringvoice.org/2013/12/night-vision/.

Nancy Ward

Nancy Ward is one of the leaders of the self-advocacy movement, which is an advocacy and rights campaign led by people with intellectual and developmental disabilities (IDD).

Ward first became active in the early days of the self-advocacy movement in Lincoln, Nebraska. Her friends encouraged her to join the movement after Ward became enraged about a Special Olympics commercial. She recalled, "The image they portrayed was, 'Pity us because we have a disability.' This made me mad so I yelled at the TV. A lot of good it does to yell at the TV! This is when my friends talked to me about joining People First of Lincoln. There I learned how to direct my feelings in a positive way" (Ward, n.d.). Through People First, Ward experienced significant personal growth. She noted, "I didn't see myself as a person because of all the labels that were placed on me. Now I see myself as a person. People First taught me how to say 'Yes, I have a disability and that's okay' " (Ward, n.d.).

After contributing to the growth of People First, Ward went on to cofound Self Advocates Becoming Empowered (SABE), the largest self-advocacy organization for and by people with IDD. She also served as the first chair of SABE.

Today, Ward continues to be active in self-advocacy. She is one of the leaders of SABE's Vote Project, which encourages people with IDD to exercise their rights to vote. The Vote Project also works to address inaccessibility and break down many of the barriers that make it more difficult for people with disabilities to vote.

Further Reading

Ward, Nancy. n.d. "Nancy Ward: What Self-Advocacy Means to Me." http://mn.gov/mnddc/parallels/seven/7d5/1.html.

Liz Weintraub

Liz Weintraub is one of the leaders of the self-advocacy movement, which is an advocacy and rights campaign led by people with intellectual and developmental disabilities (IDD). Weintraub works at the state and national level and is currently the advocacy specialist for the Association of University Centers on Disability (AUCD). She is also a quality-enhancement specialist with the Council on Quality and Leadership, an organization that works to improve quality of services and quality of life for people with disabilities.

Weintraub credits the self-advocacy movement with her sense of disability pride and her interest in disability rights and activism. She observes, "I am proud of my disability, although I wouldn't say that I was always very proud, until in my twenties, I discovered self-advocacy. I thought of myself as someone who needed to be 'taken care of' and 'needy.'" She also was terrified her parents would give up on her if she told them no. Now that she's become more comfortable with advocacy, she explains, "I feel very strongly that I can't just advocate for myself, I need to advocate for others" (Weintraub n.d.).

Weintraub hosts a video Web series for AUCD, *Tuesdays with Liz: Disability Policy for All*, in which she interviews policy makers and advocates about issues that matter to people with disabilities. Liz was also appointed to the President's Committee for People with Intellectual Disabilities under the Obama administration.

Further Reading

Weintraub, Liz. n.d. "Liz Weintraub." http://www.boldbeautyproject.com/portfolio-item/liz-weintraub/.

Stevie Wonder (1950–)

Stevie Wonder, originally Stevland Hardaway Judkins, is an acclaimed musician, singer, and music producer. He is one of the

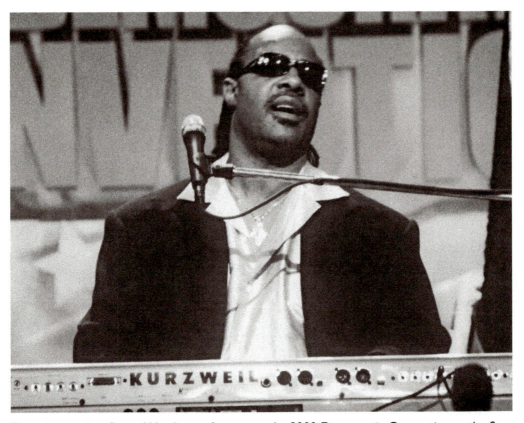

Singer-songwriter Stevie Wonder performing at the 2000 Democratic Convention at the Staples Center in Los Angeles, California. In addition to his musical career, Wonder is known for his international cross-disability activism. (American Spirit/Dreamstime.com)

most commercially successful musicians of all time and is an accomplished civil rights and disability activist.

Born prematurely, Wonder became blind shortly after birth. By age 9, he had learned to play the piano, harmonica, and drums. By age 12, his musical talent had become well known locally, and the owners of Motown Records offered him a recording contract (Library of Congress, n.d.). His legacy is connected with his pioneering work in the music industry, such as becoming only the second African American musician to win the Academy award for Best Original Song. Over the course of his career, he has produced more than 25 albums and won 25

Grammy Awards. He also was awarded the Grammy Lifetime Achievement Award in 1996 (Library of Congress, n.d.).

In addition to being a music prodigy, Wonder has used his influence to advocate for political causes. He rallied to have Martin Luther King Jr.'s birthday become a national holiday, fought apartheid in South Africa, and supported the organization Mothers Against Drunk Driving.

Wonder has also advocated for accessibility for people with disabilities. He made a political statement at the 2016 Grammy Awards while announcing Song of the Year. After joking that his co-presenter could not read the winner because it was in Braille, he stated, "I just want to say—before saying the winner—that we need to make every single thing accessible to every single person with a disability" (Vinh Tien Trinh 2016).

In 2009, Wonder was appointed as a United Nations Messenger of Peace. In 2014, President Barack Obama presented Wonder with a Presidential Medal of Freedom for his civil rights work.

Further Reading

Library of Congress. n.d. "Featured Profile: Stevie Wonder." https://www.loc.gov/disability awareness/profiles/wonder.html.

Vinh Tien Trinh, Brian. 2016. "Stevie Wonder's Joke at 2016 Grammys Turns into Statement on Accessibility." http://www.huffingtonpost.ca/2016/02/15/stevie-wonder-grammys-2016-accessibility_n_9240248.html.

Alice Wong (1974–)

Alice Wong is a disability rights activist and the founder and project coordinator of the Disability Visibility Project. Wong was born in 1974 with spinal muscular atrophy. She was 16 years old when the Americans with Disabilities Act of 1990 passed. The ADA had a significant impact on Wong. Not only did it provide her with increased opportunities and accessibility, but it also led her to understand people with disabilities as a minority group. Wong stated, "Learning about disability history and realizing I was a member of a protected class encouraged me to imagine and create the life that I want" (Wong 2017).

Wong earned a master's degree in medical sociology from the University of California, San Francisco (UCSF). Wong also worked as a staff research associate at UCSF for more than 15 years, conducting qualitative research and developing curricula for the Community Living Policy Center (Disability Visibility Project, n.d.).

In 2014, Wong started the Disability Visibility Project (DVP). The DVP is "an online community dedicated to recording, amplifying, and sharing disability stories and culture" (Disability Visibility Project, n.d.). The DVP partners with StoryCorps to collect oral histories of disabled people. The DVP also works with #CripTheVote, a nonpartisan effort to engage voters with disabilities and encourage politicians and voters to consider and discuss disability issues.

As an Asian American woman with a disability and a daughter of Chinese immigrants, Wong is particularly concerned with how disability intersects with race, ethnicity, immigrant status, gender, sexuality, and other social identities. She serves as an advisory board member of Asians and Pacific Islanders with Disabilities of California. Through the Disability Visibility Project, she has also uplifted the voices and stories of disabled people of color and hosted Twitter chats on topics related to intersectionality.

President Barack Obama appointed Wong to the National Council on Disability, which she served on from 2013 to 2015. In 2015, Wong was the first person in history to visit the White House via telepresence robot. Using the telepresence robot, she attended a reception for the 25th anniversary of the Americans with Disabilities Act and met with President Obama.

Wong was recognized with the American Association of People with Disabilities Paul G. Hearne Leadership Award in 2016.

Further Reading

Disability Visibility Project. n.d. "About." https://disabilityvisibilityproject.com/about/.

Wong, Alice. 2017. "My Medicaid, My Life." *New York Times*, May 3. https://www .nytimes.com/2017/05/03/opinion/my -medicaid-my-life.html?mcubz=0.

Irving Zola (1935–1994)

Irving Zola was an activist and academic, revered for his contributions to the fields of medical sociology and disability studies. Zola used braces and canes to assist his mobility after recovering from polio at the age of 16. At age 19, a car accident further reduced the mobility of his right leg. Zola graduated with a doctorate from Harvard in 1962, and he was a professor at Brandeis University from 1963 until his passing.

Zola founded and worked at the Boston Self-Help Center, which acted as a support center for people with chronic diseases and disabilities and addressed concerns surrounding independence. Zola later authored articles on independent living, its relationship to rehabilitation, and the challenges within rehabilitation processes. Zola also recognized and explained how the personal-tragedy framework of disability undermined efforts of the disability community in his papers. He advocated for inclusivity with the U.S. disability rights movement and openly criticized exclusive language and sectarianism. Throughout his academic work, Zola consistently framed disability as a universal experience—one that is experienced across a spectrum in almost all people—and considered the overmedicalization of such human conditions to be dangerous.

Zola also authored an autobiography, *Missing Pieces: A Chronicle of Living with Disability* (1982) and edited an anthology of short stories, *Ordinary Lives: Voices of Disability and Disease* (1982). Both of these books included personal accounts, Zola openly grappled with disability identity. He is quoted as saying, "Until we own our disability as an important part, though not necessarily all, of our identity, any attempt to create a meaningful pride, social movement or culture is doomed" (Pace 1994). The autobiographical nature of these writings was strengthened by the academic frameworks he previously established in sociology. Zola was a founding member of the Society for Disability Studies and the first editor of the *Disability Studies Quarterly*. A collection of his work can be found at Brandeis University's Samuel Gridley Howe Library.

Further Reading
Pace, Eric. 1994. "Irving Kenneth Zola Dies at 59; Sociologist Aided the Disabled." *The New York Times*, December 8.

Primary Documents

I. Act for the Relief of Sick and Disabled Seamen (1798)

Introduction

In 1798, President John Adams signed the Act for the Relief of Sick and Disabled Seamen, which was implemented to provide sick and disabled seamen with health care. Under the act, seamen had 20 cents deducted from their wages each month, which was used to fund medical care and the construction of additional hospitals. The act was one of the earliest disability-specific policies in the United States.

SEC. 3. And be it further enacted, That it shall be the duty of the several collectors to make a quarterly return of the sums collected by them, respectively, by virtue of this act, to the Secretary of the Treasury; and the President of the United States is hereby authorized, out of the same, to provide for the temporary relief and maintenance of sick or disabled seamen, in the hospitals or other proper institutions now established in the several ports of the United States, or, in ports where no such institutions exist, then in such other manner as he shall direct:
Provided, that the monies collected in any one district, shall be expended within the same.

SEC. 4. And be it further enacted, That if any surplus shall remain of the monies to be collected by virtue of this act, after defraying the expense of such temporary relief and support, that the same, together, with such private donations as may be made for that purpose (which the President is hereby authorized to receive) shall be invested in the stock of the United States, under the direction of the President; and when, in his opinion, a sufficient fund shall be accumulated, he is hereby authorized to purchase or receive cessions or donations of ground or buildings, in the name of the United States, and to cause buildings, when necessary, to be erected as hospitals for the accommodation of sick and disabled seamen.

SEC. 5. And be it further enacted, That the President of the United States be, and he is hereby authorized to nominate and appoint, in such ports of the United States, as he may think proper, one or more persons, to be called directors of the marine hospital of the United States, whose duty it shall be to direct the expenditure of the fund assigned for their respective ports, according to the third section of this act; to provide for the accommodation of sick and disabled seamen, under such general instructions as shall be given by the President of the United States, for that purpose, and also subject to the like general instructions, to direct and govern such hospitals as the President may direct to be built in the respective ports; and that the said directors shall hold their offices during the pleasure of the President, who is authorized to fill up all vacancies that may be occasioned by the death or removal of any of the persons so to be appointed. And the said directors shall render an account of the monies received and expended by them, once in every quarter of a year, to the Secretary of the Treasury, or such other person as the President shall direct; but no other allowance or compensation shall be made to the said directors, except the payment of such expenses as they may incur in the actual discharge of the duties required by this act.

APPROVED, July 16, 1798.

Source: *Congressional Record.* 1798. Fifth Congress, Session II, Chapter 77. https://history.nih.gov/research/downloads/1StatL605.pdf.

2. Article on "Drapetomania" in Dr. Samuel Cartwright's *Diseases and Peculiarities of the Negro* (1851)

Introduction

Throughout history, disability has been used as a justification for the oppression of racial and ethnic minorities. In the antebellum era, white supremacists often defended and promoted slavery by categorizing black people as disabled. In 1851, Dr. Samuel Cartwright hypothesized that runaway slaves suffered from a condition he termed "drapetomania." Cartwright claimed that this "disease of the mind" was most common in slaves with masters who "made themselves too familiar with them, treating
them as equals." Cartwright further argued that drapetomania was cured by ensuring slaves were kept in a submissive state. Although Cartwright's ideas have long been discredited, race and disability continue to intersect in rationalizations of inequality.

Drapetomania, or the Disease Causing Negroes to Run Away

It is unknown to our medical authorities, although its diagnostic symptom, the absconding from service, is well known to our planters and overseers . . . .

In noticing a disease not heretofore classed among the long list of maladies that man is subject to, it was necessary to have a new term to express it. The cause in the most of cases, that induces the negro to run away from service, is as much a disease of the mind as any other species of mental alienation, and much more curable, as a general rule. With the advantages of proper medical advice, strictly followed, this troublesome practice that many negroes have of running away, can be almost entirely prevented, although the slaves be located on the borders of a free state, within a stone's throw of the abolitionists.

If the white man attempts to oppose the Deity's will, by trying to make the negro anything else than "the submissive knee-bender," (which the Almighty declared he should be,) by trying to raise him to a level with himself, or by putting himself on an equality with the negro; or if he abuses the power which God has given him over his fellow-man, by being cruel to him, or punishing him in anger, or by neglecting to protect him from the wanton abuses of his fellow-servants and all others, or by denying him the usual comforts and necessaries of life, the negro will run away; but if he keeps him in the position that we learn from the Scriptures he was intended to occupy, that is, the position of submission; and if his master or overseer be kind and gracious in his hearing towards him, without conde-scension, and at the same time ministers to his physical wants, and protects him from abuses, the negro is spell-bound, and cannot run away.

According to my experience, the "genu flexit"—the awe and reverence, must be exacted from them, or they will despise their masters, become rude and ungovern-able, and run away. On Mason and Dixon's line, two classes of persons were apt to lose their negroes: those who made themselves too familiar with them, treating them as equals, and making little or no distinction in regard to color; and, on the other hand, those who treated them cruelly, denied them the common necessaries of life, neglected to protect them against the abuses of oth-ers, or frightened them by a blustering man-ner of approach, when about to punish them for misdemeanors. Before the negroes run away, unless they are frightened or panic-struck, they become sulky and dissatisfied. The cause of this sulkiness and dissatisfac-tion should be inquired into and removed, or they are apt to run away or fall into the negro consumption. When sulky and dis-satisfied without cause, the experience of those on the line and elsewhere, was decid-edly in favor of whipping them out of it, as a preventive measure against absconding, or other bad conduct. It was called whipping the devil out of them.

If treated kindly, well fed and clothed, with fuel enough to keep a small fire burn-ing all night—separated into families, each family having its own house—not permit-ted to run about at night to visit their neigh-bors, to receive visits or use intoxicating liquors, and not overworked or exposed too much to the weather, they are very easily

governed—more so than any other people in the world. When all this is done, if any one or more of them, at any time, are inclined to raise their heads to a level with their master or overseer, humanity and their own good require that they should be punished until they fall into that submissive state which it was intended for them to occupy in all after-time, when their progenitor received the name of Canaan or "submissive knee-bender." They have only to be kept in that state and treated like children, with care, kindness, attention and humanity, to pre-vent and cure them from running away.

Source: Cartwright, Samuel A. 1851. *Diseases and Peculiarities of the Negro. De Bow's Review: Southern and Western States.* Volume XI. New Orleans: n.p.

3. Patent for Improved Invalid-Chair (First Wheelchair) (1869)

Introduction

In 1869, a patent was filed for an "improved invalid-chair," which marked the creation of the modern wheelchair. Unlike previous iter-ations of wheelchairs, the improved invalid-chair had large wheels in the back and was able to be self-propelled. These develop-ments significantly increased the mobility and independence of wheelchair users.

UNITED STATES PATENT OFFICE
A. P. BLUNT AND JACOB S. SMITH, OF WASHINGTON, DISTRICT OF COLUMBIA.
Letters Patent No. 86,899, dated February 16, 1869.
IMPROVED INVALID-CHAIR

The Schedule referred to in these Letters Patent and making part of the same.

To all whom it may concern:

Be it known that we, A. P. BLUNT and JACOB S. SMITH, of Washington city, in the District of Columbia, have invented new and useful Improvements in Adjustable Invalid-Chairs; and we do declare that the following is a full and exact description thereof, reference being had to the accompanying drawings, and to the letters marked thereon.

8. The nature of our invention consists in making an upholstered chair, with back that may incline backward to any given point, by means of steel catches in socket-joints at foot of back posts; with having two wheels, instead of back legs, attached to the back part of the seat by means of springs; also, in having a foot-rest, which is elevated and lowered independently of all the rest, by means of a cogged quadrant attached to either side, and worked by two small cog-wheels turned by a small crank, all so adjusted that it may be an upright chair, or a flat lounge, as the occupant may desire.

Source: Blunt, A. P., and Jacob S. Smith. "Patent for Improved Invalid-Chair." Disability History Museum. http://www.disabilitymuseum.org/dhm/lib/detail.html?id=2108.

4. Letter from Alexander Graham Bell to Annie M. Sullivan (1903)

Introduction

Although Alexander Graham Bell is best known for inventing the telephone, he also played a significant role in deaf education in the United States. His work with deaf students connected him with one of the most well-known disabled figures in history, Helen Keller. In 1886, Captain Arthur Keller and Kate Adams Keller contacted Alexander Graham Bell, requesting assistance with educating their deaf-blind daughter, Helen. Bell referred the parents to the Perkins School for the Blind, who suggested they hire Anne Mansfield Sullivan as Helen's teacher. After learning about Helen's incredible progress, Bell praised Sullivan for her pedagogical abilities and urged her, in a letter written on April 2, 1903, to instruct others on how to teach deaf and disabled students.

Although Bell, Keller, and Sullivan each played a significant role in disability history, they are controversial figures. Sullivan discouraged Keller from marrying and starting a family, believing Keller would not be able to care for children because of her disabilities. Bell forwarded oralism, which is a form of deaf education that seeks to normalize deaf students by teaching them to lip-read and speak rather than use sign language. Additionally, Bell and Keller were both known to defend eugenic theory and practice.

April 2nd, 1903.
Miss Annie Sullivan,
73 Dana Street,
Cambridge, Mass.

Dear Miss Sullivan: I have read Helen's book with interest and delight, and have written to Mr. Macey congratulating him upon the part he has played in the production of the book. . . .

You must be placed in a position to impress your ideas upon other teachers. YOU MUST TRAIN TEACHERS so that the deaf as a whole may get the benefit of your instruction. Please keep this matter in mind. What you have done with Helen can surely be done with some of the deaf who are not blind. It is a fallacy to suppose that blindness is an ADVANTAGE to a deaf child—it is a fallacy to suppose that language can be intuitively acquired. Once we realize that language is acquired by imitation—it becomes obvious that language comes from without, not from within. The most startling demonstration of this fact was contained in the Frost King incident. We all do what Helen did. Our most original compositions are composed exclusively of expressions derived from others. The fact that the language presented to Helen was in the early days, so largely taken from books, has enabled us in many cases to trace the origin of her expressions but they are none the less original with Helen for all that. We do the very same thing. Our forms of expression are copied—verbatim et literatim—in our earlier years from the expressions of others which we have heard in childhood. It is difficult for us to trace the origin of our expressions because the language addressed to us in infancy has been given by word of mouth, and not permanently recorded in books so that investigators—being unable to examine printed records of the language addressed to us in childhood—are unable to charge us with plagiarism. We are all of us however, nevertheless unconscious plagiarists, especially in childhood. As we grow older and read books the language we absorb through the eye, unconsciously affects our style. Books however do not affect our language to the same extent that they affected Helen because our habits of language, have already been formed before we come to read books. Nevertheless our style IS affected, hence the very great importance of selecting with care, the kinds of books to be read by children.

It is ridiculous to expect that a deaf child—or a hearing child for that matter—shall talk or write good English, unless good English has been PREVIOUSLY presented to the child in spoken or written form—and in sufficient quantity to impress Good English expressions upon his mind.

Then—and then only will he spontaneously use good English in expressing his own thoughts. This thought lies at the ROOT of the instruction of the deaf. Once we clearly grasp this conception we can see the cause of the poor English used by the deaf. It makes one sad to see how this principle is persistently violated in all of our schools for the deaf—but you have pointed out the remedy and have clearly demonstrated the truth of your position by an illustrious example.

My best wishes go with you and Helen, and in conclusion allow me to repeat—what I began with—YOU MUST TRAIN TEACHERS.

Yours sincerely, Alexander Graham Bell

P. S. Dr. Bell asked me to say that he wanted to write Miss Helen, but he was unexpectedly called away, and will write later. Private Secretary

Source: "Image 2 of Letter from Alexander Graham Bell to Annie Sullivan, April 2, 1903." Library of Congress. https://www.loc.gov/resource/magbell.12800108/?sp=2.

5. Preface to Henry H. Goddard's *The Kallikak Family: A Study in the Heredity of Feeble-Mindedness* (1912)

Introduction

The Kallikak Family: A Study in the Heredity of Feeble-Mindedness *was written by American psychologist and eugenicist Henry H. Goddard in 1912. Feeble-mindedness was a general category used for people labeled as "mentally deficient." Goddard was the director of research at the Training School for Backward and Feeble-Minded Children in Vineland, New Jersey, an institution for people diagnosed with mental disabilities. In his text, he claimed to have studied the genealogy of one of the patients at the training school, a woman he called Deborah Kallikak. He claimed that Deborah's great-great-grandfather had reproduced with two women—one "feeble-minded" and one "normal." Goddard reported that the descendants of the feeble-minded woman, which included Deborah, were poor, unintelligent, and insane. Conversely, the descendants of the normal woman were intelligent, successful, and moral. Goddard used this family history to argue that feeble-mindedness was heredity and that steps needed to be taken to ensure feeble-minded people did not reproduce, to improve the human race. Scholars eventually found that Goddard had fabricated the case study, but* The Kallikak Family *was extremely popular at the time and was used to further eugenic beliefs and practices.*

On September 15, 1906, the Training School for Backward and Feeble-minded Children at Vineland, New Jersey, opened a laboratory and a Department of Research for the study of feeble-mindedness.

A beginning was made in studying the mental condition of the children who lived in the Institution, with a view to determining the mental and physical peculiarities of the different grades and types, to getting an accurate record of what deficiencies each child had and what he was capable of doing, with the hope that in time these records could be correlated with the condition of the nervous system of the child, if he should die while in the Institution and an autopsy should be allowed.

As soon as possible after the beginning of this work, a definite start was made toward determining the cause of feeble-mindedness. After some preliminary work, it was concluded that the only way to get the information needed was by sending trained workers to the homes of the children, to learn by careful and wise questioning the facts that could be obtained. It was a great surprise to us to discover so much mental defect in the families of so many of these children. The results of the study of more than 300 families will soon be published, showing that about 65 per cent of these children have the hereditary taint.

The present study of the Kallikak family is a genuine story of real people. The name is, of course, fictitious, as are all of the names throughout the story. The results here presented come after two years of constant work, investigating the conditions of this family.

Some readers may question how it has been possible to get such definite data in regard to people who lived so long ago.

A word of explanation is hence in order. In the first place, the family itself proved to be a notorious one, so the people, in the community where the present generations are living, know of them; they knew their parents and grandparents; and the older members knew them farther back, because of the reputation they had always borne. Secondly, the reputation which the Training School has in the State is such that all have been willing to cooperate as soon as they understood the purpose and plan of the work. This has been of great help. Thirdly, the time devoted to this investigation must not be over-looked. A hasty investigation could never have produced the results which we have reached. Oftentimes a second, a third, a fifth, or a sixth visit has been necessary in order to develop an acquaintance and relationship with these families which induced them gradually to relate things which they otherwise had not recalled or did not care to tell. Many an important item has been gathered after several visits to these homes.

Chapter IV will throw still more light on the method used.

If the reader is inclined to the view that we must have called a great many people feeble-minded who were not so, let him be assured that this is not the case. On the contrary, we have preferred to err on the other side, and we have not marked people feeble-minded unless the case was such that we could substantiate it beyond a reasonable doubt. If there was good reason to call them normal, we have so marked them. If not, and we are unable to decide in our own minds, we have generally left them unmarked. In a few cases, we have marked them normal or feeble-minded, with a question mark. By this is meant that we have studied the case and after deliberation are still in doubt, but the probabilities are "N" or "F" as indicated. The mere fact of the doubt shows, however, that they are at least border-line cases.

To the scientific reader we would say that the data here presented are, we believe, accurate to a high degree. It is true that we have made rather dogmatic statements and have drawn conclusions that do not seem scientifically warranted from the data. We have done this because it seems necessary to make these statements and conclusions for the benefit of the lay reader, and it was impossible to present in this book all of the data that would substantiate them. We have, as a matter of fact, drawn upon the material which is soon to be presented in a larger book. The reference to Mendelism is an illustration of what we mean. It is, as it is given here, meager and inadequate, and the assumption that the given law applies to human heredity is an assumption so far as the data presented are concerned. We would ask that the scientist reserve judgment and wait for the larger book for the proof of these statements and for an adequate discussion of Mendelism in relation to the problem.

The necessary expense for this study, as well as for all of the work of the Research Laboratory, has been met by voluntary contributions from philanthropic men and women, who believe that here is an opportunity to benefit humanity, such as is hardly equaled elsewhere.

We take this means of expressing to them our deep appreciation of their sympathy and generosity. I wish also to make special mention of the indefatigable industry, wisdom, tact, and judgment of our field workers who have gathered these facts and whose results, although continually checked up, have stood every test put upon them as to their accuracy and value.

The work on this particular family has been done by Elizabeth S. Kite, to whom I am also indebted for practically all of Chapter IV.

I am also greatly indebted to my assistants in the laboratory, for help in preparing the charts, keeping the records, and correcting manuscript and proof.

To Superintendent Edward R. Johnstone, whose wisdom and foresight led to the establishment of this Department of Research, whose help, sympathy, and encouragement have been constant throughout the work of preparing this study, the thanks and gratitude of the entire group of readers who find in these facts any help toward the solution of the problems that they are facing, are due.

HENRY H. GODDARD.
VINELAND, N.J.,
SEPTEMBER, 1912.

Source: Goddard, Henry Herbert. 1912. *The Kallikak Family: A Study in the Heredity of Feeble-Mindedness.* New York: Macmillan. Available online at https://archive.org/stream/kallikakfamilyst00godduoft/kallikakfamilyst00godduoft_djvu.txt.

6. Virginia Sterilization Act (1924)

Introduction

Eugenics is an ideological and scientific movement that seeks to reportedly improve the human race through controlled and selective breeding. Eugenicists forwarded the belief that a wide variety of traits that they labeled as desirable or undesirable were genetic. According to eugenicists, desirable traits (e.g., intelligence, morality, and ambition) could be increased and undesirable traits (e.g., disability, criminality, and poverty) could be eradicated in the human population by regulating who could reproduce. In 1924, Virginia passed the Sterilization Act, which was heavily based on eugenics. The act permitted the involuntary sterilization of disabled inmates in state institutions who were labeled "mentally defective." Although the act was challenged in the Supreme Court case of Buck v. Bell, *the Supreme Court upheld the act as constitutional. Justice Oliver Wendell Holmes Jr. wrote in the court's ruling, "Three generations of imbeciles are enough." Consequently, more than 7,000 disabled people in Virginia were sterilized against their will, and the act became a model for other sterilization laws throughout the United States.*

2. An emergency existing, this act shall be enforced from its passage.

Chap. 394.—An ACT to provide for the sexual sterilization of inmates of State institutions in certain cases. [S B 281] Approved March 20, 1924.

Whereas, both the health of the individual patient and the welfare of society may be promoted in certain cases by the sterilization of mental defectives under careful safeguard and by competent and conscientious authority, and

Whereas, such sterilization may be effected in males by the operation of vasectomy and in females by the operation of salpingectomy, both of which said operations may be performed without serious pain or substantial danger to the life of the patient, and

Whereas, the Commonwealth has in custodial care and is supporting in various State institutions many defective persons who if now discharged or paroled would likely become by the propagation of their kind a menace to society but who if incapable of procreating might properly and safely be discharged or paroled and become self-supporting with benefit both to themselves and to society, and

Whereas, human experience has demonstrated that heredity plays an important part in the transmission of sanity, idiocy, imbecility, epilepsy and crime, now, therefore

1. Be it enacted by the general assembly of Virginia, That whenever the superintendent of the Western State Hospital, or of the Eastern State Hospital, or of the Southwestern State Hospital, or of the Central State Hospital, or the State Colony for Epileptics and Feeble-Minded, shall be of opinion that it is for the best interests of the patients and of society that any inmate of the institution under his care should be sexually sterilized, such superintendent is hereby authorized to perform, or cause to be performed by some capable physicians or surgeon, the operation of sterilization on any such patient confined in such institution afflicted with hereditary forms of insanity that are recurrent, idiocy, imbecility, feeble-mindedness or epilepsy; provided that such superintendent shall have first complied with the requirements of this act.

2. Such superintendent shall first present to the special board of directors of his hospital or colony a petition stating the facts of the case and the grounds of his opinion, verified by his affidavit to the best of his knowledge and belief, and praying that an order may be entered by said board requiring him to perform or have performed by some competent physician to be designated by him in his said petition or by said board in its order, upon the inmate of his institution named in such petition, the operation of vasectomy if upon a male and of salpingectomy if upon a female.

A copy of said petition must be served upon the inmate together with a notice in writing designating the time and place in the said institution, not less than thirty days before the presentation of such petition to said special board of directors when and where said board may hear and act upon such petition.

Source: Virginia General Assembly. March 20, 1924. https://www.dnalc.org/view/11213-Virginia-Sterilization-Act-of-3-20-1924.html

7. Flyer Distributed by the League of the Physically Handicapped (1935)

Introduction

In May 1935, a group of six disabled people formed the League of the Physically Handicapped (LPH), which eventually grew to several hundred members. This early disability rights group sought economic and social justice for disabled people, with a particular emphasis on employment. In their first action, LPH occupied the Emergency Relief Bureau in New York City to challenge its refusal to refer disabled people to the Works Progress Administration

for employment. After the sit-in lasted nine days, the Works Progress Administration pledged it would no longer discriminate against disabled workers, but the administration did not fulfill its promise. The LPH then launched another demonstration, which it called a death watch. This protest was a weekend-long sit-in to "honor the dead promises of the administration." It also encouraged other people to get involved by writing, telegraphing, and phoning the Works Progress Administration to demand an end to disability discrimination. Eventually, the group's efforts generated several thousand jobs nationwide for disabled workers. LPH was a pioneer and early precursor to the Disability Rights Movement of the 1970s.

"DEATH WATCH"

On December 6th, Mr. Ridder announced to the press that within ten days jobs will be given to the unemployed members of THE LEAGUE FOR THE PHYSICALLY HANDICAPPED. There was to be no more discrimination against handicapped workers.

WE ACCEPTED THIS PLEDGE OF THE ADMINISTRATION.

WE WITHDREW OUR PICKET LINES FROM W.P.A. HEADQUARTERS

at 111 - 8th Ave.

BUT THE ADMINISTRATION DELIBERATELY BROKE ITS PROMISE !!

WE ACCUSE !!!

The Administration of

UNJUST DISCRIMINATION AGAINST THE HANDICAPPED.

DISREGARDING THE NEEDS OF THE HANDICAPPED EVEN AFTER OUR PROBLEM HAD BEEN BROUGHT TO THEIR ATTENTION. ASSUMING A CALLOUSED AND INHUMAN ATTITUDE TOWARD US. DEPRIVING US OF WHAT IS RIGHTFULLY OURS —THE RIGHT TO LIVE.

OUR NEEDS ARE DESPERATE !!!

****
****

We will honor the dead promises of the administration with a "DEATH WATCH" at 111 - 8th Ave. starting on Friday, Dec. 20th at 4 P.M. and continue through the night.

WE WILL FIGHT UNTIL WE WIN -- WE WANT JOBS !!

****
****

Since the Administration has ignored our problem, we appeal now to the highest law of the land —PUBLIC OPINION.

WRITE-WIRE-OR-PHONE YOUR PROTESTS DEMANDING

That Discrimination Be Stopped !!

That the Promised Jobs be Given !!

YOU AND YOUR FRIENDS CAN HELP US.

Phone Watkins 9-3500.

LEAGUE FOR THE PHYSICALLY HANDICAPPED

929 Broadway—New York City

UNEMPLOYED SECTION MEETS EVERY MON. 7:30 P.M.

Source: "Disability Militancy—the 1930s." Disability Social History Project. http://www.disabilityhistory.org/dw_text.html.

8. President Franklin Delano Roosevelt's Statement on the Signing of the Social Security Act (1935)

Introduction

The Social Security Act was signed into law by President Franklin D. Roosevelt on August 14, 1935. The act was part of Roosevelt's Second New Deal programs, which aimed to alleviate poverty and stimulate the economy during the Great Depression. The Social Security Act established Social Security Insurance, which is an old-age pension system that protects elders from experiencing poverty. It also provided unemployment compensation, support for low-income families with children, and aid for blind people. This legislation provided the foundation for the provision of social welfare in the United States. It also served as the precursor for Social Security Disability Insurance, which provides benefits to disabled people who are unable to work.

August 14, 1935

Today a hope of many years' standing is in large part fulfilled. The civilization of the past hundred years, with its startling industrial changes, has tended more and more to make life insecure. Young people have come to wonder what would be their lot when they came to old age. The man with a job has wondered how long the job would last.

This social security measure gives at least some protection to thirty millions of our citizens who will reap direct benefits through unemployment compensation, through old-age pensions and through increased services for the protection of children and the prevention of ill health.

We can never insure one hundred percent of the population against one hundred percent of the hazards and vicissitudes of life, but we have tried to frame a law which will give some measure of protection to the average citizen and to his family against the loss of a job and against poverty-ridden old age.

This law, too, represents a cornerstone in a structure which is being built but is by no means complete. It is a structure intended to lessen the force of possible future depressions. It will act as a protection to future Administrations against the necessity of going deeply into debt to furnish relief to the needy. The law will flatten out the peaks and valleys of deflation and of inflation. It is, in short, a law that will take care of human needs and at the same time provide for the United States an economic structure of vastly greater soundness.

I congratulate all of you ladies and gentlemen, all of you in the Congress, in the executive departments and all of you who come from private life, and I thank you for your splendid efforts in behalf of this sound, needed and patriotic legislation.

If the Senate and the House of Representatives in this long and arduous session had done nothing more than pass this Bill, the session would be regarded as historic for all time.

Source: Franklin D. Roosevelt. 1935. "Statement on Signing the Social Security Act." August 14. Online by Gerhard Peters and John T. Woolley, The American Presidency Project. http://www.presidency.ucsb.edu/ws/?pid=14916.

9. President Franklin Delano Roosevelt's Announcement on the Founding of the National Foundation for Infantile Paralysis (1937)

Introduction

President Franklin D. Roosevelt was diagnosed with polio in 1921, and he experienced paralysis. This personal experience with disability informed his approach to medical care, research, and philanthropy. In 1938, he founded the National Foundation for Infantile Paralysis. Roosevelt tasked the NIIP with leading, directing, and unifying the people and entities seeking to prevent polio, treat and cure polio, and care for people with polio. The organization ultimately raised enough money to support the development of Salk's polio vaccine. After polio was largely eradicated, the NIIP changed its focus from polio to birth defects, arthritis, and virus diseases. The NIIP later changed its name to the March of Dimes, and it is now one of the largest nonprofit organizations in the United States. The present focus of the March of Dimes is to support the health of mothers and children to prevent birth defects, premature birth, and infant mortality.

On September 23, 1937, President Roosevelt made the following announcement:

"I have been very much concerned over the epidemics of infantile paralysis which have been prevalent in many cities in different parts of the country. I have had reports from many areas in which this disease is again spreading its destruction. And once again there is brought forcibly to my mind the constantly increasing accumulation of ruined lives—which must continue unless this disease can be brought under control and its after-effects properly treated.

"My own personal experience in the work that we have been doing at the Georgia Warm Springs Foundation for over ten years leads me to the very definite conclusion that the best results in attempting to eradicate this disease cannot be secured by approaching the problem through any single one of its aspects, whether that be preventive studies in the laboratory, emergency work during epidemics, or after-treatment. For over ten years at the Foundation at Warm Springs, Georgia, we have devoted our effort almost entirely to the study of improved treatment of the aftereffects of the illness. During these years other agencies, which we have from time to time assisted, have devoted their energies to other phases of the fight. I firmly believe that the time has now arrived when the whole attack on this plague should be led and directed, though not controlled, by one national body. And it is for this purpose that a new National Foundation for Infantile Paralysis is being created.

"As I have said, the general purpose of the new Foundation will be to lead, direct and unify the fight on every phase of this sickness. It will make every effort to ensure that every responsible research agency in this country is adequately financed to carry on investigations into the cause of infantile paralysis and the methods by which it may be prevented. It will endeavor to eliminate much of the needless aftereffect of this disease—wreckage caused by the failure to make early and accurate diagnosis of its presence. We all know that improper care during the acute stage of the disease, and the use of antiquated treatment, or downright neglect of any treatment, are the cause of thousands of crippled, twisted, powerless bodies now. Much can be done along these lines right now. The new Foundation will carry on a broad-gauged educational campaign, prepared under expert medical supervision, and this will be placed within the reach of the doctors and the hospitals of the country. The practising physician is in reality the front line fighter of the sickness, and there is much existing valuable knowledge that should be disseminated to him.

"And then there is also the tremendous problem as to what is to be done with those hundreds of thousands already ruined by the aftereffects of this affliction. To investigate, to study, to develop every medical possibility of enabling those so afflicted to become economically independent in their local communities will be one of the chief aims of the new Foundation.

"Those who today are fortunate in being in full possession of their muscular power naturally do not understand what it means to a human being paralyzed by this disease to have that powerlessness lifted even to a small degree. It means the difference between a human being dependent on others, and an individual who can be wholly independent. The public has little conception of the patience and time and expense necessary to accomplish such results. But the results are of the utmost importance to the individual.

"The work of the new organization must start immediately. It cannot be delayed. Its activities will include among many others those of the Georgia Warm Springs Foundation, of which I have been president since its inception. I shall continue as president of that Foundation. But, in fairness to my official responsibilities, I cannot at this time take a very active part in the much broader work that will be carried out by the new Foundation, and I therefore do not feel that I should now hold any official position in it. However, because I am wholeheartedly in this cause, I have enlisted the sincere interest of several representative and outstanding individuals who are willing to initiate and carry on the work of the new Foundation."

In December President Roosevelt selected thirty-four trustees to take over administration of The National Foundation for Infantile Paralysis. Announcing the creation of the Foundation, the President, on October 18 last, wrote Basil O'Connor of

New York, treasurer of the Georgia Warm Springs Foundation:

"I have your letter with respect to using again my birthday in 1938 in the cause of infantile paralysis.

"As you know, I am very much interested in the steps that are being taken to perfect the organization of the new National Foundation for Infantile Paralysis about which I made a public announcement on September 23rd of this year.

"As I said in that statement, it is the desire of everyone interested in this cause that the work of the new Foundation be carried forward as expeditiously as possible. Nevertheless we all realize that plans of such importance and magnitude must at the same time be worked out carefully and soundly, and that undue haste may be as fatal to the cause as delay. To pick the personnel of the new Foundation wisely and to project its purposes properly must of necessity consume some time.

"Against this is the fact, as I stated on September 23rd, that it is my opinion that all fund-raising should be under the control and supervision of the new Foundation, including the activity for raising money in connection with the celebration of my birthday in January, 1938. Heretofore we have for one reason or another, over which no one had control, always been crowded for time in which to make arrangements for properly permitting the public to participate in those occasions for the benefit of the cause of infantile paralysis. You have advised me that if the plans for that event in 1938 are delayed until the perfection of the organization of the new Foundation, we will again find ourselves handicapped by lack of time in making the proper arrangements for the 1938 birthday celebration.

"In these circumstances, and in view of the fact that the past birthday celebrations have to a very large extent been organized and supervised by individuals officially connected with Georgia Warm Springs Foundation, I feel that we should not take any chance of delay, particularly in view of the much larger work to be done by the new Foundation. I therefore wish that, as an officer of Georgia Warm Springs Foundation, you would undertake to define and carry out plans for the 1938 celebration. The funds received from that occasion will, of course, go to the new Foundation, and when its organization is complete it will take over the supervision of that event as well as any other fund-raising activity.

Very sincerely yours, FRANKLIN D. ROOSEVELT."

Source: "The Dawn of the National Foundation for Infantile Paralysis." Disability History Museum. http://www.disabilitymuseum.org/dhm/lib/detail.html?id=2153&print=1.

10. Section 14(c) of the Fair Labor Standards Act (FLSA) (1938)

Introduction

People with disabilities face numerous forms of discrimination in employment, including access to fair and equal wages. Presently, Section 14(c) of the Fair Labor Standards Act permits certified employers to pay individuals with disabilities a subminimum wage, or a wage below minimum wage. Under the law, the exact rate of the wage is determined on the basis of how productive a disabled person is compared to a nondisabled person. Some disabled people have reported earning as little as under $1 an hour. Advocates of subminimum wage claim that it expands employment opportunities for disabled people and provides a way for disabled people to receive training, occupy their time, and earn money.

However, many disability activists contest subminimum wage, noting that it is legalized discrimination that forces disabled people to live in poverty.

(c) Handicapped workers

    (1) The Secretary, to the extent necessary to prevent curtailment of opportunities for employment, shall by regulation or order provide for the employment, under special certificates, of individuals (including individuals employed in agriculture) whose earning or productive capacity is impaired by age, physical or mental deficiency, or injury, at wages which are—

        (A) lower than the minimum wage applicable under section 206 of this title,

        (B) commensurate with those paid to nonhandicapped workers, employed in the vicinity in which the individuals under the certificates are employed, for essentially the same type, quality, and quantity of work, and

        (C) related to the individual's productivity.

    (2) The Secretary shall not issue a certificate under paragraph (1) unless the employer provides written assurances to the Secretary that—

        (A) in the case of individuals paid on an hourly rate basis, wages paid in accordance with paragraph (1) will be reviewed by the employer at periodic intervals at least once every six months, and

        (B) wages paid in accordance with paragraph (1) will be adjusted by the employer at periodic intervals, at least once each year, to reflect changes in the prevailing wage paid to experienced nonhandicapped individuals employed in the locality for essentially the same type of work.

    (3) Notwithstanding paragraph (1), no employer shall be permitted to reduce the hourly wage rate prescribed by certificate under this subsection in effect on June 1, 1986, of any handicapped individual for a period of two years from such date without prior authorization of the Secretary.

    (4) Nothing in this subsection shall be construed to prohibit an employer from maintaining or establishing work activities centers to provide therapeutic activities for handicapped clients.

    (5)

        (A) Notwithstanding any other provision of this subsection, any employee receiving a special minimum wage at a rate specified pursuant to this subsection or the parent or guardian of such an employee may petition the Secretary to obtain a review of such special minimum wage rate. An employee or the employee's parent or guardian may file such a petition for and in behalf of the employee or in behalf of the employee and other employees similarly situated. No employee may be a party to any such action unless the employee or the employee's parent or guardian gives consent in writing to become such a party and such consent is filed with the Secretary.

(B) Upon receipt of a petition filed in accordance with subparagraph (A), the Secretary within ten days shall assign the petition to an administrative law judge appointed pursuant to section 3105 of Title 5. The administrative law judge shall conduct a hearing on the record in accordance with section 554 of Title 5 with respect to such petition within thirty days after assignment.

(C) In any such proceeding, the employer shall have the burden of demonstrating that the special minimum wage rate is justified as necessary in order to prevent curtailment of opportunities for employment.

(D) In determining whether any special minimum wage rate is justified pursuant to subparagraph (C), the administrative law judge shall consider—
  (i) the productivity of the employee or employees identified in the petition and the conditions under which such productivity was measured; and
  (ii) the productivity of other employees performing work of essentially the same type and quality for other employers in the same vicinity.

(E) The administrative law judge shall issue a decision within thirty days after the hearing provided for in subparagraph (B). Such action shall be deemed to be a final agency action unless within thirty days the Secretary grants a request to review the decision of the administrative law judge. Either the petitioner or the employer may request review by the Secretary within fifteen days of the date of issuance of the decision by the administrative law judge.

(F) The Secretary, within thirty days after receiving a request for review, shall review the record and either adopt the decision of the administrative law judge or issue exceptions. The decision of the administrative law judge, together with any exceptions, shall be deemed to be a final agency action.

(G) A final agency action shall be subject to judicial review pursuant to chapter 7 of Title 5. An action seeking such review shall be brought within thirty days of a final agency action described in subparagraph (F).

Source: The Fair Labor Standards Act of 1938, as Amended. May 2011. https://www.dol.gov/whd/regs/statutes/FairLaborStandAct.pdf.

II. President Harry S. Truman's Proclamation of National Employ the Physically Handicapped Week (1945)

Introduction

People with disabilities experience significant barriers to obtaining and retaining gainful employment. Although disabled people report a number of impediments in securing employment, such as inadequate education and training and lack of accessible transportation, one of the greatest challenges is prejudice and the associated discrimination. Employment began to receive national attention as a disability rights issue shortly after World War II, when many disabled veterans who returned to the United States struggled to find work. In 1945, President Harry S. Truman issued a proclamation to establish "National Employ the Physically Handicapped Week," which aimed to educate people about the employment needs of people with disabilities and raise awareness regarding the contributions disabled employees make to the economy. In 1988, Congress expanded this effort and declared October to be National Disability Employment Awareness Month.

September 21, 1945

By the President of the United States of America

A Proclamation

Whereas the people of this Nation are determined to foster an environment in which those of their fellow citizens who have become physically handicapped can continue to make their rightful contribution to the work of the world and can continue to enjoy the opportunities and rewards of that work; and

Whereas Public Resolution No. 176, 79th Congress, approved August 11, 1945, provides in part:

"That hereafter the first week in October of each year shall be designated as National Employ the Physically Handicapped Week. During said week, appropriate ceremonies are to be held throughout the Nation, the purpose of which will be to enlist public support for and interest in the employment of otherwise qualified but physically handicapped workers":

Now, Therefore, I, Harry S. Truman, President of the United States of America, do hereby call upon the people of the United States to observe the week of October 7–13, 1945 as National Employ the Physically Handicapped Week. I ask the governors of States, mayors of cities, heads of the various agencies of the Government, and other public officials, as well as leaders in industry, education, religion, and every other aspect of our common life, during this week and at all other suitable times, to exercise every appropriate effort to enlist public support of a sustained program for the employment and development of the abilities and capacities of those who are physically handicapped.

In Witness Whereof, I have hereunto set my hand and caused the seal of the United States of America to be affixed.

Done at the City of Washington this 21st day of September, in the year of our Lord nineteen hundred and forty-five and of the Independence of the United States of America the one hundred and seventieth.

HARRY S. TRUMAN
By the President:
DEAN ACHESON,
Acting Secretary of State.

Source: Harry S. Truman. 1945. "Proclamation 2664—National Employ the Physically Handicapped Week, 1945," September 21. Online by Gerhard Peters and John T. Woolley, The American Presidency Project. http://www.presidency.ucsb.edu/ws/?pid=87042.

I2. Excerpt from the President's Panel on Mental Retardation, Report of the Task Force on Law (1963)

Introduction

In 1961, President John F. Kennedy created the President's Panel on Mental

Retardation. He appointed 26 members to the panel, including experts in medicine, science, education, psychology, sociology, and law. The majority of the panel had little to no direct experience with people with intellectual disabilities. However, one member, Dr. Elizabeth Boggs, was closely connected with the parents' movement, which was an advocacy group of parents of children with intellectual disabilities. The panel was tasked with researching and proposing solutions to the issues affecting people with intellectual disabilities. The resulting report provided 112 recommendations in various areas, including education, medical care, social services, and care facilities. The panel's report prompted new legislation, such as the Mental Retardation and Community Mental Health Centers Construction Act of 1963.

Judge David L. Bazelon, *Chairman*

Dr. Elizabeth M. Boggs, *Vice-Chairman*

Law and the Retarded: The Social Context

Growing understanding of a broad disability such as retardation usually sets off three altogether different processes, each of which affects the others, and has a bearing on practical decisions.

First, general understandings, the presumptions on which people operate every day, are altered so that human behavior comes to be seen in a substantially different light. This has occurred in relation to what we have learned both about mental disease and mental retardation. Second, important institutions such as school, church and home alter their views, doctrines and practices in the light of new knowledge. Lastly, new, specialized social institutions and services designed to deal with the problem are brought into being.

Ours is a society in flux. It accommodates the mentally retarded in changing ways, both in its ordinary social institutions and by special provisions for the retarded. These provisions and accommodations—present and projected—are the subject of much of the full Report of the President's Panel, to which this Task Force study is an adjunct. The law must consider not only new knowledge concerning the retarded but also the new contexts in which such knowledge is found.

What especially needs discussion is the bearing on our problem of changes in our ordinary social institutions. These institutions are of two kinds: those addressed to other social problems such as delinquency, dependency, chronic disability, etc., and those not concerned with "problems" as such, but with wider aspects of living, such as the church, the school and the law generally.

Thus, what the public school system does, or leaves undone, influences what it means to be or to have a mentally retarded child. It also affects the burden laid on more specialized institutions.

A major principle of the American school system is free education for all children. Many state constitutions guarantee each child the right to basic educational opportunities at public expense. These mandates do not specifically exclude children because of physical or mental handicapping conditions. Obviously, retarded children require special educational services and programs if they are to receive opportunities equal in value, if not in kind, to those received by normal children. The responsibility for applying this principle has been placed upon the local school systems with stimulation and support being provided from the state and federal governments.

In varying degrees, and with more or less success, local school boards have tackled the problem of providing services for educable, mildly retarded children. But on the whole, they have fallen short of what we conceive to be their obligation to moderately and severely retarded children. To the extent that the moderately retarded can learn academic skills, they may be provided for. But they, and the severely retarded, can profit by training both in personal habits and in simple unskilled occupations. The moderately retarded, for instance, may sometimes be trained to undertake semi-skilled work. It is in providing for these trainable retarded children that our public school systems have generally failed.

The emergence of governmental and non-governmental service programs, not specifically addressed to retardation, profoundly affects the context of the retardation problem. The various social security and disability insurance programs have already had a notable effect. Even things as seemingly remote as the formation or extension of a Boy Scout troop, a family service association, a factory inspections service, or a state program to provide visual aids in schools, are all relevant.

The richer these general services, and the more easily available they are, the less the need for special services for the retarded. (It should be noted, however, that even where general services exist, they may in practice be "unavailable" to the lower classes simply because their procedures are not adapted to lower-class life, and their vocabulary and way of looking at things may be incomprehensible to lower-class people.) The general services remove from the special services for the retarded only that part of their burden which the special services were not organized to bear, but are required to bear if others will not. The optimum condition obtains only when each fulfills its proper function, e.g., when mental hospitals have

to accept non-psychotic retarded persons because waiting lists are too long at residential care facilities, both the mentally ill and the retarded are hurt, and the hospital is crippled because it is trying to perform a function for which it was not intended.

What is true for general services and institutions is also true for general law. For instance, to the extent that the law protecting minors generally is adequate, the burden of providing special legislation for the retarded minor is reduced. Such general protective legislation is like the salt in a body of water; its presence is helpful to all swimmers, but especially so for the weaker and less skilled. Similarly, general improvements in social conditions, such as higher levels of affluence, education, wisdom or morality, are likely to ameliorate the lot of the mentally retarded. The higher the level of education, the more likely it is that disabilities will be seen and treated for what they are.

Next in importance to these changes in general conditions is the enormous multiplication of programs, services and personnel designed to aid individuals and groups in society. An index of the new professions and services is sizable—visiting nurses, psychiatric social workers, remedial reading specialists, group therapy leaders, participant observers in youth programs, guidance specialists, marriage counselors, to name a few. They not only deal with the problems of retardation, they also represent resources for dealing with the problems which the retarded provoke in their immediate environment, e.g., the family distress that may spring from caring for the retarded. To some degree their presence also helps ameliorate the social causes of retardation.

Many studies have shown that the vast bulk of social work, money and effort goes into so-called "multi-problem" families. Such families frequently exhibit crime, delinquency, mental illness, physical defects, "excessive drinking," broken family relations, physical sickness, sometimes in different members of the family, but quite commonly in the same members. This is at least partially because, both for the individual and the family, one misfortune generally reduces capacity to fend off others. The same aggregation of defects and disabilities frequently affects the retarded. Here as elsewhere each additional misfortune exacerbates the effect of the previous one, and each additional misfortune helps pave the way for the next. Thus to the extent that the community successfully attacks the other social problems, the burden of mental retardation will become easier to bear.

In dealing with these problems, there is, lately, a tendency to increase the individual's mobility between institutions and services. Such mobility is as vital in this context as the physician's freedom to change his patient's prescription as the patient's condition changes. Effective coordination between services permits the disabled person to move between various levels of support or security as his needs vary.

There is also a recognition of the need to spread as far down the line as possible responsibility and initiative in handling the person. This means moving away from the formal towards the informal, from the organized towards the spontaneous, from higher levels of government towards the local, from the mandatory towards the encouraged, from "strangers" towards "kin," from the specialist towards the non-specialist—in general, as far as possible towards the resources of the person himself, his family, friends, neighbors, etc., strengthened and buttressed, as need be, by more formalized resources.

Laws and their administration influence the extent to which the mentally retarded are permitted to benefit from these trends and advances.

Source: The President's Panel on Mental Retardation. "Report of the Task Force on Law." https://mn.gov/mnddc/parallels2/pdf/60s/63/63-ROT-PPMR.pdf.

13. Declaration of Objectives from the Older Americans Act (1965)

Introduction

The Older Americans Act was signed into law on July 14, 1965, by President Lyndon B. Johnson. This landmark legislation was designed to ensure older adults in the United States had access to employment, income in retirement, housing, nutrition, medical and personal care, social support, and community participation. Through the establishment of the Administration on Aging and the Area Agencies on Aging, the Older Americans Act supports home and community-based social services for individuals aged 60 and older and their caregivers. During the signing of the act, President Johnson stated:

No longer will older Americans be denied the healing miracle of modern medicine. No longer will illness crush and destroy the savings that they have so carefully put away over a lifetime so that they might enjoy dignity in their later years. No longer will young families see their own incomes, and their own hopes, eaten away simply because they are carrying out their deep moral obligations to their parents, and to their uncles, and to their aunts. And no longer will this nation refuse the hand of justice to those who have given a lifetime of service and wisdom and labor to the progress of this progressive country.

The Older Americans Act has been reauthorized numerous times since 1965, and continues to provide essential home and community-based services and supports for elders, particularly those with disabilities.

Declaration of Objectives for Older Americans

Se. 101. The Congress hereby finds and declares that, in keeping with the traditional American concept of the inherent dignity of the individual in our democratic society, the older people of our Nation are entitled to, and it is the joint and several duty and responsibility of the governments of the United States and of the several States and their political subdivisions to assist our older people to secure equal opportunity to the full and free enjoyment of the following objectives:

(1) An adequate income in retirement in accordance with the American standard of living.
(2) The best possible physical and mental health which science can make available and without regard to economic status.
(3) Suitable housing, independently selected, designed and located with reference to special needs and available at costs which older citizens can afford.
(4) Full restorative services for those who require institutional care.
(5) Opportunity for employment with no discriminatory personnel practices because of age.
(6) Retirement in health, honor, dignity— after years of contribution to the economy.
(7) Pursuit of meaningful activity within the widest range of civic, cultural. And recreational opportunities.

(8) Efficient community services which provide social assistance in a coordinated manner and which are readily available when needed.
(9) Immediate benefit from proven research knowledge which can sustain and improve health and happiness.
(10) Freedom, independence, and the free exercise of individual initiative in planning and managing their own lives.

Source: Government Publishing Office. "Public Law 89-73." https://www.gpo.gov/fdsys/pkg/STATUTE-79/pdf/STATUTE-79-Pg218.pdf.

14. Excerpt from the Rehabilitation Act (1973)

Introduction

In 1973, President Richard Nixon signed the Rehabilitation Act into law. Section 504 of the Rehabilitation Act prohibited discrimination on the basis of disability in federal and federally funded programs. This law was a significant victory for the disability rights movement, as it was the first civil rights law for people with disabilities.

Sec. 2. Findings; Purpose; Policy.

(a) Findings.—Congress finds that—
  (1) millions of Americans have one or more physical or mental disabilities and the number of Americans with such disabilities is increasing;
  (2) individuals with disabilities constitute one of the most disadvantaged groups in society;
  (3) disability is a natural part of the human experience and in no way diminishes the right of individuals to—
    (A) live independently;

(B) enjoy self-determination;

(C) make choices;

(D) contribute to society;

(E) pursue meaningful careers; and

(F) enjoy full inclusion and integration in the economic, political, social, cultural, and educational mainstream of American society;

(4) increased employment of individuals with disabilities can be achieved through implementation of statewide workforce development systems defined in section 3 of the Workforce Innovation and Opportunity Act that provide meaningful and effective participation for individuals with disabilities in workforce investment activities carried out under the vocational rehabilitation program established under title I, and through the provision of independent living services, support service, and meaningful opportunities for employment in integrated work settings through the provision of reasonable accommodations;

(5) individuals with disabilities continually encounter various forms of discrimination in such critical areas as employment, housing, public accommodations, education, transportation, communication, recreation, institutionalization, health services, voting, and public services;

(6) the goals of the Nation properly include the goal of providing individuals with disabilities with the tools necessary to—

(A) make informed choices and decisions; and

(B) achieve equality of opportunity, full inclusion and integration in society, employment, independent living, and economic and social self-sufficiency, for such individuals; and

(7) (A) a high proportion of students with disabilities is leaving secondary education without being employed in competitive integrated employment, or being enrolled in postsecondary education; and

(B) there is a substantial need to support such students as they transition from school to postsecondary life.

Source: U.S. House. Legal Counsel. https://legcounsel.house.gov/Comps/Rehabilitation%20Act%20Of%201973.pdf.

---

15. Excerpt from *In re Marriage of Carney* Decision by the California State Supreme Court (1979)

Introduction

Carney v. Carney *is a landmark California Supreme Court case that established that disabled parents have rights equal to those of nondisabled parents. In the 1970s, William T. Carney separated from his wife, Ellen J. Carney, and moved with their two sons from New York to California. William cared for the boys for the next four years. Ellen was largely uninvolved, and she never contributed financially to the boys' care or visited them. William was then in a serious car accident and became a quadriplegic. About a year after the accident, Ellen requested a change in custody, which was granted solely on the basis of William's disability. William contested the decision, and the California Supreme Court ruled in his favor, noting that prejudicial stereotypes about disability should not determine child custody decisions and that disabled parents have the right to be involved in their children's lives.*

In re the Marriage of ELLEN J. and WILLIAM T. CARNEY. WILLIAM T. CARNEY, Appellant, v. ELLEN J. CARNEY, Respondent

(Opinion by Mosk, J., expressing the unanimous view of the court.)

. . . It is erroneous to presume that a parent in a wheelchair cannot share to a meaningful degree in the physical activities of his child, should both desire it. On the one hand, modern technology has made the handicapped increasingly mobile, as demonstrated by William's purchase of a van and his plans to drive it by means of hand controls. In the past decade the widespread availability of such vans, together with sophisticated and reliable wheelchair lifts and driving control systems, have brought about a quiet revolution in the mobility of the severely handicapped. No longer are they confined to home or institution, unable to travel except by special vehicle or with the assistance of others; today such persons use the streets and highways in ever-growing numbers for both business and pleasure. Again as Dr. Share explained, the capacity to drive such a vehicle "opens more vistas, greater alternatives" for the handicapped person.

At the same time the physically handicapped have made the public more aware of the many unnecessary obstacles to their participation in community life. Among the evidence of the public's change in attitude is a growing body of legislation intended to reduce or eliminate the physical impediments to that participation, i.e., the "architectural barriers" against access by the handicapped to buildings, facilities, and transportation systems used by the public at large. (See, e.g., Gov. Code, §4450 et seq. [requires handicapped access to buildings and facilities constructed with public funds]; Health & Saf. Code, §19955 et seq. [access to private buildings open to the general public]; Gov. Code, §4500 [access to public transit systems]; Pub. Resources Code, §5070.5, subd. (c) [access to public recreational trails]; see also Veh. Code, §§22507.8, 22511.5 et seq. [special parking privileges for handicapped drivers].) fn. 10 [24 Cal. 3d 739]

While there is obviously much room for continued progress in removing these barriers, the handicapped person today need not remain a shut-in. Although William cannot actually play on his children's baseball team, he may nevertheless be able to take them to the game, participate as a fan, a coach, or even an umpire—and treat them to ice cream on the way home. Nor is this companionship limited to athletic events: such a parent is no less capable of accompanying his children to theaters or libraries, shops or restaurants, schools or churches, afternoon picnics or long vacation trips. Thus it is not true that, as the court herein assumed, William will be unable "to actively go places with [his children], take them places, . . ."

On a deeper level, finally, the stereotype is false because it fails to reach the heart of the parent-child relationship. Contemporary psychology confirms what wise families have perhaps always known—that the essence of parenting is not to be found in the harried rounds of daily carpooling endemic to modern suburban life, or even in the doggedly dutiful acts of "togetherness" committed every weekend by well-meaning fathers and mothers across America. Rather, its essence lies in the ethical, emotional, and intellectual guidance the parent gives to the child throughout his formative years, and often beyond. The source of this guidance is the adult's own experience of life; its motive power is parental love and concern for the child's well-being; and its teachings deal with such fundamental matters as the child's feelings about himself, his relationships with others, his system of values, his standards of conduct, and his goals and priorities in life. Even if it were true, as the court herein asserted, that William cannot do "anything" for his sons except "talk to them and teach them, be a tutor," that would not only be "enough"—contrary to the court's conclusion—it would be the most valuable service a parent can render. Yet his capacity to do so is entirely unrelated to his physical prowess: however limited his bodily strength may be, a handicapped parent is a whole person to the child who needs his affection, sympathy, and wisdom to deal with the problems of growing up. Indeed, in such matters his handicap may well be an asset: few can pass through the crucible of a severe physical disability without learning enduring lessons in patience and tolerance.

Source: Supreme Court of California. 1979. *In re Marriage of Carney.* L.A. No. 31064. August 7. Available online at Justia.com. http://law.justia .com/cases/california/supreme-court/3d/24/725 .html.

16. The Introduction from *Toward Independence*, a National Council on Disability Report to the President and the Congress of the United States (1986)

Introduction

In February 1986, the National Council on the Handicapped (now known as the National Council on Disability) released the report Toward Independence: An Assessment of Federal Laws and Programs Affecting Persons with Disabilities. *The report focused on ten major areas identified as relevant to disabled people in the United States: equal opportunity laws, employment, disincentives to work under Social Security laws, prevention of disabilities, transportation, housing, community-based services for independent living, education, personal assistance services, and service coordination. Numerous stakeholders, including disabled people, disability advocates, experts in disability services and supports, family members, policy advisors, and business owners, provided input to the council as they developed the report. In the report, the council identified key issues faced by disabled people and provided legislative recommendations. One of the most significant recommendations was the need for a comprehensive equal opportunity and civil rights law. The council suggested that such as law might be called the* "Americans with Disabilities Act of 1986." *Although it took four years, their recommendation became a reality when President George H. W. Bush signed the Americans with Disabilities Act into law in 1990.*

Our country calls not for the life of ease, but for the life of strenuous endeavor.
President Theodore Roosevelt, 1899

As for other Americans, life for people with disabilities involves striving, working, taking risks, failing, teaming, and overcoming obstacles. We have all had the experience of seeking something that eludes us, of trying to reach a goal that seems to dance just out of reach. Most of us have also had the rewarding experience of surmounting obstacles to achieve a goal or accomplish a task, succeeding even though someone else or even we ourselves doubted we could do it.

A major difference between persons with disabilities and other individuals is the number, degree, and complexity of the barriers they face in trying to achieve their personal goals and fulfillment. Some of these barriers result from the disabilities themselves—a disability may be considered to be the lack of some mental, physical, or emotional "tool" which most other people can call upon in addressing life's tasks. A person with a physical disability, for example, may be unable to perform certain physical movements or functions that other people take for granted. A person with a sensory disability may lack or have significant impairment of one of the major senses, such as sight or hearing, which for other people provide important channels for receiving information about the world around them. An individual with a mental or emotional impairment may have a reduced ability to deal with the stresses of life or to sort out the real from the imagined. And people with cognitive impairments, such as learning disabilities and mental retardation, have disorders in the ability or rate of accepting, processing, storing, and recalling information.

But whatever the limitations associated with particular disabilities, people with disabilities have been saying for years that their major obstacles are not inherent in their disabilities, but arise from barriers that have been imposed externally and unnecessarily. As an international group of experts concluded:

> *Despite everything we can do, or hope to do, to assist each physically or mentally disabled person achieve his or her maximum potential in life, our efforts will not succeed until we have found the way to remove the obstacles to this goal directed by*

human society—the physical barriers we have created in public buildings, housing, transportation, houses of worship, centers of social life, and other community facilities—the social barriers we have evolved and accepted against those who vary more than a certain degree from what we have been conditioned to regard as normal. More people are forced into limited lives and made to suffer by these man-made obstacles than by any specific physical or mental disability.

Report of the United Nations Expert Group Meeting on Barrier-Free Design, International Rehabilitation Review, vol. 26, p. 3 (1975).

As detailed subsequently in this report, our Nation's current annual Federal expenditure on disability benefits and programs is more than $60 billion. Overall Federal spending associated with disability can be expected to mushroom as the "baby boom" generation grows older and age-related disabilities increase. The present and future costs of disability to our nation are directly related to the degree of success we attain in reducing existing barriers, both structural and attitudinal, and in providing appropriate services to individuals with disabilities so that they may realize their full potential and become more independent and self-sufficient. If we are unsuccessful, dependency will increase and be accompanied by increasing costs for services and care as they become more custodial in nature.

The time is ripe for a careful assessment of disability-related expenditures and programs to see how effective they are in enhancing independence and equality of opportunity for people with disabilities. To this end, Congress has directed the National Council on the Handicapped to assess the extent to which Federal programs serving people with disabilities:

> *provide incentives or disincentives to the establishment of community-based services for handicapped individuals, promote the full integration of such individuals in the community, in schools, and in the workplace, and contribute to the independence and dignity of such individuals.*
>
> *(Section 401 of the Rehabilitation Act of 1973, as amended)*

In response to this mandate, the Council has engaged in a variety of efforts to collect pertinent information and viewpoints. It has:

- Examined current legislation and programs,
- Collected and analyzed information about exemplary programs,
- Consulted with experts on programs for persons with disabilities and consumers of disability services,
- Conducted special seminars and hearings, and
- Conducted forums with persons with disabilities and their families throughout the country.

Based upon such information, the Council selected ten topic areas of critical importance for in-depth analysis and recommendations. The resulting topic papers are presented in a separate appendix to this report. The major conclusions of the detailed topic papers, along with an overview of the population with disabilities and a listing and summary review of Federal programs providing services to individuals with disabilities, are presented in the body of this report.

Source: "Toward Independence: An Assessment of Federal Laws and Programs Affecting Persons with Disabilities—With Legislative Recommendations." National Council on Disability (NCD). http://www.ncd.gov/publications/1986/February1986#5.

17. Flyer for a Rally Calling for the Appointment of a Deaf President for Gallaudet University, Issued by the Deaf President Now Committee (DPN) (1988)

Introduction

Gallaudet University is the only university in the world designed to be barrier free for Deaf and hard of hearing students, staff, and faculty. Although it was established by Congress in 1857, Gallaudet had never been led by a Deaf president prior to 1988. During a search for a new president in 1988, the Board of Trustees, under the leadership of Jane Bassett Spilman, initially selected Elisabeth Zinser, a hearing woman, despite having a candidate pool with two qualified Deaf individuals. A large-scale demonstration referred to as the Deaf President Now protest ensued. Students barricaded access to the Gallaudet campus, and supporters marched on Capitol Hill. Such high-powered politicians as George H. W. Bush, Bob Dole, and Tom Harkin endorsed the protest. The protest lasted six days, at which point Elisabeth Zinser and Jane Bassett Spilman resigned, the Board of Trustees agreed to reconstitute to have a majority of Deaf members, and I. King Jordan was selected as the first Deaf president in Gallaudet University's history.

It's time! In 1842, a Roman Catholic became president of the University of Notre Dame. In 1875, a woman became president of Wellesley College. In 1875, a Jew became president of Yeshiva University. In 1926, a Black person became president of Howard University.

AND in 1988, the Gallaudet University presidency belongs to a DEAF person. To show OUR solidarity behind OUR mandate for a deaf president of OUR university, you are invited to participate in a historical RALLY!

DEAF PRESIDENT NOW DEAF PRESIDENT NOW DEAF PRESIDENT NOW WHAT IS THE RALLY ALL ABOUT?

The purpose of the rally is to indicate support for choosing a deaf president of Gallaudet University for the first time in the 124-year history of the university.

WHO IS RESPONSIBLE FOR THE RALLY?

The Deaf President Now Committee (DPN) which consists of Gallaudet students, alumni, faculty and staff members.

WHY A DEAF PRESIDENT?

It is time for Gallaudet University, the only liberal arts university for the deaf in the WORLD, to become sensitive to the needs of deaf people of Gallaudet and of the United States. Here are a few examples of the lack of sensitivity shown towards the needs of the deaf by Gallaudet University.

1. Only 22% of Gallaudet employees are deaf. only 18% of the employees in administrative positions are deaf.
2. The Gallaudet Board of Trustees has twenty-one (21) members of only which four (4) are deaf.
3. There are faculty members who can't sign very well but meet the minimal requirements needed to teach at the university. some of those teachers have been teaching at the university for many years. Needless to say, this deprives students of a good education.

4. Senators Bob Dole and Bob Graham, among many other legislators have a Telecommunications Device for the Deaf (TDD) in their office and yet, Senator Dan Inouye, member of the Gallaudet Board of Trustees has no such machine in his office.

We do not accuse the people responsible for the conditions mentioned above of callousness. It is merely a lack of awareness on their part. With a deaf person in the position of leadership, one that has the same views, experiences, and needs that we do, people will become more informed of the needs of deaf people.

The remaining deaf candidates for the office of the Gallaudet presidency have a prodigious background in deaf education as compared to the remaining hearing candidates. The position is considered the highest office, possibly attained in the world of deaf education, one that indicates leadership of the deaf educational world. The remaining deaf candidates also have the administrative and financial abilities needed to manage the office of the presidency as indicated by their past experiences.

HAS THE DPN RECEIVED SUPPORT FROM OUTSIDE SOURCES?

Senators Bob Dole (R) of Kansas and Bob Graham (D) of Florida have each sent a letter to the Board of Trustees indicating support for a deaf president. The National Association of the Deaf (NAD) has sent individually addressed letters to each Congressman, Congresswoman, and Senators urging them to send letters to the Board of Trustees or call the Gallaudet President's office in support of a deaf president.

Deafpride, Inc., a social service agency in the Washington, D.C. area has contributed the use of four American Sign Language interpreters to today's rally.

HOW CAN I HELP GET A DEAF PRESIDENT OF GALLAUDET?

You are helping by showing your support at this rally. You can also contribute further by giving just five minutes of your time to call your congressperson and senators.

CONGRESS HAS A CENTRAL TDD-RELAY NUMBER, IT IS (202) 224-1904. BE SURE TO HAVE THE NAMES OF YOUR CONGRESSPERSON AND SENATORS READY.

The message should be brief and to the point. Say that you are in support of a deaf president of Gallaudet University and WANT your congressperson and senators to send a letter to the Gallaudet Board of Trustees as soon as possible. Also add that the NAD has sent a letter to your legislator and that the legislator can refer to it for further information. DO THIS AS SOON AS POSSIBLE. Remember, the number is (202) 224- 1904. Share this number with as many people as possible. Time is-short but only five minutes of your and their time will make a WORLD OF A DIFFERENCE. Also call the Gallaudet President's office and leave a message to the Board of Trustees in support of a deaf president, the number is (202) 651-5005.

WHAT WILL THE DPN DO IF A HEARING PERSON IS SELECTED?

The DPN's work is just beginning. Regardless of the outcome, our next goal is to get a majority of deaf people on the Gallaudet Board of Trustees. The Commission on Education of the Deaf has recommended this and we wholeheartedly support this.

AGAIN, PLEASE CALL YOUR CONGRESSPERSON AND SENATORS, THE NUMBER IS (202) 224-1904. ALSO CALL THE PRESIDENT'S OFFICE, THE NUMBER IS (202) 651-5005. UNITED WE STAND, DIVIDED WE FALL.

Thank you for coming today, your support counts.

Source: "Rally Flyers." Gallaudet University. https://www.gallaudet.edu/about/history-and-traditions/rally-flyers.

18. Preamble of the Americans with Disabilities Act (1990)

Introduction

Many disabled activists in the disability rights and independent living movements of the 1970s and 1980s were inspired by the civil rights movement to seek antidiscrimination legislation and equal rights for people with disabilities. Although the Rehabilitation Act of 1973 prohibited discrimination on the basis of disability in federal or federally funded programs, agencies, and projects, people with disabilities did not achieve a comprehensive antidiscrimination law until the Americans with Disabilities Act of 1990 (ADA). Consequently, the ADA represents a significant victory for disability rights in the United States. The Preamble to the ADA outlines its purpose and establishes its importance.

TITLE 42—THE PUBLIC HEALTH AND WELFARE
CHAPTER 126—EQUAL OPPORTUNITY FOR INDIVIDUALS WITH DISABILITIES
Sec. 12101. Findings and purpose
(a) Findings
　　The Congress finds that
　　　　(1) some 43,000,000 Americans have one or more physical or mental disabilities, and this number is increasing as the population as a whole is growing older;
　　　　(2) historically, society has tended to isolate and segregate

individuals with disabilities, and, despite some improvements, such forms of discrimination against individuals with disabilities continue to be a serious and pervasive social problem;

(3) discrimination against individuals with disabilities persists in such critical areas as employment, housing, public accommodations, education, transportation, communication, recreation, institutionalization, health services, voting, and access to public services;

(4) unlike individuals who have experienced discrimination on the basis of race, color, sex, national origin, religion, or age, individuals who have experienced discrimination on the basis of disability have often had no legal recourse to redress such discrimination;

(5) individuals with disabilities continually encounter various forms of discrimination, including outright intentional exclusion, the discriminatory effects of architectural, transportation, and communication barriers, overprotective rules and policies, failure to make modifications to existing facilities and practices, exclusionary qualification standards and criteria, segregation, and relegation to lesser services, programs, activities, benefits, jobs, or other opportunities;

(6) census data, national polls, and other studies have documented that people with disabilities, as a group, occupy an inferior status in our society, and are severely disadvantaged socially, vocationally, economically, and educationally;

(7) individuals with disabilities are a discrete and insular minority who have been faced with restrictions and limitations, subjected to a history of purposeful unequal treatment, and relegated to a position of political powerlessness in our society, based on characteristics that are beyond the control of such individuals and resulting from stereotypic assumptions not truly indicative of the individual ability of such individuals to participate in, and contribute to, society;

(8) the Nation's proper goals regarding individuals with disabilities are to assure equality of opportunity, full participation, independent living, and economic self-sufficiency for such individuals; and

(9) the continuing existence of unfair and unnecessary discrimination and prejudice denies people with disabilities the opportunity to compete on an equal basis and to pursue those opportunities for which our free society is justifiably famous, and costs the United States billions of dollars in unnecessary expenses resulting from dependency and nonproductivity.

(b) Purpose

It is the purpose of this chapter

(1) to provide a clear and comprehensive national mandate for

the elimination of discrimination against individuals with disabilities;

(2) to provide clear, strong, consistent, enforceable standards addressing discrimination against individuals with disabilities;

(3) to ensure that the Federal Government plays a central role in enforcing the standards established in this chapter on behalf of individuals with disabilities; and

(4) to invoke the sweep of congressional authority, including the power to enforce the fourteenth amendment and to regulate commerce, in order to address the major areas of discrimination faced day-to-day by people with disabilities.

Source: Information and Technical Assistance on the Americans with Disabilities Act. United States Department of Justice. Civil Rights Division. ADA.gov. https://www.ada.gov/archive/adastat91 .htm#Anchor-Sec-49575.

19. Cheryl Marie Wade's "Disability Culture Rap" (1994)

Introduction

Disability culture consists of beliefs, values, expressions, and artifacts that emerge from disabled people's shared experiences. Cheryl Marie Wade, a key leader in the disability arts and culture movement, wrote "Disability Culture Rap" to emphasize the importance of disability culture and highlight its roots in disability history, community, politics, humor, and pride.

Disability culture. *Say what?* Aren't disabled people just isolated victims of nature or circumstance?

Yes and no. True, we are far too often isolated. Locked away in the pits, closets and institutions of enlightened societies everywhere. But there is a growing consciousness among us: "that is not acceptable." Because there is always an underground. Notes get passed among survivors. And the notes we're passing these days say, "there's power in difference. Power. Pass the word."

Culture. It's about passing the word. And disability culture is passing the word that there's a new definition of disability and it includes *power*.

Culture. New definitions, new inflections. No longer just "poor cripple." Now also "CRIPPLE" and, yes, just "cripple." A body happening. But on a real good day, why not C*R*I*P*P*L*E; a hap-pen-ing. (**Dig it or not**).

Culture. It's finding a history, naming and claiming ancestors, heroes. As "invisibles," our history is hidden from us, our heroes buried in the pages, unnamed, unrecognized. Disability culture is about naming, about recognizing.

Naming and claiming our heroes. Like Helen Keller. Oh, not the miracle-worker version we're all so familiar with, but the social reformer, the activist who tried so desperately to use her celebrity to tell the truth of disability: that it has far more to do with poverty, oppression and the restriction of choices than it has to do with wilted muscles or milky eyes. And for her efforts to tell this truth, she was ridiculed, demeaned as revolutionaries often are. And because Helen Keller was a survivor, and that is the first thing any culture needs— survivors who live long enough so that some part of the truth makes it to the next generation.

Helen Keller was a survivor, so she pulled back from telling the fuller truth; that's often what survivors have to do: they have to swallow the rage, wear the mask, and, yes, pull back from telling it exactly like it is so that there might be a next generation. And so, Helen Keller, a survivor, we honor you as our ancestor, our hero.

Naming and claiming our hidden history, our ancestors. Like the thousands of mental and physical "defectives," singled out for "special treatment" by the Nazis. Yes, disability culture is recognizing that we were the first victims of the Holocaust, that we are the people the Nazis refined their methods of torture on. So we must honor these unnamed victims as our ancestors, we must raise their unmarked graves into our consciousness, into the consciousness of America so it never happens again. And just as Native Americans insist the true name of discovery is genocide, more and more of us insist that the true name of "right to die with dignity" (without opportunities to live with dignity) is murder, the first syllable of genocide.

Naming and claiming our ancestors, our heroes. Like all those circus and carnival freaks, the first disability performance artists. Those rowdy outcasts who learned to emphasize their Otherness, turn it into work, a career, a life. Oh, it may have been a harsh life, sometimes even brutal, but a life: they kept themselves from being locked away in those institutions designed for the excessively different that have always been such a prominent part of the American economy. And so we claim these survivors & our ancestors and we honor them.

Naming and claiming our ancestors, our heroes. Now most of you probably know the story of James Meredith, freedom fighter, African American, who helped break the color barrier, the racial barrier to higher learning by insisting he had a right to an education; *insisting*.

And without that insistence, the doors of Ole Miss would have remained closed. But do you know the story of Ed Roberts, cripple freedom fighter, disabled man, who, armed with self-esteem and a portable respirator, broke the disability barrier to higher learning by insisting he had a right to an education, by insisting that the doors to the University of California at Berkeley be opened, and by doing so, laid a significant brick onto the foundation of the independent Living Movement? Independent! Living! Movement! The language of it!—that revolution of identity and possibilities for disabled people. The independent living movement. Oh, you may never have heard of it. It never made it onto prime time. Norman Mailer did not rush out to capture its essence in 30,000 words.

Yet it took root; it grew; it spread all across this country, all around the world—because there is always an underground. Notes get passed among survivors. And the notes we're passing these days say: there's power in difference. Power. Pass the word.

So what's this disability culture stuff all about? It's simple; it's just "This is disability. From the inside out."

Culture. Pass the word. Now maybe the word is the moan and wail of a blues. Maybe it's the fierce rhythms and clicking heels and castanets of flamenco. Maybe it's outsider art. Passing the word. Maybe the word is authentic movement, that dance that flows from the real body notes of cripples. Maybe it's the way pieces of cloth are stitched together to commemorate a life, to remember a name. Maybe it's American Sign Language, a language that formed the foundation of a cultural identity for a people, Deaf people, and bloomed into ASL performance art and ASL mime.

Culture. Sometimes it happens over coffee or on a picket line. A poem gets said and passed along. And passed back. Amended. Embellished. And passed along again. Language gets claimed. Ms. Gay. Crip. Guerrilla theater becomes theater with a soul. Teatro Campesino. The Dance Theater of Harlem. And, of course, WRY CRIPS Disabled Women's Theater. Radical. True. Passing the word.

Culture. Maybe so far you've been deprived. Maybe right now the primary image you have of disability is that of victim. Perhaps all of you know of us is Jerry's Kids, those doom-drenched poster children hauled out once each year to wring our charitable pockets dry.

But I promise you: you will also come to know us as Jerry's Orphans. No longer the grateful recipients of tear-filled handouts we are more and more proud freedom fighters, talking to the streets, picket signs strapped to our chairs.

No longer the polite tin-cuppers waiting for your generous inclusion, we are more and more proud freedom fighters taking to the stages, raising our speech-impaired voices in celebration of who we are. No longer the invisible people with no definition beyond "Other," we are more and more proud, we are freedom fighters, taking to the streets and to the stages, raising our gnarly fists in defiance of the narrow, bloodless image of our complex humanity shoved down the American consciousness daily.

And these changes, they will happen, just as the Independent Living Movement happened, just as the Rehabilitation Act's 504 regulations for access happened; just as the Americans with Disabilities Act—the most comprehensive civil rights law ever written—happened.

Because there is always an underground. Notes will be passed among survivors.

And the notes we're passing these days say, "There's power in difference. Power. Pass the word."

Disability culture. What is it really all about?

It's this
And *this*.
And **this.**
Yeah, this—
COMING AT YOU FROM
THE INSIDE OUT.

Source: Wade, Cheryl Marie. "Disability Culture Rap." 1994. In *The Ragged Edge: The Disability Experience from the Pages of the First Fifteen Years of the Disability Rag*, edited by Barrett Shaw, 15–18. Louisville, KY: Advocado Press.

20. Lisa Blumberg's "Public Stripping" (1994)

Introduction

Public stripping is an abusive and objectifying practice in which disabled people are stripped down to their underwear and examined by a group of doctors, residents, students, and other onlookers. Disabled activist Lisa Blumberg critiqued this practice in The Disability Rag, *noting that while nondisabled people expect to be examined in medical settings in private, this is not the norm for disabled people, particularly children with disabilities.*

At a recent disability rights conference, a 30-year old woman with spina bifida described her medical experiences in a voice shaking with pain and anger. All through childhood and adolescence, Anne told us, the semi-annual orthopedic examinations her doctors required her to have took place in a large hospital room, with 20 or more doctors, residents and physical therapists looking on. After the hospital acquired videotaping equipment, the examinations were videotaped. During the sessions, Anne was permitted to wear only underpants.

When she was 12, she said, she tried to keep on her training bra. The head doctor, in order to explain something about her back to the residents, took it off without saying anything to her, but with noticeable irritation. A nurse quickly apologized—not to Anne but to the doctor.

Anne knew that when her sisters and classmates went to the doctor, they were seen by just one doctor, in a small, private room. No one ever explained to Anne why she had to be examined in front of a group. No one ever considered whether she found it embarrassing or upsetting to be viewed nearly naked by so many people. No one ever acknowledged to her that she was being used as a teaching tool. No one ever told her or her parents that she had any choice in the matter.

Anne grew up thinking that what she called "public stripping," a crude phrase to describe a crude practice, was a periodic humiliation inflicted upon her because she was, as one young doctor called her, "significantly deformed and handicapped." Anne's experiences are not unique. Privacy in medical examinations may be the norm for ordinary persons, but they're not the norm for disabled people—particularly not for disabled children. Doctors at hospitals and clinics which specialize in "pediatric handicapping conditions" such as spina bifida, cerebral palsy, muscular dystrophy, brittle bone disease and dwarfism have traditionally displayed their patients in front of colleagues, residents, therapists and other professionals. Although it may be slightly less extensive than a decade ago, the degrading practice continues today.

The individual is almost always examined without a hospital gown. Other procedures vary: she may be told to undress in the examining area; or he may be forced to disrobe with others in a hall.

My friend Joe, who has cerebral palsy, was repeatedly examined in an amphitheater where residents and medical students could line up to see and feel for themselves exactly how
tight the muscles of a "spastic c.p." really were. Social workers, invited not for any clinical reason but just so they could feel "part of the team," looked on attentively.

The public strippings went on for Joe until he was 18, at which time he told his parents he'd never again go to any doctor for his disability. He never has.

It was only happenstance that I avoided public stripping myself. My first orthopedist, a consultant to a rehabilitation center, had both disabled and nondisabled patients, children
and adults, whom he treated with equal respect and courtesy. He always examined patients in a private room, with only a parent present. Since the aim of the examination was solely to provide
the patient with information, rather than to provide learning experience for other people, there was time when very little clothing removal was necessary.

My second orthopedist, associated with the esteemed Boston Children's Hospital, was a monster. He operated on me (as he did on almost all of his patients) with the result that my awkward but functional gait was turned into a snail-paced stagger. However, since Boston Children's Hospital, unlike some perhaps more egalitarian hospitals, allowed the parents to "buy" the right for their child to be examined in private—and my parents could afford to do so—public stripping was the one indignity he was unable to inflict on me. Whenever I talk to someone who has had their privacy so incredibly violated, though, my stomach churns and I feel as though it has happened to me.

Doctors seem to find it hard to understand why anyone "suffering" from something so supposedly terrible as a "life long handicap" would be interested in anything so trivial as modesty and privacy. To them, the examination procedures they use on disabled children seem reasonable and efficient because they facilitate teaching and the exchange of medical knowledge. Why wouldn't "the handicapped" be eager to help in the development of cures and new treatments?

What the medical profession and perhaps the larger community does not comprehend is that disabled people who seek medical advice are like anyone else seeking such advice. By and large, we want to be provided with a medical service—not *render* one.

Examining a patient in front of and with the participation of an audience should be regarded as bad medical practice even when considered from a purely clinical viewpoint. A person may be so upset and intimidated that he/she will not disclose all the information the doctor would need to know in order to provide effective treatment. Indeed, it is virtually impossible for a patient to develop any rapport with a medical professional in such a situation. The actual results of the examination may be influenced as well; even at 4 years old, Joe was so uptight from the experience, he says, that he believes it was not possible for anyone to determine how tight his muscles were in a typical situation—or what should be done about it.

Public stripping also presents quality-of-life concerns. People who have been required to submit to the experience repeatedly say they have been traumatized by it. The trauma stems not only from being viewed naked or nearly naked by so many people, with videotaping or photography frequently included, but also from listening to oneself being discussed—often in quite derogatory medical terms—as though one were a defective machine.

Susan, who has a form of muscular dystrophy, was driven to hysteria and nightmares by hearing a large group of people, oblivious to her views, dispassionately debate the multiple orthopedic surgeries she should have and the order in which she should have them.

Yet medical ethicists and others in the medical community who profess to be so concerned about "quality of life" when it comes to deciding whether it is worthwhile for a disabled person to live do not seem to be offended by public stripping.

Left unanswered is this question: If a person who's disabled can be subjected to medical examination procedures not designed for her benefit, can she not also be subjected to other things at the hands of doctors not to her direct benefit? Does a hospital's interest in giving practical experience to residents, for example, not play a role in recommendations for surgery?

Public stripping, of course, does not occur in isolation. Society's prejudices against disabled people are played out in medical settings in many virulent ways, ranging from indiscriminate surgery to unnecessary hospitalization to the denial of basic health care.

There are to be sure some health care professionals like my first orthopedist and my present physical therapist who will sincerely do their best for persons with disabilities who come to them for services. However, too often such individuals are found only by luck.

Both children and adults are victims of medical discrimination against disabled people. Children are the more vulnerable, though, since they lack the power to give and refuse consent. Moreover, parents who are slow to grasp the way the system works and who may be coping with their own prejudices may not always be able to act as effective advocates.

Unlike the women's movement, where health care concerns are high on the agenda, we in the disability movement spend very little time on medical issues. Our apathy in this area is amazing. We have not even begun to consider questions as basic as whether medical care given in segregated settings such as hospitals "for crippled children" can ever be equal. Not even deliberate medical murder galvanizes us into action.

As a movement, we seem to buy into the prevailing social myth that any problem a person has with the medical establishment is a personal problem—and probably the person's own

fault. However, equal access to medical care—that is, the right to receive the same health care one would receive if one were not disabled—is as important and as vital to our interests as is equal access to transportation. Equal access to health care, like equal access to transportation, is a political issue.

Many health care issues will be difficult to resolve because they involve money and the readjustment of social priorities. We would be able to go far, though, in obtaining the right to privacy in medical examination by simply discussing the issue whenever and wherever we can. When publicly confronted with our views, doctors will find that public stripping is a practice impossible to defend.

January/February 1990

Source: Blumberg, Lisa. "Public Stripping." 1994. In *The Ragged Edge: The Disability Experience from the Pages of the First Fifteen Years of the* Disability Rag, edited by Barrett Shaw, 73–77. Louisville, KY: Advocado Press.

21. Table of the Medals Won in the Atlanta Paralympics (1996)

Introduction

The Paralympic Games is an international multisport event that highlights the athletic achievements of people with disabilities. During the Paralympics, people with physical disabilities, sensory disabilities, and intellectual and developmental disabilities come together to compete. Like the Olympics, the Paralympics occur every four years, with summer and winter competitions, and feature diverse sports such as track and field, swimming, cycling, wheelchair tennis, wheelchair basketball, skiing, hockey, and snowboarding. Although the Paralympics strive for equality with the Olympics, they are less well funded, receive less media coverage, and are less celebrated. Despite this, the accomplishments of Paralympian athletes demonstrate how disabled people have strived to overcome social, environmental, and attitudinal barriers to engage in athletics. The 1996 Paralympics in Atlanta were the first to obtain widespread corporate sponsorship and more significant media coverage.

1996 Atlanta Paralympic Games
USA 16–25 August, 1996

Countries	104
Athletes	3,259
Men	2,469
Women	790
World Records	269
Paralympic Games Records	508
Medal Events	508
Sports	19
Volunteers	12,000

Top 5 Medals Table

Position	Country	Gold	Silver	Bronze
1	USA	46	46	65
2	Australia	42	37	27
3	Germany	40	58	51
4	Great Britain	39	42	41
5	Spain	39	31	36

Source: "Atlanta 1996." Paralympic Movement. https://www.paralympic.org/atlanta-1996.

22. Remarks of Judith E. Heumann, Assistant Secretary, U.S. Department of Education, at the White House upon the Signing of the Individuals with Disabilities Education Act (IDEA) (1997)

Introduction

On June 4, 1997, Judith "Judy" Heumann, the assistant secretary of the Office of Special Education and Rehabilitation Services in the U.S. Department of Education, delivered a powerful speech at the bill-signing ceremony for the Individuals with Disabilities Education Act (IDEA). The IDEA meant a great deal to Heumann, personally and politically. As a disabled child, she had been denied access to public education because school officials claimed that her wheelchair was a fire hazard. Years later, as a young disability activist, Heumann assisted in the drafting of the Education for All Handicapped Children Act of 1975, which was the original version of the IDEA. As Heumann observed in her speech, the IDEA is a critical step toward providing all disabled children with the right to a free and high-quality public education.

Mr. President, Secretary Riley, distinguished members of Congress, students, parents, friends, and colleagues—Mr. President, one month ago you spoke at the dedication of the Franklin Delano Roosevelt Memorial here in Washington. On that proud and sun-filled day, you spoke about President Roosevelt's great faith in our nation and the American people. And you also spoke about his faith in himself. You said—"It was that faith in his own extraordinary potential that enabled him to guide his country from his wheelchair . . . and from that wheelchair . . . he set America to march toward its destiny."

Mr. President, today we come together to celebrate the extraordinary potential of millions of disabled young people who are ready to help America move toward our common destiny in the 21st century.

It was, however, one of the great ironies of this century that President Roosevelt, who was so sure and resolute in his leadership, often felt the need to hide his disability. Today we understand why. He lived at a time when disabled people were segregated, hidden away, and ignored.

I was born in the midst of that period. When it was time for me to go to school, the school officials did see me—they only saw my wheelchair. And they barred me from class. I was a fire hazard, they said. Well, it was pretty easy for them to push around a kindergarten kid, but my mother was something else again. She is one of the toughest kinds of woman you'll ever meet—a housewife from Brooklyn, New York. Without experience, she and my father became activists and my strong advocates. And I finally did get my education. Thank you, mom. Years later, when I applied for my teacher's license, the Board of Education of the City of New York refused me again. I was still a fire hazard. But this time I could fend for myself. I sued them. And I got my license, and taught elementary school for three years.

Today, thanks to the Individuals with Disabilities Education Act, those days have been replaced by the light of hope and opportunity. And this light has given us a brand new vision.

Today, we can see a future where no child is denied his or her civil right to get a quality education. We can see a future where young people learn in different ways—but all are expected to learn to higher standards. And I am talking about young people like these—Josh Bailey, Danielle Boustos, Lamar Lawson, Will McCarthy, and Cecilia Pauley—and all the others here today and in our nation's schools.

We can see a future where we finally put an end to the divisive, false argument that goes, "something for your child means something less for my child." If the American experience tells us anything, it is that expanding opportunity lifts us all up. Let us be a proud nation that takes responsibility for all our children.

Today, we can also see a brighter future for the parents of children with disabilities—parents like my mother and those here today, like Mary Samosa, Penny Ford, Paul Guzzo, Connie Garner, Barbara Ramondo, and so many others. The new I.D.E.A. helps make sure that parents won't have to resort to superhuman means to get what they need for their children.

Most importantly, we can see a future where the tyranny of low expectations is overthrown once and for all—and that's really what this I.D.E.A. reauthorization is all about. So to all the young people here today, I say—You have a great opportunity—but also a great responsibility. We can open the door for you, but it won't mean a thing unless you study hard and make the most of your education. Be proud and have high expectations for yourselves. Join with your classmates and build America's accessible house

together, as equal partners. As we moved forward on reauthorizing the I.D.E.A., we were guided by the goals the President has identified for all disability programs and policies—inclusion, not exclusion; independence, not dependence; and empowerment, not paternalism.

Today, we are closer to achieving these goals than ever before. I want to thank those who helped to make this happen: President Clinton, who has worked so tirelessly to give all our citizens the tools they need to make the most of their lives; Secretary Riley, whose support and counsel means so much—it is such a great honor to work for this caring and committed leader, who believes that "all means all."

My colleagues at the U.S. Department of Education, including Tom Hehir, Patty Guard, Joleta Reynolds, Carol Cichowski, Susan Craig, Suzanne Sheridan, Theda Zawaiza, Charlotte Fraas, and everyone else who worked so hard.

The members of Congress and their staffs who worked in the finest spirit of bipartisanship and openness, and taught me so much. And the members of the education and disabled communities and their advocates, who worked fairly and in the spirit of cooperation and collaboration. There are so many that I cannot mention all of you by name, but we thank you so much.

We have come a long way, but we know that we can and must do better. Making progress will require continued partnership, aggressive collaboration, and a love for all children. This Act will give disabled young people more opportunities for quality education and meaningful employment than ever before in our nation's history.

This is a splendid day of reaffirmation and promise. I thank everyone who worked so hard to allow this day to finally arrive.

Thank you. Now the real work begins.

Source: "IDEA '97 Speeches—Remarks by Assistant Secretary of Education, OSERS." U.S. Department of Education. https://www2.ed.gov/policy/speced/leg/idea/speech-2.html.

23. Kitty Cone's "Short History of the 504 Sit In" for the Twentieth Anniversary of the Sit In (1997)

Introduction

Section 504 of the Rehabilitation Act of 1973 was a significant victory for the Disability Rights Movement, as it was the first antidiscrimination legislation specific to disability. However, the law could not be enforced until the U.S. Secretary of Health, Education, and Welfare signed regulations outlining how the law would be enforced. Despite efforts from disability activists and advocates, the regulations were still not signed four years later. On April 5, 1977, more than 150 disabled and deaf activists and allies occupied the San Francisco Office of the U.S. Department of Health, Education, and Welfare. They refused to leave until Joseph Califano, U.S. Secretary of Health, Education, and Welfare, signed the regulations. The protest lasted 28 days, and it was the longest occupation of a federal building in U.S. history. Kitty Cone, one of the key organizers of the 504 Sit-in, discusses the importance of the sit-in for the disability rights movement and the significance of Section 504 for disabled people.

In 1973 the first federal civil rights protection for people with disabilities, Section 504 of the Rehabilitation Act was signed into law. What section 504 says is "no otherwise qualified handicapped individual in the United States shall solely on the basis of his handicap, be excluded from the participation, be denied the benefits of, or be subjected to discrimination under any program or activity receiving federal financial assistance." Essentially it said no program receiving federal funds could discriminate against a person with a disability.

Section 504 was based on the language of previous civil rights laws that protected women and minorities. It recognized that society has historically treated people with disabilities as second-class citizens based on deeply held fears and stereotypes that go way back. Those attitudes had translated into pity and persecution, and later into policies that were based on paternalism.

People with disabilities ourselves didn't think the issues we faced in our daily lives were the product of prejudice and discrimination. Disability had been defined by the medical model of rehabilitation, charity and paternalism. If I thought about why I couldn't attend a university that was inaccessible, I would have said it was because I couldn't walk, my own personal problem. Before section 504, responsibility for the consequences of disability rested only on the shoulders of the person with a disability rather than being understood as a societal responsibility. Section 504 dramatically changed that societal and legal perception.

Only with section 504 was the role of discrimination finally legally acknowledged. Sen. Hubert Humphrey, who had attempted in earlier years to pass civil rights legislation covering people with disabilities said about Section 504:

> *the time has come to firmly establish the right of disabled Americans to dignity and self-respect as equal and contributing members of society and to end the virtual isolation of millions of children and adults.*

At that time, discrimination existed in education, employment, housing, transportation, access to public buildings and other facilities, access to equal medical care and in many other areas.

So, after the law was passed, in order for it to become effective, regulations had to be issued defining who was a disabled person, what did otherwise qualified mean, what constituted discrimination and nondiscrimination in the context of disability etc. Enforcement timelines had to be developed as well as an administrative enforcement mechanism. The regulations would provide a consistent, coherent interpretation of 504's legal intent rather than leaving it up to any judge who heard a 504 case to interpret what the law meant.

There were contradictory rulings being handed down by courts. There was one case involving the right of a wheelchair user to use public buses in which the decision was that if a driver stopped and opened the doors that constituted nondiscrimination. Another case acknowledged that steps prevented a wheelchair user from boarding. These cases illustrated the need to define nondiscrimination, and also to define differences as well as similarities with race and gender discrimination.

The Department of Health, Education, and Welfare (HEW) was the lead agency, and their regulations would become the guidelines for all the other federal agencies—Department of Transportation, HUD etc. It was crucial that the regulations be strong, because ultimately 504 would cover every area that received federal financial assistance.

Between 1973 and 1977 no regulations were issued. During that period strong regulations were drafted by attorneys in the Office for Civil Rights, sent to the Secretary of HEW with a recommendation to publish them in proposed form in the Federal Register for public comment.

By this time, opposition was developing on the part of covered entities—hospitals, universities, state and county governments—and the regulations were not published. There was much delay; the disability community filed a lawsuit in federal court; the judge ruled that they must be issued but not when.

HEW sent the regulations to Congress which was totally unusual and Congress sent them back. HEW published an intent to propose regulations in the Federal Register.

There were a few actions taken by the disability community, and finally, HEW printed the proposed regs; there was extensive public comment, and a final compromise set of regs was waiting on HEW Secretary Califano's desk when the Carter administration came into office.

During this time, the American Coalition of Citizens with Disabilities (ACCD) a national cross disability was formed. ACCD became deeply involved in leading the effort to get regulations out.

Once the Carter administration was an office, instead of signing the regulations, HEW set up a task force with no representation from the disability community to "study" them. It became clear, through delays and leaks from inside, that the regulations were being seriously weakened in coverage, enforcement, and the whole integration mandate.

There was a list of issues that included consortia: this would have meant that all the universities in a locale could form a consortium and thereby offer a full curriculum. Attending classes at a variety of universities would be absurd for a nondisabled person, but for a person with a disability it was absurd and patently unequal. The list of issues also included whether alcoholics and drug addicts were to be covered by the regulations. A case that occurred later concerned whether a coach who was a recovering alcoholic could be fired, although he had been sober for years. The list started out as short and grew to be about 20 issues.

Although most of the leadership of ACCD supported the Democrats, they understood that even as they were being told that the changes were cosmetic, the changes were so profound that would put us in direct confrontation with the administration.

ACCD, realizing our civil rights protections were being gutted, demanded HEW issue the regulations unchanged by April 4, or action would occur. They called for sit ins at eight HEW regional headquarters, April 5th if HEW didn't comply.

I think this was brilliant, because rather than waiting until watered-down regulations were issued publicly and then responding, issue by issue, this meant the government would have to respond to the demonstrators. Additionally, it was not that easy to organize people, particularly people with physical disabilities, in those days, due to lack of transit, support services and so on. A sit in meant people would go and stay, until the issue was resolved definitively.

The San Francisco federal building sit in, the only one that endured, lasted 28 days and was critical in forcing the signing of the regulations almost unchanged. It began with a rally outside the federal building, then we marched inside where between 1 and 200 people would remain until the end. The composition of the sit in represented the spectrum of the disability community with participation from people with a wide variety of disabilities, from different racial, social and economic backgrounds, and ages from adults to kids with disabilities and their parents.

We all felt that we were acting on behalf of hundreds of thousands of people who were not able to participate, people all over the country who were institutionalized or stuck in other dependency situations.

In the Bay Area, a broad cross disability coalition, the Emergency 504 Coalition, began building for a rally on April 5th, knowing we'd sit in afterwards. We set up committees to take on different tasks such as rally speakers, media, fund-raising, medics, monitors, publicity, and outreach.

The outreach committee was very successful in garnering broad community support: from churches, unions, civil rights organizations, gay groups, elected politicians, radical parties and others.

The work of that committee proved to be invaluable once we were inside the building. Those organizations built support rallies outside the building and the breath of the support made it more difficult to move against us. The International Association of Machinists facilitated our sending a delegation to Washington. Politicians sent mattresses and a shower hose to attach to the sink.

Glide Memorial Church and the Black Panther party sent many delicious meals that nourished us between days of coffee and doughnuts.

The other committees also continued inside the building. The media committee met regularly to review the coverage and discuss how to make our purpose more clear, how to use the press to get particular issues across. It directed reporters to appropriate spokespeople, called news conferences and so on.

The committees had a great deal of work to do and kept many people involved. This was good, because the conditions were physically grueling, sleeping sometimes three or four hours a night on the floor and everyone was under stress about their families, jobs, our health, the fact that we were all filthy and so on.

All the participants met daily to make tactical decisions. These were flowing, creative meetings but they often went on for hours, which meant very little sleep. But they were important in developing consensus and arriving at a course of action.

Some of the issues taken up in the mass meetings were: what to do if we were arrested, a hunger strike in sympathy with the Washington demonstrators who had been starved out, which we decided would be voluntary, how to deal with the bomb scare, the decision to have congressional hearings in the building on HEW's list of proposed changes, who would speak at the hearing, who would speak at the rallies outside, the decision to send a contingent from the building to Washington DC, a process for choosing the 12 or so people who would go.

At every moment, we felt ourselves the descendants of the civil rights movement of the '60s. We learned about sit ins from the civil rights movement, we sang freedom songs to keep up morale, and consciously show the connection between the two movements. We always drew the parallels. About public transportation we said we can't even get on the back of the bus. A high point was Julian Bond's visit to the building.

A congressional hearing was held in the building that was extremely dramatic. The testimony of Judy Heumann, Ed Roberts, Debby Kaplan, Phil Newmark and others was so compelling, that the representative from HEW got up and locked himself in an office. Congressman Phil Burton leapt up and ran after him and kicked on the door insisting he come out.

After about two weeks, a contingent was chosen to go to Washington to lend the moral authority and the leadership of the sit in to the efforts there to pressure the administration. We really wanted to break open the East Coast press and we wanted some more demonstrations that would mobilize people, and we were striving to get a meeting at the White House.

The machinists union, the IAM rented a large U-Haul truck with a lift on the back, and all the demonstrators who were wheelchair riders were transported in that vehicle. They held a large reception for us at their international headquarters, and after we had eaten, we were asked to speak and I believe we all sang "We Shall Overcome." An international vice president became very involved in assisting us in anything we needed. They allowed us to use their union headquarters to organize demonstrations, so we had access to telephone lines, copy machines and other things necessary for organizing.

One of the first things was hold meetings in the capital with senators Alan Cranston and Harrison Williams. Sen. Cranston was one of the original sponsors of the legislation. Up until we met with him, he had been supporting the administration position. Cranston, at that time possibly the most important man in Congress, raised the administration's objections to the "unchanged" 504 regulations, one by one. Each objection was answered by a different member of our delegation, and answered very thoroughly.

It was a testament to the group's self-confidence and total understanding of the contested issues, that issue by issue, Cranston was turned around, in front of national TV cameras and other media. We were all extremely tired and sleep deprived and yet everyone managed to marshal their wits to carry out this extremely important political discussion. Frank Bowe, who was the director of ACCD, a deaf man, spoke last. He made such eloquent remarks, in which he said, "Senator, we are not even second-class citizens, we are third class citizens," that we all began to cry.

An important tactic when we got to Washington was challenging Carter on having an open door administration. Each administration defines itself by a slogan such as The Great Society. The Carter administration presented itself as accessible to people and they called it the Open Door Administration, so we demonstrated wherever Carter and Califano went, forcing them to go out backdoors. At Carter's church, when Califano spoke to the press club, holding vigils and prayers outside of Califano's home was all about getting East Coast coverage. And that was important in getting us a meeting at the White House.

The sit in and contingent it sent to Washington were pivotal in getting strong 504 regulations signed that embodied concepts of equality and integration, and the affirmative steps that must be taken to achieve that for people with disabilities. 504 has never enforced as it should be. The Department of Transportation 504 regulations which called for reasonable, phased in measures to make public transportation accessible turned into a bitter fight between the American Public Transit Association and the disability community and were overturned in federal court in 1980. Those measures became part of the ADA 10 years later.

The HEW Section 504 regulations established the basic operational principles that became the basis for legal compliance with the ADA. Nondiscrimination is the fundamental right established by 504. Discrimination can occur through exclusionary practices as well as an inaccessible environment. Affirmative conduct may be required to remove architectural or communication barriers or to provide reasonable accommodations. People with disabilities experience discrimination as a class, irrespective of diagnosis.

504 established the three pronged legal definition of disability as opposed to a medical one. The definition includes people with physical or mental impairments that substantially limit one or more major life activity, those who have a record of such an impairment, and those who are regarded as having such an impairment. Another 504 principal that is particular to disability civil rights is the balancing of the individual's right to be free from discrimination with the cost to society to effect a remedy. It established the right of an individual who has experienced discrimination to pursue an administrative remedy with the appropriate federal agency as well as to go to court.

Even though 504 wasn't strongly enforced, the sit in was of historic importance. For the first time we had concrete federal civil rights protection. We had shown ourselves and the country through network TV that we, the most hidden, impoverished, pitied group of people in the nation were capable of waging a deadly serious struggle that brought about profound social change. The sit in was a truly transforming experience the likes of which most of us had never seen before or ever saw again. Those of us with disabilities were imbued with a new sense of pride, strength, community and confidence. For the first time, many of us felt proud of who we were. And we understood that our isolation and segregation stemmed from societal policy, not from some personal defects on our part and our experiences with segregation and discrimination were not just our own personal problems.

Without 504—its coverage and example and the disability civil rights principles contained in the regulations we fought so hard for, and the empowerment of tens of thousands of disability activists through 504 trainings, and activities and mobilizations— there might well be no Americans with Disabilities Act, that finally brought us up to parity with federal civil rights laws covering gender and race.

Source: Cone, Kitty. "Short History of the 504 Sit in." Disability Rights Education and Defense Fund (DREDF). https://dredf.org/504 -sit-in-20th-anniversary/short-history-of-the-504 -sit-in/.

24. Excerpt from the U.S. Supreme Court Decision in *Olmstead v. L. C.* (1999)

Introduction

Throughout U.S. history, disabled people have been forced to live in institutions, which has denied them independence, autonomy, and societal inclusion. Although a significant number of institutions were closed in the 1960s, many disabled people continued to be confined in psychiatric hospitals, nursing homes, and other types of institutions. In 1995, Lois Curtis and Elaine Wilson, two women with cognitive and psychiatric disabilities institutionalized in Georgia, sued the state for their right to live in the community. Although their doctors had acknowledged that their needs could be met outside of the institution, the two women were still not released. Lawyers representing Curtis and Wilson argued that the state's failure to provide community-based services violated the Americans with Disabilities Act. The case was eventually heard by the U.S. Supreme Court. The Supreme Court ruled in Olmstead v. L. C. *that unjustified segregation of people with disabilities constitutes discrimination in violation of Title II of the Americans with Disabilities Act. Although many states are still in violation of the* Olmstead *decree, the ruling has had a significant impact on disabled people's right to community integration.*

In the Americans with Disabilities Act of 1990 (ADA), Congress described the isolation and segregation of individuals with disabilities as a serious and pervasive form of discrimination. 42 U.S.C. §12101(a)(2), (5). Title II of the ADA, which proscribes discrimination in the provision of public services, specifies, *inter alia*, that no qualified individual with a disability shall, "by reason of such disability," be excluded from participation in, or be denied the benefits of, a public entity's services, programs, or activities. §12132. Congress instructed the Attorney General to issue regulations implementing Title II's discrimination proscription. See §12134(a). One such regulation, known as the "integration regulation," requires a "public entity [to] administer . . . programs . . . in the most integrated setting appropriate to the needs of qualified individuals with disabilities." 28 CFR §35.130(d). A further prescription, here called the "reasonable-modifications regulation," requires public entities to "make reasonable modifications" to avoid "discrimination on the basis of disability," but does not require measures that would "fundamentally alter" the nature of the entity's programs. §35.130(b)(7).

Respondents L. C. and E. W. are mentally retarded women; L. C. has also been diagnosed with schizophrenia, and E. W., with a personality disorder. Both women were voluntarily admitted to Georgia Regional Hospital at Atlanta (GRH), where they were confined for treatment in a psychiatric unit. Although their treatment professionals eventually concluded that each of the women could be cared for appropriately in a community-based program, the women remained institutionalized at GRH. Seeking placement in community care, L. C. filed this suit against petitioner state officials (collectively, the State) under 42 U.S.C. §1983 and Title II. She alleged that the State violated Title II in failing to place her in a community-based program once her treating professionals determined that such placement was appropriate. E. W. intervened, stating an identical claim. The District Court granted partial summary judgment for the women, ordering their placement in an appropriate community-based treatment program. The court rejected the State's argument that inadequate funding, not discrimination against L. C. and E. W. "by reason of [their] disabilit[ies]," accounted for their retention at GRH. Under Title II, the court concluded, unnecessary institutional segregation constitutes discrimination *per se*, which cannot be justified by a lack of funding. The court also rejected the State's defense that requiring immediate transfers in such cases would "fundamentally alter" the State's programs. The Eleventh Circuit affirmed the District Court's judgment, but remanded for reassessment of the State's cost-based defense. The District Court had left virtually no room for such a defense. The appeals court read the statute and regulations to allow the defense, but only in tightly limited circumstances. Accordingly, the Eleventh Circuit instructed the District Court to consider, as a key factor, whether the additional cost for treatment of L. C. and E. W. in community-based care would be unreasonable given the demands of the State's mental health budget.

Held: The judgment is affirmed in part and vacated in part, and the case is remanded.

138 F.3d 893, affirmed in part, vacated in part, and remanded.

Justice Ginsburg delivered the opinion of the Court with respect to Parts I, II, and III—A, concluding that, under Title II of the ADA, States are required to place persons with mental disabilities in community settings rather than in institutions when the State's treatment professionals have determined that community placement is appropriate, the transfer from institutional care to a less restrictive setting is not opposed by the affected individual, and the placement can be reasonably accommodated, taking into account the resources available to the State and the needs of others with mental disabilities. Pp. 11–18.

(a) The integration and reasonable-modifications regulations issued by the Attorney General rest on two key determinations: (1) Unjustified placement or retention of persons in institutions severely limits their exposure to the outside community, and therefore constitutes a form of discrimination based on disability prohibited by Title II, and (2) qualifying their obligation to avoid unjustified isolation of individuals with disabilities, States can resist modifications that would fundamentally alter the nature of their services and programs. The Eleventh Circuit essentially upheld the Attorney General's construction of the ADA. This Court affirms the Court of Appeals decision in substantial part. Pp. 11–12.

(b) Undue institutionalization qualifies as discrimination "by reason of . . . disability." The Department of Justice has consistently advocated that it does. Because the Department is the agency directed by Congress to issue Title II regulations, its views warrant respect. This Court need not inquire whether the degree of deference described in *Chevron U.S.A. Inc.* v. *Natural Resources Defense Council, Inc.,* 467 U.S. 837, 844, is in order; the well-reasoned views of the agencies implementing a statute constitute a body of experience and informed judgment to which courts and litigants may properly resort for guidance. *E.g., Bragdon* v. *Abbott,* 524 U.S. 624, 642. According to the State, L. C. and E. W. encountered no discrimination "by reason of" their disabilities because they were not denied community placement on account of those disabilities, nor were they subjected to "discrimination," for they identified no comparison class of similarly situated individuals given preferential treatment. In rejecting these positions, the Court recognizes that Congress had a more comprehensive view of the concept of discrimination advanced in the ADA. The ADA stepped up earlier efforts in the Developmentally Disabled Assistance and Bill of Rights Act and the Rehabilitation Act of 1973 to secure opportunities for people with developmental disabilities to enjoy the benefits of community living. The ADA both requires all public entities to refrain from discrimination, see §12132, and specifically identifies unjustified "segregation" of persons with disabilities as a "for[m] of discrimination," see §§12101(a)(2), 12101(a)(5). The identification of unjustified segregation as discrimination reflects two evident judgments: Institutional placement of persons who can handle and benefit from community settings perpetuates unwarranted assumptions that persons so isolated are incapable or unworthy of participating in community life, cf., *e.g., Allen* v. *Wright,* 468 U.S. 737, 755; and institutional confinement severely diminishes individuals' everyday life activities. Dissimilar treatment correspondingly exists in this key respect: In order to receive needed medical services, persons with mental disabilities must, because of those disabilities, relinquish participation in community life they could enjoy given reasonable accommodations, while persons without mental disabilities can receive the medical services they need without similar sacrifice. The State correctly uses the past tense to frame its argument that, despite Congress' ADA findings, the Medicaid statute "reflected"

a congressional policy preference for institutional treatment over treatment in the community. Since 1981, Medicaid has in fact provided funding for state-run home and community-based care through a waiver program. This Court emphasizes that nothing in the ADA or its implementing regulations condones termination of institutional settings for persons unable to handle or benefit from community settings. Nor is there any federal requirement that community-based treatment be imposed on patients who do not desire it. In this case, however, it is not genuinely disputed that L. C. and E. W. are individuals "qualified" for noninstitutional care: The State's own professionals determined that community-based treatment would be appropriate for L. C. and E. W., and neither woman opposed such treatment. Pp. 12–18.

Justice Ginsburg, joined by Justice O'Connor, Justice Souter, and Justice Breyer, concluded in Part III—B that the State's responsibility, once it provides community-based treatment to qualified persons with disabilities, is not boundless. The reasonable-modifications regulation speaks of "reasonable modifications" to avoid discrimination, and allows States to resist modifications that entail a "fundamenta[l] alter[ation]" of the States' services and programs. If, as the Eleventh Circuit indicated, the expense entailed in placing one or two people in a community-based treatment program is properly measured for reasonableness against the State's entire mental health budget, it is unlikely that a State, relying on the fundamental-alteration defense, could ever prevail. Sensibly construed, the fundamental-alteration component of the reasonable-modifications regulation would allow the State to show that, in the allocation of available resources, immediate relief for the plaintiffs would be inequitable, given the responsibility the State has undertaken for the care and treatment of a large and diverse population of persons with mental disabilities. The ADA is not reasonably read to impel States to phase out institutions, placing patients in need of close care at risk. Nor is it the ADA's mission to drive States to move institutionalized patients into an inappropriate setting, such as a homeless shelter, a placement the State proposed, then retracted, for E. W. Some individuals, like L. C. and E. W. in prior years, may need institutional care from time to time to stabilize acute psychiatric symptoms. For others, no placement outside the institution may ever be appropriate. To maintain a range of facilities and to administer services with an even hand, the State must have more leeway than the courts below understood the fundamental-alteration defense to allow. If, for example, the State were to demonstrate that it had a comprehensive, effectively working plan for placing qualified persons with mental disabilities in less restrictive settings, and a waiting list that moved at a reasonable pace not controlled by the State's endeavors to keep its institutions fully populated, the reasonable-modifications standard would be met. In such circumstances, a court would have no warrant effectively to order displacement of persons at the top of the community-based treatment waiting list by individuals lower down who commenced civil actions. The case is remanded for further consideration of the appropriate relief, given the range of the State's facilities for the care of persons with diverse mental disabilities, and its obligation to administer services with an even hand. Pp. 18–22.

Justice Stevens would affirm the judgment of the Court of Appeals, but because there are not five votes for that disposition, joined Justice Ginsburg's judgment and Parts I, II, and III—A of her opinion. Pp. 1–2.

Justice Kennedy concluded that the case must be remanded for a determination of the questions the Court poses and for a determination whether respondents can show a violation of 42 U.S.C. §12132's ban on discrimination based on the summary judgment materials on file or any further pleadings and materials properly allowed. On the ordinary interpretation and meaning of the term, one who alleges discrimination must show that she received differential treatment vis-à-vis members of a different group on the basis of a statutorily described characteristic. Thus, respondents could demonstrate discrimination by showing that Georgia (i) provides treatment to individuals suffering from medical problems of comparable seriousness, (ii) as a general matter, does so in the most integrated setting appropriate for the treatment of those problems (taking medical and other practical considerations into account), but (iii) without adequate justification, fails to do so for a group of mentally disabled persons (treating them instead in separate, locked institutional facilities). This inquiry would not be simple. Comparisons of different medical conditions and the corresponding treatment regimens might be difficult, as would be assessments of the degree of integration of various settings in which medical treatment is offered. Thus far, respondents have identified no class of similarly situated individuals, let alone shown them to have been given preferential treatment. Without additional information, the Court cannot address the issue in the way the statute demands. As a consequence, the partial summary judgment granted respondents ought not to be sustained. In addition, it was error in the earlier proceedings to restrict the relevance and force of the State's evidence regarding the comparative costs of treatment. The State is entitled to wide discretion in adopting its own systems of cost analysis, and, if it chooses, to allocate health care resources based on fixed and overhead costs for whole institutions and programs. The lower courts should determine in the first instance whether a statutory violation is sufficiently alleged and supported in respondents' summary judgment materials and, if not, whether they should be given leave to replead and to introduce evidence and argument along the lines suggested. Pp. 1–10.

Ginsburg, J., announced the judgment of the Court and delivered the opinion of the Court with respect to Parts I, II, and III—A, in which Stevens, O'Connor, Souter, and Breyer, JJ., joined, and an opinion with respect to Part III—B, in which O'Connor, Souter, and Breyer, JJ., joined. Stevens, J., filed an opinion concurring in part and concurring in the judgment. Kennedy, J., filed an opinion concurring in the judgment, in which Breyer, J., joined as to Part I. Thomas, J., filed a dissenting opinion, in which Rehnquist, C. J., and Scalia, J., joined.

Source: Legal Information Institute. 1999. *Olmstead v. L. C.* (98-536) 527 U.S. 581. https://www .law.cornell.edu/supct/html/98-536.ZS.html.

25. Findings and Purpose from the Developmental Disabilities Assistance and Bill of Rights Act (DD Act) (2000)

Introduction

The Developmental Disabilities Assistance and Bill of Rights Act of 2000 supports more than 5 million children and people with developmental disabilities and their families in the United States. It is critical to the operation of the developmental disability service network, which provides community-based services and supports that aim to enhance the education, self-determination, and independence of people with developmental disabilities.

TITLE I—PROGRAMS FOR INDIVIDUALS WITH DEVELOPMENTAL DISABILITIES
Subtitle A—General Provisions
SEC. 101. FINDINGS, PURPOSES, AND POLICY.

(a) Findings.—Congress finds that—

(1) disability is a natural part of the human experience that does not diminish the right of individuals with developmental disabilities to live independently, to exert control and choice over their own lives, and to fully participate in and contribute to their communities through full integration and inclusion in the economic, political, social, cultural, and educational mainstream of United States society;

(2) in 1999, there were between 3,200,000 and 4,500,000 individuals with developmental disabilities in the United States, and recent studies indicate that individuals with developmental disabilities comprise between 1.2 and 1.65 percent of the United States population;

(3) individuals whose disabilities occur during their developmental period frequently have severe disabilities that are likely to continue indefinitely;

(4) individuals with developmental disabilities often encounter discrimination in the provision of critical services, such as services in the areas of emphasis (as defined in section 102);

(5) individuals with developmental disabilities are at greater risk than the general population of abuse, neglect, financial and sexual exploitation, and the violation of their legal and human rights;

(6) a substantial portion of individuals with developmental disabilities and their families do not have access to appropriate support and services, including access to assistive technology, from generic and specialized service systems, and remain unserved or underserved;

(7) individuals with developmental disabilities often require lifelong community services, individualized supports, and other forms of assistance, that are most effective when provided in a coordinated manner;

(8) there is a need to ensure that services, supports, and other assistance are provided in a culturally competent manner, that ensures that individuals from racial and ethnic minority backgrounds are fully included in all activities provided under this title;

(9) family members, friends, and members of the community can play an important role in enhancing the lives of individuals with developmental disabilities, especially when the family members, friends, and community members are provided with the necessary community services, individualized supports, and other forms of assistance;

(10) current research indicates that 88 percent of individuals with developmental disabilities live with their families or in their own households;

(11) many service delivery systems and communities are not prepared to meet the impending needs of the 479,862 adults with developmental disabilities who are living at home with parents who are 60 years old or older and who serve as the primary caregivers of the adults;

(12) in almost every State, individuals with developmental disabilities are waiting for appropriate services in their communities, in the areas of emphasis;

(13) the public needs to be made more aware of the capabilities and competencies of individuals with developmental disabilities, particularly in cases in which the individuals are provided with necessary services, supports, and other assistance;

(14) as increasing numbers of individuals with developmental disabilities are living, learning, working, and participating in all aspects of community life, there is an increasing need for a well trained workforce that is able to provide the services, supports, and other forms of direct assistance required to enable the individuals to carry out those activities;

(15) there needs to be greater effort to recruit individuals from minority backgrounds into professions serving individuals with developmental disabilities and their families;

(16) the goals of the Nation properly include a goal of providing individuals with developmental disabilities with the information, skills, opportunities, and support to—

(A) make informed choices and decisions about their lives;

(B) live in homes and communities in which such individuals can exercise their full rights and responsibilities as citizens;

(C) pursue meaningful and productive lives;

(D) contribute to their families, communities, and States, and the Nation;

(E) have interdependent friendships and relationships with other persons;

(F) live free of abuse, neglect, financial and sexual exploitation, and violations of their legal and human rights; and

(G) achieve full integration and inclusion in society, in an individualized manner, consistent with the unique strengths, resources, priorities, concerns, abilities, and capabilities of each individual; and

(17) as the Nation, States, and communities maintain and expand community living options for individuals with developmental disabilities, there is a need to evaluate the access to those options by individuals with developmental disabilities and the effects of those options on individuals with developmental disabilities.

(b) Purpose.--The purpose of this title is to assure that individuals with developmental disabilities and their families participate in the design of and have access to needed community services, individualized supports, and other forms of assistance that promote self-determination, independence, productivity, and integration and inclusion in all facets of community life, through culturally competent programs authorized under this title, including specifically—

(1) State Councils on Developmental Disabilities in each State to engage in advocacy, capacity building, and systemic change activities that—

(A) are consistent with the purpose described in this subsection and the policy described in subsection (c); and

(B) contribute to a coordinated, consumer- and family-centered, consumer- and family-directed, comprehensive system that includes needed community services, individualized supports, and other forms of assistance that promote self-determination for individuals with developmental disabilities and their families;

(2) protection and advocacy systems in each State to protect the legal and human rights of individuals with developmental disabilities;

(3) University Centers for Excellence in Developmental Disabilities Education, Research, and Service—

(A) to provide interdisciplinary preservice preparation and continuing education of students and fellows, which may include the preparation and continuing education of leadership, direct service, clinical, or other personnel to strengthen and increase the capacity of States and communities to achieve the purpose of this title;

(B) to provide community services—

(i) that provide training and technical assistance for individuals with developmental disabilities, their families, professionals, paraprofessionals, policymakers, students, and other members of the community; and

(ii) that may provide services, supports, and assistance for the persons described in clause (i) through demonstration and model activities;

(C) to conduct research, which may include basic or applied research, evaluation, and the analysis of public policy in areas that affect or could affect, either positively or negatively, individuals with developmental disabilities and their families; and

(D) to disseminate information related to activities undertaken to address the purpose of this title, especially dissemination of information that demonstrates that the network authorized under this subtitle is a national and international resource that includes specific substantive areas of expertise that may be accessed and applied in diverse settings and circumstances; and

(4) funding for—

(A) national initiatives to collect necessary data on issues that are directly or indirectly relevant to the lives of individuals with developmental disabilities;

(B) technical assistance to entities who engage in or intend to engage in activities consistent with the purpose described in this subsection or the policy described in subsection (c); and (C) other nationally significant activities.

Source: Public Law 106-402. Government Publishing Office. https://www.gpo.gov/fdsys/pkg /PLAW-106publ402/html/PLAW-106publ402.htm.

26. Executive Summary from "The ADA, 20 Years Later," a National Report on a Survey Conducted for the Kessler Foundation and the National Organization on Disability (NOD) (2010)

Introduction

In 2010, the Kessler Foundation and National Organization on Disability released a report titled "The ADA, 20 Years Later," which focused on the progress that had occurred since the passage of the Americans with Disabilities Act of 1990 (ADA). The report explored the quality of life of people with disabilities, with a particular emphasis on the indicators of employment, finances, education, health care, access to mental health services, transportation, socialization, trips to restaurants, attendance at religious services, technology, political participation, and satisfaction with life. Using longitudinal data collected between 1986 and 2010, the report demonstrated that while there had been advancements in a few areas since the ADA, significant improvements were still needed to enhance the lives of disabled Americans.

Executive Summary

The Kessler Foundation/National Organization on Disability 2010 Survey of Americans with Disabilities marks the sixth effort over the past 24 years (since 1986) to assess the quality of life of people with disabilities on a wide range of critical dimensions, to measure the differences, or "gaps," between people with and without disabilities on these indicators, and to track them over time. The National Organization on Disability and Kessler Foundation, working with Harris Interactive, have established a series of

10 measures of significant life activities of Americans with disabilities. These indicators, which have been tracked over the course of six surveys, are: employment, poverty, education, health care, transportation, socializing, going to restaurants, attendance at religious services, political participation, and satisfaction with life. This year, three new indicators were added, which include: technology, access to mental health services, and overall financial situation.

While there has been modest improvement among a few indicators, the general trend of the measures is that twenty years after the passage of the Americans with Disabilities Act (ADA), there has yet to be significant progress in many areas. For instance, although there has been substantial improvement reported in education attainment and political participation since 1986, large gaps still exist between people with and without disabilities with regard to: employment, household income, access to transportation, health care, socializing, going to restaurants, and satisfaction with life. In some instances, the spread has actually gotten worse since the inception of the survey in 1986.

Since this survey was last conducted in 2004, America has undergone a significant economic downturn. Some areas measured in the survey, such as employment, poverty, and going to restaurants were negatively impacted by the state of the economy. However, the consistency of the size of the gaps this year suggests that people with disabilities and without disabilities were affected as much, or more, by the recession.

The 2010 survey continues to underscore the notion that there is no single indicator of the quality of lives of people with disabilities. They face a range of challenges, and have varied experiences and aspirations. This diversity is characterized not only by a broad spectrum of disability characteristics, specifically type and severity, but also by a range of personal characteristics and circumstances. Understanding this heterogeneity will be crucial toward properly equipping people with disabilities with the tools, skills, and opportunities they need to succeed.

In addition to the gap measures that have been included in this and previous research, the survey includes an expanded section on employment, and selected questions on financial independence. These items add further texture to the disadvantages faced by people with disabilities and point to the potential of accommodations and programs that can be designed to facilitate and improve the employment outcomes of more people with disabilities.

There have been some improvements measured over the years that may be in part attributable to the implementation of the ADA of 1990. However, there is clearly much work to be done in order to narrow the very substantial gaps that still exist. Hopefully policymakers, employers, and the disability community will work together to translate these findings into actions and policies that will improve the lives of millions of Americans with disabilities in the future.

Source: Kessler Foundation/NOD Survey of Americans with Disabilities. 2010. Survey conducted by Harris Interactive for Kessler Foundation and NOD. http://www.2010disabilitysurveys.org/pdfs/surveyresults.pdf.

---

27. Excerpt from the National Council on Disability Report "Rocking the Cradle: Ensuring the Rights of Parents with Disabilities and Their Children" (2012)

Introduction

Parents with disabilities face a significant amount of prejudice and discrimination.

Numerous state policies exist that marginalize disabled parents. In approximately 35 states, disability can be used as grounds for terminating parental rights, and in every state, a parent's disability status can be considered when determining the best interests of a child. In 2012, the National Council on Disability released "Rocking the Cradle: Ensuring the Rights of Parents with Disabilities and Their Children." The report discusses how parents and prospective parents with disabilities are viewed and treated, reviews federal and state policies that may interfere with disabled people's right to parent, and assesses state and federal agencies that interface with parents with disabilities and their children. The report illustrates the barriers that exist for parents and prospective parents with disabilities and provides recommendations on how these barriers can be reduced or eliminated.

The Evolution of Parenting in the Disability Community

The desire to become a parent traverses all cultural, physical, and political boundaries. However, for people with disabilities—including intellectual and developmental, psychiatric, sensory, and physical disabilities—this innate desire has long been forestalled by societal bias. Today, people with disabilities continue to encounter significant legal, medical, and familial resistance to their decision to become parents. This opposition has profound and disconcerting roots.

Parenting with a Disability in the 20th Century

The first half of the 20th century was characterized by the eugenics movement, during which more than 30 states legalized involuntary sterilization. This legislative trend was premised on the belief that people with disabilities and other "socially inadequate" populations would produce offspring who would be burdensome to society. Because of these state statutes, more than 65,000 Americans were involuntarily sterilized by 1970.

Forced sterilization gained the blessing of the U.S. Supreme Court in the 1927 *Buck v. Bell* decision. Carrie Buck was an institutionalized woman in Virginia who was deemed "feebleminded." She was the daughter of a "feebleminded" mother who was committed to the same institution. At age 17, Buck became pregnant after being raped; her daughter Vivian allegedly also had an intellectual disability and was also deemed feebleminded. After the birth of Vivian, the institution sought to sterilize Buck in accordance with Virginia's sterilization statute. Following a series of appeals, Virginia's sterilization statute was upheld on the premise that it served "the best interests of the patient and of society." Concluding this historical decision, Justice Oliver Wendell Holmes, Jr., declared, "Three generations of imbeciles are enough."

Despite receiving severe criticism, *Bell* has never been overruled. In fact, in 1995, the Supreme Court denied the petition for certiorari of a woman with an intellectual disability challenging Pennsylvania's involuntary sterilization statute. Bell was cited by a federal appeals court as recently as 2001, in *Vaughn v. Ruoff.* In this case, the plaintiff had a "mild" intellectual disability and both of her children were removed by the state. Immediately following the birth of her second child, the social worker told the mother that if she agreed to be sterilized, her chances of regaining custody of her children would improve. The mother agreed to sterilization, but approximately three months later, the state informed her that it would recommend termination of parental rights. The district court found that the plaintiff had a protected liberty interest in the 14th Amendment and that the social worker's conduct violated her due process rights. The judgment was affirmed by the U.S. Court of Appeals for the Eighth Circuit. However, the appeals court, citing *Bell*, acknowledged that "involuntary sterilization is not always unconstitutional if it is a narrowly tailored means to achieve a compelling government interest."

Parenting with a Disability Today: The Eugenics Movement's Backdoor?

Even today, 22 years after the passage of the ADA, several states still have some form of involuntary sterilization laws on their books. A few even retain the original statutory language, which labels the targets of these procedures as possessing hereditary forms of "idiocy" and "imbecility," and state that the best interests of society would be served by preventing them from procreating.

In fact, there appears to be a growing trend nationally and internationally toward sterilizing people with intellectual or psychiatric disabilities. Five years ago, a nine-year-old American girl with developmental disabilities was forced to undergo a procedure to, among other things, stunt her growth and remove her reproductive organs. Since then, more than 100 families have reportedly subjected their disabled children to similar treatment, while thousands more have considered doing so.

In the fall of 2011, the Massachusetts Department of Mental Health filed a petition to have the parents of a woman with a psychiatric disability appointed as temporary guardians for the purpose of consenting to an abortion, despite the fact that the woman had refused such a procedure, citing her religious beliefs. The court ordered that the woman's parents be appointed as co-guardians and said she could be "coaxed, bribed, or even enticed . . . by ruse" into a hospital where she would be sedated and an abortion would be performed. The judge also ordered the facility that performed the abortion to sterilize the woman "to avoid this painful situation from recurring in the future." The decision was reversed on appeal. With regard to the sterilization order, the appeals court ruled, "No party requested this measure, none of the attendant procedural requirements has been met, and the judge appears to have simply produced the requirement out of thin air." In overturning the order to terminate the pregnancy, the court stated, "The personal decision whether to bear or beget a child is a right so fundamental that it must be extended to all persons, including those who are incompetent." The appropriate result of the proceedings does not erase its troubling genesis—a state agency that intervened to terminate a pregnancy on the basis of the disability of the pregnant woman, despite her objection to having an abortion.

The familial rights of people with disabilities appear to be declining rapidly. In 1989, 29 states restricted the rights of people with psychiatric disabilities to marry. Ten years later, this number had increased to 33. Further, in 1989, 23 states restricted the parenting rights of people with psychiatric disabilities; by 1999, 27 states had enacted restrictions.

Unquestionably, the power of eugenics ideology persists. Today, women with disabilities contend with coercive tactics designed to encourage sterilization or abortions because they are deemed not fit for motherhood. Similarly, there is a pervasive myth that people with disabilities are either sexually unwilling or unable. According to

Michael Stein, internationally recognized expert on disability law and policy, "Mainstream society's discomfort with the notion of people with disabilities' relational intimacy is well documented. One poll found that 46 percent of nondisabled people stated they 'would be concerned' if their teenage son or daughter dated a person with a disability, and 34 percent 'would be concerned' if a friend or relative married a person with a disability." Stein says, "The main consequences of the disabled non-sexuality myth are (1) difficulty in the formation of intimate interpersonal relationships between disabled and nondisabled people; (2) limited awareness and availability of health care services to women with disabilities; and (3) as a corollary to the myth, severe misperceptions about and often prejudices against individuals with disabilities acting in parental or guardianship capacities."

Indeed, despite the increasing numbers of people with disabilities becoming parents, most still struggle with family, community, and social ambivalence about this choice. According to Corbett Joan O'Toole and Tanis Doe, international disability activists, "In general, with rare exceptions, people with disabilities do not get asked if they want to have children. They don't get asked if they want to be sexual. The silence around sexuality includes their parents, their counselors, their teachers, and most health professionals. Yet these same people sometimes counsel in favor of involuntary sterilization." Lindsay, a woman with physical and cognitive disabilities and a mother of two, reflects on this: "I was first discouraged from being a mother by family and community's attitudes toward sex and disability, especially by their belief, which I internalized, that my difference (my scarred face and starfish-shaped hands) made me ugly, and therefore less desirable."

As Carrie Killoran, a mother with a physical disability, recalls, "Before I got pregnant, I was told by my father that it would be irresponsible of me to have a baby because I would be an unfit mother. This is the view of most of society. . . . On the contrary, I turned out to be one of the fittest mothers I know. The ability to be a good mother does not reside in the ability to chase around after a toddler, nor in the ability to teach your child how to ride a bike. Neither does it include protecting your child from being teased about her parent's disability; all children find something to tease each other about and a sturdy, self-confident child will emerge unscathed."

People with disabilities face these negative attitudes even after becoming parents. O'Toole and Doe state, "If we do have a child we get asked if it is ours, 'Who is the parent?' 'Where is the parent?' or 'Why are you holding it?' " When Jessica, a woman with cerebral palsy, told her mother that she was pregnant with twins, her mother responded, "Now your husband has three babies." Cassandra, a woman with significant physical disabilities and a mother of one, frequently has strangers approach her and question her ability to be a parent.

According to another mother with a physical disability, "The most difficult preparations were those to mentally ready ourselves for the likely probability that there would be—and will always be—people who doubted our abilities and worth as parents." The mother recalls, "I learned long ago that the stereotypes and judgments held by people about [my husband] and me aren't usually encased in their words. It's often what is not said. Several of our friends were married around the same time we were. Almost immediately after our celebrations, my fellow brides would complain about the annoyance they felt when people peppered them with questions about when they were going to have a baby. That certainly wasn't a question that people lined up to ask us."

People with disabilities also face resistance to procreate if their disability is hereditary. Ora Prilletensky, professor, author, and mother with a disability, writes:

> In addition to the myth of asexuality and skepticism regarding their ability to attract partners, women with disabilities have been discouraged from having children for a variety of other reasons. Concerns that they will give birth to "defective" babies and prejudicial assumptions about their capacity to care for children often underpin the resistance that they may encounter. The growing sophistication of prenatal tests, coupled with societal disdain for imperfection, translates into increased pressure on all women to ensure the infallibility of their offspring. Women choosing to forgo prenatal testing often have to contend with the clear disapproval of their doctors and may even run the risk of losing their medical insurance if they choose to bring to term rather than abort the 'flawed' (and expensive) fetus. Indeed, there is an estimated 80 percent rate of abortion of fetuses diagnosed as having a condition that could result in a significant disability.

Kathryn, a wheelchair user and little person, reports that she and her husband, who has a similar disability, were encouraged to adopt because there was a chance their child could have their disability. In fact, many people did not express happiness regarding Kathryn's pregnancy until tests revealed that their baby did not have their disability.

Although the right to be a parent is generally regarded as fundamental, this right is not always assumed for people with disabilities. According to Megan Kirshbaum and Rhoda Olkin of Through the Looking Glass (TLG), "Parenting has been the last frontier for people with disabilities and an arena in which parents are likely to encounter prejudice." Indeed, carrying on a shameful tradition of discrimination against people with disabilities, states continue to erect legislative, administrative, and judicial obstacles to impede people with disabilities from creating and maintaining families.

As discussed in this report, the rate of removal of children from families with parental disability—particularly psychiatric, intellectual, or developmental disability—is ominously higher than rates for children whose parents are not disabled. And this removal is carried out with far less cause, owing to specific, preventable problems in the child welfare system. Further, parents with disabilities are more likely to lose custody of their children after divorce, have more difficulty in accessing reproductive health care, and face significant barriers to adopting children.

Source: "Rocking the Cradle: Ensuring the Rights of Parents of with Disabilities and Their Children." National Council on Disability. https://www.ncd.gov/publications/2012/Sep272012/Ch1.

28. The Toronto Declaration on Bridging Knowledge, Policy and Practice in Aging and Disabilities (2012)

Introduction

Historically, individuals, institutions, and public policies constructed aging and disability as distinct experiences, and consequently, education, research, and services and supports for older adults and people with disabilities have remained separate.

Although it is important not to conflate aging and disability, older adults and people with disabilities experience many shared needs and concerns, including affordable health care, caregiving and family support, consumer-directed services, and physically and socially accessible communities. The Toronto Declaration on Bridging Knowledge, Policy and Practice in Aging and Disability calls on governmental, nongovernmental, professional, and consumer stakeholders to support the bridging of aging and disability to better meet the challenges of the growing numbers of people aging into disability and aging with disability.

Authors: Jerome Bickenbach, Christine Bigby, Luis Salvador-Carulla, Tamar Heller, Matilde Leonardi, Barbara LeRoy, Jennifer Mendez, Michelle Putnam, and Andria Spindel We, as organizers and participants of the 2011 Growing Older with a Disability (GOWD) Conference, a part of the Festival of International Conferences on Caregiving, Disability, Aging and Technology (FICCDAT), held in Toronto, Canada June 5–8, 2011 forward this declaration and invite governmental, non-governmental, professional, and consumer stakeholders to join us in supporting and implementing this plan of action.

The 2011 World Report on disability, produced jointly by the World Health Organization (WHO) and the World Bank, estimates that there are over one billion people with disabilities in the world today, of whom nearly 200 million experience significant difficulties. At the same time, in almost every country, the proportion of people aged over 60 years is growing faster than any other age group, forecast to reach 1.5 billion by 2050, according to

the Global Health and Aging Report, also released in 2011 by WHO in partnership with US National Institute on Aging. This means that in the years ahead disability will be an even greater concern to developed and developing nations due to aging populations, higher risk of disability in older people, as well as the global increase in chronic health conditions, such as diabetes, cardiovascular disease, cancer and mental health disorders. Taken together, the dual phenomena of global aging and increased longevity for individuals with disabilities represent significant advances in public health and education.

However, along with these positive trends come new challenges for the 21st century. These include: strains on pension and social security systems; preparing health providers and societies to meet the needs of populations aging with and aging into disability; preventing and managing age and disability associated secondary conditions and chronic diseases; designing sustainable policies to support healthy aging and community-living as well as long-term and palliative care; and developing disability and age-friendly services and settings.

Bridging the fields of aging and disability research, policy, and practice is critical for meeting these challenges. All of us aspire to healthy aging, regardless of the presence of age-related impairments or disabling conditions. The experience of growing older with a disability and growing older into a disability may differ—in part because of the different dynamics of ageism and ableism and the differences in economic and social conditions that result—but these life course trajectories present similar challenges and opportunities. In this document we seek common ground, in terms of the modern conception of active aging and of disability, defined as difficulty in functioning at the body, person or societal levels experienced by an individual with a health condition in interaction with the person's physical, social and attitudinal environment. Moreover, we firmly believe that, despite the distinctions between aging and disability created by professionals, academics, advocacy NGOs, public policies and government agencies, the time has come to emphasize similarities in experiences and needed supports, services and policies rather than focusing on differences. Distinctions between early and late onset of disability are to a large extent a reflection of policy issues—with various utilities across nations—but they do provide a picture of the parameters of practice and research that can inform bridging and consequences of this distinction.

This declaration builds upon the Barcelona Declaration on Bridging Knowledge in Long-Term Care and Support, March 5–7, 2009, the Graz Declaration on Disability and Ageing, 9th June, 2006, the Linz Declaration as well as United Nations Conventions (in particular the United Nations Convention on the Rights of Persons with Disabilities and the United Nations 2002 Political Declaration from the Madrid World Assembly on Aging II) and international directives that recognize the human rights and the biopsychosocial approach to disability. Bridging encompasses a range of concepts, tasks, technologies and practices aimed at improving knowledge sharing and collaboration across stakeholders, organizations and fields in care and support for persons with disabilities, their families, and the aging population. Bridging tasks include activities of dissemination, coordination, assessment, empowerment, service delivery, management, financing and policy. The overall purpose of bridging is to improve efficiency, equity of care, inclusion and support at all levels, from the person to the society. It is also an issue of recognition of the complexity of the human condition from birth to death, the capabilities of all people, and the need for a conceptual vision that takes into consideration planning for a society where participation of all citizens is the ultimate goal.

Based on the findings of the GOWD and larger FICCDAT meetings, we assert that:

National and international bridging of aging and disability knowledge, policy and practice must be actively promoted. Aging with and aging into disability are global population trends. Cross-national and international collaborations can support effective and efficient knowledge development and transfer, implementation of best practices, and facilitate information exchange among and empowerment of persons with disabilities and their families.

Bridging is composed of several activities which must occur simultaneously, at multiple levels of knowledge development, policy and practice, and include disability and aging stakeholder groups. The scope of required bridging activities is broad, including the analysis of public policies, interdisciplinary research, the development of professional best practices, and coalition building across advocacy groups and among individual stakeholders. Older adults and people with disabilities and their families must be meaningfully included in bridging activities in recognition of their rights to self-determination and social inclusion.

Building effective bridges across aging and disability knowledge, policy and practice requires

interdisciplinary collaboration and engagement with national and international decision-makers. Development of effective models of bridging and successful bridging practices requires engagement of professional and citizen stakeholders bringing together relevant knowledge and experience. Decision leaders must engage knowledge brokers to pursue program and policy changes that support bridging activities.

Connecting the field of aging and disability will require development of a clear model of bridging. Research at all levels will support the science of bridging as it develops. However, research must give immediate and persistent attention to the pace of bridging to assure that it aligns with the needs of the person aging with disability in order for them to negotiate and make life choices, navigate support and service systems, and engage in opportunities for full inclusion and participation in society.

Bridging requires developing a common terminology and knowledge base. Tasks include activities of dissemination, coordination, assessment, empowerment, service delivery, management, financing and policy. Technologies include various Information Technologies, assessment instruments and guidelines. Bridging practices should be catalogued and incorporated to open-access repositories for use by aging and disability networks.

Therefore we identify the following priority areas for bridging aging and disability knowledge, policies, and practice:

Health and well-being: Improved access to healthcare services; improved diagnosis and treatment of secondary conditions and diseases; care coordination; health literacy; health promotion and wellness; prevention of age-related chronic conditions; prevention of abuse and neglect; reduction in pre-mature mortality and training of health professionals in aging and disability.

Inclusion, participation and community: Accessible societies, including age and disability friendly communities, removal of barriers of any kind: architectural, cultural, legislative. Impact and implications of aging and disability on civic and community engagement, and the role of technology and universal design in fostering inclusion, participation and knowledge management.

Long-term supports and services: Support for families and caregivers, training and education of direct support professionals; self-determination, access, availability, and affordability of supports and services; ethical issue related to non-discrimination, such as in palliative care, end of life issues.

Income security: Employment, retirement security, asset development; accommodation and accessibility in the work setting; value of non-paid social and community contributions.

Science of bridging: Research on bridging aging and disability and on ways to transfer this knowledge locally, nationally, and internationally to policy development.

We therefore recommend that:

An international agenda for bridging aging and disability be formally developed through the involvement of researchers, practice professionals, policy-makers, older adults, persons with disabilities and their families.

Public and private funders provide financial support for research and scholarship that advances the science of bridging aging and disability knowledge, practice and policies.

Health and social policy-makers incorporate bridging and knowledge transfer as key strategies in policy planning for building a society where all citizens can fully participate including persons with disabilities of all ages.

We invite endorsement and implementation of this declaration

The authors, all of whom were participants at the Growing Older with a Disability conference at FICCDAT 2011, endorse this Declaration and invite feedback.

Response can be sent to the attention of Toronto Declaration@marchofdimes.ca.

Individuals and organizations which have endorsed this declaration are listed below. Others are invited to add their endorsement by sending an email with your full contact information to TorontoDeclaration@marchofdimes.ca, adding 'TD Endorsement' in the subject line.

Most importantly, we call upon governments, practitioners, policy-makers and academics to work together with consumers and their families to ensure attention and implementation of the preceding recommendations.

Co-Chairs of Growing Older with a Disability (GOWD) conference, Festival of International Conferences on Caregiving, Disability, Aging and Technology (FICCDAT), 2011 Margaret Campbell, PhD, Jennifer Mendez, PhD, Sandy Keshen

Endorsement by the Authors

Jerome E. Bickenbach, PhD. Department of Health Sciences and Health Policy, University of Lucerne and Schweizer Paraplegiker-Forschung, Nottwil, Switzerland

Christine Bigby, PhD. Department of Social Work and Social Policy, La Trobe University, Bundoora, Victoria, Australia

Luis Salvador-Carulla, MD PhD. Faculty of Health Sciences, University of Sydney, Sydney, Australia

Tamar Heller, PhD. Rehabilitation Research and Training Center on Aging with Developmental Disabilities, University of Illinois at Chicago, Chicago, IL, USA

Matilde Leonardi, PhD. Head Neurology, Public Health, Disability Unit Foundation IRCCS Istituto Neurologico Carlo Besta, Milan, Italy

Barbara LeRoy, PhD. Developmental Disabilities Institute, Wayne State University, Detroit, Michigan, USA

Jennifer Mendez, PhD. School of Medicine, Wayne State University, Detroit, Michigan, USA

Michelle Putnam, PhD. School of Social Work, Simmons College, Boston, USA

Andria Spindel, MSW. March of Dimes Canada, Toronto, Canada

References

European Association of Service Providers for Persons with Disabilities (EASPD).

The Graz Declaration on Disability and Ageing. Graz, Austria, June 9, 2006. (Joint Publication of the European Disability Forum, AGE: The European Older People's Platform, European Federation of Older Persons, Inclusion Europe, Association on Research and Training in Europe, Lebenshilfe Österreich, Die Steirische Behindertenhilfe.): http://www.easpd.eu/LinkClick.aspx?fileticket=eDUBIDI0HSU%3D&tabid=3531.

Salvador-Carulla, L., Balot, J., Weber, G., Zelderloo, L., Parent, A.S., McDaid, D., Solans, J., Knapp, M., Mestheneos, L., Wolfmayr, F. Participants at the Conference. (2010).

The Barcelona Declaration on bridging knowledge in long-term care and support. Barcelona (Spain), March 7, 2009. International Journal of Integrated Care, April 12:

http://www.ijic.org/index.php/ijic/articl
e/viewArticle/521/1035

European Association of Service Providers
for Persons with Disabilities (EASPD).
The Linz Declaration: Independent living for ageing persons with disabilities.
Linz, Austria, January, 2012: http://www
.poraka.org.mk/en/2012/EASPD%20
Linz%20Declaration%202011.pdf.

World Health Organization. World
Report on Disability. Geneva, Switzerland, 2011. (Joint Publication of The
World Bank: http://whqlibdoc.who.int
/publications/2011/9789240685215_eng.pdf.

United Nations. Convention on the Rights of
Persons with Disabilities. New York, USA.
December 13, 2006: http://www.un.org
/disabilities/convention/conventionfull
.shtml.

United Nations. Political Declaration and
Madrid International Plan of Action on
Ageing. Madrid, Spain, 2002: http://social
.un.org/index/Portals/0/ageing/docu
ments/Fulltext-E.pdf.

Source: Bridging Aging and Disability International Network (BADIN)/March of Dimes. http://
www.badinetwork.org/uploads/6/2/2/7/62278365
/toronto_declaration.pdf.

29. "Social Security Disability: Times for Reform," Comment of Peter Blanck to the Social Security Advisory Board (SSAB) (2013)

Introduction

Social Security Disability Insurance (SSDI) was enacted in 1956 as an amendment to the Social Security Act. Policy makers forwarded SSDI as a safety net for workers who become disabled and can no longer work. Recipients of SSDI receive a monthly benefit that is based on their previous wages. In 2017, the average monthly benefit was $1,171. Recipients are also enrolled in Medicare. Numerous scholars and activists, including Dr. Peter Blanck, university professor and chair of the Burton Blatt Institute at Syracuse University, have called for SSDI to be restructured and improved. Dr. Blanck is an expert on disability law and policy issues. On March 8, 2013, Blanck participated as a discussant in a Social Security Advisory Board (SSAB) forum titled "Social Security Disability: Time for Reform." Following the forum, Dr. Blanck provided supplemental comments for the SSAB to consider. He urged the SSAB to preserve the financial benefits of SSDI while expanding training programs and work incentives, with the ultimate goal of supporting the economic self-sufficiency of people with disabilities.

Dear Acting Chair Kennelly and Members of the Social Security Advisory Board:

Thank you for the opportunity to serve as a discussant at your March 8, 2013, forum on "Social Security Disability: Time for Reform." It was an honor to participate. Below, I present my supplemental comments, which are based on my remarks to be included in the record of the forum. I thank you for your consideration of these points as you deliberate recommendations on this important topic.

My comments focus on the following:

(1) The definitions of disability under the Social Security Act and under the Americans with Disabilities Act (ADA) serve different important, yet complementary, national policy goals.

(2) To further the goals of a comprehensive national disability policy, additional study and dialogue on the Social Security disability programs should focus

on supporting the economic security, stability, and productivity of people with disabilities.

1. The definitions of disability under SSI/SSDI and under the ADA serve different important, yet complementary, national policy goals.

At the SSAB March 8 forum, several panelists drew conclusions from comparison of the definitions of disability under SSI/SSDI and under the ADA, suggesting that there is a need to align the SSI/SSDI definition with the ADA definition. In my opinion, these two definitions serve different important, yet complementary, national policy goals.

The Social Security Act provides monetary benefits to eligible participants with a disability. The definition of disability for an adult in the SSI/SSDI programs is based upon the individual's inability to engage in substantial work. Eligibility for these programs requires that an individual cannot perform substantial gainful activity (SGA) due to a medically determinable physical or mental impairment that is expected to either result in death or to last not less than a continuous period of 12 months.[1]

The ADA seeks to eliminate discrimination against individuals with disabilities.[2] The ADA defines disability as a physical or mental impairment that substantially limits one or more major life activities.[3] The ADA prohibits discrimination by covered employers against a "qualified individual" with a disability—that is, a person who is able to perform the essential functions of the job, with or without reasonable accommodations.[4]

The definitions of disability under SSI/SSDI and the ADA thereby reflect different statutory purposes.[5] As the United States stated in its amicus brief in the Cleveland case (which logic was adopted by the Supreme Court in its decision):

Social security benefits and the ADA are not necessarily alternative remedies between which people with disabilities must choose. Rather they are complementary measures that provide financial support to people with physical or mental impairments who face practical barriers to work while at the same time encouraging and facilitating their efforts to move off the benefit rolls and return to work.[6]

Primary among the statutory differences is that when the Social Security Administration determines an individual is disabled for purposes of the SSI or SSDI programs, it does not consider the possibility of reasonable accommodation.[7] The U.S. Supreme Court has concluded in its 1999 Cleveland v. Policy Management Systems Corp. decision:

[The difference in the SSI/SSDI and ADA definition of disability] reflects the facts that the SSI/SSDI receives more than 2.5 million claims for disability benefits each year; its administrative resources are limited; the matter of reasonable accommodation may turn on highly disputed workplace-specific matters; and an SSI/SSDI misjudgment about that detailed, and often fact-specific matter would deprive a seriously disabled person of the critical financial support the statute seeks to provide.[8]

For these reasons, the determination of reasonable accommodation under the ADA cannot be transferred to the determination of disability eligibility under SSI/SSDI. Additional information on my views on this topic is available in 2002 testimony that I delivered before the U.S. House of Representatives.[9] Please note that my testimony preceded enactment of the ADA Amendments Act of 2008. Regulations and Interpretive Guidance on the equal employment provisions of Title I of the ADA, as amended by the ADA Amendments Act of 2008, provide additional information on the reasonable accommodation analysis under the ADA, highlighting the differences in purpose and process between the ADA analysis and the SSI/SSDI eligibility determination.[10]

2. To further the goals of a comprehensive national disability policy, additional study and dialogue on the Social Security disability programs should focus on supporting the economic security, stability, and productivity of people with disabilities.

Since the passage of the ADA in 1990,[11] there has been unprecedented change brought to public policy that recognizes "disability as a natural part of life experience," no longer defined purely in a medical context, but now explained by social and environmental barriers and facilitators.[12] The prior paradigm of disability often viewed people with disabilities as "defective and in need of fixing."[13] The modern paradigm embodies a "disability policy framework,"[14] as articulated in the ADA, and sets forth the goals of "equality of opportunity, individualization, full participation, independent living and economic self-sufficiency."[15]

By providing cash assistance that includes work incentives, the Social Security disability programs support the participation of people with disabilities in our American democracy and community life. Importantly, these programs play a vital role in advancing the goal of fostering economic self-sufficiency, defined as "economic security, stability, and productivity of persons with disabilities."[16]

The Social Security disability programs should not be viewed as a problem to be fixed, but rather as a solution to be strengthened in support of the shared national disability policy goals. In developing recommendations, the SSAB should adopt a critical view of the assumptions of those who view modernization as a strictly intellectual exercise. This is particularly true for assumptions about the adoption of international models in the U.S. and about the best ways to achieve economic self-sufficiency among people with disabilities.

International systems differ markedly from the U.S. system. Some panelists at the SSAB forum suggested that the U.S. adopt models such as experience rating that are used in other nations, for instance, in the Netherlands. However, monetary benefit systems in other developed nations operate within often vastly different geographies, legal frameworks, and social assistance systems.

Geographies. As I pointed out at the SSAB forum, countries such as the Netherlands are significantly smaller than the vast majority of states in the U.S. The challenges associated with administering a cash benefit for people with disabilities across the entire U.S. likely are qualitatively different and quantitatively much larger than those that confront smaller nations.

Legal frameworks. Major differences exist in the structure and evolution of disability rights laws in other nations, as compared to the U.S. The ADA and other U.S. disability rights laws focus primarily on negative rights to be free from future interference or discrimination,[17] whereas many other developed nations have focused more on positive rights to overcome the existing unequal position of people with disabilities resulting from past discrimination.[18] For example, Japan has in the past largely focused on providing protection through vocational rehabilitation and services, and has an employment quota for people with disabilities set at 1.8% for the private sector and 2.1% for the public sector.

Social assistance systems. Compared with the U.S., other developed nations typically spend a much higher percentage of their Gross Domestic Product on social assistance ("social protection programs"),[20] use much less stringent definitions of "disability" to determine eligibility for monetary benefits,[21] and regulate their labor markets in ways that offer significantly greater protections for workers.[22] For example, developed nations like the Netherlands provide universal health care and have established important rights and safeguards for most workers in areas such as hiring, termination and compensation.

These vast differences suggest that attempts to replicate in the U.S. reforms to government operated social insurance systems in other developed nations are likely to carry significant implementation challenges as well as serious risks for people with disabilities. The SSAB should not accept such replication proposals.

SSI/SSDI benefits play a vital role in the economic self-sufficiency of people with disabilities. Any reforms to the Social Security disability programs must continue to open up opportunities for employment, while recognizing that even with increased employment many people will continue to require SSI/SSDI benefits due to limited earnings.

The SSAB should adopt recommendations that build on the strong foundation of the Social Security Act in ways that preserve cash assistance for current and future beneficiaries while continuing to expand the SSI/SSDI work incentives. For example, the SSAB should encourage implementation of promising practices from existing demonstration programs, and should call for research on additional work incentive enhancements such as increasing the SGA level, simplifying the SSDI work incentives, and providing permanent eligibility for Medicare for individuals who no longer receive SSDI cash benefits. This last recommendation would be similar to the provision in P.L. 99-643, the Employment Opportunities for Disabled Americans Act of 1986, which made permanent section 1619 of the Social Security Act—a provision that benefitted from the essential support of then-Commissioner of Social Security Dorcas Hardy.[23]

In closing, thank you for the opportunity to participate in the March 8, 2013, SSAB forum and to submit these supplemental comments for the record.

Sincerely,
Peter Blanck, Ph.D., J.D.*
University Professor
& Chairman, Burton Blatt Institute
*The views expressed in this statement reflect only those of the author and do not represent the views of Syracuse University or any other entities.

Endnotes

1 See 42 U.S.C. 423(d)(1)(A).

2 See *Cleveland v. Policy Management Systems Corp.*, 526 U.S. 795, 802 (1999).

3 See 42 U.S.C. 12012(1)

4 *Supra* note 2.

5 Peter Blanck, Bruce Goldstein, & William Myhill, *Legal Rights of Persons with*

Disabilities: An Analysis of Federal Law: Second Edition, LRP Publications (2013).

6 Brief for the United States and the Equal Employment Opportunity Commission as Amici Curiae Supporting Petitioner, in Cleveland, 1998 WL 839956 at 5 (emphasis added).

7 *Cleveland*, at 803.

8 Id.

9 Peter Blanck, Statement before the Subcommittee on Social Security, House Committee on Ways and Means, Hearing on "Social Security Disability Programs' Challenges and Opportunities," July 11, 2002.

10 See 29 CFR. pt. 1630 (2011) and 29 CFR pt. 1630 Appendix (2011).

11 Pub. L. 101-336, 104 Stat. 327, (1990).

12 NIDRR Long Range Plan (64 Fed. Reg. 68608). See also Peter Blanck & Helen Schartz, Towards researching a national employment policy for persons with disabilities, in LR McConnell (ed), *Switzer Monograph Series* (July 2001); Harlan Hahn, Disability Policy and the Problem of Discrimination, 28 *Am. Behav. Sci.* 293, 294 (1985).

13 Peter Blanck & Michael Millender, Before disability civil rights: Civil War pensions and the politics of disability in America, 52 *Alabama L. Rev.* 1 (2000); Peter Blanck, Civil War pensions and disability, 62 *Ohio State L. J.* 109 (2001).

14 See Robert Silverstein, Emerging Disability Policy Framework: A Guidepost for Analyzing Public Policy, 85 *Iowa L. Rev.* 1691 (2000).

15 Id.

16 Id. See also Lisa Schur, Douglas Kruse, & Peter Blanck, *People with Disabilities: Sidelined or Mainstreamed?*, Cambridge University Press (2013).

17 Eve Hill & Peter Blanck, Future of Disability Rights Advocacy and "The Right to Live in the World", 15 *Texas Journal on Civil Liberties & Civil Rights* 1 (2009).

18 *Supra* note 23.

19 Jun Nakagawa & Peter Blanck, Future of Disability Law in Japan: Employment and Accommodation, 33 *Loy. L.A. Int'l & Comp. L. Rev.* 173 (2010).

20 For example, see Fig. 1, International Labour Office and Organisation for Economic Co-Operation and Development, Towards national social protection floors, (2011). http://www.oecd.org/els/48732216.pdf.

21 Organisation for Economic Co-Operation and Development, "Sickness, Disability, and Work: Breaking the Barriers: A Synthesis of Findings across OECD Countries" (2010), http://ec.europa.eu/health/mental _health/eu_compass/reports_studies/dis ability_synthesis_2010_en.pdf.

22 For example, see Fig. 2.1., 2.2 and 2.3, Organisation for Economic Co-Operation and Development, OECD Employment Outlook 2013, OECD Publishing (2012), http://dx.doi .org/10.1787/empl_outlook-2013-en.

23 Sarah G. Rocklin & David R. Mattson, The Employment Opportunities for Disabled Americans Act: Legislative History and Summary of Provisions, 50 *Social Security Bulletin* 25 (1987).

Source: *Congressional Record*, August 14, 2013. Written comments available at http://bbi.syr.edu/ _assets/docs/news_events/Blanck_to_SSAB.pdf.

30. Statement of Senator Robert J. Dole on the Convention on the Rights of Persons with Disabilities before the Senate Foreign Relations Committee (2013)

Introduction

The United Nations Convention on the Rights of Persons with Disabilities (CRPD) is an international treaty that provides disabled people with human rights, including the right to be protected from prejudice and discrimination, the right to education, the right to employment and economic self-sufficiency, the right to live independently and participate in society, the right to health care, and the right to vote. The CRPD was adopted on December 31, 2006, at the United Nations Headquarters in New York. Nations must first sign the CRPD and then ratify it to indicate that they consent to be bound to the treaty. As of January 2018, the CRPD had 160 signatories and 175 ratifications worldwide. Although the United States signed the CRPD on July 30, 2009, it has not yet ratified it. An attempt to ratify the CRPD occurred on December 4, 2012, but fell short by five votes. Numerous activists, scholars, and policy makers have repeatedly called on the United States to ratify the CRPD. On November 5, 2013, Senator Robert J. Dole, a disabled veteran, delivered a statement to the Senate Foreign Relations Committee. Dole called on the Committee to back the ratification of the CRPD, to further support the rights of people with disabilities in the United States.

Chairman Menendez, Ranking Member Corker, and members of this Committee.

I urge you to give your support and consent to the Convention on the Rights of Persons with Disabilities (CRPD). While I cannot stand before you in person today, I approach you in the strong hope that, on your second examination of this important treaty, you will again do the right thing and advance the rights of disabled individuals from the United States and throughout the world. In so doing, I am privileged to join with over twenty veterans' organizations, forty religious groups, more than seven hundred disability and allied groups,

dozens of you on both sides of the Senate aisles, and many other prominent Americans who recognize the imperative of U.S. leadership on this issue—a leadership that will be imperiled without U.S. ratification of the CRPD.

When this treaty came before the Senate last year, it fell just five votes short of passage. In debating the treaty's merits, treaty opponents expressed concern that the CRPD would diminish American sovereignty—that, through U.S. ratification, the United Nations would somehow be able to supersede U.S. law, even by interfering with American parents' right to home-school their children.

Along with Senator John McCain, Secretary John Kerry and others, I could not disagree more strongly with this view. This treaty contains reservations, understandings and declarations (RUDs) that explicitly describe how the treaty will and will not apply to the U.S. At the same time, I respect this institution, its provision for debate, and its tolerance of the opinions and conclusions of its one hundred members. Today, I urge all of you to keep an open mind and recognize another important characteristic of this august body: the opportunity it presents for policies to evolve and be strengthened as members work together in a bipartisan fashion for a greater good. This treaty, in a way that is both telling and unique, enjoys the support of diverse groups serving a variety of interests: Republicans and Democrats, veterans organizations and disability groups, businesses and religious organizations. Given the broad support, I hope those of you with reservations about any aspect of the treaty, will work with your colleagues, whom I know are ready to work with you, to address your concerns. If improvements to the RUDs are needed, then I urge members from both parties to work together on that.

This treaty is important for America because of who we are as a nation. It is particularly important, though, for a distinguished group of which I am a member. As I recalled in my statement to this committee last year, I left World War II having joined an exceptional group—one which no one joins by personal choice. It is a group that neither respects nor discriminates by age, gender, wealth, education, skin color, religious beliefs, political party, power, or prestige. That group, Americans with disabilities, has grown in size ever since. So, therefore, has the importance of maintaining access for people with disabilities to be part of mainstream American life, whether through access to a job, an education, or registering to vote. To me, this is not about extending a privilege to a special category of people; it is instead about civil rights.

When Congress passed the Americans with Disabilities Act (ADA) in 1990, it was not only one of the proudest moments of my career, it was a remarkable bipartisan achievement that made an impact on millions of Americans. The simple goal was to foster independence and dignity, and its reasonable accommodations enabled Americans with disabilities to contribute more readily to this great country.

If not before the ADA, then certainly after its passage, our nation led the world in developing disability public policy and equality. In recent years, many countries—including our allies in Australia, Britain, Canada, France, Germany, Israel, Mexico, and South Korea—have followed our lead. In 2006, President George W. Bush took U.S. leadership on this issue to a new level by negotiating and supporting approval of the CRPD. On the anniversary of the ADA in 2009, President Barack Obama signed the treaty—a landmark document that commits countries around the world to affirm what are essentially core American values of equality, justice, and dignity.

U.S. ratification of the CRPD will increase the ability of the United States to improve physical, technological and communication access in other countries, thereby helping to ensure that Americans—particularly, many thousands of disabled American veterans—have equal opportunities to live, work, and travel abroad. In addition, the treaty comes at no net cost to the United States. In fact, it will create a new global market for accessibility goods. An active U.S. presence in implementation of global disability rights will promote the market for devices such as wheelchairs, smart phones, and other new technologies engineered, made, and sold by U.S. corporations.

With the traditional reservations, understandings, and declarations that the Senate has adopted in the past, current U.S. law satisfies the requirements of the CRPD. Indeed, as President George H. W. Bush informed this committee last year, the treaty "would not require any changes to U.S. law." It would extend protections pioneered in the United States to the more than one billion people with disabilities throughout the world.

President Obama has again submitted the treaty to you for your advice and consent. I urge you to seize this critical opportunity to continue the proud American tradition of supporting the rights and inclusion of people with disabilities.

Years ago, in dedicating the National World War II Memorial, I tried to capture what makes America worth fighting for, indeed, dying for. "This is the golden thread that runs throughout the tapestry of our nationhood," I said, "the dignity of every life, the possibility of every mind, the divinity of every soul." I know many of you share this sentiment and hope you will consider this treaty through that lens. In ratifying this treaty, we can affirm these goals for Americans with disabilities.

I urge you to support U.S. ratification of this important treaty and I thank you for the courtesy of your consideration. God Bless America.

Source: *Congressional Record.* 2013. Statement of Senator Robert J. Dole on the Convention on the Rights of Persons with Disabilities before the Senate Foreign Relations Committee November 5, 2013. https://www.foreign.senate.gov/imo/media/doc/Senator_Dole_Testimony.pdf.

31. Senator Tom Harkin's Congressional Farewell Speech (2014)

Introduction

Tom Harkin is a celebrated former Democratic senator of Iowa who accomplished much in his 40-year career in the U.S. Congress, particularly for disability rights. Harkin introduced to the Senate the Americans with Disabilities Act of 1990 (ADA), which is heralded as the first comprehensive civil rights law for disabled people in the United States. He was also an outspoken critic of the institutional bias in Medicaid, which forces many disabled people to live in nursing homes or other care facilities rather than in the community. In 2014, Harkin called on his colleagues in the Senate to vote to ratify the United Nations Convention on the Rights of Persons with Disabilities (CRPD), although the vote was prevented from taking place. In his congressional farewell speech on December 12, 2014, Harkin reflected on his long career and the status of disabled people in the United States. He urged Congress to ratify the CRPD, and he pledged that although he was retiring from Congress, he would never retire from the fight for disability rights.

Almost two years ago I announced I was not going to seek a sixth term in the United States Senate. That decision and announcement did not seem all that difficult or hard at that time. Two years was a long time off. And since then I have been busy working, having hearings, meeting constituents, getting legislation through the HELP Committee, working on Appropriations.

But now—knowing this will be my final, formal speech on the floor of the U.S. Senate; Now—knowing that in a few days a semi-truck will pull up to the Hart Senate Office Building and load hundreds of boxes containing forty years of my Senate and House records and haul them off to Drake University and the Harkin Institute of Public Policy and Civic Engagement in Des Moines;

Now—seeing my office in 731 Hart stripped nearly bare; Now—when I will soon cast my last vote; Now—when I will no longer be engaged in legislative battle, when I will no longer be summoned by the Senate bells, now—when I will soon just be number 1,763 of all the Senators who have ever served in the U.S. Senate.

Now—the leaving becomes hard and wrenching and yes, emotional. That's because I love this U.S. Senate. I love this work. It has been said that the Senate is broken. No, it's not broken. Oh, a few dents here and there. Some scrapes. Banged up a little. But, there is still no other place in America where one person can do big things—for good or for ill—for our people and our nation.

I love the people with whom I work: Senators, staff, clerks, Congressional Research Service, doorkeepers, cloakroom, police, restaurant employees . . . and yes, pages. Especially to those who labor outside the lights and cameras and news stories: who make the Senate function on a daily basis, I thank you.

I particularly want to thank my wonderful, hardworking, dedicated staff, both present and past, both personal and committee staff. And when I say committee staff, I mean the Appropriations sub-committee on Labor, Health and Human Services, which I have been privileged to chair or be ranking member since 1989. I mean also the Committee on Agriculture, which I chaired twice for two farm bills, once in 2001–2002, and in 2007–2009, and I mean the Committee on Health, Education, Labor and Pensions which I have chaired since the untimely death of Senator Ted Kennedy in 2009.

I first heard Senator Pat Leahy say this, so I always attribute it to him: that we Senators are just a constitutional impediment to the smooth functioning of staff! This is truer than most of us would like to admit. Also, in thanking my staff, I don't just mean those who work in Washington.

I would never have been re-elected four times without the hands on, day in, day out, constituent service of my Iowa staff. The casework they have done in helping people with problems is every bit as important as any legislative work done here in Washington.

In 2012, our office marked a milestone. The 100,000 constituent service case we have processed since 1985. I cannot count the number of times Iowans have personally thanked me for something my staff had done to help them. I didn't get here by myself. My staff helped.

So, I thank my staff of past and present who have so strongly supported me when I was right, so diplomatically corrected me when I was wrong, and who all labored in a shared commitment to provide a hand up, a ladder of opportunity, to those who had been dealt a bad hand in the lottery of life. I ask consent to list the names of my present staff, so they will forever be enshrined in the history of the U.S. Senate.

But most of all, I thank Ruth, the love of my life, my wife of forty-six years. You have been my constant companion, my soul-mate, my strongest supporter, and my most honest critic. You have been my joy in happy times, and my solace when things just didn't go right. I'm looking forward to more adventures, love, and excitement with you in the years ahead.

To our two beautiful, smart, caring and compassionate daughters, Amy and Jenny: I thank you for always being there for your dad, for giving me such wondrous joy in being a part of your growing up. I am so proud of both of you. And to my son-in-law Steve, and my grandkids McQuaid, Daisy, and Luke—look out—because here comes grandpa!

There is so much I want to say, but I want to be respectful of those who have come to share this moment with me—my staff, family, friends, fellow Senators. I want to state as briefly as I can why I'm here, my guiding philosophy for the past forty years. It has to do with that ladder of opportunity I mentioned. A ladder—not escalator. A ramp—not a moving walkway.

Not one nickel or dime in the ADA is given to a person with a disability. But we broke down barriers, opened doors of accessibility and accommodation, and said to people with disabilities—Now go on, follow your dreams, and in the words of the Army motto, "be all you can be."

Government must not be just an observant bystander, it must be a force for good, for lifting people up, for giving hope to the hopeless.

I've never had an "I love me" wall in my office. What I did have were two items on the wall by the door so I would see them when I walked out to go vote, or to a hearing, or working on a bill. One was a drawing of the house in which my mother was born and lived to the age of twenty-five when she came to America. It was a small house in the village of Suha, Yugoslavia, now Suha, Slovenia. That house had a dirt floor, no running water.

The second item on my wall is this—my father's WPA card from 1939. My father had a 6th grade education, worked many years in coal mines, was 53 years old in 1939, out of work with five kids and one on the way: me. There were no jobs. Things looked hopeless. Then dad, as he related to me years later, got the letter from Franklin Roosevelt giving him a job. So dad got some income, and the dignity of meaningful work. But most importantly, our government gave him hope. Hope that tomorrow would be better. That his family would be okay. That his kids would have a better future.

Every federal judge takes an oath to "do equal right to the poor and to the rich." Can we here in the Congress say we do that? That we provide equal right to the poor and rich alike? Our growing inequality proves we are not. Maybe we should be taking that oath.

There are four overriding issues that I hope this Senate will address in the coming session. Number one, as I mentioned, the growing economic inequality in America. It is destructive of lives, it slows our progress as a nation, and it will doom broad support for representative government. When people at the bottom of the economic ladder feel the government is not helping them and in fact may be stacked against them, they will cease to vote, or will turn to the siren song of extreme elements in our society. History proves this to be true.

I don't have a cookie-cutter answer or solution, but it must include more fair tax laws and trade laws, more job training and retraining, rebuilding our physical infrastructure, and manufacturing. And I believe it must include some things, seemingly unrelated, like quality, free, early education for every child in America.

The answer to closing the inequality gap must include rebuilding labor unions and collective bargaining. If you trace the line over the last 40 years of our growing economic inequality and put that over another line showing the loss in the number of union workers, they are almost identical. I do not believe it is a stretch to say that organized labor, unions, built the middle class in America, and they are a part of the answer in strengthening and rebuilding our middle class.

Another part of the answer is raising the minimum wage to above the poverty line and inflation indexing it for the future. We also need new flex time laws especially for women in the workforce. We need to strengthen Social Security as in Senator Brown's bill. We need a new retirement system for all workers. Not another 401(k), but a system in which employers and employees contribute, which can only be withdrawn as an annuity for life after one retires, like the Netherlands has. Lack of a reliable retirement is one of the most under reported, unexamined crises on our national horizon, and is a big part of our growing inequality.

Finally, we must continue to build on the Affordable Care Act. The cost and availability of good health care has in the past widened the inequality gap. We are now starting to close that element of inequality. We need to add a public option to the exchange as another choice for people. And we must continue support for prevention and public health—moving us more and more away from "sick care" to real "health care."

I believe that the second overriding issue is the destruction of the family of man's only home—planet earth—through the continued use of fossil fuels. We know what's happening. The science is irrefutable, the data is clear, the warning signs are flashing in bright neon red: "stop what you are doing with fossil fuels." We must shift massively and quickly to renewable energy, a new smart electric grid, retro fitting our buildings for energy efficiency, and moving rapidly to a hydrogen based energy cycle.

The third issue I commend to the Senate for further development and changes in existing laws is the under employment of people with disabilities. As you all know, ensuring equal rights and opportunities for people with disabilities has been the major part of my work in the Senate for the past 30 years. We have made significant strides forward in changing America to fulfill two of the four goals of the Americans with Disabilities Act. These two are full participation and equal opportunity. The other two goals—independent living and economic self-sufficiency—need more development.

I ask you all in the next Congress to do two things to advance these two goals of independent living and economic self-sufficiency.

First, help states to fully implement the Supreme Court's *Olmstead* decision, to more rapidly de-institutionalize people with disabilities and provide true independent living with support services. This will save money, and the lives of people with disabilities will be better and more truly independent.

Secondly, we must do more on employment of people with disabilities in competitive, integrated employment.

We all get the monthly unemployment figures every month. Last month unemployment held steady at 5.8% officially, but Leo Hindery has better calculations to show the real rate is twice that figure. Also, we know that unemployment among young African-Americans is 11.1%.

But how many of us know that the unemployment rate among adult Americans with disabilities who want to work and can work is over 60%?! Yes, you heard me right: almost two out of three people with disabilities cannot find a job. That is a blot on our national character.

Thankfully, some enlightened employers have affirmative action plans to hire more people with disabilities. Employers are finding that many times these become their best employees—they are more productive, the hardest working, most reliable workers.

I ask you to meet with Greg Wasson, CEO of Walgreens, and Randy Lewis, who was Senior V.P., now retired. Walgreens has hired many people with disabilities in Walgreens' distribution centers, and now has set a goal of 10% of their store employees will be people with disabilities. There are others making strides in this area: Best Buy, Lowes, Home Depot, IBM, and Marriott—to mention some other large companies moving forward in hiring people with disabilities. We need to learn from them what we—the federal and perhaps state government—can do to help in this area. We also need to implement policies to help small businesses employ more people with disabilities.

I dwell on this because perhaps I feel I haven't done enough on this issue of employment for people with disabilities, and we just have to do better. I will say, however, that our HELP Committee passed this year and President Obama signed into law, a new re-authorization of the old Workforce Investment Act, now named the Workforce Investment and Opportunity Act. In the law, there is a new provision I worked on to get more intervention in high school for kids with disabilities to prepare for the workplace through summer jobs, job coaching, and internships.

However, this is just starting, and funding is tight, but it will do much for young people with disabilities to enter competitive, integrated employment. I want to thank all members of the HELP Committee for their support of this bill, but especially Senator Murray and Senator Isakson for taking the lead to get the bill done—along with Senator Enzi, Senator Alexander, and me.

And while I am mentioning the HELP Committee, let me thank all members for a very productive last two years, during which we passed 24 bills signed into law by the President. Important bills dealing with drug track and tracing, compounding drugs, WIAO—which I mentioned, Child Care Development Block grant, among others.

I want to thank Senator Alexander for being a great partner in these efforts. He will be taking the helm of this great committee in the next Congress. Senator Alexander certainly has the background to lead the committee, combined with a keen mind and a good heart. I wish him continued success as the new Chairman of HELP.

The fourth issue concerns the U.N. Convention on the Rights of People with Disabilities.

I don't think anything has saddened me more in my 30 years here than the failure of the Senate to ratify the CRPD. This convention was modeled after our own Americans with Disabilities Act. It has been ratified by 150 nations. It has broad and deep support in our country, supported by the U.S. Chamber of Commerce, the Business Roundtable, veterans groups, every disability organization, every former living President, every former Republican leader of the Senate: Senator Dole, Senator Lott, and Senator Frist. In November, we received a letter of support from the National Association of Evangelicals. I also want to point out that Senator Dole has worked his heart out on this. I hope the next Senate will take this up and join with the rest of the world in helping make changes globally for people with disabilities.

So, I came to Congress—the House—in 1974 as one of the "Watergate Babies." With my retirement and the retirement in the House of Congressman George Miller and Congressman Henry Waxman, we are the last of the "Watergate Babies," with 2 exceptions. Among all the Democrats elected in 1974 there were a few Republicans, and one is left: my senior colleague from Iowa, Senator Chuck Grassley. I have great respect for and friendship with Chuck. Several weeks ago, here on the floor, he said some gracious things about me. I especially appreciated his observation that, though he and I are like night and day when it comes to our political views, there is no light between us when it comes to Iowa. We have collaborated on so many important initiatives for the people of Iowa, and we made a heck of a good tag team on behalf of our state. So again, I salute and thank my friend and colleague of nearly 40 years, Chuck Grassley. The other exception is my dear friend Rick Nolan, who was in the 1974 class, voluntarily left Congress after 3 terms, then returned to the House in 2012 and was recently re-elected.

So, 40 years later this "Watergate baby" is grown up and grey. I came to the Senate 30 years ago as a proud progressive, determined to get things done. And as I depart the Senate, I can say in good conscience that I remained true to my progressive roots. I have worked faithfully to leave behind a more vibrant Iowa, a more just and inclusive America, and a stronger ladder—and ramp—of opportunity for the disadvantaged in this great country.

You might say that my career in Congress is the story of a poor kid from Cumming, Iowa trying his best to "pay it forward", saying thank you for the opportunities I was given by leaving that ladder and ramp of opportunity stronger for those who follow.

If I have accomplished this in any small way, if many Americans are able to lead better lives because of my work, I leave office a satisfied man.

So, I am retiring from the Senate but I'm not retiring from the fight. I will never retire from the fight to ensure equal opportunity, full participation, independent living, and economic self-sufficiency for people with disabilities.

I will never retire from the fight to give a hand up—and hope to those who have experienced disadvantage and adversity. And I will never retire from the fight to make this a land of social and economic justice for all Americans.

Let me close with a single word from American sign language that has a powerful message for all of us. Let me teach it to you. (PAUSE to sign "America" in American Sign language). This is the sign for America. All of us, inter connected, bound together in a single circle of inclusion with no one left out. This is the ideal America toward which we must always aspire.

And with that Mr. President, for the last time, I yield the floor.

Source: *Congressional Record*. December 12, 2014.

32. Excerpt from the Individuals with Disabilities Education Act (2015)

Introduction

The Individuals with Disabilities Education Act (IDEA) was originally passed as the Education for All Handicapped Children Act in 1975. This policy establishes education as a civil right for students with disabilities. Under the law, all students with disabilities are entitled to a free appropriate public education. Additionally, their education must be individualized to fit their specific needs. The IDEA is essential for ensuring that children with disabilities receive the same educational opportunities as their nondisabled peers.

(c) Findings.—Congress finds the following:

(1) Disability is a natural part of the human experience and in no way diminishes the right of individuals to participate in or contribute to society. Improving educational results for children with disabilities is an essential element of our national policy of ensuring equality of opportunity, full participation, independent living, and economic self-sufficiency for individuals with disabilities.

(2) Before the date of the enactment of the Education for All Handicapped Children Act of 1975 (Public Law 94-142), the educational needs of millions of children with disabilities were not being fully met because—

(A) the children did not receive appropriate educational services;

(B) the children were excluded entirely from the public school system and from being educated with their peers;

(C) undiagnosed disabilities prevented the children from having a successful educational experience; or

(D) a lack of adequate resources within the public school system forced families to find services outside the public school system.

(3) Since the enactment and implementation of the Education for All Handicapped Children Act of 1975, this title has been successful in ensuring children with disabilities and the families of such children access to a free appropriate public education and in improving educational results for children with disabilities.

(4) However, the implementation of this title has been impeded by low expectations, and an insufficient focus on applying replicable research on proven methods of teaching and learning for children with disabilities.

(5) Almost 30 years of research and experience has demonstrated that the education of children with disabilities can be made more effective by—

(A) having high expectations for such children and ensuring access to the general education curriculum in the regular classroom, to the maximum extent possible, in order to—
   (i) meet developmental goals and, to the maximum extent possible, the challenging expectations that have been established for all children; and
   (ii) be prepared to lead productive and independent adult lives, to the maximum extent possible;

(B) strengthening the role and responsibility of parents and ensuring the families of such children have meaningful opportunities to participate in the education of their children at school and at home;

(C) coordinating this title with other local, educational service agency, including improvement efforts under the Elementary and Secondary Education Act of 1965, in order to ensure that such children benefit from such efforts and that special education can become a service for such children rather than a place where such children are sent;

(D) providing appropriate special education and related services, and aids and supports in the regular classroom, to such children, whenever appropriate;

(E) supporting high-quality, intensive preservice preparation and professional development for all personnel who work with children with disabilities in order to ensure that such personnel have the skills and knowledge necessary to improve the academic achievement and functional performance of children with disabilities, including the use of scientifically based instructional practices, to the maximum extent possible;

(F) providing incentives for whole-school approaches, scientifically based early reading programs, positive behavioral interventions and supports, and early intervening services to reduce the need to label children as disabled in order to address the learning and behavioral needs of such children;

(G) focusing resources on teaching and learning whiles reducing paperwork and requirements that do not assist in improving educational results; and

(H) supporting the development and use of technology, including assistive technology devices and assistive technology services, to maximize accessibility for children with disabilities.

(6) While States, local educational agencies, and educational service agencies are primarily responsible for providing an education for all children with disabilities, it is in the national interest that the Federal Government have a supporting role in assisting State and local efforts to educate children with disabilities in order to improve results for such children and to ensure equal protection of the law.

(7) A more equitable allocation of resources is essential for the Federal Government to meet its responsibility to provide an equal educational opportunity for all individuals.

(8) Parents and schools should be given expanded opportunities to resolve their disagreements in positive and constructive ways.

(9) Teachers, schools, local educational agencies, and States should be relieved of irrelevant and unnecessary paperwork burdens that do not lead to improved educational outcomes.

(10)(A) The Federal Government must be responsive to the growing needs of an increasingly diverse society.

(B) America's ethnic profile is rapidly changing. In 2000, 1 of every 3 persons in the United

States was a member of a minority group or was limited English proficient.

(C) Minority children comprise an increasing percentage of public school students.

(D) With such changing demographics, recruitment efforts for special education personnel should focus on increasing the participation of minorities in the teaching profession in order to provide appropriate role models with sufficient knowledge to address the special education needs of these students.

(11)(A) The limited English proficient population is the fastest growing in our Nation, and the growth is occurring in the many parts of the Nation.

(B) Studies have documented apparent discrepancies in the levels or referral and placement of limited English proficient children in special education.

(C) Such discrepancies pose a special challenge for special education in the referral of, assessment of, and provision of service for, our Nation's students from non-English language backgrounds.

(12)(A) Greater efforts are needed to prevent the intensification of problems connected with mislabeling and high dropout rates among minority children with disabilities.

(B) More minority children continue to be served in special education than would be expected from the percentage of minority students in the general school population.

(C) African-American children are identified as having intellectual disabilities and emotional disturbance at rates greater than their White counterparts.

(D) In the 1998–1999 school year, African-American children represented just 14.8 percent of the population aged 6 through 21, but comprised 20.2 percent of all children with disabilities.

(E) Studies have found that schools with predominantly White students and teachers have placed disproportionately high numbers of their minority students into special education.

(13)(A) As the number of minority students in special education increases, the number of minority teachers and related services personnel produced in colleges and universities continues to decrease.

(B) The opportunity for full participation by minority individuals, minority organizations, and Historically Black Colleges and Universities in awards for grants and contracts, boards of organizations receiving assistance under this title, peer review panels, and training of professionals in the area of special education is essential to obtain greater success in the education of minority children with disabilities.

(14) As the graduation rates for children with disabilities continue to climb, providing effective transition services to promote successful

post-school employment or education is an important measure of accountability for children with disabilities.

Source: U.S. House Legal Counsel. https://legcounsel.house.gov/Comps/Individuals%20With%20Disabilities%20Education%20Act.pdf.

33. Executive Summary from the National Council on Disability Report "Breaking the School-to-Prison Pipeline for Students with Disabilities" (2015)

Introduction

The school-to-prison pipeline refers to a national trend in which children are increasingly removed from public education, often through suspension and expulsion, and transitioned into the criminal legal system. A significant amount of research and activism has highlighted that students marginalized by race and class are disproportionately affected by the school-to-prison pipeline. However, even though up to 85 percent of youth in juvenile detention facilities are disabled, the role of disability in the school-to-prison pipeline has received less attention. In 2015, the National Council on Disability released a report titled "Breaking the School-to-Prison Pipeline for Students with Disabilities." The report considers the role of special education in the school-to-prison pipeline and discusses how the Individuals with Disabilities in Education Act (IDEA) can be used as one way to address this growing national crisis.

Studies show that up to 85 percent of youth in juvenile detention facilities have disabilities that make them eligible for special education services, yet only 37 percent receive these services while in school. A disproportionate percentage of these detained youth are youth of color. These statistics should lead to the conclusion that many disabled youth in the juvenile justice and criminal justice systems are deprived of an appropriate education that could have changed their School-to-Prison Pipeline trajectory. The School-to-Prison Pipeline refers to policies and practices that push our nation's schoolchildren, especially those most at risk, out of classrooms and into the juvenile and criminal justice systems. This pipeline reflects the prioritization of incarceration over education. Yet the benefits of special education are in question. Students with disabilities who receive special education services in school have poorer outcomes and are suspended and expelled more often than their peers without disabilities. These dire statistics are even worse for students of color with disabilities, who are disproportionately classified as having an emotional disturbance or an intellectual disability and disproportionately segregated. These realities are often contradictory and confounding:

(1) Many students with disabilities, including students of color, go through general education with unidentified and unaddressed academic, behavioral, or mental health needs;

(2) Students of color are overrepresented in special education and experience more segregation and worse outcomes; and

(3) Students who qualify for special education too often receive inferior services in segregated settings and incur repeated suspensions and expulsions.

In conjunction with its fall quarterly meeting, the National Council on Disability

(NCD) convened a stakeholder forum in Atlanta on October 6, 2014, to receive testimony on the role of special education in the School-to-Prison Pipeline and to confront these issues. The meeting began with the following facts, principles, and questions:

FACTS:
- All races have members with disabilities.
- Among incarcerated youth, 85 percent have learning and/or emotional disabilities, yet only 37 percent receive special education in school. Most were either undiagnosed or not properly served in school.
- Many students have invisible disabilities, such as specific learning disability (SLD), emotional disturbance, posttraumatic stress disorder, or attention deficit/hyperactivity disorder (ADHD).
- Schools suspended students with disabilities and students of color at many times the rate of their white counterparts.
- Schools suspend students of color with individualized education plans (IEPs), whether they have disabilities or not, to the most disproportionate degree.

PRINCIPLES:
- We cannot address the School-to-Prison Pipeline without a disability lens.
- Special education is not a place. We are talking about a system of services and supports for inclusion in general education.
- Special educators have developed tools for teaching students with a variety of disabilities, including learning, behavioral, and emotional disabilities.
- A referral for special education assessments can help identify learning, behavior, and emotional needs.
- Students with disabilities and their families need information, training, and

leadership development to effectively use the Individuals with Disabilities Education Act (IDEA) as a tool to secure better educational services.

- There is a need for advocates to assist students with disabilities and their families in securing services and providing oversight to the delivery of services.
- An investment in IDEA, Section 504 of the Rehabilitation Act, and the Americans with Disabilities Act (ADA) is necessary to ensure that youth of color reap the benefits of disability laws.
- Students of color should have access to the benefits of IDEA/504/ADA services to the same extent as white students.

QUESTIONS

- Does IDEA offer important tools to infuse better educational services for students of color with disabilities who are currently suspended or expelled?
- Can the proper implementation of IDEA help disrupt the School-to-Prison Pipeline for these students?

NCD has concluded that IDEA can and should be an important part of the solution to the School-to-Prison Pipeline crisis. Thus, the recommendations in this report focus on ways to improve existing special education delivery and enforcement systems to better meet the needs of students with disabilities who risk entering the Pipeline.

First and foremost, NCD would like to see a unified system of education with all students educated in the regular education classrooms with special education supports. But improved implementation of disability laws in this manner alone will not eradicate the persistent racial and ethnic disparities within the class of students with disabilities caught in the Pipeline. Thus, the

recommendations acknowledge that efforts to break the School-to-Prison Pipeline for students with disabilities must address both conscious and unconscious racial biases that combine with disability discrimination to contribute to the crisis.

Summary of Key Findings and Recommendations
Key Findings

- The confusing disciplinary provisions added and refined in the last two IDEA reauthorizations have allowed schools to ignore their overarching obligation to provide a free appropriate public education (FAPE), particularly the requirement to consider behavioral supports in the IEP.
- Persistent racial and ethnic disparities in identification, discipline, placement, and other key categories show IDEA implementation breakdowns disproportionately affect students of color with disabilities.
- Although the overall inclusion of students with disabilities in the general education classroom has increased over the last decade, statistics shows that students of color with disabilities remain disproportionately segregated from their peers without disabilities.
- Reports of both overrepresentation and underrepresentation of students of color in special education suggest that child find enforcement does not ensure schools refer and assess these students in a non-discriminatory manner.
- Racial and ethnic disparities in suspensions and expulsions suggest the presence of unconscious or implicit biases that combine with discrimination on the basis of disability to contribute to the School-to-Prison Pipeline crisis.

- Schoolwide positive behavior interventions and supports (SWPBIS) and response to intervention (RTI) do not reduce racial and ethnic disparities in discipline without specific attention to issues of race and culture.
- State and local government entities often fail to enforce and comply with mandatory data collection and reporting laws.

Key Recommendations

- The U.S. Departments of Education (ED) and Justice (DOJ) should issue joint guidance on the discipline of students with disabilities under IDEA and Section 504 that reconciles the obligation to provide a FAPE with the 10-day suspension rule and focuses on how special education supports and services in the general education classroom can support students who are at risk of academic failure and suspensions.
- Schools should develop data-driven early warning systems to identify students whose academic and behavioral issues put them at risk of suspensions and expulsions that lead to entry into the juvenile justice and criminal justice systems and refer these students for more intensive general or special education services and supports.
- ED and DOJ should bolster efforts to monitor and enforce the provision of FAPE to students with disabilities in the least restrictive environment.
- ED should issue guidance setting forth minimum substantive standards for the quality and delivery of special education and related services, particularly as they relate to behavioral supports.
- Federal and state enforcement activities must directly address race to remedy longstanding racial disparities in

the placement and discipline of students with disabilities.
- ED should fund the development of systems for evaluating implicit racial and disability bias in schools where minorities are overrepresented in identification, discipline, or placement, and implement implicit bias training in enforcement agreements and compliance reviews.
- ED should take affirmative steps to enforce mandatory data collection and reporting requirements and ensure the validation of data submitted.
- Federal and state enforcement agencies should coordinate enforcement of disability rights laws and other civil rights laws such as Title VI of the Civil Rights Act of 1964 and bolster enforcement efforts on the specific issue of disproportionality in school discipline and juvenile justice referrals, including initiating litigation.

Conclusion

There is no question that the statistical picture of special education is bleak. But after its meeting of stakeholders, interviews with experts, and review of the research, NCD believes that IDEA and other related disability laws, with improved enforcement, can and should benefit at-risk students who are properly referred and served. In fact, the interventions and supports developed in special education are the key recommendations in the My Brother's Keeper Task Force report and other initiatives to curb the School-to-Prison Pipeline in general education. Special educators and the Office of Special Education and Rehabilitative Services (OSERS) should play a leading role in both special and general education reform. However, improved implementation of disability laws alone will not eliminate persistent racial disparities in special education. Enforcement activities must also address race head on to finally ameliorate the problem of disproportionality in special education.

Source: National Council on Disability. 2015. "Breaking the School-to-Prison Pipeline for Students with Disabilities." https://www.ncd.gov /publications/2015/06182015.

34. "Disability and Health" from Healthy People 2020 on the Office of Disease Prevention and Health Promotion (ODPHP) Website (2017)

Introduction

In 2010, the U.S. Department of Health and Human Services launched Healthy People 2020, a national plan for health promotion and disease prevention. Healthy People 2020's objective is to work toward a society in which all people live long, healthy lives. For people with disabilities, Healthy People 2020 aims to eliminate barriers to health care, create more accessible environments, promote community living and participation, and establish more inclusive health care systems and policies.

Goal

Maximize health, prevent chronic disease, improve social and environmental living conditions, and promote full community participation, choice, health equity, and quality of life among individuals with disabilities of all ages.

Overview

Individuals with disabilities represent 18.7% (about 56.7 million people) of the U.S. population. Disability is part of human existence, occurring at any point in life, with conditions ranging from mild to severe even among those with the same diagnosis. A diagnosis of impairment or disabling condition does not define individuals, their talents and abilities, or health behaviors and health status. Consistent with the World Health Organization's (WHO) model of social determinants of health, Healthy People 2020 recognizes that what defines individuals with disabilities, their abilities, and their health outcomes more often depends on their community, including social and environmental circumstances. To be healthy, all individuals with or without disabilities must have opportunities to take part in meaningful daily activities that add to their growth, development, fulfillment, and community contribution. This principle is central to all objectives outlined in this topic area. Meeting the Disability and Health objectives over the decade will require that all public health programs develop and implement ways to include individuals with disabilities in program activities.

Why Is Disability and Health Important?

The first objective in this topic area, DH-1, is critical for understanding why disability and health is important. DH-1 calls for including measures of disability in all health data collection systems as well as analyzing and publishing the data in a standard demographic format to help monitor progress toward reducing health disparities and achieving health equity. Until recently, people with disabilities have been overlooked in public health surveys, data analyses, and health reports, making it difficult to raise awareness about their health status and existing disparities. Emerging data indicate that individuals with disabilities, as a group, experience health disparities in routine public health arenas such as health behaviors, clinical preventive services, and chronic conditions. Compared with individuals without disabilities, individuals with disabilities are:

- Less likely to receive recommended preventive health care services, such as routine teeth cleanings and cancer screenings
- At a high risk for poor health outcomes such as obesity, hypertension, falls-related injuries, and mood disorders such as depression
- More likely to engage in unhealthy behaviors that put their health at risk, such as cigarette smoking and inadequate physical activity

Understanding Disability and Health

There are many factors that determine or influence one's health. Healthy People 2020 organizes the social determinants of health around 5 key domains: (1) Economic Stability, (2) Education, (3) Health and Health Care, (4) Neighborhood and Built Environment, and (5) Social and Community Context. Within each of these domains, compared to individuals without disabilities, individuals with disabilities are more likely to experience challenges finding a job, being included in regular educational classrooms or attending college, receiving preventive health care services, being able to visit homes in the neighborhood, using fitness facilities, using health information technology, and obtaining sufficient social-emotional support.

To address these and other health determinants, the following WHO principles of action are recommended to achieve health equity among individuals with disabilities.

1. Improving the conditions of daily life by:

- Encouraging communities to be accessible so all can live in, move through, and interact with their environment
- Encouraging community living
- Removing barriers in the environment using both physical universal design concepts and operational policy shifts

2. Addressing the inequitable distribution of resources among individuals with disabilities and those without disabilities by increasing:

- Appropriate health care for individuals with disabilities
- Education and work opportunities
- Social participation
- Access to needed technologies and assistive supports

3. Expanding the knowledge base and raising awareness about determinants of health for individuals with disabilities by increasing:

- The inclusion of individuals with disabilities in public health data collection efforts across the lifespan
- The inclusion of individuals with disabilities in health promotion activities
- The expansion of disability and health training opportunities for public health and health care professionals
- Emerging Issues in Disability and Health

There are three critical emerging issues in disability and health:

The first is the need for better disability health data to inform policy and program development regarding critical issues of health disparities and health equity.

A solution is to ensure that standard disability items are included in all public health surveillance instruments and that data is analyzed for individuals with disabilities where disability is in the data source.

The second is the need to increase the implementation of evidence-based health and wellness programs that have been demonstrated to be effective among people with disabilities in community settings, including adequate strategies for preparedness and response for individuals with disabilities. Related to this is the need to translate existing evidence-based interventions demonstrated to be effective in clinical settings for people with disabilities to community programs. A solution is to add individuals with disabilities to community-based health promotion efforts where possible.

The third is the need to improve environmental designs and public infrastructure. Solutions include:

- Ensuring the accessibility of technology, health information technology tools and systems, broadly defined, for people with physical, sensory, and cognitive disabilities. This includes electronic health records and personal health records as well as wearable technologies and home monitoring systems.
- Designing homes and community spaces that are fully accessible to individuals with disabilities.
- Ensuring that professional degree programs offer coursework in disability and health.

Source: Healthy People 2020. Office of Disease Prevention and Health Promotion (ODPHP). https://www.healthypeople.gov/2020/topics-objectives/topic/disability-and-health.

35. Laura Hershey's Poem "You Get Proud by Practicing"

Introduction

Laura Hershey was a disabled poet, journalist, and activist. One of her most cherished poems is "You Get Proud by Practicing." Ableism in society often leads disabled people to feel shame and doubt. However, "You Get Proud by Practicing" asserts that pride is a characteristic that one achieves through continuous effort, self-love, and empowerment. Written in 1990, the poem has been published in numerous forums; read at disability pride parades; featured at feminist, LGBT, and disability events; and even adapted into a choral arrangement.

If you are not proud
For who you are, for what you say, for how you look;
If every time you stop
To think of yourself, you do not see yourself glowing
With golden light; do not, therefore, give up on yourself.
You can get proud.

You do not need
A better body, a purer spirit, or a Ph.D.
To be proud.
You do not need
A lot of money, a handsome boyfriend, or a nice car.
You do not need
To be able to walk, or see, or hear,
Or use big, complicated words,
Or do any of those things that you just can't do
To be proud. A caseworker
Cannot make you proud,
Or a doctor.

You only need more practice.
You get proud by practicing.

There are many many ways to get proud.
You can try riding a horse, or skiing on
one leg,
Or playing guitar,
And do well or not so well,
And be glad you tried
Either way.
You can show
Something you've made
To someone you respect
And be happy with it no matter
What they say.
You can say
What you think, though you know
Other people do not think the same way,
and you can
keep saying it, even if they tell you
You are crazy.

You can add your voice
All night to the voices
Of a hundred and fifty others
In a circle
Around a jailhouse
Where your brothers and sisters are
being held
For blocking buses with no lifts,
Or you can be one of the ones
Inside the jailhouse,
Knowing of the circle outside.
You can speak your love
To a friend
Without fear.
You can find someone who will listen
to you
Without judging you or doubting you or
being
Afraid of you
And let you hear yourself perhaps
For the very first time.

These are all ways
Of getting proud.
None of them
Are easy, but all of them
Are possible. You can do all of these things,
Or just one of them again and again.
You get proud
By practicing.

Power makes you proud, and power
Comes in many fine forms
Supple and rich as butterfly wings.
It is music
when you practice opening your mouth
And liking what you hear
Because it is the sound of your own
True voice.

It is sunlight
When you practice seeing
Strength and beauty in everyone,
Including yourself.
It is dance
when you practice knowing
That what you do
And the way you do it
Is the right way for you
And cannot be called wrong.
All these hold
More power than weapons or money
Or lies.
All these practices bring power, and power
Makes you proud.
You get proud
By practicing.

Remember, you weren't the one
Who made you ashamed,
But you are the one
Who can make you proud.
Just practice,
Practice until you get proud, and once you
are proud,

Keep practicing so you won't forget.
You get proud
By practicing.

Source: Estate of Laura Hershey, Denver, CO.

---

36. An Overview of the International Classification of Functioning, Disability, and Health (ICF)

Introduction

The International Classification of Functioning, Disability, and Health (ICF) is a framework for understanding and categorizing disability as it relates to health and functioning. The World Health Organization's (WHO) original framework was the International Classification of Impairments, Disabilities, and Handicaps (ICIDH), which was approved in 1980. However, ICIDH was heavily criticized for its emphasis on the medical aspects of disability and its lack of attention to attitudinal, environmental, and structural barriers experienced by disabled people. On May 22, 2001, all 191 nations belonging to the World Health Organization voted to approve the ICF. The ICF draws from multiple models of disability. It examines the impairments and functioning of disabled people's bodies and minds, the activities of disabled people and the limitations they experience, the participation of disabled people in society, and the environmental facilitators or barriers that influence disabled people's experiences.

THE MODEL OF ICF

Two major conceptual models of disability have been proposed. The *medical model* views disability as a feature of the person, directly caused by disease, trauma or other health condition, which requires medical care provided in the form of individual treatment by professionals. Disability, on this model, calls for medical or other treatment or intervention, to 'correct' the problem with the individual.

The *social model* of disability, on the other hand, sees disability as a socially created problem and not at all an attribute of an individual. On the social model, disability demands a political response, since the problem is created by an unaccommodating physical environment brought about by attitudes and other features of the social environment.

On their own, neither model is adequate, although both are partially valid. Disability is a complex phenomena that is both a problem at the level of a person's body, and a complex and primarily social phenomena. Disability is always an interaction between features of the person and features of the overall context in which the person lives, but some aspects of disability are almost entirely internal to the person, while another aspect is almost entirely external. In other words, both medical and social responses are appropriate to the problems associated with disability; we cannot wholly reject either kind of intervention.

A better model of disability, in short, is one that synthesizes what is true in the medical and social models, without making the mistake each makes in reducing the

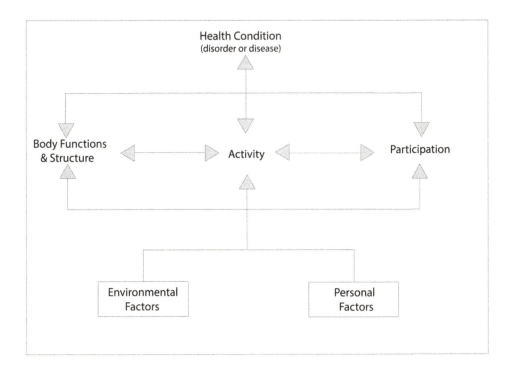

whole, complex notion of disability to one of its aspects.

This more useful model of disability might be called the *biopsychosocial model*. ICF is based on this model, an integration of medical and social. ICF provides, by this synthesis, a coherent view of different perspectives of health: biological, individual and social.

The diagram above is one representation of the model of disability that is the basis for ICF.

Concepts of functioning and disability

As the diagram indicates, in ICF disability and functioning are viewed as outcomes of interactions between *health conditions* (diseases, disorders and injuries) and *contextual factors*.

Among contextual factors are external *environmental factors* (for example,

social attitudes, architectural characteristics, legal and social structures, as well as climate, terrain and so forth); and internal *personal factors*, which include gender, age, coping styles, social background, education, profession, past and current experience, overall behaviour pattern, character and other factors that influence how disability is experienced by the individual.

The diagram identifies the three levels of human functioning classified by ICF: functioning at the level of body or body part, the whole person, and the whole person in a social context. Disability therefore involves dysfunctioning at one or more of these same levels: impairments, activity limitations and participation restrictions. The formal definitions of these components of ICF are provided . . . [on the next page].

Body Functions are physiological functions of body systems (including psychological functions).

Body Structures are anatomical parts of the body such as organs, limbs and their components.

Impairments are problems in body function or structure such as a significant deviation or loss.

Activity is the execution of a task or action by an individual. Participation is involvement in a life situation.

Activity Limitations are difficulties an individual may have in executing activities.

Participation Restrictions are problems an individual may experience in involvement in life situations.

Environmental Factors make up the physical, social and attitudinal environment in which people live and conduct their lives.

Source: Centers for Disease Control and Prevention (CDC). https://www.cdc.gov/nchs/data/icd/icfoverview_finalforwho10sept.pdf.

Glossary

Ableism: Ableism is the systemic oppression of people with disabilities. It centers on the belief that able-bodiedness and able-mindedness are the "norm" or "ideal," thereby casting disability as a diminished state of being. Ableism encompasses prejudice and discrimination against people with disabilities.

Accessibility: Accessibility refers to the extent to which people with disabilities can enter and move within a space, use an object or product, or participate in an event or activity. Accessibility occurs when an environment, building, or event is designed or modified so that it can be used by the greatest number of people. Accessibility allows people with disabilities to fully participate in society.

Accommodation: Accommodations are individualized modifications or adjustments that reduce barriers people with disabilities may face in education or employment.

Activism: Activism involves taking action to create economic, political, and social change. Activism typically occurs within the context of social movements, in which people come together to work toward a desired change. People engage in activism in diverse ways, such as educating others, collecting signatures for petitions, writing letters to newspapers, campaigning for political causes or politicians, boycotting companies, and participating in or organizing protests.

Activities of daily living: Activities of daily living, or ADLs, are self-care tasks that are fundamental to daily functioning, such as eating, bathing, dressing, and toileting.

Advocacy: Advocacy refers to supporting a person or group of people, policy, or cause. While nondisabled people may serve as advocates for disabled people, the disability rights and self-advocacy movements have established the importance of disabled people advocating for themselves.

Assistive technology: Assistive technology comprises devices, equipment, and systems that maintain or improve disabled people's functionality and ability to accomplish tasks or engage in activities. Examples of assistive technology include wheelchairs, ramps, hearing aids, magnifiers, Braille or tactile letters, and computerized speech synthesizers.

Deinstitutionalization: Deinstitutionalization refers to the transition of people with disabilities out of institutions, asylums, psychiatric hospitals, nursing homes, and other spaces of confinement and into community-based settings.

Disability: Disability is a social construction in which people with actual or perceived socially meaningful differences in their bodies or minds experience economic, political, social, legal, and cultural forms of oppression. Disability also serves as a source of personal and minority group identity, individual and social experience, community, and culture.

Disability culture: Disability culture consists of beliefs, values, expressions, and artifacts that emerge from disabled people's shared experiences of marginalization and resilience. Disability culture celebrates disabled people's unique experiences and fosters group solidarity, pride, and community.

Disability studies: Disability studies is an academic discipline that analyzes disability and the lived experiences of disabled people through social, cultural, economic, and political lenses. It is a highly interdisciplinary field that integrates perspectives from the social sciences, arts, and humanities. Disability studies is closely aligned with disability activism and is committed to creating social change and enacting social justice.

Discrimination: Discrimination is differential, biased, and unjust treatment of people on the basis of their perceived or actual membership in a marginalized social group. People may be discriminated against on the basis of disability, race, sex, gender, class, age, sexuality, religion, or other social identities. Discrimination occurs at individual, institutional, and societal levels.

Diversity: Diversity represents the wide range of individual differences between people. Such differences encompass background, life experiences, culture, race, ethnicity, gender, class, disability, age, sexuality, religion, political beliefs, and other aspects of human identity and experience.

Empowerment: Empowerment is an emancipatory process in which disabled people assert their ability to make decisions about and control their lives and claim their civil and human rights.

Ethics: Ethics is the branch of philosophy that explores what is moral (i.e., right) and immoral (i.e., wrong). Individuals use ethics to make decisions regarding their own behavior and the behavior of others. Ethics are often complex and vary based on situation, context, and culture. (As defined in "Ethics.")

Gender: Gender is the socially constructed characteristics, expectations, and norms assigned to masculinity and femininity. Gender encompasses identity, expression, and roles.

Globalization: Globalization is the complex process of interaction, and consequently integration, between people, corporations, governments, and cultures on an international scale. Globalization is driven by economic growth, rapidly developing technologies, and business and corporate interests. Critics of globalization note that it is connected to human exploitation and environmental destruction, as well as erasure of local traditions and cultures.

Health: Health involves achieving and maintaining optimal physical, mental, and social wellness, based on a person's individual capabilities and access to resources.

Identity: Identity is a complex process that encompasses personal identity (i.e., how individuals view and understand themselves) and social identity (i.e., individuals' perceived or actual membership in social groups). Personal and social identities are evolving and contextual, and they influence each other. Due to inequalities, social identities, such as disability, gender, and race, often determine how we are viewed and treated.

Impairment: An impairment is a sensory, psychological, cognitive, or physical difference that may affect a person's functioning.

Inclusion: Inclusion is the state or action of being included and integrated in all aspects of society. Inclusion occurs for disabled people when they have the opportunity to participate in education, employment, social networks, community activities, politics, and other areas of everyday life.

Independent living: Independent living is a movement of people with disabilities aiming at emancipatory participation in the community and ability to control every aspect of their life (as defined in "Independent Living").

Individualized Education Program: An Individualized Education Program (IEP) is a legal document for K–12 students with disabilities that details their present level of performance; their annual educational goals; their least restrictive setting; the accommodations, supports, and services they will receive; and a plan for measuring their progress. Each student receives a unique IEP based on his or her capabilities and needs.

Intersectionality: Intersectionality is a framework for understanding how multiple systems of oppression intersect to affect people's lived experiences. It originated from the work of black feminists, who called attention to the ways racism and sexism interconnect to affect black women's lives.

Least restrictive environment: The least restrictive environment is a setting that is as integrated with people without disabilities as possible, based on a person's capabilities and needs.

Life course: Life course is a framework that understands aging as a lifelong process, from birth until death, that is influenced by individual psychological and developmental factors as well as social, political, and cultural factors.

Medical model: The medical model of disability is a framework for understanding disability that regards disability as an impairment, abnormality, or defect. Under the medical model, a disability is a problem that must be rehabilitated, treated, fixed, or cured if possible.

Normal: Normal refers to a person, place, object, or condition that is considered typical, usual, or natural. Normality is a social construction, meaning that what is considered normal versus abnormal or pathological is socially, historically, and politically determined.

Oppression: Oppression refers to systems of power that maintain unjust treatment and disadvantage based on social group membership, such as race, class, gender, sexuality, and disability. Oppression operates on individual, institutional, and societal/cultural levels.

Participation: Participation is the act of taking part in aspects of everyday life and society.

Performance: Performance is the practice of presenting oneself and acting in certain ways that form and represent an identity, such as gender or disability. Understanding identities such as gender or disability as performed, rather than innate, highlights the ways such identities are constructed through social situations and everyday human interaction.

Poverty: Poverty is the state of being poor and having inadequate financial resources to meet basic needs related to shelter, housing, food, health, and safety. Poverty makes it difficult to maintain one's physical, mental, and social well-being. People with disabilities experience poverty at much higher rates than people without disabilities.

Pride: Pride is the practice of embracing and celebrating marginalized identities and cultures and rejecting the cultural and societal narratives that label those identities and cultures as inferior or negative. Pride can be a personal feeling related to oneself, or it can be community based. Disability pride has been an important aspect of the disability rights movement.

Race and ethnicity: Race is a social construction used to categorize human beings and justify inequality based on actual or perceived differences in physical traits, ancestry, and social practices. Ethnicity is ancestral and cultural identity and heritage, which encompasses language, customs, social norms, history, and other aspects of culture.

Rehabilitation: Rehabilitation is the practice of restoring people to their typical level of functioning after they have experienced a change in functioning due to injury, illness, or impairment. Rehabilitation most often occurs through education, training, and therapy.

Representation: Representation refers to (1) the inclusion of people with disabilities in the political arena, activism, and advocacy and (2) the portrayal or description of people with disabilities in film, stories, literature, media, and other cultural products.

Rights: Rights are legal or moral entitlements. Human rights are rights that people are entitled to simply because they are human, such as the rights to life, liberty, and security. Civil rights are freedoms and protections granted to citizens of a nation-state that allow full participation in civil and social aspects of society, such as the right to vote, the right to free speech, and the right to protection from violence and discrimination. Economic, social, and cultural rights are rights to material goods or social benefits necessary to facilitate a person's well-being, such as the rights to employment, education, health care, and housing.

Self-determination: Self-determination is the level of control individuals have over the direction of their life and the extent to which they are the ones deciding on and making changes to improve their quality of life (as defined in "Self-Determination, Concept and Policy").

Sexuality: Sexuality refers to the ways people express themselves sexually and romantically. It varies from person to person and encompasses sexual and romantic preferences, desires, and activities.

Social justice: Social justice is a concept in which all people in society are treated equitably and fairly and provided with equal access to opportunities and resources.

Social model: The social model of disability is a framework for understanding disability that regards disability as socially constructed, meaning that disability is created through the interaction between an individual's body/mind and society. Under the social model, disabled people are limited, not by their impairments, but rather by attitudinal, environmental, and structural barriers. These barriers must be eliminated for disabled people to have equal rights and fully participate in society.

Social movements: A social movement represents a group of people who come together with the goals of empowering oppressed people, challenging oppressive attitudes and practices, and creating social change.

Stigma: Stigma is a social construct that involves the recognition of an individual's difference based on some distinguishing characteristic and that results in the devaluation of that individual (as defined in "Stigma").

Supports: Supports are devices, programs, and services that assist people with disabilities in completing self-care tasks and participating in society. Supports include personal care attendants, assistive technology, transportation services, and employment programs.

Transition: Transition refers to the process of students with disabilities progressing from K–12 education to postschool life, which may include postsecondary education or employment and community living. There are numerous services, supports, and programs that assist students with disabilities during the transition process.

Welfare: Welfare refers to government benefits and services provided to people in need. There are a variety of federal and state welfare programs, which may consist of cash and food assistance, medical care, subsidies for housing and utilities, education, child care, and other services. Welfare may be granted on the basis of old age, disability, income level, and other factors.

Work: Work, or employment, is the process of engaging in activities or completing tasks to earn income.

Annotated Resource List

U.S. Government Organizations

Administration for Children and Families

Address:
U.S. Department of Health & Human Services
330 C Street SW
Washington, DC 20201

Web site:
https://www.acf.hhs.gov/

The Administration for Children and Families manages a group of federal programs serving families, children, and community members. Overall, these programs provide financial and organizational support to promote economic and social well-being. Some programs specifically address the adoption of children with disabilities.

Administration for Community Living

Address:
330 C Street SW
Washington, DC 20201

Web site:
https://www.acl.gov/

The Administration for Community Living (ACL) funds and supports research initiatives, as well as community-based organizations, to assist people with disabilities in choosing where to live, whom to live with, and how to engage with the community. In addition to these specific program operations, the ACL oversees units such as the Administration on Aging (AoA), the Administration on Disabilities (AoD), and the National Institute on Disability, Independent Living, and Rehabilitation Research (NIDILRR). An organizational chart demonstrating how the Administration for Community Living relates to these units can be found at the following Web address: https://www.acl.gov/sites/default/files/about-acl/2016-10/OrgChart-large.png.

Administration on Aging

Address:
Administration for Community Living
330 C Street SW
Washington, DC 20201

Web site:
https://www.acl.gov/node/915

The Administration on Aging (AoA) is a unit within the Administration for Community Living and is responsible for upholding the amended Older Americans Act of 1965. AoA protects the welfare and dignity of older individuals and also supports multiple programs specifically related to the well-being of older adults with disabilities.

Administration on Disabilities

Address:
Administration for Community Living
330 C Street SW
Washington, DC 20201

Web site:
https://www.acl.gov/node/916

The Administration on Disabilities (AoD) is an additional unit within the Administration for Community Living. This administration works with states and local partners to support the independence, productivity, and integration of people with disabilities into their communities. The AoD also oversees the Administration on Intellectual and Developmental Disabilities (AIDD).

Administration on Intellectual and Developmental Disabilities

Address:
Administration for Community Living
330 C Street SW
Washington, DC 20201

Web site:
https://www.acl.gov/node/916

The Administration on Intellectual and Developmental Disabilities (AIDD) provides grants that stipulate the formation of developmental disabilities networks in each state. These networks consist of state councils on developmental disabilities, university centers for excellence in developmental disabilities, and state protection and advocacy systems. The goals of these networks vary.

Aging and Disability Resource Centers

Address:
National Association of Area Agencies on Aging
1730 Rhode Island Avenue NW, Suite 1200
Washington, DC 20036

Web site:
https://www.acl.gov/programs/
aging-and-disability-networks/
aging-and-disability-resource-centers

Aging and Disability Resource Centers (ADRC) are part of the Administration for Community Living's (ACL) Aging and Disability Network program. Associated ADRCs support older adults with disabilities as they navigate and acquire long-term services and supports. ADRCS contribute to the "No Wrong Door" system model and provide counseling and information to all people. Contact information for local ADRCs can be identified via ACL's "Eldercare Locator."

Centers for Disease Control and Prevention: Disability and Health Branch

Address:
1600 Clifton Rd., MS-E88
Atlanta, GA 30333
Phone: 800-CDC-INFO (232-4636)

Web site:
https://www.cdc.gov/ncbddd/
disabilityandhealth/index.html

The Disability and Health branch of the Centers for Disease Control and Prevention monitors the health of people with disabilities, promotes public health and inclusion of people with disabilities, supports the development of policy that integrates disability into broader health programming, and endows research/intervention strategies to mitigate secondary conditions that can accompany disability.

Department of Education: Office of Special Education and Rehabilitative Services

Address:
Office of Special Education and
Rehabilitative Services
U.S. Department of Education
400 Maryland Avenue SW
Washington, DC 20202-7100
Phone: 202-245-7468

Web site:
https://www2.ed.gov/about/offices/list/osers/index.html

Under the general Department of Education, the Office of Special Education and Rehabilitative Services (OSERS) oversees the Office of Special Education Programs and the Rehabilitation Services Administration. The OSERS mission is to help educate youth with disabilities and provide rehabilitation for youth and adults with disabilities by supporting states, school districts, and families.

Department of Health and Human Services

Address:
200 Independence Avenue SW
Washington, DC 20201
Phone: 877-696-6775

Web site:
https://www.hhs.gov/

The Department of Health and Human Services (HHS) works to promote the health of all Americans. In doing so, HHS oversees a number of operating divisions including, but not limited to, the Administration for Children and Families (ACF), the Administration for Community Living (ACL), and the Centers for Disease Control and Prevention (CDC). Each of these administrations has a disability-specific component.

Department of Labor: Office of Disability Employment Policy

Address:
200 Constitution Avenue NW
Washington, DC 20210
Phone: 866-4-USA-DOL

Web site:
https://www.dol.gov/odep/

The Office of Disability Employment Policy (ODEP) promotes the quantity and quality of work opportunities for people with disabilities by shaping policy and delivering credible, evidence-based information on the subject. The ODEP Web page also hosts resources that were previously available on the disability.gov Web site.

National Council on Disability

Address:
1331 F Street NW, Suite 850
Washington, DC 20004
Phone: 202-272-2004

Web site:
https://www.ncd.gov/

The National Council on Disability (NCD) functions as an independent, federal advisory agency that provides input to the president, Congress, and other federal organizations on programs and policies that affect people with disabilities.

National Institute of Child Health and Human Development

Address:
P.O. Box 3006
Rockville, MD 20847
Phone: 800-370-2943

Web site:
https://www.nichd.nih.gov/

The Eunice Kennedy Shriver National Institute of Child Health and Human Development (NICHHD) conducts research relating to the health of children and families but places a particular emphasis on understanding disabilities that are diagnosed during pregnancy. NICHHD aims to reduce infant and mother mortality and benefit the well-being of people with disabilities throughout their life course.

National Institute of Child Health and Human Development: Intellectual and Developmental Disabilities Branch

Address:
P.O. Box 3006
Rockville, MD 20847
Phone: 800-370-2943

Web site:
https://www.nichd.nih.gov/about/org/der/branches/iddb

The Intellectual and Developmental Disabilities Branch (IDDB) is 1 of 16 factions with the division of extramural research of the NICHHD. The IDDB supports research and training related to the prevention of, and reduction of challenges related to, intellectual and developmental disabilities.

National Institute on Aging

Address:
National Institute on Aging
Building 31, Room 5C27
31 Center Drive, MSC 2292
Bethesda, MD 20892
Phone: 800-222-2225

Web site:
https://www.nia.nih.gov

The National Institute on Aging (NIA) produces research on the aging process, conditions related to aging, and the needs of older Americans. The NIA promotes discourse around aging and disseminates evidence-based information on the topic to the general public.

National Institute on Deafness and Other Communication Disorders

Address:
31 Center Drive, MSC 2320
Bethesda, MD 20892-2320
Phone: 800-241-1044

Web site:
https://www.nidcd.nih.gov/

The National Institute on Deafness and Other Communication Disorders (NIDCD) supports research on sensory process, including hearing, tasting, speaking, and smelling, as well as related topics of balance, voice, and language. This knowledge is used to help detect and address communication disabilities.

National Institute on Health Clinical Center: Rehabilitation Medicine

Address:
10 Center Drive
Bethesda, MD 20892
Phone: 301-496-4114

Web site:
https://clinicalcenter.nih.gov/welcome.html

The National Institute on Health Clinical Center hosts a Physical and Rehabilitation Medicine branch. This branch offers high-quality patient care for persons affected by neuromuscular impairments, functional limitations, pain, and other disabilities. This branch of the NIH center also supports other health care professionals by assisting with clinical research studies.

National Institute on Mental Health

Address:
6001 Executive Boulevard, Room 6200,
MSC 9663
Bethesda, MD 20892-9663
Phone: 866-615-6464

Web site https://www.nimh.nih.gov/index.shtml
The National Institute on Mental Health (NIMH) is the national leader in conducting and supporting research related to mental health and illness. Research topics including prevention, diagnosis, and treatment of mental illness are emphasized.

National Institutes of Health

Address:
9000 Rockville Pike
Bethesda, Maryland 20892
Phone: 301-496-4000

Web site:
https://www.nih.gov/

The National Institutes of Health (NIH) is the primary federal agency responsible for conducting national medical research. This agency falls under the U.S. Department of Health and Human Services and oversees 27 various institutes on specific medical subjects. Some of these institutes have disability-specific focuses, such as the National Institute on Aging, the National Institute on Deafness and Other Communications Disorders, the National Institute on Child Health and Human Development, and the National Institute on Mental Health.

State Units on Aging

Address:
Administration for Community Living
330 C Street SW
Washington, DC, 20201

Web site:
https://www.acl.gov/programs/
aging-and-disability-networks/
state-units-aging

State Units on Aging (SUAs) are Administration for Community Living (ACL)–sponsored agencies that support advocacy at the state level. SUAs support aging individuals and, in some states, aging individuals with physical disabilities. There are 56 SUAs, with one in every state as well as D.C., Guam, Puerto Rico, American Samoa, the Mariana Islands, and the Virgin Islands. Each SUA develops and administers multi-year plans for its respective territory.

Substance Abuse and Mental Health Services Administration

Address:
5600 Fishers Lane
Rockville, MD 20857
Phone: 877-726-4727

Web site:
https://www.samhsa.gov/

The Substance Abuse and Mental Health Services Administration (SAMHSA) is a federal agency that supports efforts to address and improve the impact substance abuse and mental illness have in the United States. SAMHSA oversees the Center for Mental Health Services, the Center for Substance Abuse Prevention, and the Center for Substance Abuse Treatment.

Nongovernmental Organizations and University Programs

Access Living

Address:
115 West Chicago Avenue
Chicago, IL 60654
Phone: 312-640-2100

Web site:
https://www.accessliving.org/

Access Living is a Chicago-based organization that is run largely by people with disabilities, for people with disabilities. Access Living offers peer-oriented and independent living services, as well as public education. In addition, Access Living promotes individual and systemic advocacy regarding civil rights. These supports all contribute to its mission of enhancing the options available to people with disabilities so they can live a satisfying life. Access Living's Web site offers a wealth of links to relevant articles, brochures, a referral directory, and legal documents.

ADA National Network

Address:
N/A
Phone: 800-949-4232

Web site:
https://adata.org/

The ADA National Network provides information, guidance, and training on the Americans with Disabilities Act (ADA). Ten regional ADA centers disseminate this information and training. Each regional network has its own address and specific contact information. This network is funded through a grant provided by the Department of Health and Humans Services, National Institute on Disability, Independent Living, and Rehabilitation Research.

ADAPT

Addresses:
1208 South Logan Street
Denver, CO 80210
1640-A E. Second Street, Suite 100
Austin, TX 78702
Phone: 512-442-0252

Web site:
http://adapt.org/

ADAPT, formerly known as the American Disabled for Attendant Programs Today, is a national grassroots organization that supports the engagement of disability rights activists in nonviolent action to fight for the human rights of people with disabilities. In particular, ADAPT supports the transition of people with disabilities from institutions and nursing homes into community living.

Alzheimer's Association

Address:
Alzheimer's Association National Office
225 N. Michigan Avenue, Floor 17
Chicago, IL 60601
Phone: 800-272-3900

Web site:
https://www.alz.org/

The Alzheimer's Association has the mission of promoting advancement of research relating to Alzheimer's disease, supporting the provision of quality care for people and families affected, and educating the public about brain health.

American Association of Health and Disability

Address:
110 N. Washington Street, Suite 328-J
Rockville, MD 20850
Phone: (301) 545-6140

Web site:
https://www.aahd.us/

The American Association of Health and Disability (AAHD) is a national nonprofit organization that is dedicated to reducing the existing health disparities between people with and without disabilities. AAHD maintains an online resource center, partners with federal and local organizations relating to disability, shares evidence-based research through its various platforms, and advocates for intervention programs that improve the lives of people with disabilities.

American Association of People with Disabilities

Address:
2013 H Street NW, 5th Floor
Washington, DC 20006
Phone: 202-521-4316

Web site:
https://www.aapd.com/

The American Association of People with Disabilities (AAPD) is built upon the membership of people with a variety of disabilities. AAPD aims to use a unified voice to take a stance on political, economic, and social issues that affect people with disabilities. Some of its advocacy initiatives include voting access, technology development, and adherence to the Americans with Disabilities Act.

American Association of Retired Persons (AARP)

Address:
601 E Street NW
Washington, DC 20049
Phone: 888-687-2277

Web site:
https://www.aarp.org/

The AARP is a nonprofit group that supports older Americans by providing resources. AARP also developed the associated charity, the AARP Foundation, which supports low-income older Americans and provides training and resources around pertinent topics, such as employment and retirement.

American Association on Intellectual and Developmental Disabilities

Address:
501 Third Street NW, Suite 200
Washington, DC 20001
Phone: 202-387-1968

Web site:
https://aaidd.org/

The American Association on Intellectual and Developmental Disabilities (AAIDD) promotes the universal human rights of people with intellectual and developmental disabilities. Specifically, AAIDD focuses on supporting progressive policy, sharing effective practices, and disseminating evidence-based research. In addition to highlighting people with disabilities, AAIDD works with professionals to increase its capacity to provide quality care for the community of people with intellectual or developmental disabilities.

APSE: The Association of People Supporting Employment First

Address:
414 Hungerford Drive, Suite 224
Rockville, MD 20850
Phone: 301-279-0060

Web site:
http://apse.org/

The Association of People Supporting Employment First (APSE) is a national nonprofit organization that exclusively focuses on integrated employment and meaningful career advancement for people with disabilities. APSE has chapters in 38 states and Washington, D.C., and hosts an annual conference on employment and disability.

The Arc of the United States

Address:
1825 K Street NW, Suite 1200
Washington, DC 20006
Phone: 800-433-5255

Web site:
http://www.thearc.org/

The Arc of the United States (The Arc) is the largest community-based organization that supports people with intellectual or developmental disabilities and their families in the United States. There are more than 700 local Arc chapters, and all of them prioritize a "people first" perspective. The Arc has a mission of enabling all individuals and families to fully participate in their larger communities and the U.S. democracy.

Association of Assistive Technology Act Programs (ATAP)

Address:
1020 S. Spring
Springfield, IL 62704
Phone: 217-522-7985, 217-522-9966 (TTY)

Web site:
https://www.ataporg.org/

The Association of Assistive Technology Act Programs (ATAP) is a nonprofit organization that encompasses 54 state assistive technology (AT) programs. ATAP works to coordinate these state programs and provides them with technical assistance so that they can best serve their community members. In addition, ATAP streamlines the communication and joint action among these programs and provides a forum to address national concerns relating to assistive technology.

Association of University Centers on Disabilities

Address:
1100 Wayne Avenue, Suite 1000
Silver Spring, MD 20910
Phone: 301-588-8252

Web site:
https://www.aucd.org/template/index.cfm

The Association of University Centers on Disabilities (AUCD) is a national network that includes 67 University Center for Excellence in Developmental Disabilities (UCEDD), 52 Leadership Education in Neurodevelopmental Disabilities programs (LEND), and 14 Developmental Disability Research Centers (IDDRC). These programs use university resources and research to support the needs of the surrounding community.

Association on Higher Education and Disability

Address:
8015 West Kenton Circle, Suite 230
Huntersville, NC 28078
Phone: 704-947-7779

Web site:
https://www.ahead.org/

The Association on Higher Education and Disability (AHEAD) is a professional membership organization that advocates for quality service and supportive policy in relation to people with disabilities and their participation in higher education.

Autism Society of America

Address:
4340 East-West Highway, Suite 350
Bethesda, MD 20814
Phone: 800-328-8476

Web site:
http://www.autism-society.org/

The Autism Society of America is a grassroots organization devoted to raising public awareness about the challenges people on the autism spectrum may face in their daily lives. The Autism Society advocates for the expansion of appropriate and quality services so that all people on the autism spectrum can receive support.

Autism Speaks

Address:
1 East 33rd Street, 4th Floor
New York, NY 10016
Phone: 212-252-8584

Web site:
https://www.autismspeaks.org/

Autism Speaks is a nonprofit organization that sponsors scientific research and organizes awareness and outreach initiatives relating to autism. This organization has faced criticism in the past for framing autism as a disease, presenting autism in a negative light, and prioritizing research related to vaccinations and increased risk of autism. In response to these critiques, Autism Speaks has reshaped its mission so it does not mention finding a "cure" for autism and clarified that vaccines do not cause autism. Autism Speaks allocates the majority of its funds to scientific research investigating the cause of autism.

Autistic Self Advocacy Network (ASAN)

Address:
P.O. Box 66122
Washington, DC 20035

Web site:
http://autisticadvocacy.org/

The Autistic Self Advocacy Network (ASAN) is a national nonprofit organization, run by autistic people, with the goal of furthering the disability rights movement and empowering autistic people to take control of the direction of their own lives. ASAN participates in public policy advocacy, provides leadership training for self-advocates, and works to improve public perceptions of autism.

Brain Injury Association of America

Address:
1608 Spring Hill Road, Suite 110
Vienna, VA 22182
Phone: 703-761-0750

Web site:
https://www.biausa.org/

The Brain Injury Association of America (BIAA) aims to advance research and treatment for all people affected by brain injury. They promote a vision in which everyone in the United States who has a brain injury is appropriately diagnosed, supported to receive treatment, and accepted into their communities.

Burton Blatt Institute

Address:
900 S. Crouse Avenue
Crouse-Hinds Hall, Suite 300
Syracuse, NY 13244
Phone: 315-443-2863

Web site:
http://bbi.syr.edu/

The Burton Blatt Institute (BBI) at Syracuse University seeks to advance the rights of people with disabilities and their social participation at a local, national, and international level. BBI provides an environment in which collaboration between private and public sectors can take place and benefit their mission of human rights advancement.

Center for Disability Studies, University of Hawaii at Manoa

Address:
1410 Lower Campus Road, 171F
Honolulu, HI 96826

Web site:
http://www.cds.hawaii.edu/

The Center for Disability Studies (CDS) is a research unit within the University of Hawaii network. The CDS provides training for community members and professionals, conducts research and evaluation projects, and shares findings and evidence-based information.

Center for Independent Living Inc.

Address:
3075 Adeline Street, Suite 100
Berkeley, CA 94703
Phone: 510-841-4776

Web site:
http://www.thecil.org/

The Center for Independent Living Inc. (CIL) provides programs that assist people to build skills, knowledge, and resources related to the empowerment of people with disabilities. The CIL developed from the independent living movement in Berkeley, California, in the 1960s and has influenced the national development of peer-based services. The CIL has an associated online blog, *The Independent*.

Center on Human Policy, Law, and Disability Studies, Syracuse University

Address:
230 Huntington Hall
Syracuse, NY 13244
Phone: 315-443-4752

Web site:
http://soeweb.syr.edu/centers_institutes/
center_human_policy/default.aspx

The Center on Human Policy, Law, and Disability Studies (CHPLDS) at Syracuse University is a network of academic programs, research centers, and organizations that aim to promote the rights of people with disabilities. Associated research centers include the Center on Huma Policy (CHP), Syracuse University Parent Advocacy Center (SUPAC), and Mid-State Early Childhood Direction Center (ECDC). The center provides print and electronic resources related to the inclusion of persons with disabilities.

Consortium for Citizens with Disabilities

Address:
820 First Street NE, Suite 740
Washington, DC 20002
Phone: 202-567-3516

Web site:
http://www.c-c-d.org/

The Consortium for Citizens with Disabilities (CCD) is a coalition of national organizations that all advocate for national policy that promotes and protects the rights of people with disabilities to have self-determination, independence, and integration within society. The CCD publishes policy recommendations, educates members of Congress, and encourages advocacy among the disability community.

Council on Quality and Leadership

Address:
100 West Road, Suite 300
Towson, MD 21204
Phone: 410-583-0060

Web site:
https://www.c-q-l.org/

The Council on Quality and Leadership (CQL) provides training as well as accreditation and certification for professionals and advocates who work with people with disabilities. CQL has the mission of improving the quality of life for people with disabilities by affecting the quality of the services they use.

Disabilities, Opportunities, Internetworking, and Technology, University of Washington

Address:
DO-IT, University of Washington
Box 354842
Seattle, WA 98195
Phone: 206-685-3648

Web site:
https://www.washington.edu/doit/

Disabilities, Opportunities, Internetworking, and Technology (DO-IT) at the University of Washington offers programs and resources related to information technology to support people with disabilities in pursuing challenging academic programs. DO-IT advocates for universal design and provides free resources for students with disabilities, educators, employers, families, and supporters. In addition to providing print and electronic resources, DO-IT facilitates workshops.

Disability Rights Education and Defense Fund

Address:
3075 Adeline Street, Suite 210
Berkeley, CA 94703
Phone: 510-644-2555

Web site:
https://dredf.org/

The Disability Rights Education and Defense Fund (DREDF) is a national center, led by people with disabilities and parents of children who have disabilities, that promotes the advancement of civil rights laws and policies. In doing so, DREDF participates in legal advocacy, training initiatives, and policy and legislative action.

Easter Seals Inc.

Address:
141 W. Jackson Boulevard, Suite 1400A
Chicago, IL 60604
Phone: 800-221-6827

Web site:
http://www.easterseals.com/

Easter Seals Inc. is an international nonprofit organization that provides such services as rehabilitation, employment training, and recreational activities for youth and adults with disabilities.

Eunice Kennedy Shriver Center, University of Massachusetts Medical School

Address:
465 Medford Street, Suite 500
Charlestown, MA 02129
Phone: 774-455-6562

Web site:
https://shriver.umassmed.edu/

The Eunice Kennedy Shriver Center at the University of Massachusetts Medical School aims to improve the quality of life of people with intellectual and developmental disabilities and their families. It performs research related to the environmental and biological processes surrounding intellectual and developmental disability. This center publishes a biannual newsletter with information about research updates, community initiatives, and resources.

Family Caregiver Alliance

Address:
235 Montgomery Street, Suite 950
San Francisco, CA 94104
Phone: 800-445-8106

Web site:
https://www.caregiver.org/

The Family Caregiver Alliance (FCA) is a community-based, nonprofit organization that is dedicated to supporting family members and friends who provide long-term care for people with disabilities or chronic health conditions.

Gallaudet University

Address:
800 Florida Avenue NE
Washington, DC 20002
Phone: 202-651-5000 (voice)

Web site:
http://www.gallaudet.edu/

Gallaudet University is a comprehensive liberal arts university that leads the world in learning, teaching, and research for students who are deaf or hard of hearing. Gallaudet offers both undergraduate and graduate programs.

Human Services Research Institute

Address:
2336 Massachusetts Avenue
Cambridge, MA 02140
Phone: 617-876-0426

Web site:
https://www.hsri.org/

The Human Services Research Institute (HSRI) develops community-based and person-centered services for people with disabilities of all ages. HSRI partners with government agencies to improve the efficiency of general service provision.

Independent Living Institute

Address:
Independent Living Institute, Storforsplan 36, 10 tr,123 47 Farsta, Sweden
Phone: 08-506-22-179

Web site:
https://www.independentliving.org/
indexen.html

The Independent Living Institute (ILI) promotes the self-determination of people with disabilities by developing consumer-driven policies. The ILI is a nonprofit organization that is largely run by people with disabilities.

Independent Living Research Utilization Program

Address:
ILRU
1333 Moursund
Houston, TX 77030
Phone: 713-520-0232

Web site:
http://www.ilru.org/

The Independent Living Research Utilization Program (ILRU) is a national center devoted to research, information provision, training, and technical assistance related to independent living for people with disabilities. The ILRU shares its compiled information with independent living centers, national rehabilitation programs, and educational institutions. A list of its projects, publications, and other resources is available on its Web site.

Institute for Community Inclusion

Address:
Institute for Community Inclusion UMass Boston
100 Morrissey Boulevard
Boston, MA 02125
Phone: 617-287-4300

Web site:
https://www.communityinclusion.org/

The Institute for Community Inclusion (ICI) is a national leader regarding the promotion of community inclusion for people with disabilities. ICI is based at the University of Massachusetts, Boston and provides training for professionals and organizations to improve the community's capacity for inclusion.

Institute on Community Integration, University of Minnesota

Address:
102 Patee Hall
150 Pillsbury Drive SE
Minneapolis, MN 55455
Phone: 612-624-6300

Web site:
https://ici.umn.edu/

The Institute on Community Integration (ICI) at University of Minnesota is part of the University Centers for Excellence in Developmental Disabilities national network. This institute oversees 70 different projects and 6 affiliated centers, all of which contribute to its mission of improving community supports and inclusion of people with developmental disabilities. The ICI provides an extensive list of print and video resources on its Web site.

Institute on Disability and Human Development

Address:
The University of Illinois at Chicago
1640 West Roosevelt Road
Chicago, Il, 60608-6904
Phone: 312-413-8833

Web site:
https://ahs.uic.edu/disability-human-development/institute-on-disability-and-human-development/

The Institute on Disability and Human Development (IDHD) is a University Center for Excellence in Developmental Disabilities based at the University of Illinois at Chicago. The IDHD leads the nation in research, clinical and community engagement activities, and disability studies training.

International Disability Alliance

Address:
205 East 42nd Street
New York, NY 10017
Phone: 646 776 0822

Web site:
http://www.internationaldisabilityalliance.org/

The International Disability Alliance (IDA) is a coalition comprising more than 1,100 organizations from eight global and six regional networks of people with disabilities. IDA directs advocacy toward the United Nations with the mission of making the world more inclusive for people with disabilities.

Job Accommodation Network

Address:
N/A
Phone: 800-526-7234; 887-781-9403 (TTY)

Web site:
https://askjan.org/

The Job Accommodation Network (JAN) is a service provided by the Office of Disability Employment Policy of the U.S. Department of Labor. JAN provides free expertise and guidance relating to workplace accommodations that are outlined in the Americans with Disabilities Act. In addition to on-demand resource provision via phone or e-mail, JAN also provides in-person training.

The Judge David L. Bazelon Center for Mental Health Law

Address:
1101 15th Street NW, Suite 1212
Washington, DC 20005
Phone: 202-467-5730

Web site:
http://www.bazelon.org/

The Judge David L. Bazelon Center for Mental Health Law (Bazelon Center) advocates for the civil rights of people with mental health concerns and psychosocial disabilities using litigation. This center influenced the passing of the Americans with Disabilities Act (ADA) and continues to set national legal precedents relating to the rights of people with disabilities.

Kennedy Center Inc.

Address:
2440 Reservoir Avenue
Trumbull, CT 06611
Phone: 203-365-8522

Web site:
http://www.thekennedycenterinc.org/

The Kennedy Center Inc. is a comprehensive rehabilitation facility that offers services and supports to people with disabilities. The Kennedy Center offers independent living skills training, supported living services, specialized job training, and transportation services.

Kessler Foundation

Address:
120 Eagle Rock Avenue
East Hanover, NJ 07936
Phone: 973-324-8362

Web site:
https://kesslerfoundation.org/

The Kessler Foundation is a public, charitable organization that endows rehabilitation research relating to both intellectual and physical disabilities. The Kessler Foundation's stated mission is to improve the quality of life for people with disabilities.

Leadership Education in Neurodevelopmental and Related Disabilities (LEND)

Address:
1100 Wayne Avenue, Suite 1000
Silver Spring, MD 20910
Phone: 301-588-8252

Web site:
https://www.aucd.org/template/page.cfm?id=473

Leadership Education in Neurodevelopmental and Related Disabilities (LEND) programs provide training, in addition to services, aimed at improving the health of infants and youth with disabilities. A significant portion of this training is provided for health care professionals. LEND programs operate in partnerships with University Centers for Excellence on Developmental Disabilities (UCEDD); there are currently 52 LEND programs across 44 U.S. states.

Little People of America

Address:
617 Broadway, Suite 518
Sonoma, CA 95476

Web site:
https://lpa.memberclicks.net/

Little People of America (LPA) is a national nonprofit organization that supports people of short stature by offering educational information on topics such as employment, education, disability rights, and clothing (among others). LPA has more than 6,000 members across 70 chapters in the United States. These chapters are distributed across 13 districts, each of which has its own contact information.

NADD: An Association for Persons with Developmental Disabilities and Mental Health Needs

Address:
The NADD
132 Fair Street
Kingston, NY 12401
Phone: 845-331-4336

Web site:
http://thenadd.org/

NADD: An Association for Persons with Developmental Disabilities and Mental Health Needs is a nonprofit organization for professionals, care providers, and families. NADD relies on health promotion and educational training to promote understanding of the mental health needs of people with developmental disabilities. NADD's Web site offers resources, as well as news updates on upcoming conferences and trainings.

National Alliance for Caregiving

Address:
4720 Montgomery Lane, Suite 205
Bethesda, MD 20814
Phone: 301-718-8444

Web site:
http://www.caregiving.org/

The National Alliance for Caregiving (NAC) is a nonprofit, network of organizations across the United States that focus on the subject of family caregiving. The NAC recognizes that caregivers play an important social and financial role in assisting their loved ones; in order to improve the quality of life for these caregivers, the NAC supports research and advocacy in this area.

National Alliance on Mental Illness (NAMI)

Address:
3803 N. Fairfax Drive, Suite 100
Arlington, VA 22203
Phone: 703-524-7600

Web site:
https://www.nami.org/

The National Alliance on Mental Illness (NAMI) is a national organization with a mission to improve the lives of Americans affected by mental illness. NAMI oversees numerous affiliated organizations that provide education on mental health. In addition, NAMI advocates for public policy reform, maintains a free helpline for people seeking support, and leads national awareness events like Mental Illness Awareness Weeks.

National Association of Councils on Developmental Disabilities

Address:
1825 K Street NW, Suite 600
Washington, DC 20006
Phone: 202-506-5813

Web site:
https://nacdd.org/

The National Association of Councils on Developmental Disabilities (NACDD) consists of 56 Councils on Developmental Disabilities across the United States. Each of these councils receives federal funding to support programs and initiatives for people with developmental disabilities in their respective state.

National Association of Rehabilitation Research and Training Centers

Web site:
http://narrtc.org/

The National Association of Rehabilitation Research and Training Centers (NARRTC) promotes the inclusion of persons with disabilities by endowing applied research and training programs. NARRTC believes such research and training can benefit the integration, participation, and self-determination of people with disabilities in the larger community.

National Association of the Deaf

Address:
8630 Fenton Street, Suite 820
Silver Spring, MD 20910
Phone: 301-587-1789 (TTY); 301-587-1788

Web site:
https://www.nad.org/

The National Association of the Deaf (NAD) is a civil rights association established by hard of hearing individuals in the United States. The NAD promotes the rights of Deaf and hard of hearing people by advocating for the use of American Sign Language and engaging with legislative processes at the federal level.

National Center for Learning Disabilities

Address:
32 Laight Street, Second Floor
New York, NY 10013
Phone: 888-575-7373

Web site:
https://www.ncld.org/

The National Center for Learning Disabilities (NCLD) aims to improve the opportunities for people with learning disabilities. The NCLD offers specific programs for parents (Understood), for young adults (Friends of Quinn), for professionals (Navigator), and for educators (Get Ready to Read; RTI Action Network).

National Center on Health, Physical Activity, and Disability (NCPAD)

Address:
4000 Ridgeway Drive
Birmingham, AL 35209
Phone: 800-900-8086

Web site:
https://www.nchpad.org/

The National Center on Health, Physical Activity, and Disability (NCHPAD) is a public health practice and resource center for people with disabilities. NCHPAD conducts training initiatives to educate service providers about health inclusion. A variety of resources can be found on NCHPAD's Web site.

National Center on Secondary Education and Transition

Address:
Institute on Community Integration
University of Minnesota
6 Pattee Hall
150 Pillsbury Drive SE
Minneapolis, MN 55455
Phone: 612-624-5659

Web site:
http://www.ncset.org/

The National Center on Secondary Education and Transition (NCSET) was funded by the U.S. Department of Education, Office of Special Education until 2008 and has since continued to disseminate on its Web site resources related to the transition of youth with disabilities from secondary education.

National Council on Aging

Address:
251 18th Street South, Suite 500
Arlington, VA 22202
Phone: 571-527-3900

Web site:
https://www.ncoa.org/

The National Council on Aging (NCOA) is a nonprofit organization that advocates for service provision to older Americans. NCOA partners with other organizations, the government, and business to develop innovative and influential community programs.

National Council on Independent Living

Address:
2013 H Street NW, 6th Floor
Washington, DC 20006
Phone: 202-207-0334

Web site:
https://www.ncil.org/

The National Council on Independent Living (NCIL) has the mission of advancing the rights, and specifically the right to independent living, of people with disabilities. The NCIL is a grassroots organization run by people with disabilities that promotes national advocacy around this independent living movement.

National Disability Rights Network

Address:
820 1st Street NE, Suite 740
Washington, DC 20002
Phone: 202-408-9514

Web site:
http://www.ndrn.org/index.php

The National Disability Rights Network (NDRN) is a nonprofit membership organization that promotes the integrity of the Protection and Advocacy as well as the Client Assistance Programs federal mandates. The NDRN provides legal support, training, and legislative advocacy to benefit progress toward the full recognition of the human rights of people with disabilities.

National Federation of the Blind

Address:
200 East Wells Street, Jernigan Place
Baltimore, MD, 21230
Phone: 410-659-9314

Web site:
https://nfb.org/

The National Federation of the Blind is a national organization with affiliations across every state. The National Federation of the Blind provides members with resources and works to educate the general public about vision loss.

National Organization on Disability

Address:
77 Water Street, Suite 204
New York, NY 10005
Phone: 646-505-1191

Web site:
https://www.nod.org/

The National Organization on Disability (NOD) is a nonprofit organization that promotes the full participation of people with disabilities in society. NOD specifically works to increase participation of people with disabilities in the workforce. In order to do so, NOD develops and evaluates pilot programs and shares these findings with policy makers, researchers, and service providers.

National Rehabilitation Information Center (NARIC)

Address:
N/A
Phone: 800-346-2742; 301-459-5984 (TTY)

Web site:
http://www.naric.com/?q=en

The National Rehabilitation Information Center (NARIC) has the mission of collecting and disseminating research related to disability and rehabilitation. The National Institute on Disability, Independent Living, and Rehabilitation Research (NIDILRR) has provided funding and expertise to support NARIC. NARIC has built an online repository of these resources and also offers opportunities to subscribe to e-mail lists.

National Trends in Disability Employment (nTIDE)

Address:
Research on Disability
10 West Edge Drive, Suite 101
Durham, NH 03824

Web site:
https://researchondisability.org/home/ntide

The National Trends in Disability Employment (nTIDE) is an information dissemination initiative funded by the Rehabilitation Research and Training Center on Employment Policy and Measurement (EPM-RRTC) and undertaken in partnership with the Institute on Disability at the University of New Hampshire and the Kessler Foundation. nTIDE provides monthly reports and monthly Webcasts.

Not Dead Yet: The Resistance

Address:
497 State Street
Rochester, NY 14608
Phone: 708-420-0539

Web site:
http://notdeadyet.org/

Not Dead Yet is a national grassroots organization devoted to opposing the legalization of assisted suicide and euthanasia. Not Dead Yet organizes opposition and crafts social justice arguments on the premise that these practices are extreme forms of discrimination.

Paralyzed Veterans of America

Address:
801 18th Street NW
Washington, DC 20006-3517
Phone: 800-424-8200

Web site:
http://www.pva.org/

Paralyzed Veterans of America (PVA) is a service organization that was founded by veterans of World War II in 1946. The PVA supports research and education related to spinal cord injury and dysfunction, and advocates for quality health care for veteran members. In addition, the PVA assists members in filing for benefits and services from the Department of Veterans Affairs and engages in legislative debates related to the civil rights of paralyzed veterans.

Parent to Parent USA (P2P)

Address:
1825 K Street NW, Suite 250
Washington, DC 20006
Phone: 717-503-8992

Web site:
http://www.p2pusa.org/

Parent to Parent USA (P2P) is a national nonprofit organization that oversees P2P programs across the United States. The mission of P2P is to ensure that all families with children with developmental disabilities receive emotional and informational support. Thirty-seven states have P2P programs, and new statewide P2P programs are currently being developed.

RESNA Rehabilitation Engineering and Assistive Technology Society of North America

Address:
1560 Wilson Boulevard, Suite 850
Arlington, VA 22209
Phone: 703-524-6686

Website:
http://www.resna.org/

RESNA, the Rehabilitation Engineering and Assistive Technology Society of North America, is the premier professional organization dedicated to promoting the health and well-being of people with disabilities through increasing access to technology solutions. RESNA advances the field by offering certification, continuing education, and professional development; developing assistive technology standards; promoting research and public policy; and sponsoring forums for the exchange of information and ideas to meet the needs of our multidisciplinary constituency.

Self Advocates Becoming Empowered

Address:
P.O. Box 872
Mason, OH 45040

Web site:
http://www.sabeusa.org/meet-sabe/

Self Advocates Becoming Empowered (SABE) is a self-advocacy organization that has members in every state and that acts as a national board. SABE addresses a number of concerns in the disability community, such as institutionalization, health care access, and employment opportunities.

Sibling Leadership Network

Address:
332 S. Michigan Avenue 1032-S240
Chicago, IL 60604
Phone: 312-996-1002

Web site:
http://siblingleadership.org/

The Sibling Leadership Network (SLN) is a national nonprofit organization that is dedicated to supporting siblings of people with disabilities and their larger family. SLN has chapters in 26 states, and more than 5,500 siblings and supporters are active members. The three primary focus areas of SLN are service and support provision, advocacy, and research and information dissemination. SLN provides siblings of people with disabilities with resources, training, and a wide-reaching network of support.

Sibling Support Project

Address:
The Sibling Support Project
6512 23rd Avenue NW, #322
Seattle, WA 98117
Phone: 206-297-6368

Web site:
https://www.siblingsupport.org/

The Sibling Support Project is a national program that aims to support siblings of people with disabilities as they navigate challenges they may face. The Sibling Support Project hosts "Sibshops" for school-aged youth, maintains online communities for siblings, and has created resource books.

Society for Disability Studies

Address:
SDS Executive Office
P.O. Box 5570
Eureka, CA 95502
Phone: 510-206-5767

Web site:
http://disstudies.org/

The Society for Disability Studies (SDS) is an organization dedicated to promoting the scholastic field of disability studies. SDS publishes a leading journal, *Disability Studies Quarterly*, and promotes research that advocates for social change.

Special Olympics International

Address:
1133 19th Street NW
Washington, DC 20036-3604
Phone: 202-628-3630

Web site:
https://www.specialolympics.org/

Special Olympics is an international non-profit organization that celebrates inclusion and the abilities of people with intellectual and developmental disabilities, primarily through sport. Nearly 5 million athletes from 172 countries engage in athletics via Special Olympics programs. With its international platform, Special Olympics aims to change public attitudes surrounding intellectual and developmental disabilities. Special Olympics also prioritizes health care access, research, and leadership development of its athletes.

TASH

Address:
1875 Eye Street NW, Suite 582
Washington, DC 20006
Phone: 202-429-2080

Web site:
https://tash.org/

TASH is an advocacy organization that promotes inclusion for people with disabilities. TASH supports research and community interventions that counter segregation and institutionalization.

Think College!

Web site:
https://thinkcollege.net/

Think College! is an accessible Web site with information on higher education options for people with intellectual and developmental disabilities. This online resource has a searchable database with relevant university programs sorted by state and region. In addition, Think College! publishes a newsletter and offers resources and training sessions related to transitioning to university.

Through the Looking Glass

Address:
3075 Adeline Street, Suite 120
Berkeley, CA 94703
Phone: 510-848-1112; 510-848-1005 (TTY)

Web site:
https://www.lookingglass.org/

Through the Looking Glass is a community-based, nonprofit organization that runs as a national center for families affected by disability. This training center provides trainings and resources for family members and professionals in the disability field. The funding provided from the National Institute of Disability and Rehabilitation ended in 2017, but Through the Looking Glass still provides free consultations and resources.

United Cerebral Palsy

Address:
1825 K Street NW, Suite 600
Washington, DC 20006
Phone: 800-872-5827

Web site:
http://ucp.org/

United Cerebral Palsy (UCP) connects people with a spectrum of disabilities to affiliate organizations (local service providers) that can best support their needs. UCP's mission is to promote the independence and full citizenship of people with disabilities.

University Centers for Excellence in Developmental Disabilities (UCEDD)

Address:
1100 Wayne Avenue, Suite 1000
Silver Spring, MD 20910
Phone: 301-588-8252

Web site:
https://www.aucd.org/template/page.cfm?id=24

University Centers for Excellence in Developmental Disabilities (UCEDD) is a national network of 67 centers devoted to supporting people with developmental disabilities, with at least one center in each state. UCEDDs provide preservice preparation, conduct research, disseminate evidence-based information, and develop partnerships with other local, state, and national resources. These efforts are undertaken to promote the independence, productivity, and inclusion of people with disabilities.

U.S. International Council on Disabilities

Address:
U.S. International Council on Disabilities
National Youth Transitions Center
2013 H Street NW, Suite 200
Washington, DC 20006
Phone: 202-480-2332

Web site:
http://www.usicd.org/template/index.cfm

The U.S. International Council on Disabilities (USICD) is a network of U.S.-based organizations (both nongovernmental and federal) that are dedicated to advocacy of the international disability rights movement. The USICD uses its influence to influence emerging disability rights issues at both a national and international level.

Vanderbilt Kennedy Center, University Center for Excellence in Developmental Disabilities

Address:
110 Magnolia Circle
Nashville, TN 37203
Phone: 615-322-8240

Web site:
http://vkc.mc.vanderbilt.edu/vkc/

The Vanderbilt Kennedy Center is part of the University Centers for Excellence in Developmental Disabilities national network. In addition to conducting research and providing community training, the Vanderbilt Kennedy Center maintains an extensive resource page on a wide array of topics such as employment, education, policy, spirituality, and health.

World Health Organization: Blindness and Deafness Prevention, Disability and Rehabilitation Unit

Address:
20 Avenue Appia, CH-1211 Geneva 27, Switzerland
Phone: +41-22-791-4470

Web site:
http://www.who.int/disabilities/en/

The World Health Organization (WHO) is the international authority on global health within the United Nations system. WHO oversees various programs, including the WHO Blindness and Deafness Prevention, Disability and Rehabilitation Unit (BDD). This particular team works to enhance the quality of life for people with disabilities across the globe by supporting evidence-based research, promoting community interventions, and developing technology and resources for distribution.

World Institute on Disability

Address:
3075 Adeline Street, Suite 155
Berkeley, CA 94703
Phone: 510-225-0477

Web site:
https://wid.org/

The World Institute on Disability (WID) aims to eliminate barriers that people with disabilities face when trying to achieve full social and economic integration. WID develops programs and resources and also supports research and community training to meet its goals.

Books
Adams, R., B. Reiss, and D. Serlin, eds. 2015. *Keywords for Disability Studies.* **New York: New York University Press.**

Keywords for Disability Studies is a volume of 60 essays, each relating to a pressing topic in the field of disability studies. Some of these topics include ethics, stigma, and identity. This text aims to expand the critical discourses present in disability studies to a wider audience by including perspectives from a variety of disciplines.

Albrecht, G., ed. 2006. *Encyclopedia of Disability.* **Thousand Oaks, CA: SAGE Publications.**

The *Encyclopedia of Disability* is a reference resource containing more than one thousand entries related to disability within five volumes. The first four volumes reference different topics, alphabetized from A to Z, while the fifth volume contains primary source documents for readers to explore.

Burch, S., ed. 2009. *Encyclopedia of American Disability History.* **New York: Facts on File.**

The encyclopedia was the first text of its kind with a disability focus. This book consists of more than 750 articles, authored by 350 historians, scholars, and experts, detailing disability-related events, people, and issues throughout U.S. history.

Connor, D. J., B. Ferri, and S. A. Annamma, eds. 2016. *DisCrit: Disability*

Studies and Critical Race Theory in Education. New York: Teachers College Press.

The book *DisCrit: Disability Studies and Critical Race Theory in Education* includes publications from 21 authors, all of which contribute to readers' considerations of the intersection of race and ability. The following six themes are highlighted: (1) race, class, and ability; (2) achievement/opportunity gap; (3) overrepresentation; (4) school-to-prison pipeline; (5) school reform; and (6) race, disability, and the law.

Davis, L. J., ed. 2017. *Beginning with Disability: A Primer*. New York: Routledge.

While there are many introductions to disability and disability studies, most presume an advanced academic knowledge of a range of subjects. *Beginning with Disability* is the first introductory primer for disability studies aimed at first-year students in two- and four-year colleges. This volume of essays across disciplines including education, sociology, communications, psychology, social sciences, and humanities features accessible, readable, and relatively short chapters that do not require specialized knowledge.

Davis, L. J., ed. 2017. *The Disability Studies Reader*. 5th ed. New York: Routledge.

Lennard Davis's *The Disability Studies Reader* is a comprehensive volume of essays that introduces readers to disability studies with foundational chapters, as well as essays devoted to emerging developments in the field. An interdisciplinary text, this book offers insight from the fields of law, technology, medicine, education, and more.

Iriarte, E., R. McConkey, and R. Gilligan. 2015. *Disability and Human Rights:*

Global Perspectives. London: Palgrave Macmillan.

Disability and Human Rights: Global Perspectives is an interdisciplinary text that offers a foundational understanding of disability in theory and practice. This book offers a complete evaluation of the United Nations Convention on the Rights of Persons with Disabilities and the associated international implications. A wide range of topics and regions are specifically attended to.

Longmore, P., and L. Umansky, eds. 2001. *The New Disability History: American Perspectives*. New York: New York University Press.

The New Disability History: American Perspectives is a single book within the larger History of Disability series. This volume explores the "hidden" history of disability and takes into consideration various frameworks, such as religious and cultural, rather than relying on a medical perspective. Within the pages of this text, in-depth accounts of people with disabilities from distinct time periods are revealed. These accounts are paired with empirical evidence to highlight the complex meanings of disability identity throughout American history.

Nielsen, K. E. 2012. *A Disability History of the United States*. Boston: Beacon Press.

A Disability History in the United States provides an extensive history of disability and disability-related experiences from the 15th century onward. This book places disability at the center of consideration when detailing historical accounts of such topics as slavery and immigration. Overall, this work provides a different framework to consider the history of the United States.

***The Sage Reference Series on Disability: Key Issues and Future Directions*. 2012. Thousand Oaks, CA: Sage Publications.**

The Sage Reference Series on Disability: Key Issues and Future Directions consists of eight volumes: Health and Medicine, Rehabilitation Interventions, Disability through the Life Course, Education, Assistive Technology and Science, Employment and Work, Arts and Humanities, and Ethics, Law, and Policy. Each of these books includes insight into the lives of people with disabilities and their families.

Editors and Contributors

EDITORS

Carol J. Gill is a professor emerita in the Department of Disability and Human Development (DHD) at the University of Illinois at Chicago (UIC). She has taught qualitative research methods and disability studies courses, and her research and publications focus on disability identity, health care experiences of women with disabilities, and bioethics. She directs the campus Certificate in Disability Ethics program.

Robert Gould, PhD, is the director of research for the Great Lakes ADA Center (in DHD, UIC) and is co-investigator of the ADA National Network Knowledge Translation Center. His scholarship and interests include domestic and international social policy and evaluation, employment and vocational rehabilitation, knowledge translation, and rights and social justice for people with disabilities.

Sarah Parker Harris is an associate professor and the director of graduate and undergraduate studies at DHD, UIC. Dr. Parker Harris has published and presented widely in areas of disability policy and law, entrepreneurship and disability, welfare to work, and international human rights. She is coauthor of *Disability through the Life Course.*

Tamar Heller is a distinguished professor and head of the DHD, UIC, where she directs the University Center of Excellence in Developmental Disabilities and the Rehabilitation Research and Training Center on Developmental Disabilities and Health. Her research focuses on self-directed and family supports, managed care, and health promotion interventions for individuals with disabilities. She has written more than 200 publications, including 5 books, and is one of the world's foremost scholars on bridging aging and disability.

CONTRIBUTORS

Randa Abdelrahim
University of Illinois at Chicago

Kruti Acharya
University of Illinois at Chicago

Sarah Agamah
University of Illinois at Chicago

Gary L. Albrecht
University of Illinois at Chicago

Ameen Alhaznawi
Concordia University Chicago

Khalid M. Alqahtani
Concordia University Chicago

Serenna Anan
Montclair State University

Gary Arnold
Progress Center for Independent Living

Katie Arnold
University of Illinois at Chicago, Sibling Leadership Network

Lindsay S. Athamanah
Michigan State University

Jessica Awsumb
DePaul University

Lindsey T. Back
DePaul University

Luca Badetti
DePaul University, L'Arche Chicago

Daniel Balcazar
Independent Scholar

Fabricio E. Balcazar
University of Illinois at Chicago

Sharon N. Barnartt
Gallaudet University

Alfiya Battalova
University of British Columbia

Stephanie Bay
Marianjoy Rehab Hospital

Liat Ben-Moshe
University of Toledo

Luciano Berardi
DePaul University

Jerome Bickenbach
World Health Organization

Art Blaser
Chapman University

Amanda Botticello
Kessler Foundation

Anne M. Bowers
University of Illinois at Chicago

Erik Brault
University of San Diego

Elizabeth Brewer
Central Connecticut State University

Heath K. Brosseau
Concordia University Chicago

Nili R. Broyer
University of Illinois at Chicago

Debra L. Brucker
University of New Hampshire

Molly Buren
University of Illinois at Chicago

Sheryl Burgstahler
University of Washington

Amanda Cachia
Moreno Valley College

Kate Caldwell
University of Illinois at Chicago

Allison Carey
Shippensburg University

Licia Carlson
Providence College

Eliza Chandler
Ryerson University

Jim Charlton
University of Illinois at Chicago

Vandana Chaudhry
College of Staten Island

Alarcos Cieza
World Health Organization

Cindy L. Collado
California State University-Sacramento

LaWanda H. Cook
Cornell University

Andrea Cooke
University of Illinois at Chicago

Jessica A. Cooley
University of Wisconsin–Madison

G. Thomas Couser
Hofstra University

Caitlin Meryl Crabb
University of Illinois at Chicago

Lisa S. Cushing
University of Illinois at Chicago

Shawn Dimpfl
University of Illinois at Chicago

Andrea Dinaro
Concordia University Chicago

Yochai Eisenberg
University of Illinois at Chicago

Douglas Engelman
University of South Florida

Heather Feldner
University of Washington

Jim Ferris
University of Toledo

Doris Zames Fleischer
New Jersey Institute of Technology

Anjali Forber-Pratt
Vanderbilt University

Katie Frank
Advocate Lutheran General Hospital

Angela Frederick
University of Texas at El Paso

Carli Friedman
The Council on Quality and Leadership

Kelly Fritsch
University of Toronto

Glenn T. Fujiura
University of Illinois at Chicago

Nina G
Comedian

Susan Sarno Gasber
Concordia University Chicago

Elaine Gerber
Montclair State University

Corey Goergen
Emory University

David Goldberg
University of Illinois at Chicago

Sara E. Green
University of South Florida

Alberto Guzman
University of Arizona

Gili Hammer
Hebrew University of Jerusalem

Mark Harniss
University of Washington

Elizabeth Adare Harrison
University of Illinois at Chicago

Cassandra Hartblay
Yale University

Rooshey Hasnain
University of Illinois at Chicago

Glenn Hedman
University of Illinois at Chicago

Jenna Heffron
Ithaca College

Amy Heider
University of Illinois at Chicago

Lieke van Heumen
University of Illinois at Chicago

Brian Heyburn
University of Illinois at Chicago

Willi Horner-Johnson
Oregon Health & Science University

Jessica Hovland
University of Illinois at Chicago

Alexandra Ibrahim
University of Illinois at Chicago

Katie Jajtner
Fordham University

Regina Meza Jimenez
University of Illinois at Chicago

Alisa Sheth Jordan
University of Illinois at Chicago

Thomas Jordan
Upper Iowa University

Pia Justesen
Justadvice

Stephanie Kanter
Shirley Ryan Ability Lab

Steven K. Kapp
University of Exeter

Joanna Keel
University of Illinois at Chicago

Jae Kennedy
Washington State University

Chris B. Keys
DePaul University

Richard Koenig
Housing Opportunity Development
Corporation

Nell Koneczny
University of Illinois at Chicago

Alison Kopit
University of Illinois at Chicago

F. L. Fredrik G. Langi
University of Illinois at Chicago

Sheryl A. Larson
University of Minnesota

Danbi Lee
University of Illinois at Chicago

K. M. LeFevour
University of Illinois Urbana-Champaign

Peter E. Leone
University of Maryland

Christopher Lilly
Concordia University Chicago

Amie Lulinski
University of Colorado

Kimberly Lynch
Montclair State University

Aaron A. Maass
Artfully Gifted Foundation

Romel W. Mackelprang
Eastern Washington University

Robert Maddalozzo
Ridgewood High School

Sandy Magaña
University of Texas at Austin

Lisa Mahaffey
Midwestern University

Linda Mastandrea
Federal Emergency Management Agency

Holly Matulewicz
Mathematica Policy Research

Ellyn McNamara
University of Illinois at Chicago

Michael McNicholas
University of Illinois at Chicago

Robert McRuer
George Washington University

Janie Meijas
University of Illinois at Chicago

Angel Miles
University of Illinois at Chicago

Paula M. Minihan
Tufts University

Mansha Mirza
University of Illinois at Chicago

Sophie Mitra
Fordham University

Rebekah Moras
University of Alaska at Anchorage

Shannon Moutinho
University of Illinois at Chicago

Lauren Mucha
Parents Allied with Children and Teachers
for Tomorrow (PACTT) Learning Center

Carlyn Mueller
University of Washington

Courtney Mullin
University of Illinois at Chicago

Kelly Munger
Independent Scholar

Sumithra Murthy
University of Illinois at Chicago

Michelle Nario-Redmond
Hiram College

Tia Nelis
TASH

Mallory Kay Nelson
United States Institute for Theatre
Technology

Akemi Nishida
University of Illinois at Chicago

Derek Nord
Indiana University Bloomington

Claire Nuchtern
North Start Academy

Ashmeet Kaur Oberoi
University of Miami

Bonnie O'Day
Mathematica Policy Research (Retired)

Alicia Wyche Okpareke
North Central College

Meghann O'Leary
University of Illinois at Chicago

Sarah M. Osier
Augustana College

Aleksa Owen
University of Illinois at Chicago

Randall Owen
University of Illinois at Chicago

Wendy Parent-Johnson
University of South Dakota

Michelle Parker-Katz
University of Illinois at Chicago

Ryan C. Parrey
Eastern Washington University

Alyson Patsavas
University of Illinois at Chicago

Holly Pearson
Chapman University

Jennifer Pearson
Glenbrook High Schools

Angélica Martínez Pérez
University of Illinois at Chicago

Katherine Perez
University of Illinois at Chicago

Patricia Perez
University of Illinois at Chicago

Jana J. Peterson-Besse
Pacific University

Patricia Politano
University of Illinois at Chicago

Michael Rembis
University at Buffalo

Joel Michael Reynolds
The Hastings Center

Mary Kay Rizzolo
The Council on Quality and Leadership

E. T. Russian
Artist and Author

Kristen Salkas
University of Illinois at Chicago

Linda Sandman
Illinois Imagines

Jennifer C. Sarrett
Emory College

Crom Saunders
Columbia College Chicago

Teresa A. Savage
University of Illinois at Chicago

Robert L. Schalock
Hastings College

Sarah von Schrader
Cornell University

Tina Schuh
University of Chicago

Michele Schutz
University of Illinois at Chicago

Richard K. Scotch
University of Texas at College

Haleigh M. Scott
University of Illinois at Chicago

Zoie Sheets
University of Illinois at Chicago

Carolyn Shivers
Virginia Tech

Stacy Clifford Simplican
Vanderbilt University

Nicole Sims
University of Illinois at Chicago

Kayla Smith
Independent Scholar

Natasha A. Spassiani
Napier University

Suzanne Stolz
University of San Diego

Joseph A. Stramondo
San Diego State University

Yolanda Suarez-Balcazar
University of Illinois at Chicago

Gia Super
University of Illinois at Chicago

T. J. Sutcliffe
The Arc

Kara Sutton
University of Texas at Dallas

Savneet Talwar
School of the Art Institute of Chicago

Kimberly J. The
University of Illinois at Chicago

Carolyn Theard-Griggs
Concordia University Chicago

Elizabeth Anh Thomson
University of Illinois at Chicago

Tanya Titchkosky
University of Toronto

Ashley Tomisek
Independent Scholar

Mariana Garcia Torres
University of Illinois at Chicago

Sandra Trappen
Penn State University

Shelley Tremain
University of Toronto

Agata Trzaska
University of Illinois at Chicago

Laura VanPuymbrouck
University of Illinois at Chicago

Vijay Vasudevan
University of Florida

Kelly Vaughan
Purdue University Northwest

Sara Vogt
University of Wisconsin–Whitewater

Ashley Volion
University of Illinois at Chicago

Julie Vryhof
University of Illinois at Chicago

Jess Waggoner
University of Houston

Samantha Walte
University of Illinois at Chicago

Julie Ward
The Arc

Linda Ware
State University of New York at Geneseo

Cathy Webb
University of Illinois at Chicago

Richard E. Wharton
University of Illinois at Chicago

Warren Whitaker
University of San Diego

Heather J. Williamson
Northern Arizona University

Liz Wood
Washington State University

Bernadette Wright
Meaningful Evidence LLC

Susun Xiong
University of Illinois at Chicago

Yue (Yovia) Xu
University of Illinois at Chicago

Chun-shan (Sandie) Yi
University of Illinois at Chicago

Hailee M. Yoshizaki-Gibbons
University of Illinois at Chicago

Lise M. Youngblade
Colorado State University

Jessica Zanton
Black Hills State University

Natalie Zapart
Concordia University Chicago

Jaime Zurheide
Elmhurst College

Index

Page numbers in **bold** indicate the location of main entries. Page numbers in *italics* indicate photos.